Biopsy Pathology of
the Skin

BIOPSY PATHOLOGY SERIES

General Editors

Professor Leonard S. Gottlieb, MD, MPH
Mallory Institute of Pathology,
Boston, USA

Professor A. Munro Neville, PhD, DSc, MD, FRC Path.
Ludwig Institute for Cancer Research,
Zurich, Switzerland

Professor F. Walker, MD, PhD, FRC Path.
Department of Pathology,
University of Aberdeen, UK

Other titles in the series

1. Biopsy Pathology of the Small Intestine
   F. D. Lee and P. G. Toner

2. Biopsy Pathology of the Liver
   R. S. Patrick and J. O'D. McGee

3. Brain Biopsy
   J. H. Adams, D. I. Graham and D. Doyle

4. Biopsy Pathology of the Lymphoreticular System
   D. H. Wright and P. G. Isaacson

6. Biopsy Pathology of Bone and Bone Marrow
   B. Frisch, S. M. Lewis, R. Burkhardt and R. Bartl

7. Biopsy Pathology of the Breast
   J. Sloane

8. Biopsy Pathology of the Oesophagus, Stomach and Duodenum
   D. W. Day

9. Biopsy Pathology of the Bronchi
   E. M. McDowell and T. F. Beals

10. Biopsy Pathology in Colorectal Disease
    I. C. Talbot and A. B. Price

11. Biopsy Pathology and Cytology of the Cervix
    D. V. Coleman and D. M. D. Evans

12. Biopsy Pathology of the Liver (2nd edn)
    R. S. Patrick and J. O'D. McGee

13. Biopsy Pathology of the Pulmonary Vasculature
    C. A. Wagenvoort and W. J. Mooi

14. Biopsy Pathology of the Endometrium
    C. H. Buckley and H. Fox

15. Biopsy Pathology of Muscle (2nd edn)
    M. Swash and M. S. Schwartz

16. Biopsy Pathology of the Skin
    N. Kirkham

17. Biopsy Pathology of Melanocytic Disorders
    W. J. Mooi and T. Krausz

Biopsy Pathology of the Skin

NIGEL KIRKHAM
Consultant Pathologist
Royal Sussex County Hospital, Brighton
and
Honorary Lecturer
University of Sussex

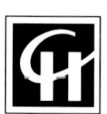

CHAPMAN & HALL MEDICAL
London · New York · Tokyo · Melbourne · Madras

UK   Chapman & Hall, 2–6 Boundary Row, London SE1 8HN
JAPAN   Chapman & Hall Japan, Thomson Publishing Japan,
            Hirakawacho Nemoto Building, 7F, 1-7-11 Hirakawa-cho,
            Chiyoda-ku, Tokyo 102
AUSTRALIA   Chapman & Hall Australia, Thomas Nelson Australia, 102
            Dodds Street, South Melbourne, Victoria 3205
INDIA   Chapman & Hall India, R. Seshadri, 32 Second Main Road, CIT
            East, Madras 600 035

First edition 1991

© 1991 Nigel Kirkham

Typeset in 10/12 pt Palatino by
Best-Set Typesetters Ltd, Hong Kong
Printed in Great Britain at the
University Press, Cambridge

ISBN 0 412 35080 7

British Library Cataloguing in Publication Data
Kirkham, N.
    Biopsy pathology of the skin.
    1. Skin. Pathology
    I. Title
    616.507

    ISBN 0-412-35080-7

Contents

Colour Plates 1–8 appear between pages 50 and 51; Plates 9–16 appear between pages 82 and 83; Plates 17–20 appear between pages 114 and 115; and Plates 21–24 appear between pages 146 and 147.

Preface		xi
Acknowledgements		xiii
1	**The Normal Skin**	1
1.1	Introduction	1
1.2	Epidermis and basement membrane	4
1.3	Dermis	5
1.4	Blood vessels and lymphatics	6
1.5	Skin associated lymphoid tissue	7
1.6	Hair follicles	8
1.7	Sweat glands	8
1.8	Nerves	9
1.9	Special stains	10
1.10	Immunohistochemical methods	11
1.11	Other special techniques	12
	References	12
2	**Biopsy methods and strategy for reporting biopsies**	15
	Dr M. L. Price and Dr N. Kirkham	
2.1	The dermatologist's point of view	15
2.2	Trimming the biopsy	21
2.3	Strategies for reporting skin biopsies	21
2.4	Examining the biopsy	22
	References	30
3	**Intraepidermal keratoses and tumours**	32
3.1	Actinic keratosis	33
3.2	Bowen's disease	34
3.3	Bowenoid papulosis	35
3.4	Flegel's disease	35
3.5	Porokeratosis	37
3.6	Disseminated superficial actinic porokeratosis (DSAP)	38

vi   Contents

3.7   Porokeratosis of Mibelli   38
3.8   Clear cell acanthoma   40
3.9   Large cell acanthoma   40
3.10 Intraepidermal epithelioma – the Jadassohn phenomenon   42
3.11 Paget's disease   43
3.12 Grover's disease   47
3.13 Darier's disease   47
3.14 Hailey-Hailey disease   47
3.15 Warty dyskeratoma   51
3.16 Acanthosis nigricans   51
      References   51

4   Warts and viral dermatoses   54
4.1   Viral warts   54
4.2   Renal allograft recipients   58
4.3   Milker's nodule   60
4.4   Seborrhoeic warts   60
4.5   Melanoacanthoma   63
4.6   Squamous cell papilloma   63
4.7   Molluscum contagiosum   63
4.8   Herpes   65
      References   65

5   Epidermal tumours   67
5.1   Basal cell carcinoma   70
5.2   Squamous cell carcinoma   77
5.3   Keratoacanthoma   78
5.4   Spindle cell squamous cell carcinoma   85
5.5   Basosquamous carcinoma   85
5.6   Adenosquamous carcinoma   87
      References   87

6   Melanocytic tumours   90
6.1   Naevi   90
6.2   Deep penetrating naevus   95
6.3   Spitz naevus   96
6.4   Pigmented spindle cell naevus of Reed   98
6.5   Blue naevus   98
6.6   Cellular blue naevus   98
6.7   Dysplastic naevus   102
6.8   Malignant melanoma   108
6.9   Regression and halo naevi   115
6.10 Lentigo maligna   119
6.11 Minimal deviation melanoma   121

6.12	Spindle cell melanoma	121
6.13	Desmoplastic melanoma	124
6.14	Balloon cell melanoma	125
6.15	Signet-ring cell melanoma	125
	References	125
7	**Adnexal tumours**	130
7.1	Eccrine sweat gland tumours	131
7.2	Apocrine gland tumours	142
7.3	Microcystic adnexal carcinoma	144
7.4	Hair follicle tumours	146
7.5	Sebaceous tumours	161
7.6	Cysts	165
	References	171
8	**Dermal tumours**	176
8.1	Mesenchymal tumours	176
8.2	Vascular tumours	188
8.3	Neural tumours	197
8.4	Neuroendocrine carcinoma	202
8.5	Smooth muscle tumours	203
8.6	Naevus lipomatosus superficialis	205
8.7	Cutaneous metastases	205
	References	212
9	**Eczematous, psoriasiform and lichenoid reactions**	218
9.1	Eczema	218
9.2	Psoriasis	221
9.3	Seborrhoeic dermatitis	225
9.4	Lichen simplex	227
9.5	Lichen planus	229
9.6	Lichen plano-pilaris	232
	References	232
10	**Benign lymphoid infiltrates**	234
10.1	Lupus erythematosus	238
10.2	Polymorphic light eruption	238
10.3	Jessner's lymphocytic infiltrate	239
10.4	Erythema multiforme	242
10.5	Lymphocytoma cutis	242
10.6	Pityriasis lichenoides acuta	244
10.7	Pityriasis lichenoides chronica	245
10.8	Pityriasis rubra pilaris	247
10.9	Gyrate erythema	247
10.10	Lyme disease – erythema chronicum migrans	247

10.11 Sweet's syndrome   250
10.12 Papular urticaria and mastocytosis   252
10.13 Incontinentia pigmenti   254
10.14 Graft versus host disease   254
10.15 Alopecia – technical note   255
10.16 Alopecia areata   258
10.17 Trichotillomania   259
10.18 Scarring alopecia   259
10.19 Follicular mucinosis   260
10.20 Erosive pustular dermatosis of the scalp   260
10.21 Subcorneal pustular dermatosis   260
      References   261

11   **Cutaneous lymphoma and other malignant lymphoid
      infiltrates**   266
11.1 Cutaneous T-cell lymphoma (CTCL)   266
11.2 Angiocentric lymphoma   272
11.3 Lymphomatoid papulosis   273
11.4 Regressing atypical histiocytosis   276
11.5 Woringer-Kolopp disease   276
11.6 Histiocytosis X   277
11.7 Cutaneous B-cell lymphoma   277
11.8 Secondary cutaneous involvement by follicular lymphoma   278
11.9 Cutaneous involvement by leukaemia   280
      References   280

12   **Vesiculo-bullous diseases**   286
12.1 Pemphigus   287
12.2 Bullous pemphigoid   291
12.3 Cicatricial pemphigoid   294
12.4 Pemphigoid gestationis   294
12.5 Linear IgA disease   295
12.6 Epidermolysis bullosa acquisita   295
12.7 Dystrophic epidermolysis bullosa   296
12.8 Dermatitis herpetiformis   297
12.9 Porphyria cutanea tarda   299
12.10 Pseudoporphyria   299
12.11 Bullous amyloidosis   300
      References   300

13   **Infective and non-infective granulomas**   304
      Dr S. Lucas and Dr N. Kirkham
13.1 Infective granulomas   305
13.2 Non-infective granulomas   318
      References   326

14	**The skin and AIDS**	328
14.1	Kaposi's sarcoma	329
14.2	Bacillary angiomatosis	333
14.3	Acute virus exanthema	334
14.4	Seborrhoeic-like dermatitis	334
14.5	Other infections	337
	References	337
15	**Vasculitis**	341
15.1	Leucocytoclastic vasculitis	342
15.2	Necrotizing vasculitis	342
15.3	Wegener's granulomatosis	342
15.4	Churg-Strauss syndrome	346
15.5	Lymphomatoid granulomatosis	348
15.6	Pyoderma gangrenosum	348
15.7	Granuloma faciale	350
15.8	Cryoglobulinaemia	350
15.9	Pigmented purpuric eruptions	352
15.10	Erythema elevatum diutinum	352
15.11	Behçet's disease	353
	References	353
16	**Panniculitis**	356
16.1	Approach to diagnosis	356
16.2	Erythema nodosum	358
16.3	Pancreatic fat necrosis	362
16.4	Lupus panniculitis	362
16.5	Eosinophilic panniculitis	363
16.6	Cytophagic histiocytic panniculitis	364
16.7	Panniculitis artefacta	364
16.8	Eosinophilic fasciitis	364
16.9	Necrotizing fasciitis	365
	References	365
17	**Dermal stromal diseases**	367
17.1	Morphoea and scleroderma	367
17.2	Lichen sclerosus	367
17.3	Mucinoses	370
17.4	Reactive perforating collagenosis	371
17.5	Chondrodermatitis nodularis	374
	References	374
18	**Artefact *et al.***	376
18.1	Drug reactions	376
18.2	Dermatitis artefacta	379

x   Contents

18.3   Panniculitis artefacta   380
18.4   Effects of heat and cold   384
       References   387

Index   388

Preface

This is intended to be a book for those engaged in the everyday task of examining skin biopsies. Particular emphasis is placed on the commoner conditions and the need for accurate differential diagnosis and for the pathologist to provide the dermatologists with the clinically relevant biopsy reports they deserve. To this end the methods of skin biopsy and the reasons for their use are described by a dermatologist, Dr Margaret Price.

The particular problems of the tropical diseases leprosy and leishmaniasis are described by Dr Sebastian Lucas, who has a wide experience of the difficulties encountered by the general pathologist in this area of dermatopathology. With international travel widely available and with widespread political and economic changes all around us the possibility of an exotic diagnosis should always be in the back of our minds.

In writing this book I have tried to give a reasonably current account of dermatopathology in everyday practice. It is not an encyclopaedic account of the subject. There are too many case reports and eponymous syndromes scattered through the literature to hope to cover them all. The text is supported with up to date references to recent reviews and papers, to act as a source of current information and to provide a starting point for further literature searches. The reference lists therefore only include selected older papers. Others will be found as references in the articles cited in the text. None of us are far away from a library. Even if you cannot go there personally it is a simple matter to request a copy of the article in question and discuss further reading possibilities with the librarian, over the phone.

With few exceptions the illustrations are taken from biopsies seen in Brighton and Worthing during the last two years. It has been my intention to avoid too much philately in selecting topics for discussion and description. So although some conditions may be missing I can say that I have attempted to include the majority of the conditions which we have seen in Sussex during that time. With few exceptions the illustrations are of haematoxylin and eosin stained sections. Where an alternative stain has been used, this is stated. In line with modern practice the original magnifications are not given: we feel that there are sufficient dermal or epidermal landmarks in them to indicate whether any individual figure is taken at low, medium or high power.

N. Kirkham

Acknowledgements

I am deeply indebted to all those who have made this book possible. Special thanks go to my dermatologist colleagues Peter Coburn, Charles Darley, Patrick Hall Smith and Meg Price, not forgetting Brent Tanner, who tackles the more challenging surgery. I would like to thank the staff of the histopathology laboratory at the Royal Sussex County Hospital, where the bulk of the sections were cut and my colleagues and locums who shared the load of other work whilst I was preoccupied in producing this. Thanks also go to Keith Roberts and Gerry O'Sullivan and their laboratory staffs for the loan of many sections.

Last but not least I must express my immense gratitude to Judy Lehmann, Martha Bush, Pat Notten, Jennifer Richards and Liisa Strong, and others who have come and gone in the last two years: the Library staff, for their untiring enthusiasm in collecting and checking references, as well as for their tea and sympathy, without which none of this would have been possible.

1 The Normal skin

1.1 Introduction

Dermatopathology was one of the first parts of histopathology to be widely practised. Indeed, the ease with which the skin can be biopsied lends itself to histopathology. However, there are two schools of thought as to how the subject should be followed. Many of the early practitioners were physicians who performed and examined their own biopsies. In many specialist dermatology departments this is still the case. The alternative approach has been for histopathologists with or without a special interest in the subject to examine the biopsies.

Both approaches have advantages and disadvantages. The dermatologist has usually seen the patient and knows the history and appearance of the lesion. By and large the pathologist receives this information second-hand, if at all, but does have the advantage of wider experience of systemic pathology. It must be remembered that dermatology as a subject is largely restricted to the epidermis and dermis and as a consequence systemic disease made manifest in the skin can cause problems.

However, the two approaches are not mutually exclusive. The best service is likely to be one where dermatologist and pathologist work together to pool the strengths of their knowledge and experience in the task of accurate diagnosis. To this end a regular dialogue is necessary. As well as frequent phone calls between clinic and laboratory, it is essential for the two to examine biopsies together and perhaps it is even more important for pathologists to venture into the clinic from time to time. Dermatologists like having clinical meetings at which their problem patients present their diseases for examination and discussion with a number of colleagues. The pathologist can learn much from such meetings and subsequent further review of the biopsies. The advent of laboratory computers has helped.

For instance in Brighton the dermatologists and pathologists meet together once a week for about half an hour, with the week's biopsies and copies of reports (produced by the computer), and the small numbers of clinical case records brought by the dermatologists for review. Once the routine has been established it is quite easy to review the week's interesting cases; revise the wrong or incomplete diagnoses in light of further clinical information; order the extra levels and special stains which could perhaps have been requested in the first place; resolve unanswered questions; and tag the interesting cases for forth-coming clinical meetings, before the first cup of tea has gone cold. This sort of feedback is essential for good practice and as a way of providing feedback on the performance of the service (Paraskeopoulos *et al.*, 1988).

In the future we may see more of the service being provided directly by family practitioners, as they are encouraged in the interests of political and economic expediency to undertake more minor surgery on their own premises (Weinstein *et al.*, 1986; Fine, 1987).

Skin biopsies themselves are rather like high board diving at the Olympic Games in that they come in varying degrees of difficulty. Table 1.1 shows an approximate breakdown of 1 year's skin biopsies in this laboratory. The figures have been derived by searching the com-puter database using the appropriate SNOMED codes.

Especially with all the recent publicity about pigmented lesions we are seeing many more biopsies of naevi. Many of these are straight-forward but a proportion are a problem, usually because they may show cytological or architectural abnormalities which raise the spectre of malignant change. Amongst tumours basal cell carcinomas are by far the most common. Perhaps the most striking feature of the table is that although many of the most obvious classes of diagnosis have been

Table 1.1 Skin biopsies from a population of 290,000 in one year

Diagnosis	Number	%
Cellular naevi	600	21
Basal cell carcinomas	508	18
Inflammatory disease	135	5
Bowen's disease and keratosis	117	4
Squamous cell carcinomas	55	2
Keratoacanthomas	44	2
Melanomas	37	1
Bullous disease	17	0.5
Cutaneous lymphomas	16	0.5
Others	1529	53
Total	2883	100

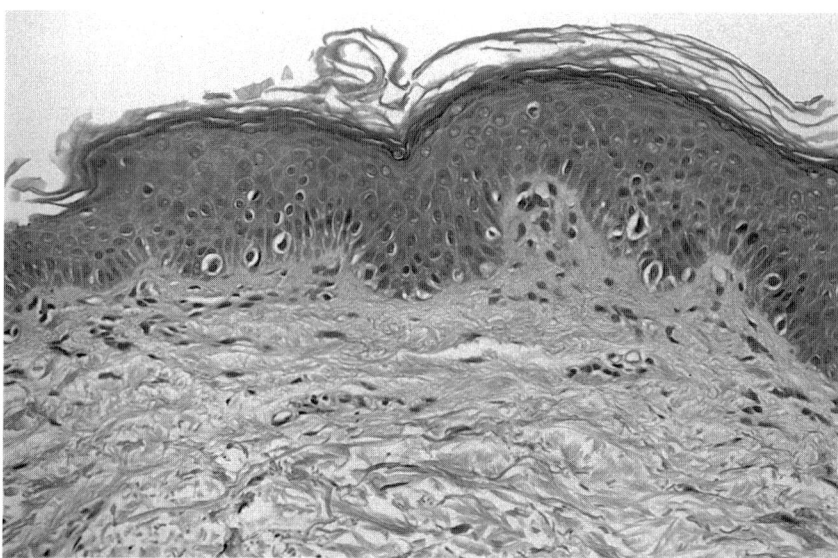

Figure 1.1 Apparently normal skin showing the various components of epidermis and dermis. This is a lesion of notalgia paraesthetica in which intraepidermal nerve fibres were, on further study, shown to be increased in number in association with hyperaesthesia.

listed, there are still 53% of cases which have been assigned miscellaneous other diagnostic codes. This is the problem of skin pathology. Although there are major groups of common disease, there are a large variety of relatively uncommon conditions which must be accurately identified and classified.

In subsequent chapters the author has attempted to describe the majority of lesions that are likely to be encountered. Almost all the illustrations are taken from biopsies seen in the routine service in Brighton and Worthing Health Districts in the past 2 years. Some hens have teeth but they are rare birds: the author hopes that there are not too many hen's teeth here (Kollar and Fisher, 1980). Finally, the author has at all times tried to concentrate on the areas of diagnostic difficulty which seem to be recurring problems for the general, non-specialist histopathologist.

The skin is the largest organ in the body and shows marked variation in appearance from one site to another. Some of the differences are obvious, such as the thick layer of keratin and absence of hair follicles on the palms of the hands and the soles of the feet. Elsewhere the variations may be more subtle, but they are variations on a theme. The

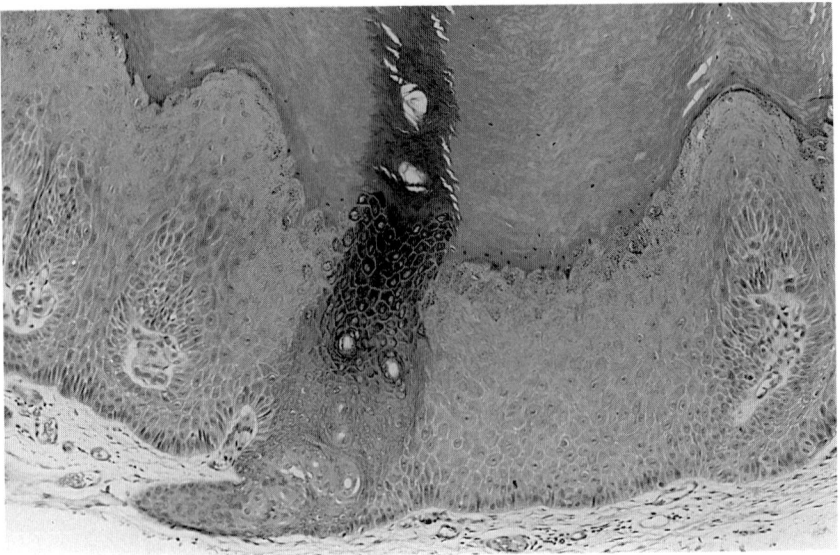

Figure 1.2   A section of epidermis with acrosyryngium, in which the basal cell, prickle cell, granular cell and keratinized layers can be clearly seen.

individual components of the skin are similar at all sites: it is the proportions that vary. In addition this variation extends with age. With increasing age the fine, regular epidermal surface patterns coarsen, with flattening of the dermal–epidermal junction and thinning of the dermis. There is also a loss of functional elasticity as elastic fibres become frayed, porous, and matted together. Blood vessels, hair follicles, sebaceous glands, and sweat glands also decrease in number and in function with increasing age (Smith, 1989).

This chapter will consider the individual components and also some of the ways in which they can be stained to investigate disease states (Urmacher, 1990).

1.2   Epidermis and basement membrane

The epidermis is a stratified squamous epithelium with proliferating cells in the basal layer which constantly replenish the epithelium as cells are in turn shed from the surface. This is a continuous process, subject to variations in rate, and so dividing the epidermis into specific layers is to a certain extent a rather artificial process. It is useful however to look at the cells in the basal layer, the prickle cell layer, the granular cell layer and the keratinized layer in a systematic way, when trying to decide what is going on in a particular biopsy.

The basal cell layer lies on the basement membrane and contains cuboidal or columnar cells, which usually show little variation. Only occasional mitotic figures will be seen in normal skin, but they may be more numerous in hyperplastic or neoplastic states. The melanocytes are also found here, their apparent number depending upon the site of the biopsy and the skin colour of the individual.

The main part of the epidermis is variously called the prickle cell layer, the spinous cell layer, the Malpighian layer or the rete Malpighii and contains cells with a greater amount of cytoplasm than basal cells. The cytoplasm is eosinophilic because of the accumulation of keratin. Between the cells the intercellular junctions are visible as 'prickles'. The cells are called keratinocytes or acanthocytes. All of these synonyms have their proponents and opponents. It is best to choose one set and use them consistently in your practice.

Above the prickle cell layer is the granular cell layer, in which specialized processing of keratin takes place, resulting in the formation of the uppermost layer of keratin. In normal epidermis all the cells in this layer are anucleate, but in hyperproliferative states nuclei may still be present: the appearance called parakeratosis.

The epidermis lies on a complex basement membrane which is difficult to see in haematoxylin and eosin (H and E) stained sections. Ultrastructural studies have shown two main layers (Katz, 1984). Immediately beneath the basal cells there is an electron lucid lamina lucida, beneath which is the electron dense lamina densa. Things are of course not so simple, because the epidermis has to be bound tightly to the dermis.

Two specialized groups of structures are associated with this function. The connection between the basal cells and basement membrane is made by hemidesmosomes, which are essentially half of the sort of complete desmosome which links the keratinocytes in the 'prickles'. The membrane is bound to the dermis by anchoring fibrils which attach to the lamina densa.

1.3 Dermis

The dermis is complex mixture of cells and extracellular matrix (Donaldson and Mahan, 1988) arranged in two layers; the upper papillary dermis and the lower reticular dermis. The former extends from the epidermal basement membrane down for about one third of the thickness of the dermis and contains relatively slender collagen and elastic fibres. In sections stained with acid orcein Giemsa (AOG), the anchoring fibrils can be seen as well as the larger elastic fibres of the dermis.

The reticular dermis occupies approximately the lower two thirds

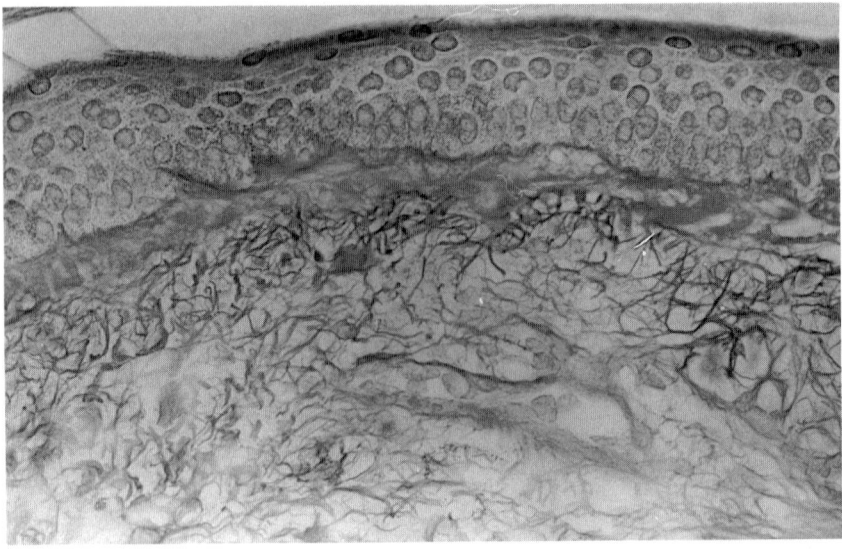

Figure 1.3   A section of skin stained for reticulin fibres, which can be seen in the dermis, with more numerous and finer fibres in the upper part of the dermis.

down to the subcutaneous fat. It has larger collagen and elastic fibres than the reticular dermis. The junction between the two can usually be seen quite clearly.

Scattered between the collagen bundles there are small numbers of poorly understood cells which are probably responsible for synthesizing and maintaining the structure. Various names are given to these cells including fibroblast, myofibroblast, histiocyte and dermal dendrocyte.

The subcutaneous fat should not be forgotten. It will not be present in any but the deepest of skin biopsies, but is arranged in a lobular fashion, with vascular septae surrounding groups of adipocytes. Small upward extensions around sweat glands will be seen in normal skin, but any substantial amount of fat seen in the dermis is a pathological abnormality.

1.4   Blood vessels and lymphatics

The blood vessels of the skin are relatively simple in their organization (Higgins and Eady, 1981a, b; Ludatscher, 1978; Ryan 1976). As seen in biopsies there are two groups or plexuses. In the papillary dermis there is the superficial plexus, which supplies the needs of the epidermis. In

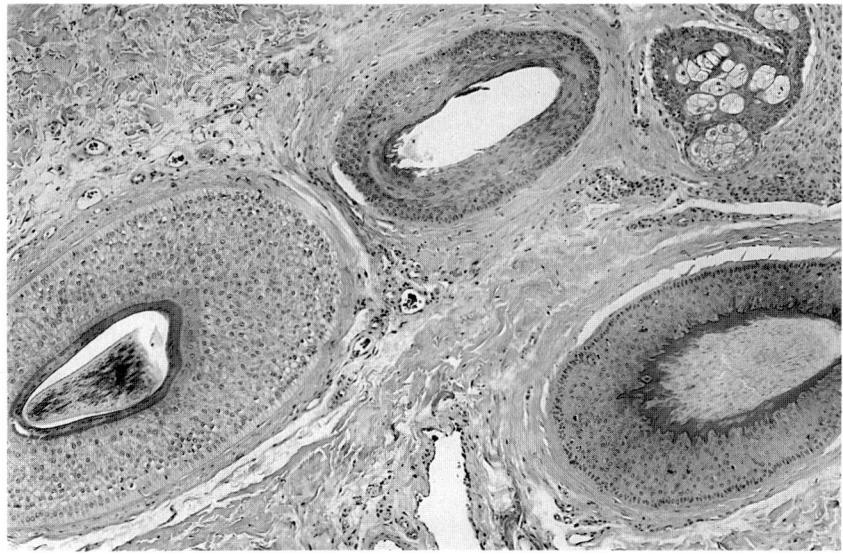

Figure 1.4 A transverse section through three hair follicles showing the outer root sheath (tricholemmal) cells, with pale cytoplasm in the lower two.

the reticular dermis there is the deep plexus. These are, of course, connected but the vertical connections are not usually very apparent. Lymphatics are present in the skin but are difficult to see except in a condition such as chronic lymphoedema, when they are ectatic.

1.5 Skin associated lymphoid tissue

Although so much time and energy has been expended in studying pathological lymphoid infiltrates of the skin it is only recently that the normal resident population of lymphocytes has been duly recognized (Streilein, 1978, 1983). There are small numbers of lymphocytes and macrophages in the skin as part of the normal process of antigen detection. The keratinocytes may also play a part in inflammatory reactions by producing lymphokines (Sauder *et al.*, 1982).

Within the epidermis there is a network of Langerhans cells, which lie in the prickle cell layer and spread dendritic processes between keratinocytes. The Langerhans cells are specialized CD1 positive macrophages, derived from bone marrow, which detect and process antigen before communicating with lymphocytes (Bieber *et al.*, 1988; Concha *et al.*, 1988; Katz *et al.*, 1985; Stingl, 1980; Silberberg *et al.*, 1975). They contain characteristic cytoplasmic granules, seen on electron microscopy (Birbeck *et al.*, 1961), which appear to be derived from the cell surface membrane and probably subserve the function of antigen processing (Takahashi and Hashimoto, 1985). There is a constant flux of Langerhans cells around the circuit made up by dermal blood vessels, epidermis, lymphatics and regional lymph nodes (Shimada and Katz, 1988).

The lymphocytes in the dermis are almost exclusively T-cells, with either the helper CD4 or suppressor/cytotoxic CD8 surface marker. B-cells are uncommon in the skin (Facchetti *et al.*, 1988). Analysis of the subsets of T-cell receptor bearing cells shows similar proportions of alpha-beta and gamma-delta cells around dermal vessels and a marginal increase of gamma-delta cells in the epidermis. The gamma-delta T cells do not appear to have a specific role in immunosurveillance in the epidermis (Bos *et al.*, 1990).

1.6   Hair follicles

The hair follicles are quite complicated structures. This complexity is sometimes acknowledged by using the description 'pilosebaceous unit' to cover the components which form the complex and which include the hair follicle itself as well as hair, sebaceous gland, arrectores pilorum muscle and sometimes the apocrine gland. From the point of view of biopsy pathology, there are two important points to consider.

The first is the distinction between the upper and lower parts of the follicle. The upper part, above the level of entry of the sebaceous gland duct, is a downward prolongation of the epidermis and is called the infundibulum. Below this level is the true mesodermally derived follicle. The infundibulum and true follicle may be involved differentially in inflammatory processes.

The second is the recognition of the various stages of the proliferative cycle of the follicle, which are important in the study of alopecias. The growth phase is anagen, the involution phase catagen and the resting phase telogen. When analysing tumours it is important to recognize the characteristics of the hair germ at the base of the follicle, and also the pale cells of the outer root sheath, as well as the appearance of tricholemmal keratinization in contrast to the keratinization associated with a granular cell layer seen in the epidermis.

1.7   Sweat glands

There are three kinds of sweat gland. The eccrine gland has a secretory coil which lies deep in the dermis, surrounded by fat which extends upwards from the subcutis. The coil is a simple tube in which two

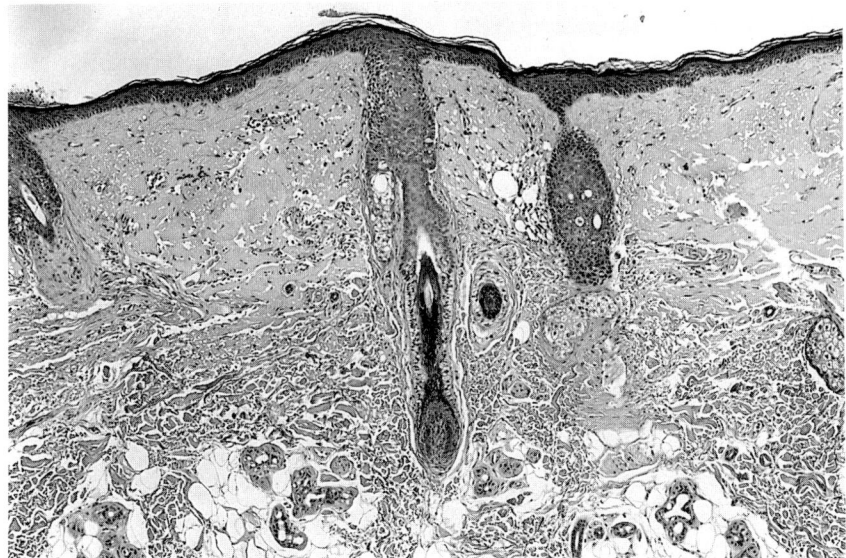

Figure 1.5 Facial skin showing hair follicles, sweat glands, dermis and subcutaneous fat. There is solar elastosis in the papillary dermis.

kinds of cells can be seen: 'dark cells' with basophilic cytoplasm and 'light cells' with eosinophilic cytoplasm. There is a layer of myoepithelial cells around the epithelial cells.

The coil leads into an excretory duct which runs relatively straight up to epidermis, where there is a specialized structure, the acrosyringium, where the duct becomes coiled and remains so until emerging on the surface of the epidermis. The cells of the acrosyringium are morphologically distinct from the surrounding epidermis and have different functional properties, such as the ability to express HLA-DR.

1.8 Nerves

There are many nerves in the skin, with trunks visible in the dermis in H and E sections. At present little is known about the neurotransmitters in cutaneous nerves and, in particular, the cutaneous sensory neurotransmitter remains unidentified. The general nerve marker protein gene product 9.5 (PGP 9.5) is a good tool for identifying nerves immunohistochemically. Nerves probably play a significant part in a number of skin diseases, the details of which remain to be studied (Levy *et al.*, 1989). Specialized neuroendocrine cells (Merkel cells) are present in the basal layer of the epidermis and hair follicle.

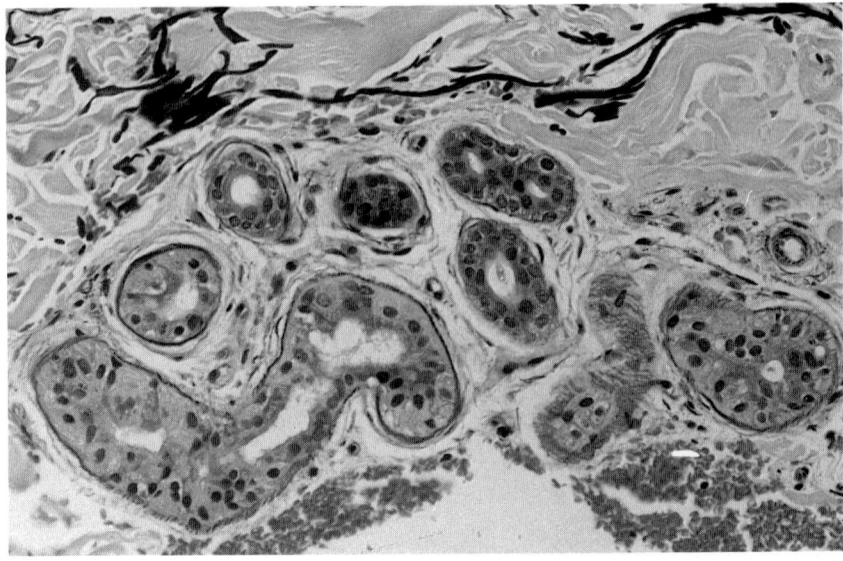

Figure 1.6   An AOG stained section showing the secretory coil and part of the excretory duct of a sweat gland. Dermal elastic fibres are also stained.

1.9   Special stains

For the vast majority of biopsies a good H and E stain on a well cut, well orientated section is more than adequate for diagnosis. Next to be considered is the AOG stain, which will demonstrate the majority of epidermal and dermal structures and changes (Pinkus and Hunter, 1960). In addition to the expected staining of nuclei and cytoplasm, mast cell granules will stain metachromatically purple, melanin dark green, haemosiderin yellowish-green and amyloid light greyish-blue to sky blue. Of particular help is the dark brown to black staining of dermal elastic tissue, which is often useful in unravelling changes in the dermal stroma.

If there is a suspicion of fungal infection then Grocott's stain has no equal in demonstrating hyphae in the upper epidermis. Periodic acid-Schiff stain (PAS) has its proponents and is a good way of demonstrating glycogen in clear cell, glycogen-rich lesions of epidermis or appendage. It is not, however, a very effective way of staining basement membrane, as has been claimed, and it is less effective at staining fungi than Grocott's stain.

The real advances have come in the use of immunohistochemistry to stain specific antigens. Many keratins have now been identified in the epidermis and their differential expression offers hope for increasing our understanding of the pathophysiology of some diseases (Lane *et al.*, 1987; Leigh *et al.*, 1987; Moll *et al.*, 1982; Morgan *et al.*, 1987a, b). Using appropriate reagents it is possible to label keratins normally expressed in basal and in suprabasal cells. These developments are only beginning to find real applications in diagnosis,but the ability to identify keratin is of use.

Antibodies to high molecular weight cytokeratin, such as LP 34, label epidermal cells, whilst low molecular weight cytokeratin antibodies, such as CAM 5.2, do not, but do label sweat glands and other internal epithelia. Lymphoid cells can now be labelled in paraffin sections, using a slowly widening panel of antibodies, including the B-cell marker L26 (Norton and Isaacson, 1987), the T-cell marker UCHL-1, and the macrophage marker MAC 387 and S100 protein which labels nerves, melanocytes and Langerhans cells (Kahn *et al.*, 1983).

1.10   Immunohistochemical methods

For those antibodies with which frozen sections must be used it is vital to receive fresh, unfixed biopsies in the laboratory, where they can be trimmed to provide blocks for section cutting which are representative of, and include tissue from, the central part of each lesion. Other parts of the biopsy can be fixed to provide paraffin sections.

Blocks may be stored in liquid nitrogen prior to cutting and should then be orientated on the cryostat chuck at a slight angle to the line of cutting. Slides must be coated with poly-l-lysine to ensure adhesion of the sections during the various stages of staining. Sections should be cut at a thickness of 10 microns, with a chuck temperature of $-40°C$ on a wedge profile knife, using the slowest speed of the motor drive of a cryostat, such as the Leitz Kryostat 1720.

For high-quality sections of epidermal lesions it is best to cut two sections, starting at the dermal side of the block, and then taking the bottom section onto the slide to avoid stripping of the epidermis from the dermis. However, it is possible to achieve good sections by cutting either the epidermal or the dermal side of the block first. Sections are fixed in dry acetone and stained using one of the available methods.

For the indirect immunoperoxidase method, primary antibody is used at an appropriate dilution, determined by dilution studies, and incubated on the sections for 30 minutes, followed by three washes of Tris buffered saline each of 2 minutes, a 30-minute incubation with horseradish peroxidase conjugated rabbit anti-mouse antibody at a titre of 1 in 50 (Dako) and three further 2-minute washes with Tris buffered saline.

A red colour reaction can be developed with aminocarbazole (Sigma) for 15 minutes, which contrasts sharply with brown melanin pigment in biopsies of pigmented lesions. In non-pigmented lesions diamino-benzidene can be used to produce brown staining. Harris's haematoxy-lin is used as a nuclear counterstain and differentiated in 1% acid alcohol. Sections using aminocarbazole must be mounted in glycerin jelly from water. Serial sections can be stained with H and E to provide morphological controls, and be processed through the immunoperoxi-dase method without primary antibody to provide negative immuno-histochemical controls.

1.11 Other special techniques

In a minority of cases other specialized techniques may be called upon to aid in the diagnosis of major problems such as cutaneous T-cell lymphoma and atypical lymphocytic infiltrates, vesiculo-bullous disorders, lupus erythematosus and collagen vascular diseases, vasculitis, poorly differentiated tumours, storage diseases, and infections (Rowden et al., 1979). Techniques which are now established for the study of morphological and functional changes include morphometric analysis, transmission electron microscopy, X-ray probe microanalysis, and digital image analysis and, more recently, molecular biological techniques (Jaworsky and Murphy, 1989).

References

Bieber, T., Ring, J. and Braun Falco, O. (1988) Comparison of different methods for enumeration of Langerhans cells in vertical cryosections of human skin. *Br. J. Dermatol.*, **118**, 385–92.

Birbeck, M. S., Breathnach, A. S. and Everall, J. D. (1961) An electron microscopic study of basal melanocytes and high-level clear cells (Langerhans cells) in vitiligo. *J. Invest. Dermatol.*, **37**, 51–64.

Bos, J. D., Teunissen, M. B. M., Cairo, I., Kreig, S. R., Kapsenberg, M. L., Das, P. K. and Borst, J. (1990) T-cell receptor gamma delta bearing cells in normal human skin. *J. Invest. Dermatol.*, **94**, 37–42.

Concha, M., Figueroa, C. D. and Caorsi, I. (1988) Ultrastructural characteristics of the contact zones between Langerhans cells and lymphocytes. *J. Pathol.*, **156**, 29–36.

Donaldson, D. J. and Mahan, J. T. (1988) Keratinocyte migration and the extracellular matrix. *J. Invest. Dermatol.*, **90**, 623–8.

Facchetti, F., de Wolf-Peeters, C., van den Oord, J. J. and Desmet, V. J. (1988) Plasmacytoid T cells in a case of lymphocytic infiltration of the skin. A component of the skin-associated lymphoid tissue? *J. Pathol.*, **155**, 295–300.

Fine, J.-D. (1987) Common office dermatoses. Approach to diagnosis and therapy. *Ala. J. Med. Sci.*, **24**, 209–15.

Higgins, J. C. and Eady, R. A. J. (1981a) Human dermal microvasculature. I. Its segmental differentiation. Light and electron microscopic study. *Br. J. Dermatol.*, **104**, 117–21.

Higgins, J. C. and Eady, R. A. J. (1981b) Human dermal microvasculature. II. Enzyme histochemical and cytochemical study. *Br. J. Dermatol.*, **104**, 521–9.

Jaworsky, C. and Murphy, G. F. (1989) Special techniques in dermatology. *Arch. Dermatol.*, **125**, 963–74.

Kahn, H. J., Marks A., Thom, H. and Baumal, R. (1983) Role of antibody to S100 protein in diagnostic pathology. *Am. J. Clin. Pathol.*, **79**, 341–7.

Katz, S. I. The epidermal basement membrane zone-structure, ontogeny, and role in disease. *J. Am. Acad. Dermatol.*, **11**, 1025–37.

Katz, S. I., Cooper, C., Ligma, M. and Tsuchida, I. (1985) The role of Langerhans cells in antigen presentation. *J. Invest. Dermatol.*, **85**, 965–85.

Kollar, E. J. and Fisher, C. (1980) Tooth induction in chick epithelium, expression of quiescent genes for enamel synthesis. *Science*, **207**, 993–5.

Lane, E. B., Bartek, J., Purkis, P. E. and Leigh, I. M. Keratin antigens in differentiating skin. *Ann. NY Acad. Sci.*, **455**, 214–58.

Leigh, I. M., Purkis, P. E. and Bruckner-Tuderman, L. (1987) LH7.2 monoclonal antibody detects type VII collagen in the sublamina densa zone of ectodermally-derived epithelia, including skin. *Epithelia*, **1**, 17–29.

Levy, D. M., Karanth, S. S., Springall, D. R. and Polak, J. M. (1989) Depletion of cutaneous nerves and neuropeptides in diabetes mellitus: an immunocytochemical study. *Diabetologia*, **32**, 427–33.

Ludatscher, R. M. (1978) Ultrastructure of human dermal blood vessels with special reference to the endothelial filaments. *Virchows Arch. B.*, **27**, 347–57.

Moll, R., Franke, W. W., Schiller, D. L., Geiger, B. and Krepler, R. (1982) The catalog of human cytokeratins, patterns of expression in normal epithelia, tumors and cultivated cells. *Cell*, **31**, 11–24.

Morgan, P. R., Leigh, I. M., Purkis, P. E., Gardner, I. D., van Muijen, G. N. P. and Lane, E. B. (1987a) Site variation in keratin expression in human oral epithelia – an immunocytochemical study of individual keratins. *Epithelia*, **1**, 31–43.

Morgan, P. R., Shirlaw, P. J., Johnson, N. W., Leigh, I. M. and Lane, E. B. (1987b) Potential applications of anti-keratin antibodies in oral diagnosis. *J. Oral Pathol.*, **16**, 212–22.

Norton, A. J. and Isaacson, P. G. (1987) Monoclonal antibody L26, an antibody that is reactive with normal and neoplastic B lymphocytes in routinely fixed and paraffin wax embedded tissues. *J. Clin. Pathol.*, **40**, 1405–12.

Paraskevopoulos, J. A., Hosking S. W. and Johnson AG. (1988) Do all minor excised lesions require histological examination? Discussion paper. *J. R. Soc. Med.*, **81**, 583–4.

Pinkus, H. and Hunter, R. (1960) Simplified acid orcein and Giemsa technique for routine staining of skin sections. *Arch. Dermatol.*, **82**, 699–700

Rowden, G., Phillips, T. M., Lewis, M. G. and Wilkinson, R. D. (1979) Target role of Langerhans cells in myocosis fungoides, transmission and immunoelectron microscopic studies. *J. Cut. Pathol.*, **6**, 364–82.

Ryan, T. J. (1976) The blood vessels of the skin. *J. Invest. Dermatol.*, **67**, 110–18.

Sauder, D. N., Carter, D., Katz, S. I. and Oppenheim, B. J. (1982) Epidermal cell production of thymocyte activating factor. *J. Invest. Dermatol.*, **79**, 34–9.

Shimada, S. and Katz, S. I. (1988) The skin as an immunologic organ. *Arch. Pathol. Lab. Med.*, **112**, 231–4.

Silberberg, J., Baer, R., Rosenthal, S., Thorbecke, J. and Berezowsky, V. (1975) Dermal and intravascular Langerhans cells at sites of passively induced allergic contact sensitivity. *Cell. Immunol.*, **18**, 435–53.

Smith, L. (1989) Histopathologic characteristics and ultrastructure of aging skin. *Cutis*, **43**, 414–24.

Stingl, G. (1980) The functional role of Langerhans cells. *J. Invest. Dermatol.*, **74**, 315–18.

Streilein, J. W. (1978) Lymphocyte traffic, T-cell malignancies and the skin. *J. Invest. Dermatol.*, **71**, 167–71.

Streilein, J. W. (1983) Skin-associated lymphoid tissue (SALT), origins and functions. *J. Invest. Dermatol.*, **80** (suppl.), 12s–16s.

Takahashi, S. and Hashimoto K. (1985) Derivation of Langerhans cell granules from cytomembrane. *J. Invest. Dermatol.*, **84**, 469–71.

Urmacher, C. (1990) Histology of normal skin. *Am. J. Surg. Pathol.*, **14**, 671–86.

Weinstein, B. R., Bernhard, J. D., Winters and T. H. (1986) Is it appropriate for primary care physicians to perform skin biopsies. *Arch. Intern. Med.*, **146**, 1293–4.

2 Biopsy methods and strategy for reporting biopsies

Dr M. L. Price and Dr N. Kirkham

In this chapter the reasons for and methods of biopsy are explained and put into context, after which the technical considerations are discussed and a strategy for producing a clinically useful histopathology report is explained.

2.1 The dermatologist's point of view

2.1.1 Types of biopsy

A biopsy is usually undertaken for one of five reasons:

i. To remove an entire dermal or epidermal growth either benign or malignant e.g. a melanocytic naevus, appendage tumour, basal cell carcinoma, or malignant melanoma. Apart from the diagnosis the clinician will wish to know if the lesion is completely excised. The degree of certainty as to excision will, of course, depend on the way the gross specimen has been sectioned in the laboratory.

ii. To check the diagnosis of a growth that is too big to remove completely by simple excision and suture, and where alternative modes of therapy, such as cryotherapy, radiotherapy or more complex surgical techniques, may be under consideration. Dermatologists will try very hard to avoid this incisional type of biopsy where the overall morphology of the lesion can be vital for assessment and diagnosis, e.g. with lesions of melanoma, Spitz naevus or keratoacanthoma. However this technique can be very helpful in confirming the diagnosis say of a large basal cell carcinoma and assessing its growth pattern before submitting the patient to definitive treatment. Bowen's disease can often cover quite a wide area and cryotherapy, rather than excision, may be more appropriate once the diagnosis and lack of invasion has been confirmed.

iii. To examine the morphology of a rash that is difficult to categorize clinically. This can take both clinician and pathologist into 'grey' areas where it is not always possible to reach a definite conclusion. Outside the teaching centres it is rare to see classical examples of, say, psoriasis, atopic eczema or lichen planus, down the microscope. The clinician does not need help with these. On the other hand he may be glad to confirm the diagnosis of conditions such as discoid lupus erythematosus, diffuse granuloma annulare or sarcoid.

Many inflammatory dermatoses do not have a specific histological appearance and it is only when the microscopic changes are considered within the clinical context that a conclusion can be reached. Thus the distinction of pityriasis rosea from a subacute dermatitis can be impossible, and while on occasion erythema multiforme will present a 'full house' appearance, more often than not the changes are subtle or atypical.

Beware also the slide that looks tantalizingly normal. Urticarial vasculitis, urticaria pigmentosa, cutaneous macular amyloid and dermatophyte infection can all be overlooked if not carefully considered.

Even if a specific diagnosis cannot be reached it is helpful to provide the clinician with the information that is available. Thus the predominant cell type and position of any infiltrate should be stated. The presence of eosinophils, for example, could suggest an exogenous cause such as unsuspected insect bites; alternatively, eosinophils may be seen in the prodromal rash preceding pemphigus or pemphigoid. The migration of lymphocytes into the epidermis in the absence of spongiosis brings early cutaneous lymphoma to mind.

The clinician will also wish to know when there is evidence of vascular damage and the extent of the changes observed. The histopathology of many vasculitic disorders can be frustrating, for although the damage to the vessels can be clearly seen, standard techniques rarely help to discover the offending antigen.

When dealing with 'grey' cases it may be that further material either for routine processing or additional techniques such as immunostaining, could be valuable and this should be discussed with the dermatologist, who may decide to watch the clinical course of the patient before repeating the biopsy, as the eruption may vary in severity or alter its nature providing more clear-cut clues to diagnosis.

Clinicians sometimes take serial biopsies over months or years to monitor the progress of a disorder. This is undertaken most frequently with cutaneous T-cell lymphomas. Early histopathology can be very subtle but provides an important baseline to further observations.

iv. For immunopathology: this is playing an ever increasing role in dermatology. Fresh specimens will be routinely sent for assessment when any of the immuno-bullous disorders are in question. Monoclonal antibodies now play an important part in the dissection of lymphocytic infiltrates and are beginning to be of importance in the study of intermediate filaments, such as cytokeratins.

v. Tissue may be supplied to the histopathologist as well as the microbiologist when an infective condition is suspected, so that organisms may be cultured from the tissue, as well as being seen in appropriately stained sections (Spencer and Callen, 1989). The recognition of deep and superficial fungi is often made on histological grounds. The same is true for diseases caused by protozoa, such as leishmaniasis. In addition, the host response to an infective agent such as leprosy may need assessing. Syphilis both a clinical and pathological mimic of other disorders may first be suggested by an alert pathologist.

2.1.2   *Biopsy techniques*

The dermatologist has the advantage of being able to see and reach the target organ easily; on the other hand, the appearance of the scar is often of considerable importance cosmetically, for instance, on the face where many biopsies are performed. Thus the material reaching the laboratory may not always be ideal from the pathologist's point of view.

Five principle forms of skin biopsy are employed, usually under local anaesthesia.

(*a*) *Excisional or incisional biopsy*   This can be used for the complete excision of a small growth, or to provide material fresh or frozen from a larger growth or more diffuse rash. From the pathologist's point of view this is usually the most satisfactory type of biopsy. It should provide adequate material that is easy to prepare and orientate. The material can be inadequate however, particularly if the specimen is too shallow. The assessment of panniculitis or scleroderma for example requires a specimen reaching beyond the fat layer to the fascia.

(*b*) *The punch biopsy*   This is obtained using a sharp punch 3 or 4 mm in diameter. The technique is quick and simple; often no sutures are required. The method is much favoured in the USA, but is less popular in the UK as frequently the quantity of material obtained is inadequate.

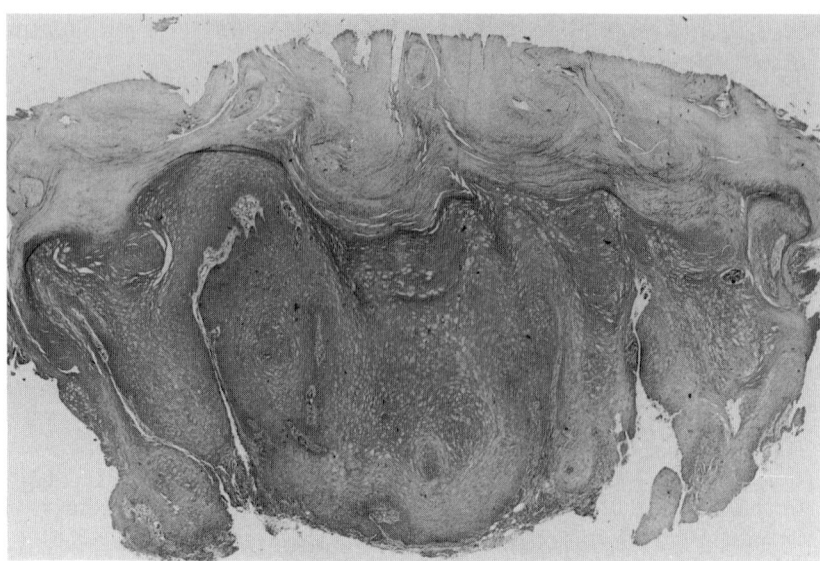

Figure 2.1   Curetting specimen of wart. The lesion is completely removed, without any accompanying dermis, and shows typical appearances of a proliferating, circumscribed epidermal lesion, without cellular atypia.

Few lesions are small enough to be completely excised in this manner; some surgeons will use the punch to excise deep, ice-pick acne scars but such lesions hold little of pathological interest.

(c)   *Curettage*   Used principally for superficial hyperkeratotic lesions, such as seborrhoeic warts or solar keratoses, this method provides the least satisfactory pathological specimens. Although considerable material can be obtained, it often consists largely of keratin with little underlying epidermis or dermis. Furthermore, the overall architecture of the lesion may have been completely disrupted by the process. Despite these drawbacks, the dermatologist may choose this method of removal because it is the most expedient for the patient. Thus a large solar keratosis on a tight scalp can be adequately dealt with by curettage, while the alternative of excision and flap rotation or even grafting is not warranted by the condition. Seborrhoeic warts are also frequently dealt with in this manner. Some clinicians advocate this technique combined with cautery for the management of small basal cell carcinomas. In this situation, the adequacy of treatment cannot always be assessed by the pathologist as further tissue is destroyed by the cautery.

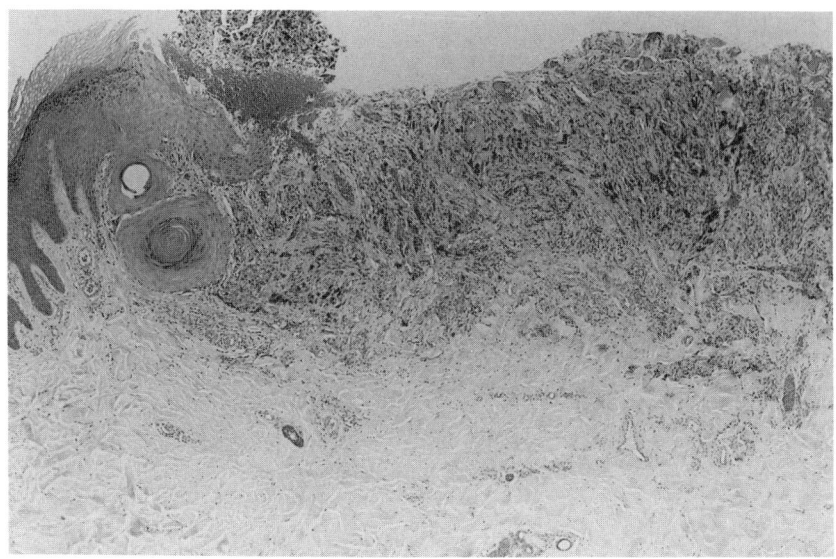

Figure 2.2 Curettage was performed on this warty lesion, but failed to remove all of the dermal pigment. Subsequent excision confirmed the presence of a blue naevus, with extension of the lesion into the lower dermis.

(*d*) *Shave biopsy* Used primarily for the removal of raised melanocytic naevi on the face. The lesion is sliced off flush with the skin using a scalpel blade. This leaves a satisfactory cosmetic result, although the lesion is often incompletely excised. This method can also be employed to obtain diagnostic biopsies. However, the amount of material obtained can be inadequate especially if the pathology is in the deeper dermis or beyond (Parkinson, 1988).

(*e*) *The snip* This is the easiest surgical procedure to perform but can only be used on pedunculated lesions such as skin tags and neurofibromas. Good, undistorted specimens are obtained.

(*f*) *Fixation* Most laboratories in the UK use some variant of formal saline fixation. Most of the biopsies illustrated in this book have been fixed in neutral buffered formal saline, which is a fail safe method but at the cost of some loss of cellular detail. Good cellular morphology can be guaranteed using the formaldehyde/mercuric chloride/acetic acid (FMA) fixation method.

The fixative is made from 100 ml of 40% formaldehyde, 20 g of mercuric chloride, 30 ml of glacial acetic acid, diluted to 1000 ml with

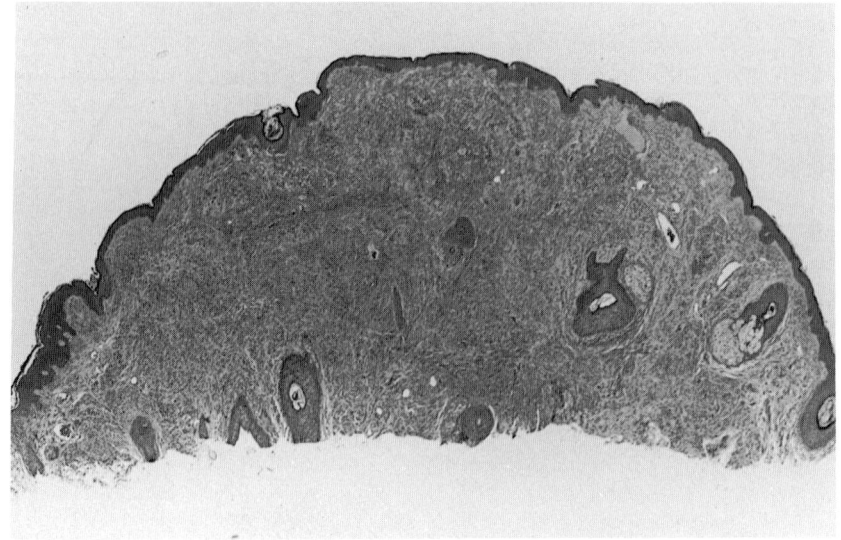

Figure 2.3   Shave biopsy is an effective way of dealing with most benign naevi. The dermis is filled with naevus cells, without atypia. Although the lesion extends to the base of the specimen recurrence is unlikely and a good cosmetic result can be expected.

distilled water. Biopsies should be fixed for 2 hr in this solution, followed by further fixation in 70% alcohol, prior to processing.

2.1.3   What the pathologist needs to know

In addition to the surgical specimen, the clinician is responsible for furnishing the pathologist with adequate clinical information. Standard forms and specimen bottles must be legibly and accurately labelled, with only one specimen per pot. The following should be recorded:

i   The site of the biopsy.
ii   The type of biopsy (excisional, incisional, punch, etc.).
iii. Brief clinical details and working diagnosis or differential diagnosis.
iv.   Appropriate requests for special stains or immunopathology.

In return the dermatologist would like a clear-cut report with a conclusion even if this is only to say that no definite diagnosis can be reached on the material supplied.

2.2   Trimming the biopsy

Most skin biopsies are small and do not need much trimming. Curettings should be put straight into the cassette, with an attempt to try and embed the larger bits on edge. Small biopsies and snips are best processed and embedded whole, with serial levels cut through the block to identify the lesion, as appropriate. Biopsies that are around 1.0 to 1.5 cm long can be bisected longitudinally. Larger biopsies and shaves are usually best cut transversely into a series of slices 1.5 to 2 mm thick, so that the best part of the whole biopsy can be examined in one block. Biopsies containing a tumour should have their bottoms painted with a pigment, such as Indian ink, so that the deep resection margin can be identified in the sections, when assessing the adequacy of the excision. Larger excisions of tumours should be sliced to ensure that the tumour and all the excision margins are represented in the sections (Hurt, 1991).

Punch biopsies usually present no problem. When these are performed for the investigation of alopecia, they must be sectioned transversely at several levels through the block to identify the changes present at different levels in the hair follicles (Headington, 1984).

2.3   Strategies for reporting skin biopsies

Dermatopathology is bedevilled with eponyms and curious names that tend to cloud the nature of the disease process. There is much to be said for analysing as many skin biopsies as possible from first principles. The abnormality should be identified and its relationship with and to the various components of the skin studied. The size of this book has been kept within reasonable bounds by excluding many less common conditions which exist as case reports in the literature, but which occur rarely and unpredictably in any individual practice.

Whilst it is true that one can only make a diagnosis if one is aware of the existence of that diagnosis, it is perhaps more important to know when one does not know the diagnosis. This could be a result of ignorance or from relying upon a short guide such as this, but it could also be because the biopsy in question is from a condition not obeying the accepted criteria. Once one is aware of the problem then there is a whole literature of published articles, case reports and reviews which may lead to the answer, especially if you ask your librarian nicely to help you to do the search, or even do the search for you.

Alternatively, it may be possible to cut further levels, or to use extra stains. Indeed, it has been said that the most important special stain is the section cut at a deeper level in the block. There is little to be gained by just letting a section lie by the side of one's microscope in the vain hope that some truth will emerge after an obscure process of incubation. It is always worth setting aside a little undisturbed time to wrestle with difficult biopsies, but if there is no result after the first round then one should cut more levels and do further stains, such as the AOG, which is highly recommended by Pinkus (Pinkus and Hunter, 1960).

Often the lesion is small and is situated at the centre of the biopsy. When the biopsy is small and is processed whole, the early cuts off the resulting block may not show the lesion. Before issuing a report concluding that the biopsy shows only normal skin or no abnormality, it is essential to examine sections from levels deeper in the block.

It may help to request immunohistochemical studies with a selection of primary antibodies appropriate to the problem in hand, in the hope of extracting further information from the tissue.

It is also worth considering whether the biopsy is truly adequate. Even after examining multiple levels it may still not be possible to see the lesion, and this may be because the lesion is not present within the biopsy. Alternatively, the biopsy may have been fixed and it may be necessary to have fresh tissue to perform immunohistochemical staining for immune complexes or lymphocyte markers. In these circumstances, it is always worth repeating the biopsy to get adequate tissue for a full investigation. If, after a good, quiet look, a phone call to the dermatologist for further information, joint review of the biopsy, examination of further levels, special stains, large books, specific articles and further biopsies there is still no conclusion, then one can always send the material away to the expert at St Elsewheres. Unless there is something extra available there to which one does not have access in the laboratory and library, then one may be disappointed by the reply. It is most important to have good biopsies dealt with adequately. This alone will lead to more accurate diagnoses in the majority of cases.

2.4   Examining the biopsy

Despite what has been said above, it is impossible to ignore the established nomenclature when describing the changes and variations from normal that are present in an individual biopsy. The vocabulary that is used is restricted to this tissue but is, in essence, a series of synonyms for the words used to describe the same general processes of pathology seen in other tissues.

We have all read, and probably written, rather unhelpful skin biopsy reports on biopsies of inflammatory or non-tumourous lesions along the lines of 'a skin biopsy showing hyperkeratosis, parakeratosis, acanthosis and dermal lymphocytic infiltration'. Each of these abnormalities

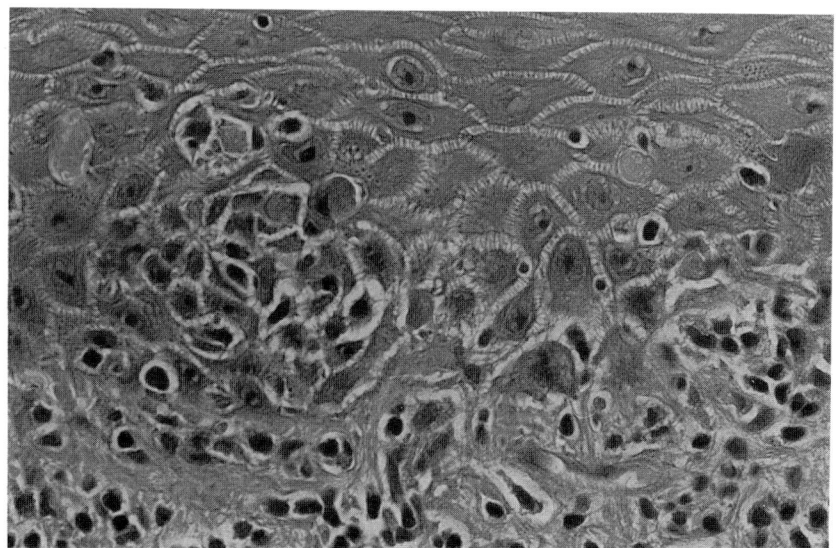

Figure 2.4 Eczema. There is exocytosis of lymphocytes and spongiosis between keratinocytes.

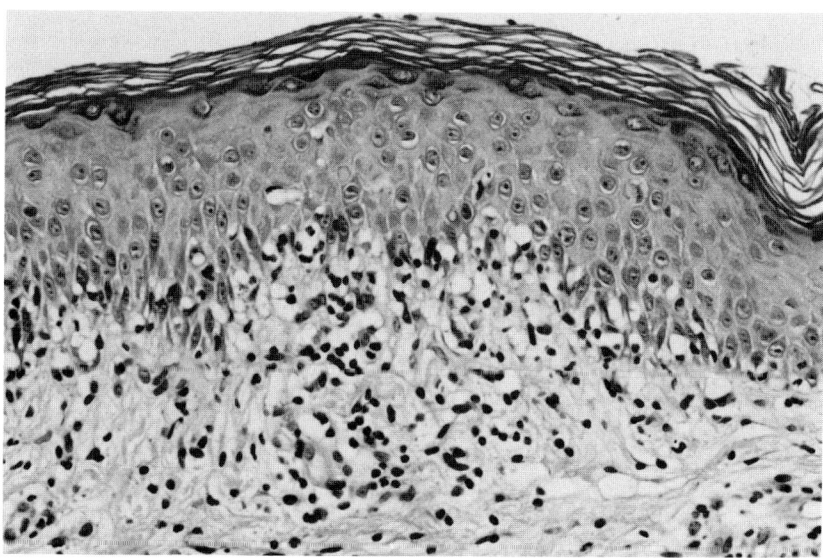

Figure 2.5 Lupus erythematosus. There is an interstitial dermal lymphocytic infiltrate with hydropic change of epidermal basal cells. The keratin is of open, basket-weave type.

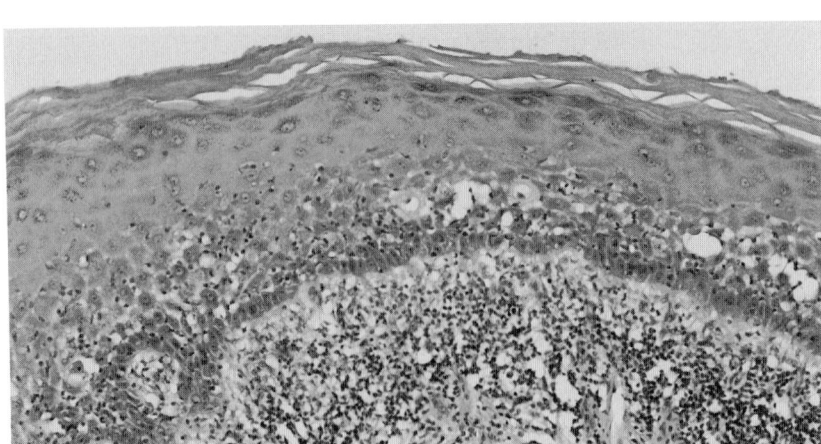

Figure 2.6   In this lichenoid infiltrate there is a band of lymphocytic infiltration in the dermis, extending into the lower epidermis, with secondary keratinocyte damage. There is also orthokeratotic hyperkeratosis.

may be present but the resulting report is meaningless. What is needed is a precise description of the abnormalities seen in the biopsy so that their relative significance can be weighed and related to the likely diagnosis or conclusion. To achieve this the biopsy must be described in a systematic way. There are various possible ways of going about this, but the author prefers to start at the top and work down.

So the first thing to look at is the keratin layer. One must decide whether this is increased or decreased in thickness for that part of the body from which the biopsy is taken. This partly depends upon experience, but by and large the keratin layer is thick where the skin is thick and thin where the skin is thin. So one can always pinch oneself in the same place if one has forgotten what the skin is like there. The range of epidermal thickness is from the palm, which is the thinnest at 1.1 mm, to the back, where it can be up to 4.0 mm thick (Goldsmith, 1990).

An increased thickness is called hyperkeratosis. This word can be modified by two further descriptors. Firstly, try to grade the degree of hyperkeratosis. Secondly, the nature of the hyperkeratosis should be described. This means saying whether the keratin is of the normal 'basket-weave' type seen in normal body skin; whether it is the dense 'orthokeratotic' keratin, densely eosinophilic but without any nuclei, seen in callosities; or whether nuclei are present, indicating 'parakeratosis'. Over a small inflammatory lesion the parakeratosis may be fairly localized, whereas an actinic keratosis should show alternating bands of orthokeratotic and parakeratotic hyperkeratosis, with the parakeratotic keratin overlying the rete ridges. There are, indeed, a whole variety of types of parakeratosis (Price *et al.*, 1984).

The presence of other cells should also be noted. Neutrophil polymorphs are the most likely cells to be present and may mean that there is fungal infection present. This can be confirmed with a special method on a serial section, such as Grocott's stain.

Next, look for the granular cell layer to see whether it is absent, present or increased in thickness, as it might be in a viral wart.

The prickle cell layer may also show variations in thickness. Increased thickness is known as 'acanthosis'. When the cells themselves start to separate and lie singly or in small groups within the epidermis the process is called 'acantholysis'.

In inflammatory lesions there is likely to be some degree of inflammatory cell infiltration or 'exocytosis'. The nature of the cells and their proportion and distribution should be assessed, together with the associated changes in the keratinocytes. These may be separated by 'spongiosis', which may be severe enough to produce a spongiotic vesicle. Other forms of vesicle may be present in association with bullous dermatoses, viral infections and lymphomas, amongst others. The reaction may result in the death of keratinocytes with the formation of eosinophilic 'Civatte' bodies.

The keratinocytes will show varying degrees of nuclear and cytoplasmic abnormality in conditions such as actinic keratosis or Bowen's disease. These also must be identified, characterized and graded. Keratinocytes which have become prematurely keratinized are known as dyskeratotic cells.

The basal layer forms the interface with the dermis, from whence the inflammatory cells spring. So various changes can occur here including 'hydropic degeneration' of lupus erythematosus (LE), and the loss of order seen in lichenoid reactions. The melanocytes also lie here so their degree of pigmentation and variation from the normal must be assessed.

The basement membrane zone cannot really be seen in H and E stained sections, but the diffuse thickening seen in LE can sometimes be made out as an acellular haze between basal cells and the nearest dermal nuclei.

Things can get even more complicated in the dermis, but if you stay calm it is not too difficult to make a reasonably comprehensive inventory of the changes present. Basically this comes down to describing

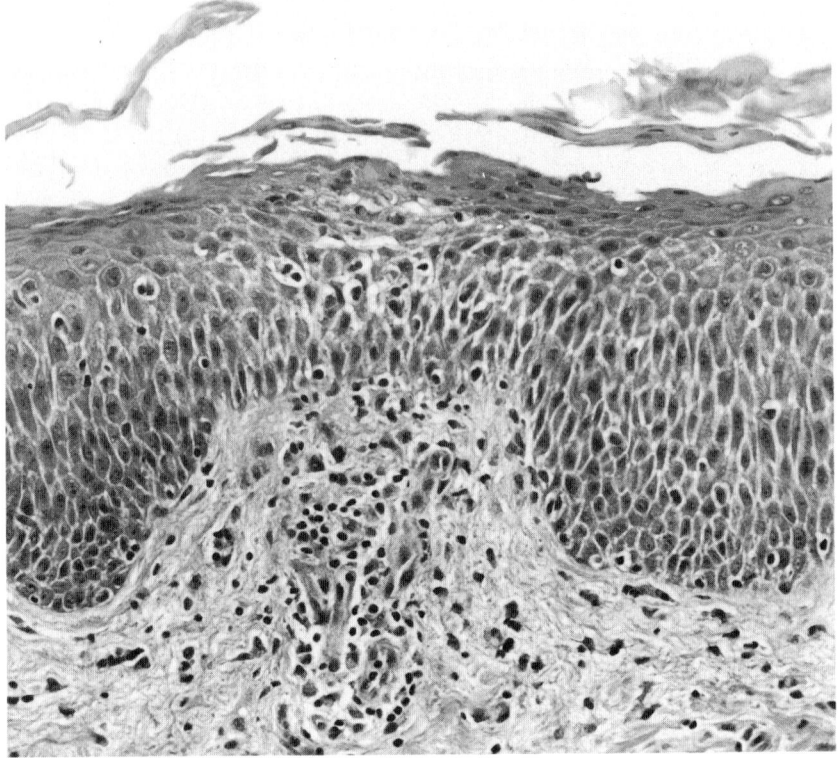

Figure 2.7   Psoriasis. Lymphocytes extend from around superficial dermal vessels into the epidermis, with interstital oedema and also with parakeratotic hyperkeratosis and loss of the granular layer.

the collagen, elastic and ground substance of the papillary and reticular parts of the dermis, together with changes in the vessels and the nature, degree and distribution of an inflammatory cell infiltrate.

These changes will be dealt with in more detail elsewhere, but it is worth remembering that polarized light shows up collagen fibres well, so filters should always be conveniently within reach, and get to know the normal appearance of collagen in the papillary and reticular dermis. The AOG stain is a good way of staining the elastic fibres.

The ground substance may sometimes be altered or increased and can be stained with Alcian blue. The diseases of dermal stroma form a rather unsatisfactory area as far as disease nomenclature is concerned, with only a few well characterized changes and many biopsies which are difficult to classify adequately.

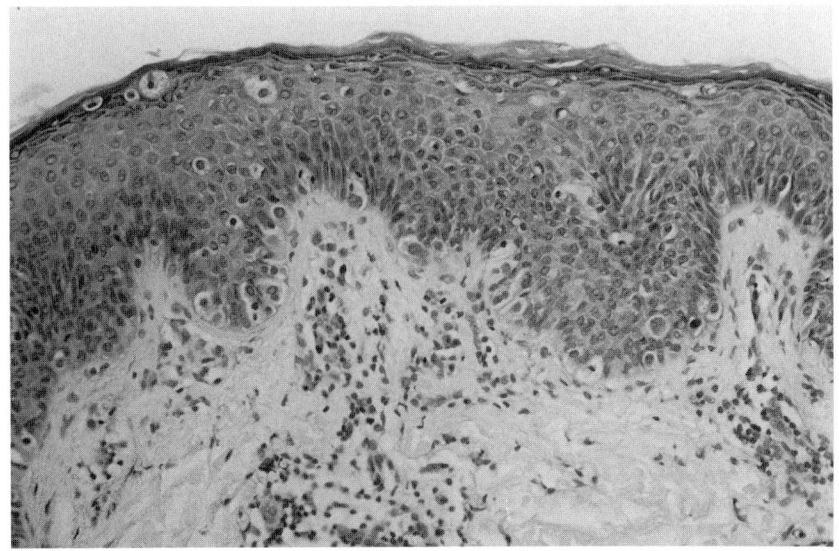

Figure 2.8 Paget's disease. Large, atypical tumour cells infiltrate the epidermis.

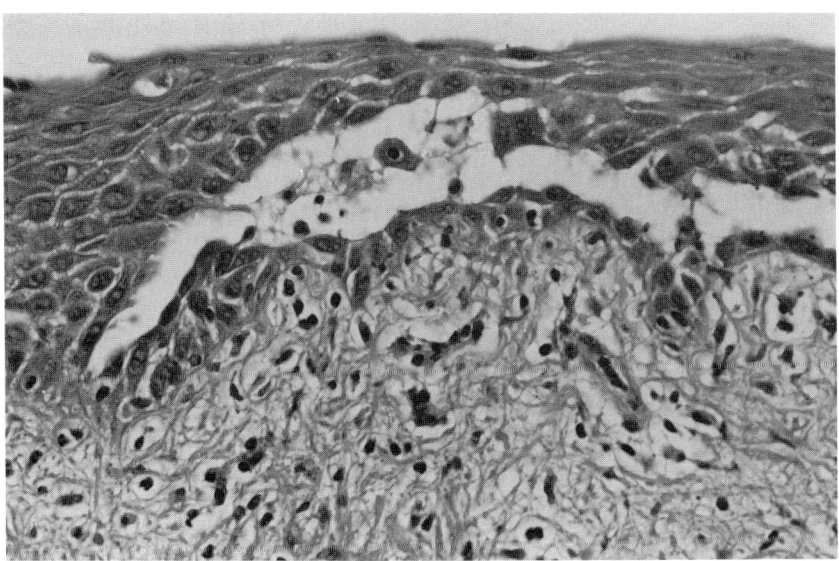

Figure 2.9 Pemphigus. An intraepidermal blister containing acantholytic cells.

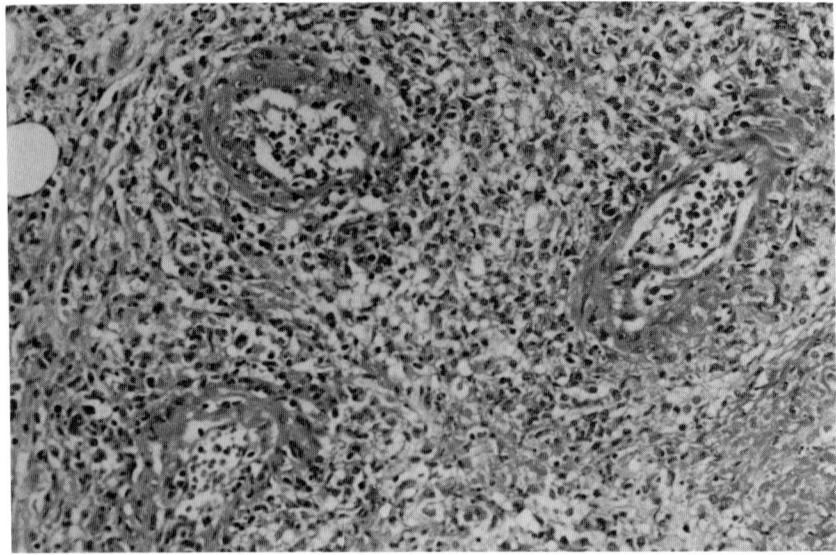

Figure 2.10   Dermal vasculitis. The vessel walls are damaged and show fibrinoid change as part of the inflammatory reaction filling the dermis.

   The blood vessels often show little change even in the presence of large numbers of lymphocytes, except for increasing size of the endothelial cells. Sometimes vessels will be seen to be occluded by thrombus, protein or some form of embolus. In cases of true vasculitis fibrinoid change or more severe manifestations of inflammatory damage may be seen.

   Last but not least, the nature and distribution of the inflammatory cell infiltrate must be determined and described. This is often the nub of the whole problem in describing and classifying biopsies of inflammatory dermatoses and will be dealt with elsewhere. In short, however, one should look out for the cell types present. Usually, small lymphocytes will predominate and immunophenotyping will show them to be T-cells, B-cells being quite rare in the skin. Macrophages may be present and will predominate in granulomas. Neutrophils may be part of an acute allergic reaction, but may also be a sign of infection (Spencer and Callen, 1989). Eosinophils may feature in insect bites or drug reactions. Also never forget the mast cell. These may not show up very well in an H and E section but their metachromatic granules are more easily seen with an AOG stain and may be especially important in the aetiology of conditions in which the biopsy shows little other apparent abnormality on the H and E.

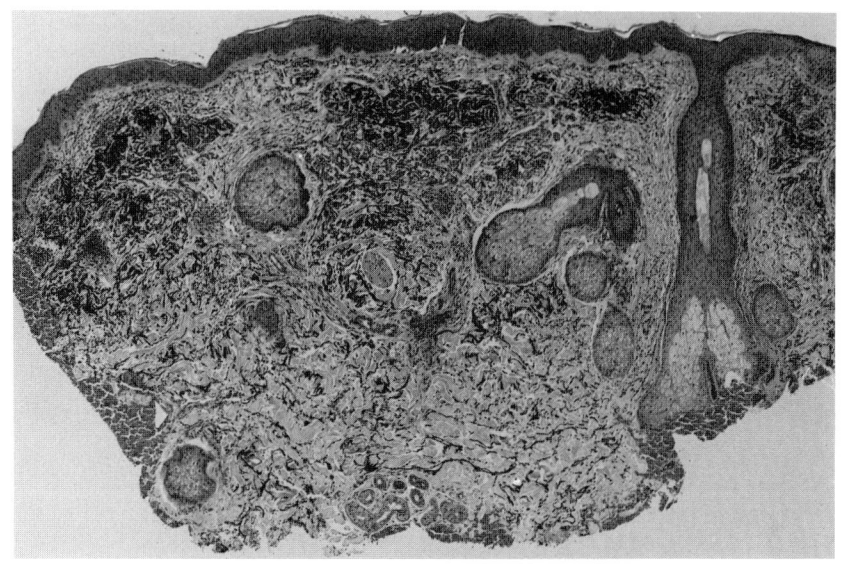

(a)

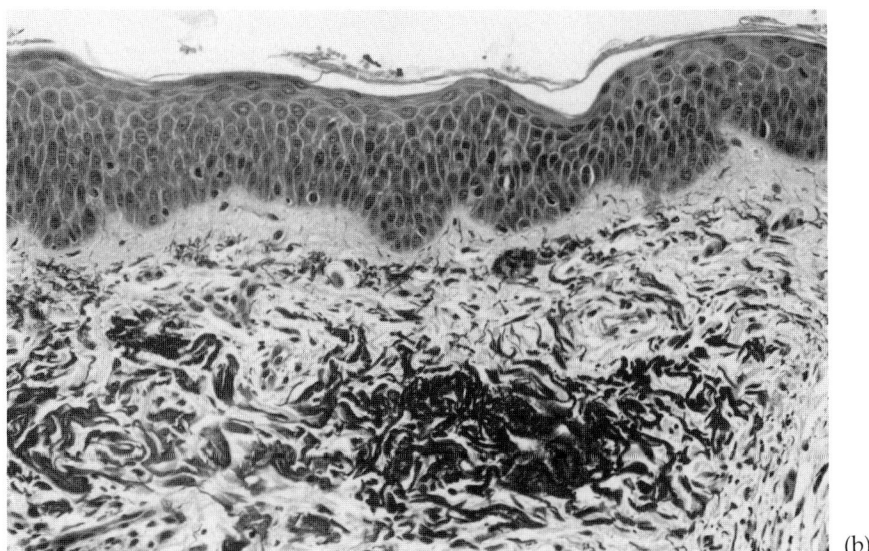

(b)

Figure 2.11 The acid orcein Giemsa stain (AOG). Elastic fibres and elastosis are easily seen in this example.

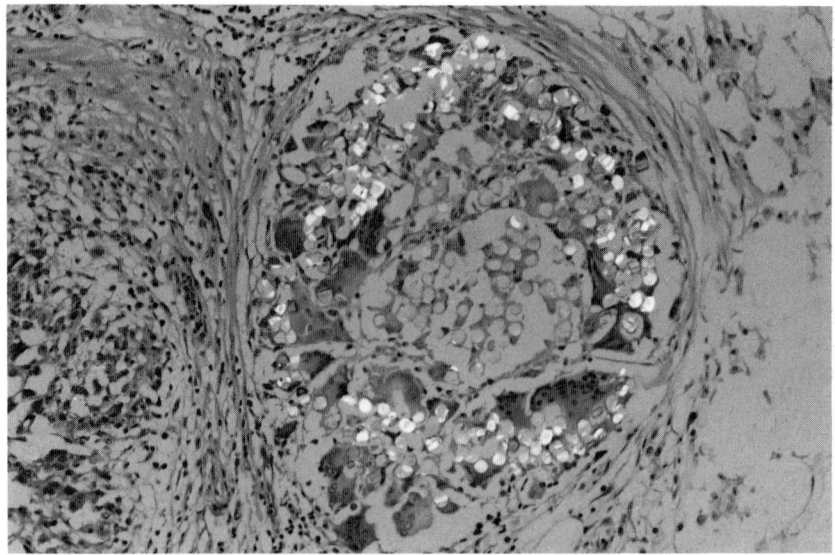

Figure 2.12 Polarizing microscopy may well show up foreign material, here a suture granuloma, or organisms, which may be inapparent on routine microscopy.

The other structures which connect the epidermis and dermis are the appendages. These may be involved in the process or may have been damaged or destroyed by it, so one must always look for the hair follicles and sweat glands to see what they show.

The subcutis is both straightforward and a problem. Straightforward because in the normal state it consists of fat separated by septae within which there are blood vessels. The changes that can take place are therefore rather limited to inflammation and necrosis, with varying degrees of granulomatous change. The problem is that the subcutis is largely beyond the remit of the dermatologist; often it is necessary to get a surgeon to perform a deep biopsy to get a good look at a subcutaneous disease process.

By adopting a systematic approach to the examination of the biopsy one should be at least half way towards the diagnosis and, failing that, at least a useful descriptive report can be produced which can then form the basis of further discussion.

References

Goldsmith, L. A. (1990) My organ is bigger than your organ. Arch. *Dermatol.*, **126**, 301–2.

Headington, J. T. (1984) Transverse microscopic anatomy of the scalp. A basis for a morphometric approach to disorders of the hair follicle. *Arch. Dermatol.*, **120**, 449–56.

Hurt, M. A. (1991) The rule of halves. A method of controlling the uniform 'cutting-in' of skin biopsies. *Am. J. Dermatopathol.*, **13**, 7–10.

Pinkus, H. and Hunter, R. (1960) Simplified acid orcein and Giemsa technique for routine staining of skin sections. *Arch. Dermatol.*, **82**, 699–700.

Parkinson, R. W. (1988) Shave biopsies – simple and useful. *Postgrad. Med.*, **84**, 161–3, 166, 169–70.

Price, M. L., Holden, C. A. and MacDonald, D. M. (1984) The diagnostic value of parakeratosis. *J. Cut. Pathol.*, **11**, 249–58.

Spencer, L. V. and Callen, J. P. (1989) Cutaneous manifestations of bacterial infections. *Dermatol. Clin.*, **7**, 579–89.

3 Intraepidermal keratoses and tumours

This chapter is concerned with abnormalities of keratinization and the epidermis, which may include atypical cytological changes, but in which the changes are still entirely intraepidermal. Epidermal tumours are dealt with in Chapter 5. This chapter considers the keratotic changes largely associated with actinic damage, a series of mainly eponymous abnormalities of keratin, a group of intraepidermal tumours and conditions featuring acantholysis and dyskeratosis.

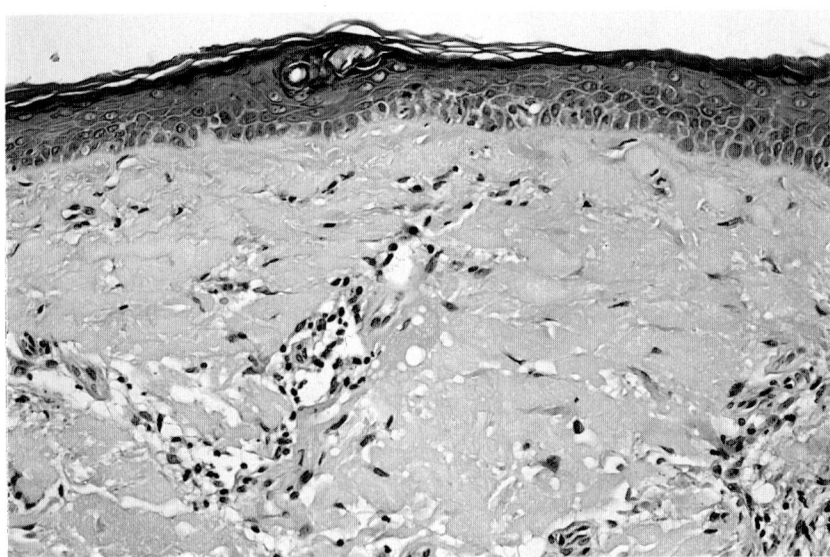

Figure 3.1 Solar elastosis. Dermal collagen bundles in the papillary dermis appear thickened and eosinophilic.

3.1   Actinic keratosis

With increasing age and exposure to the sun minor degrees of epidermal atypia become increasingly more common. These lesions are often removed, mainly for cosmetic reasons. The appearances seen in biopsies are at points on a spectrum between minor atypia and carcinoma. The average keratosis shows a mild to moderate degree of cellular atypia, mainly confined to the lower half of the epidermis. Overlying this there is a thick layer of keratin in which there are typical alternating vertical zones of hyperkeratosis and parakeratosis.

These therefore are the key points of diagnosis. The lesion must show evidence of cytological atypia in the epidermis, mainly in the form of nuclear enlargement and irregularity, and there must be parakeratosis alternating with orthokeratotic hyperkeratosis and the papillary dermis should show elastosis.

Such lesions are innocuous. There is no suggestion of dermal invasion. The underlying dermis will show a varying degree of solar elastosis: homogeneous change in the collagen which stains with eosin or orcein.

More advanced keratoses will show similar changes but of a more advanced degree. As the process advances to involve the greater part

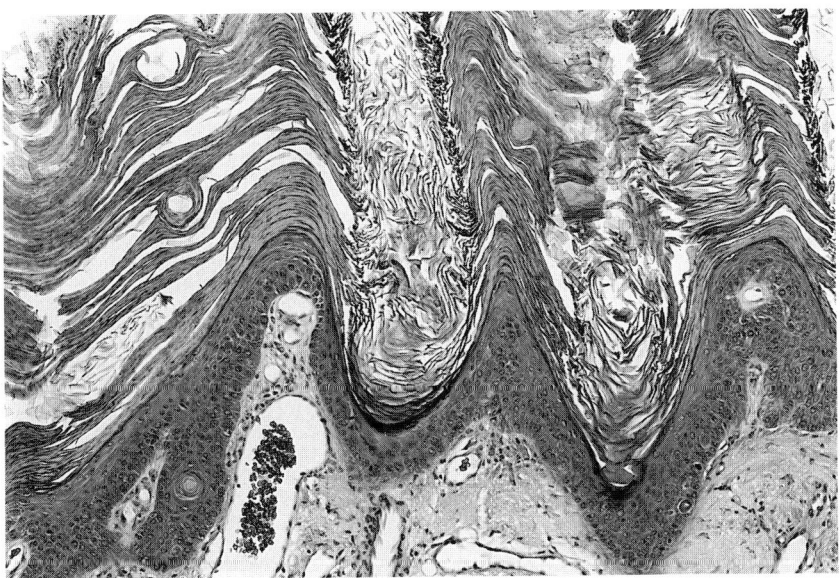

Figure 3.2   Actinic keratosis showing well-developed, alternating bands of hyperkeratosis and parakeratosis, with associated keratinocyte atypia.

of the epidermis, and the thickness of the epidermis starts to increase, then it is time to describe the lesions as 'florid keratoses'.

This sort of lesion has to be distinguished from pseudocarcinomatous hyperplasia, which is a reactive rather than a neoplastic phenomenon (Civatte, 1985). In response to an underlying inflammatory or neoplastic process it is the adnexa rather than the epidermis which undergo hyperplasia. Careful scrutiny will show that it is the infundibula of hair follicles and the eccrine ducts that are hyperplastic rather than the epidermis (Grunwald *et al.*, 1988).

Some of the more advanced keratoses show a loss of cohesion between the cells: usually the cells in the suprabasal layer. These are described as 'acantholytic keratoses'. Clinically they do not behave differently from common keratoses.

3.2   Bowen's disease

Bowen's disease is a clinical description used to describe lesions in which the whole thickness of the epidermis is atypical. In addition, there are occasional, very large atypical cells (Bowen's cells) and bizarre mitoses. The lesions are, once again, non-invasive. Sometimes it is difficult to decide between possible diagnoses of keratosis or Bowen's

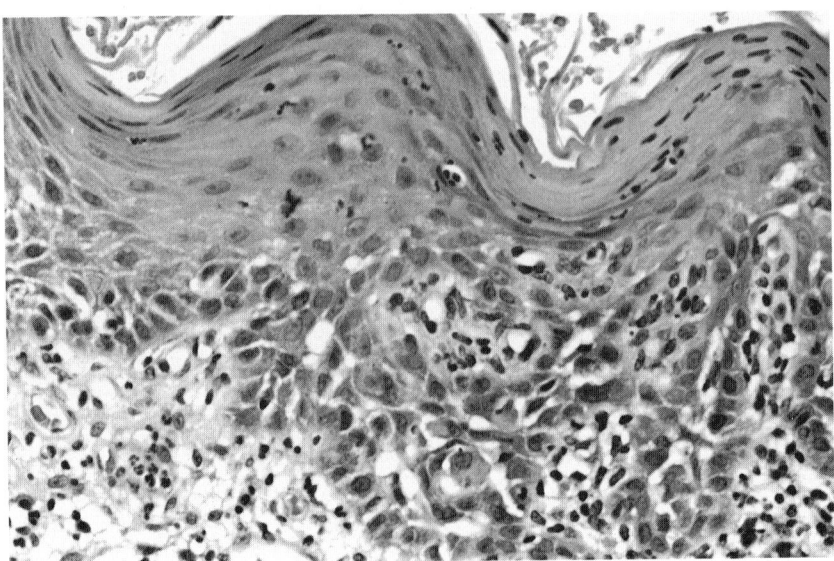

Figure 3.3   Acantholytic actinic keratosis, showing cellular atypia, acantholysis and parakeratosis.

disease, in which case the description 'Bowenoid keratosis' should be used.

3.3   Bowenoid papulosis

One should also be aware of the condition of 'Bowenoid papulosis' which occurs on the vulva or penis. The microscopic appearances are those of severe Bowenoid atypia, but the clinical behaviour is much more indolent than the biopsy appearances would suggest (Berger and Hori, 1978; Wade *et al.*, 1979). The precise association with aetiological agents, such as human papilloma virus, is uncertain, but certainly in women with this condition it is important to know that a cervical smear has been done and what the result is, as there is an increased risk of cervical carcinoma (Obalek *et al.*, 1986).

3.4   Flegel's disease

Flegel's disease is a scaly papular eruption which occurs on the lower legs, upper arms and pinnae of adults. The papules are 1 to 5 mm in

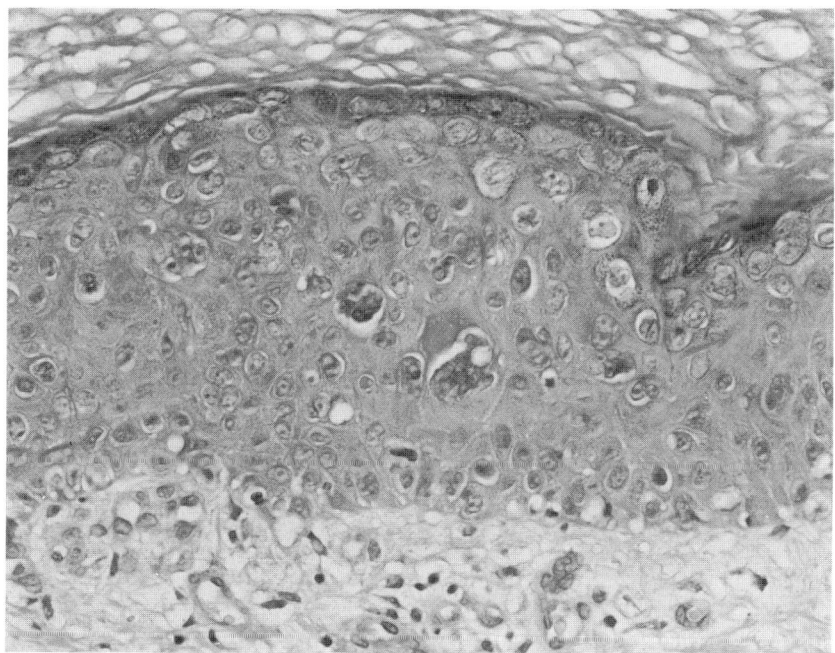

Figure 3.4   Bowen's disease. Large, atypical Bowenoid cells are present through the full thickness of the epidermis.

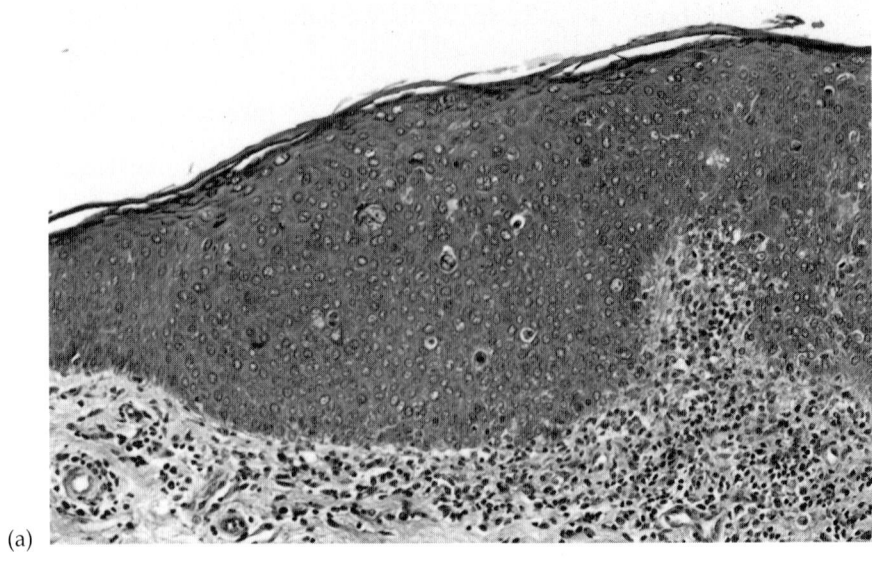

(a)

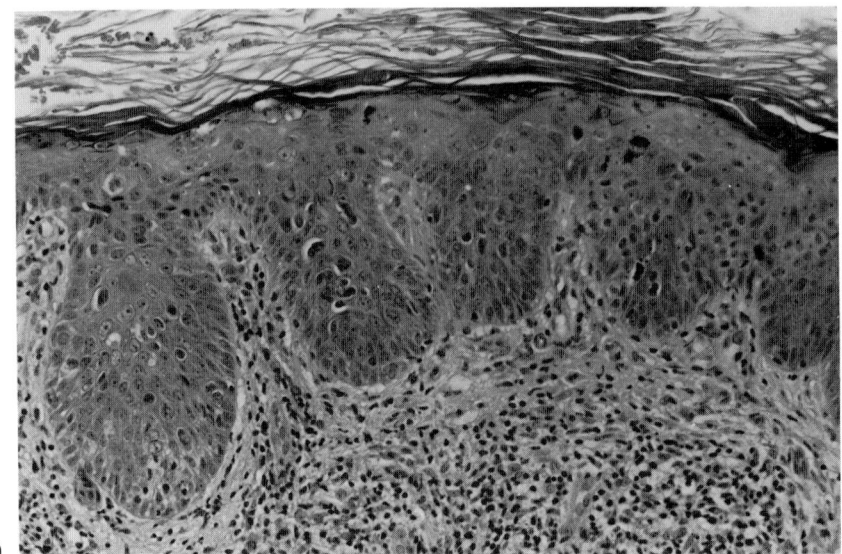

(b)

Figure 3.5 Bowenoid papulosis of the vulva (a and b). The appearance is essentially similar to cutaneous Bowen's disease.

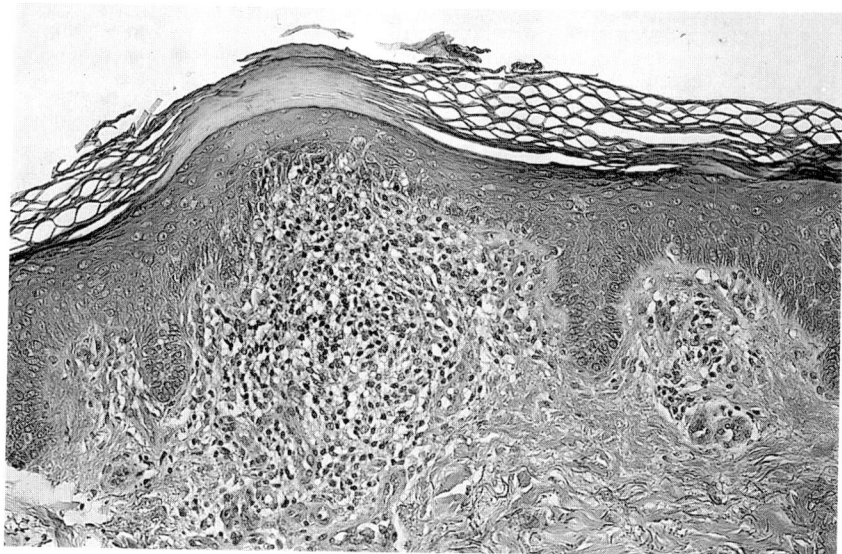

Figure 3.6   Flegel's disease. A circumscribed lesion with dermal lymphocytic reaction and peaked epidermis surmounted by dense band of hyperkeratosis.

diameter. The biopsy appearance is characteristic with a localized and piled up parakeratosis: the lens shaped lesion of hyperkeratosis lenticularis perstans. Beneath this the epidermis will shows loss of the granular layer, and a variable degree of spongiosis, in association with localized lymphocytic infiltration of the dermis at the base of the lesion.

It is uncertain whether the process is entirely inflammatory or whether there is a component of abnormal epidermal proliferation. There is some difficulty in separating this condition from Kyrle's disease, which may well be a variant of Flegel's disease (Kyrle, 1916, Tappeiner, *et al.*, 1969, Raffle and Rogers, 1969; Price *et al.*, 1987).

3.5 Porokeratosis

There is a group of conditions which have in common a distinct column of parakeratotic keratin: the so-called cornoid lamella. What appears to be a column, or pair of columns, in a section of the biopsy actually corresponds to a ring which moves centripetally as the lesion develops. Even this may not be entirely diagnostic, however, as similar appearances may be seen in a variety of conditions including viral warts and actinic keratoses (Wade and Ackerman, 1980). The clinical appearance of disseminated superficial actinic porokeratosis (DSAP) is relatively

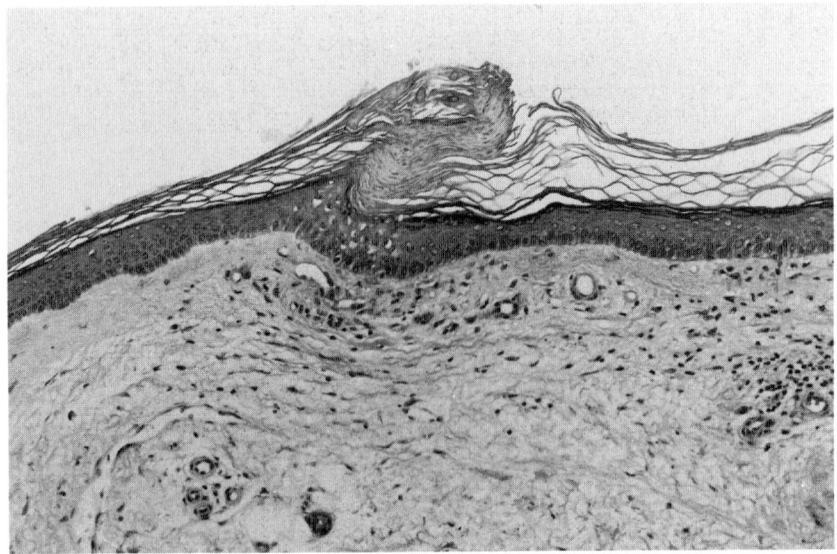

Figure 3.7   Disseminated superficial actinic porokeratosis, showing the characteristic cornoid lamella, leaning in towards the centre of the lesion.

distinct and cases are reasonably common. The other variants are rare. The biopsy must be taken from the edge of the lesion to have any chance of finding the cornoid lamella. Occasionally small lesions will be excised completely. This is another circumstance where multiple levels may need to be cut to find the lesion in the biopsy.

3.6   Disseminated superficial actinic porokeratosis (DSAP)

In this, the commonest type of porokeratosis, the lesions occur on sun exposed skin typically but not exclusively (Chernosky and Freeman, 1967). The lesions are small and thin with only a shallow furrow underlying the cornoid lamella. The epidermis at the centre of the ring may show almost any appearance from atrophic to hyperplastic.

3.7   Porokeratosis of Mibelli

This variant is usually inherited as an autosomal dominant condition in which localized areas of abnormal keratinization develop, usually in sun exposed areas of the limbs. The lesions may develop in childhood or adolescence, and have also been described as a complication of immunosuppression in renal transplant patients (Komorowski and

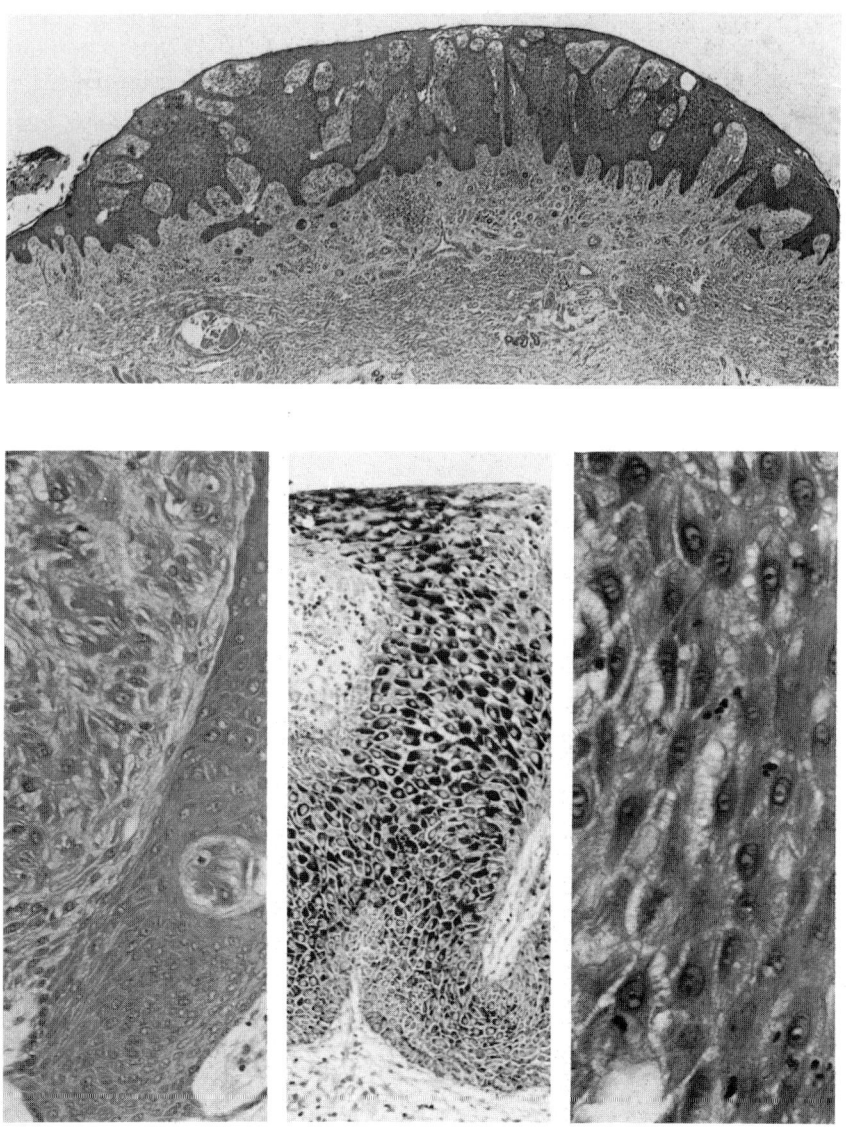

(a)

(b)   (c)   (d)

Figure 3.8   Clear cell acanthoma showing (a) rounded, radially symmetrical profile, (b) sharp demarcation from adjacent epidermis, (c) PAS-positive keratinocyte cytoplasm, and (d) neutrophils infiltrating between keratinocytes.

Clowry, 1989). They consist of plaques of variable size, from a few millimetres to a few centimetres, with well-defined borders and an atrophic or discoloured centre. In the biopsy, the well-defined border is seen to correspond to a cornoid lamella which overlies a more prominent epidermal furrow than that seen in DSAP.

The other variants are porokeratosis plantaris discreta, which occurs on the soles of young people, is painful and is associated with transepidermal elimination of dermal collagen and blood vessels (Kang and Chun, 1988); linear porokeratosis which mimics a linear epidermal naevus (Rahbari *et al.*, 1974); and punctuate porokeratosis which is characterized by small keratotic plugs on the palms or soles, with a 'music box spine' appearance (Himmelstein and Lynnfield, 1984; Friedman *et al.*, 1988).

3.8   Clear cell acanthoma

There are several benign forms of acanthoma (Brownstein, 1985). Of these the clear cell acanthoma of Degos is perhaps the commonest. Typically, the lesions occur as small, solitary, domed red plaques on the leg, usually between 5 and 20 mm in diameter (Degos and Civatte, 1970). The biopsy shows a sharply circumscribed acanthotic lesion with cells with clear PAS-positive cytoplasm. Characteristically, there is a moderate infiltrate of neutrophil polymorphs between the keratinocytes. The amount of glycogen in the cells raises the possibility of a sweat gland origin, but immunohistochemical studies show negative staining for carcinoembryonic antigen (CEA) and positive staining for involucrin. This combination is against a sweat gland origin (Hashimoto *et al.*, 1988). Occasional cases may have multiple lesions (Trau *et al.*, 1980).

3.9   Large cell acanthoma

This entity occurs as asymptomatic keratotic lesions on the face, upper limbs or back of the middle aged or elderly. It is commoner in women. The lesions may be multiple (Rabinowitz, 1983; Rahbari and Pinkus, 1978; Scholl, 1982). The biopsy should show sharply circumscribed islands of abnormal epidermis in which the keratinocytes have both large nuclei and increased cytoplasm, at least twice the usual size of cells in the epidermis or hair follicle. There is also hypergranulosis and orthokeratotic hyperkeratosis (Sanchez *et al.*, 1988).

The lesions are clinically similar to solar and seborrhoeic keratoses (Pinkus, 1970). More recently it has been reported that these lesions show nuclear and architectural atypia, dyskeratosis, suprabasal mitoses

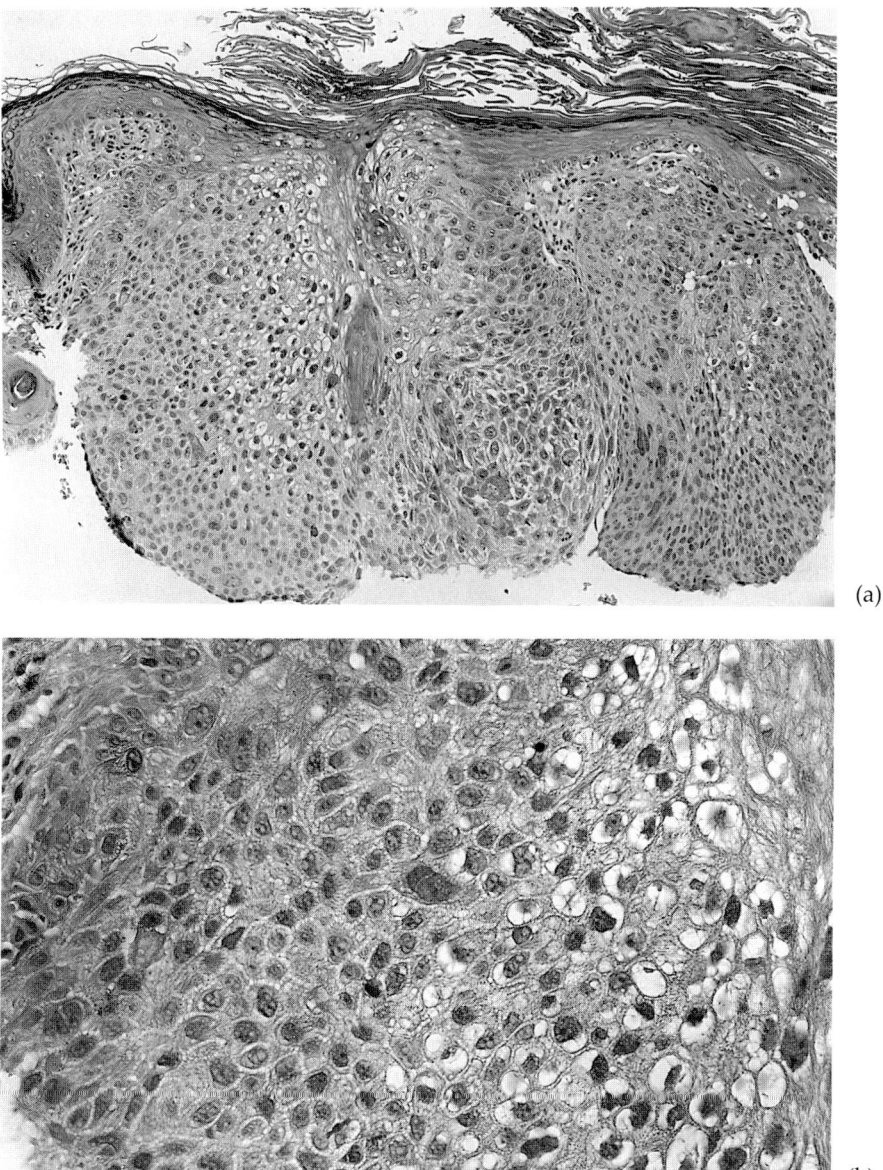

Figure 3.9 Large cell acanthoma showing (a) cytomegaly and acanthosis together with hyperkeratosis and parakeratosis, and (b) marked cytological and nuclear atypia within the lesion.

and extension to involve appendages: all features pointing towards a suggestion that the large cell acanthoma is a variant of Bowen's disease (Sanchez *et al.*, 1988).

3.10   Intraepidermal epithelioma – the Jadassohn phenomenon

There are a group of lesions characterized by intraepidermal nests of tumour cells. For a number of years pathologists have been aware of, but confused by, the *Borst-Jadassohn* phenomenon. In fact, this is an unjustified conjunction whose halves should be considered separately.

Borst described invasion of epidermis from an underlying squamous cell carcinoma of the lip. Jadassohn on the other hand described the more familiar phenomenon of nests of neoplastic keratinocytes which originate from, and remain within, the epidermis. His original description probably represented a third variation: that of pseudonests, where the border between normal and abnormal keratinocytes is not sharp. This may be seen in seborrhoeic warts. Thus the common form of intraepidermal epithelioma is best described as the Jadassohn phenomenon, and represents a variant form of seborrhoeic wart (Steffen and Ackerman, 1985).

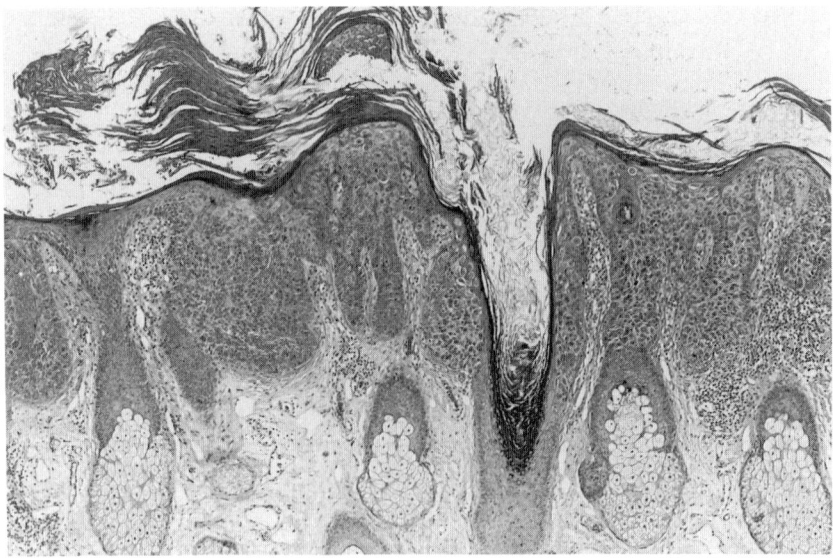

Figure 3.10 Intraepidermal epithelioma showing clonal variant of actinic keratosis, with nests of atypical cells within the epidermis and overlying bands of hyperkeratosis and parakeratosis.

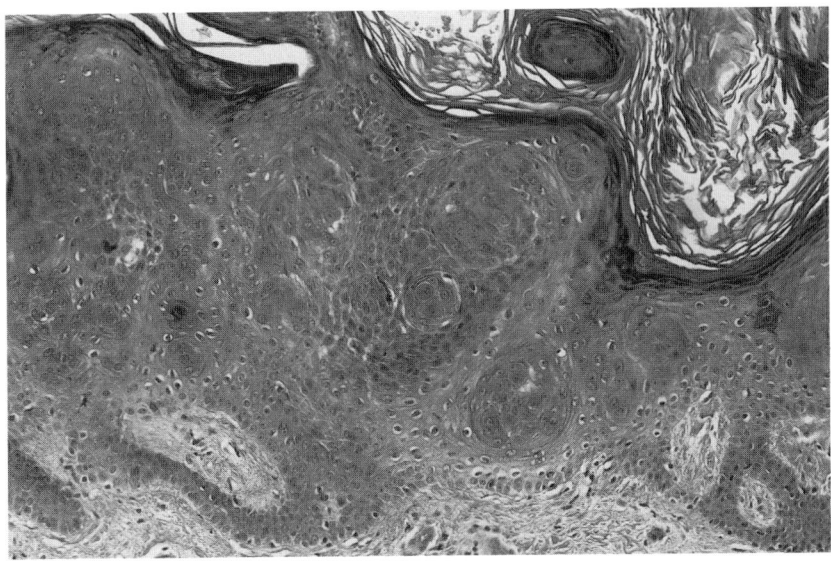

Figure 3.11 Intraepidermal epithelioma showing circumscribed nests of atypical cells within the epidermis.

3.11 Paget's disease

Paget's disease and Pagetoid malignant melanoma are separate phenomena. In mammary and extra-mammary Paget's disease the epidermis is invaded and colonized by epithelial cells which have the characteristics of simple epithelia (Kirkham *et al.*, 1985). They may be PAS positive and they stain with antibodies to low molecular weight cytokeratin and epithelial membrane antigen. Whilst mammary Paget's disease is invariably associated with a lesion in the underlying breast duct epithelium, extra-mammary Paget's appears to be a heterogeneous group of conditions (Wood and Hegedus, 1988). Using more specific antibodies, evidence of both apocrine and eccrine differentiation, and of keratin expression similar to the secretory cells of sweat glands, has been demonstrated in extra-mammary Paget's disease, suggesting the possibility of origin from pluripotent sweat gland germinative cells (Hasebe *et al.*, 1988; Cohen and DeRose, 1989; Tazawa *et al.*, 1988).

  Pagetoid melanoma is a variant of melanoma. The differential diagnosis can be made, in difficult cases, by demonstrating the presence of melanocyte markers such as HMB-45, S100 protein or NKI/C3 and the the absence of epithelial markers within the tumour cells.

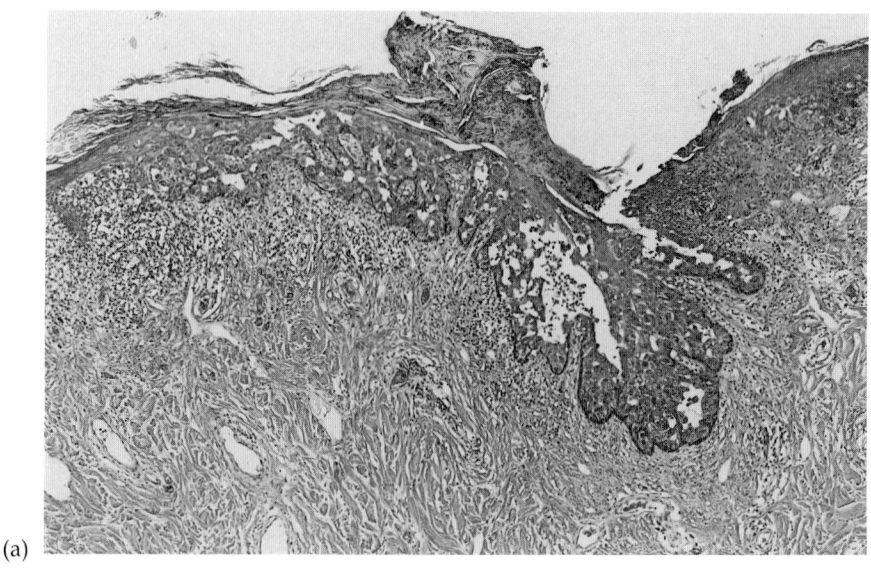

(a)

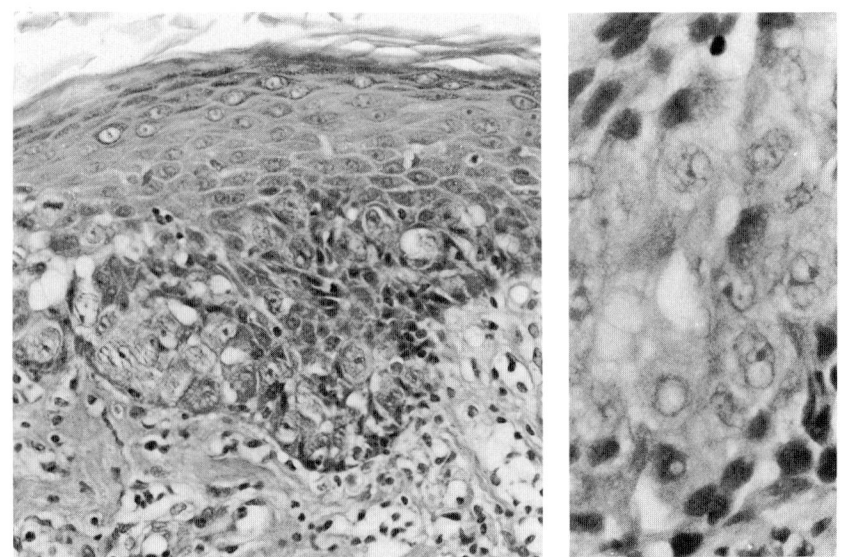

(b)

(c)

Figure 3.12 Paget's disease showing (a) epidermal thickening and hyperkeratosis, and (b) intraepidermal Paget's cells identical to (c) cells in underlying intraductal carcinoma.

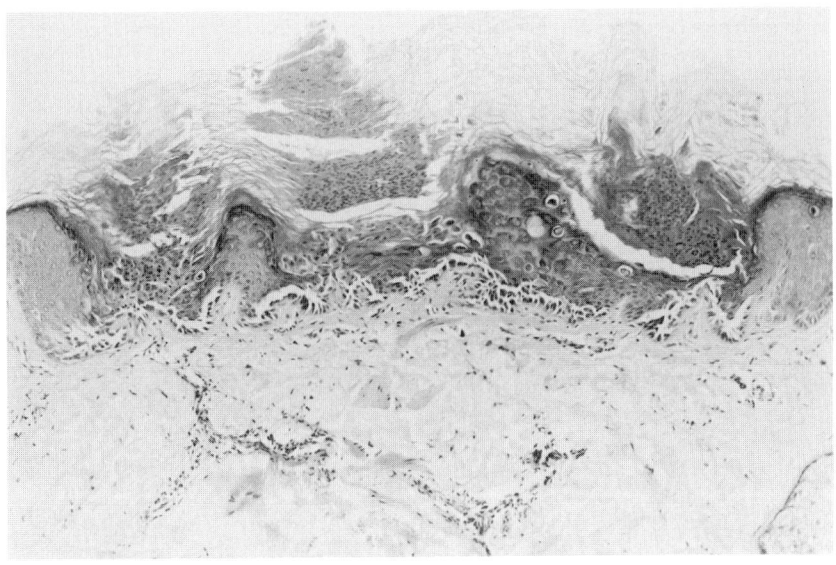

(a)

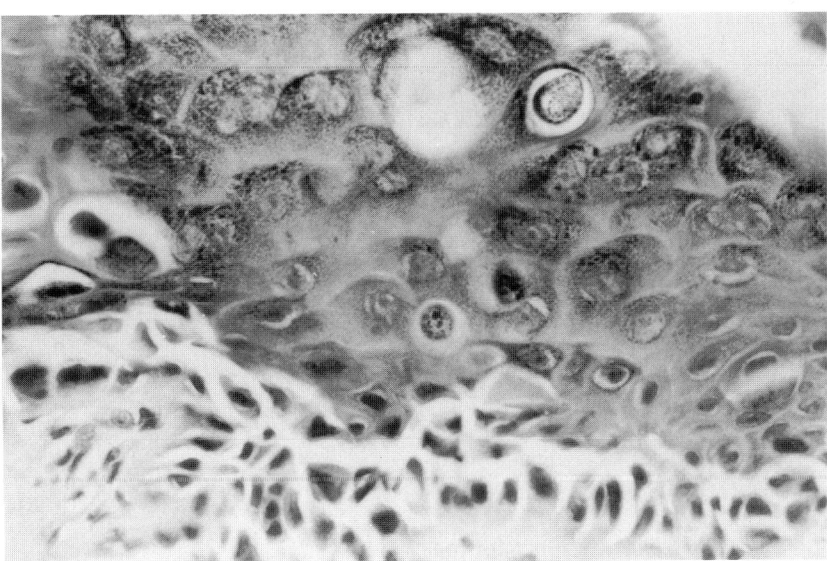

(b)

Figure 3.13 Grover's disease (a and b). A small localized acantholytic lesion with associated hyperkeratosis.

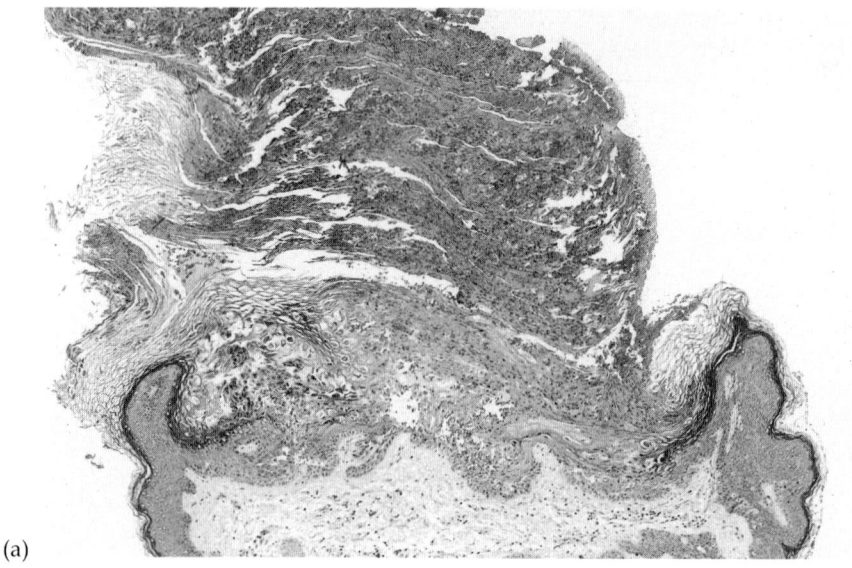

(a)

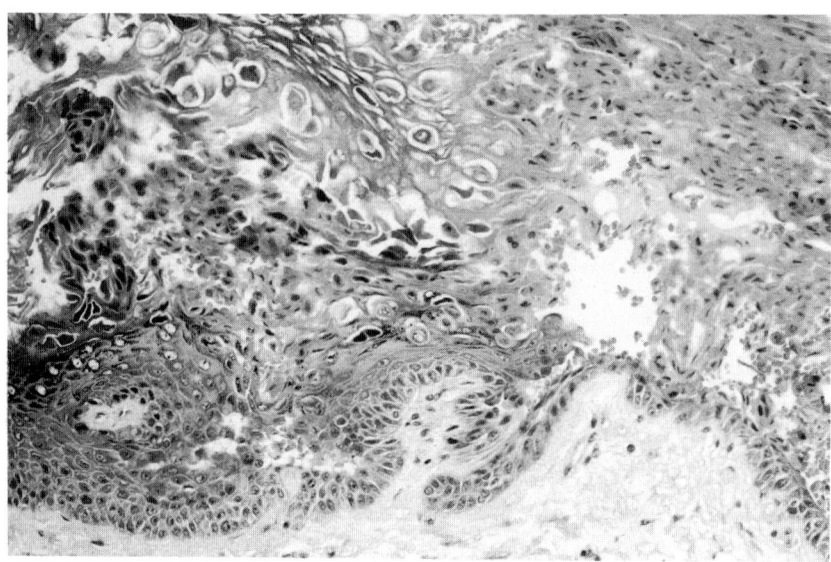

(b)

Figure 3.14 Grover's disease showing (a) a lesion with a flat base and wart-like plume of parakeratotic keratin and (b) suprabasal clefting and prominent rounded dyskeratotic cells.

3.12   Grover's Disease

Also known as transient focal acantholytic keratosis, this condition is a self-limiting, pruritic papulovesicular eruption arising on the trunk and limbs. The onset of the lesions is often associated with heat or excessive sweating, from a number of causes including the prolonged wearing of a polyester suit (Hu *et al.*, 1985).

The biopsy shows suprabasal clefts surrounding the dermal papillae and with acantholytic and dyskeratotic cells at all levels in the epidermis and overlying hyperkeratosis and parakeratosis. The appearances have much in common with Darier's disease and warty dyskeratoma and has been reported in association with pityriasis rubra pilaris (Kao and Sulica, 1989). The villi seen in Darier's disease are however, absent, as is the large crypt seen in warty dyskeratoma. Immunohistochemical studies are equivocal, with no definite evidence of immune complex deposition in the epidermis.

3.13   Darier's disease

Darier's disease is an inherited process transmitted as an autosomal dominant gene. The lesions show a characteristic appearance of suprabasal clefting, with the development of 'villi' in the base, covered by a single layer of basal cells. In the upper part of the lesion, the epidermis contains large rounded dyskeratotic cells known as 'corps ronds': Darier thought these were infective organisms (Steffen, 1988). The cytological changes resemble those of warty dyskeratoma, but that is where the resemblance ends.

Immunohistochemical studies of keratin immunoreactivity suggest that the defect is one of hyperproliferation of the suprabasal cells, resulting in abnormal keratin profiles in the keratinocytes (Burge *et al.*, 1988).

3.14   Hailey-Hailey disease

Otherwise known as benign familial pemphigus, this condition is transmitted as an autosomal dominant gene. There is a considerable overlap in morphology of the lesions with Darier's disease, although in Hailey-Hailey disease they may be larger, forming bullae rather than lacunae, there is well developed acantholysis, leading to the so-called 'dilapidated brick wall' appearance. Corps ronds are less of a feature (Schanne *et al.*, 1985).

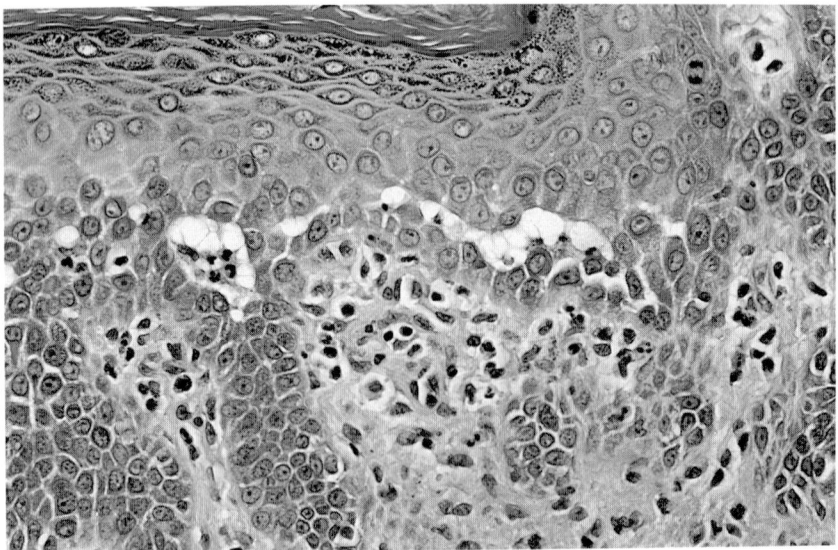

Figure 3.15   Hailey Hailey disease. There is a supra-basal cleft, with acantholytic cells lying in the cleft.

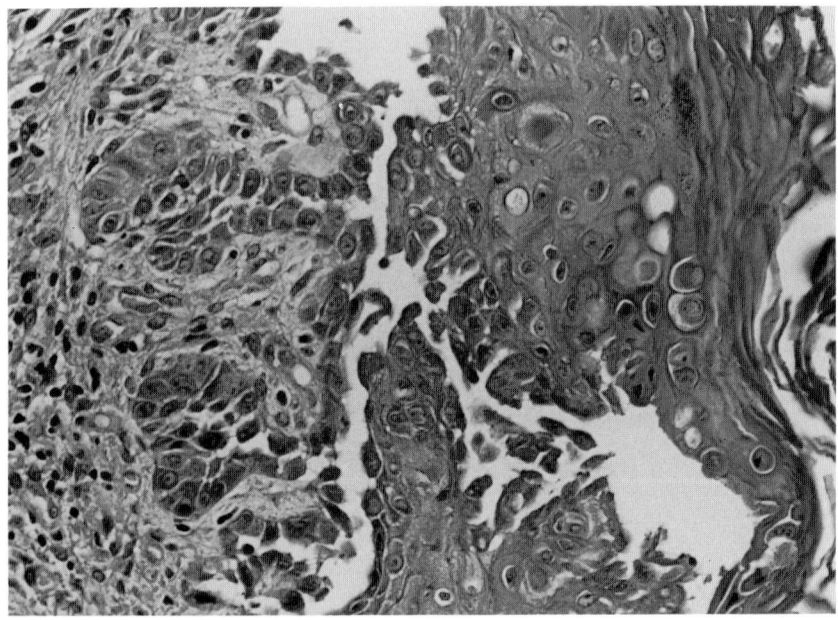

Figure 3.16   Darier's disease. Several corps ronds are present in the roof of the lesion.

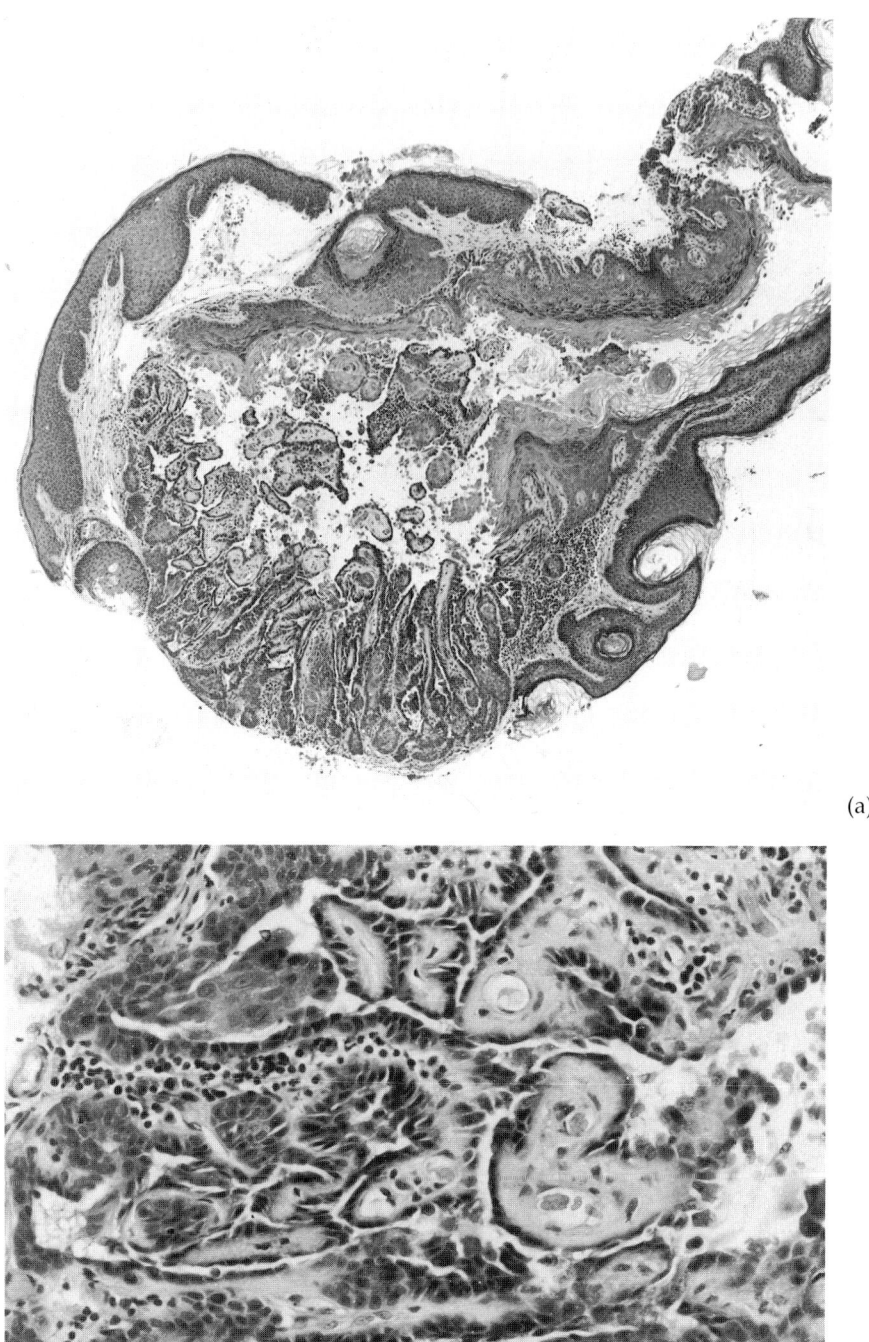

(a)

(b)

Figure 3.17 Warty dyskeratoma. (a) The dyskeratotic lesion lies at the bottom of a flask-shaped crypt, and (b) villi in the crypt base are covered by a single layer of cells.

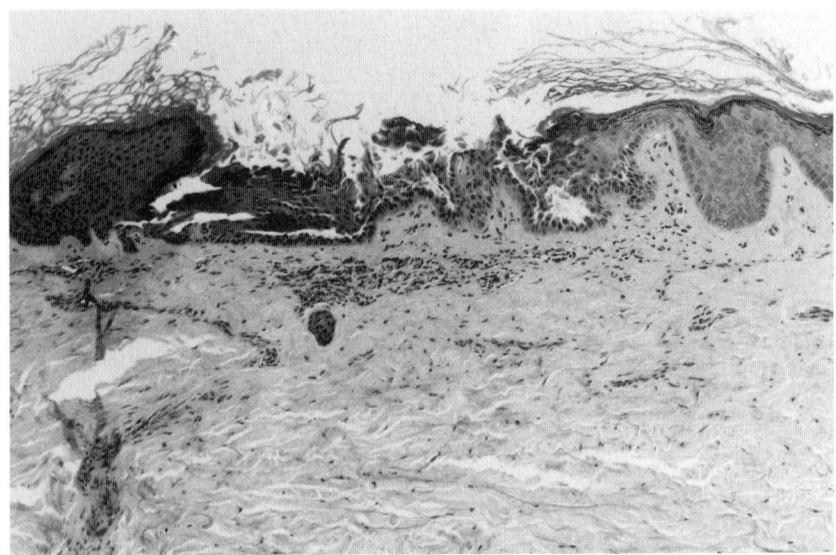

(a)

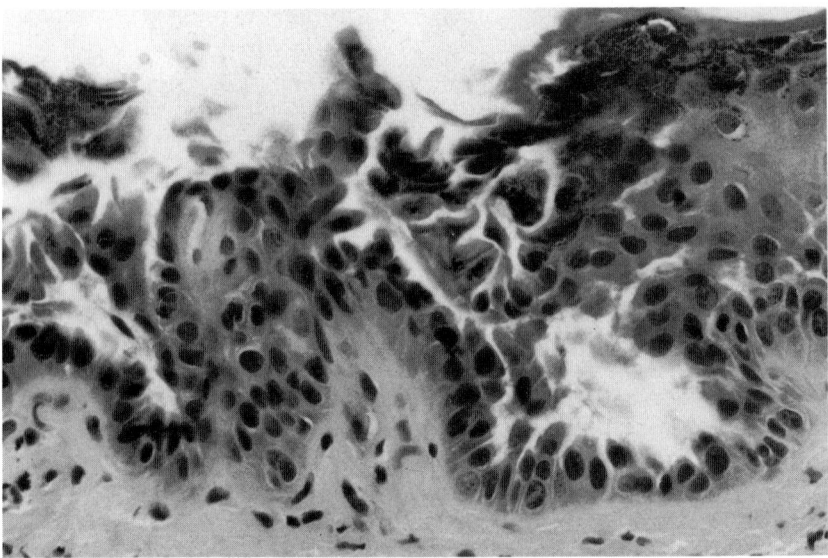

(b)

Figure 3.18 Pemphigus shows suprabasal acantholysis, but without villi and corps ronds.

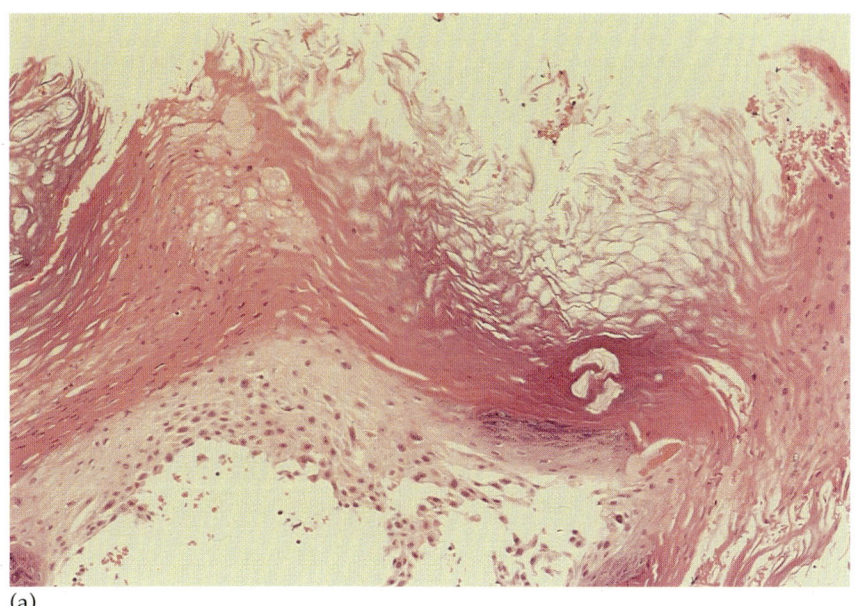

(a)

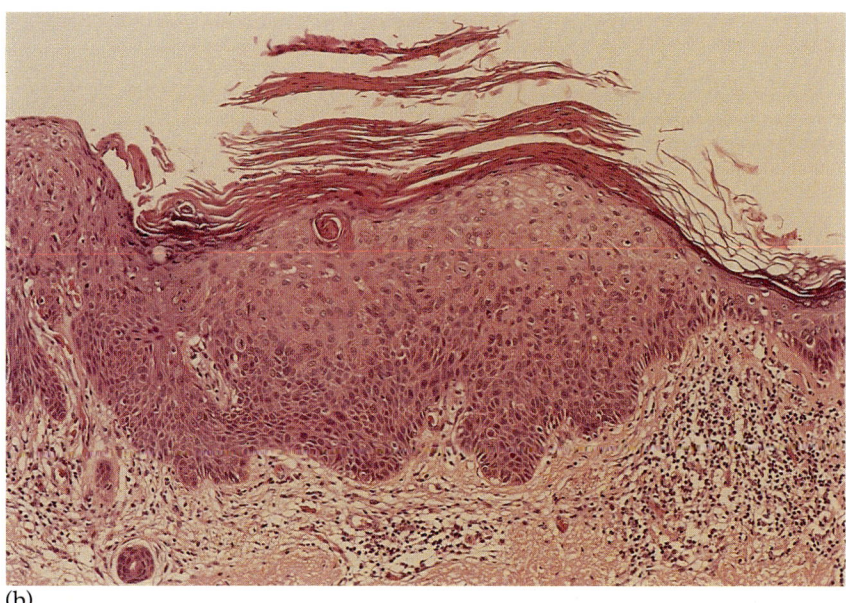

(b)

Plate 1   Actinic keratoses. (a) A curettage specimen with only mild epidermal atypia, but sufficient for diagnosis. (b) An excision biopsy showing epidermal atypia and hyperkeratosis with parakeratosis.

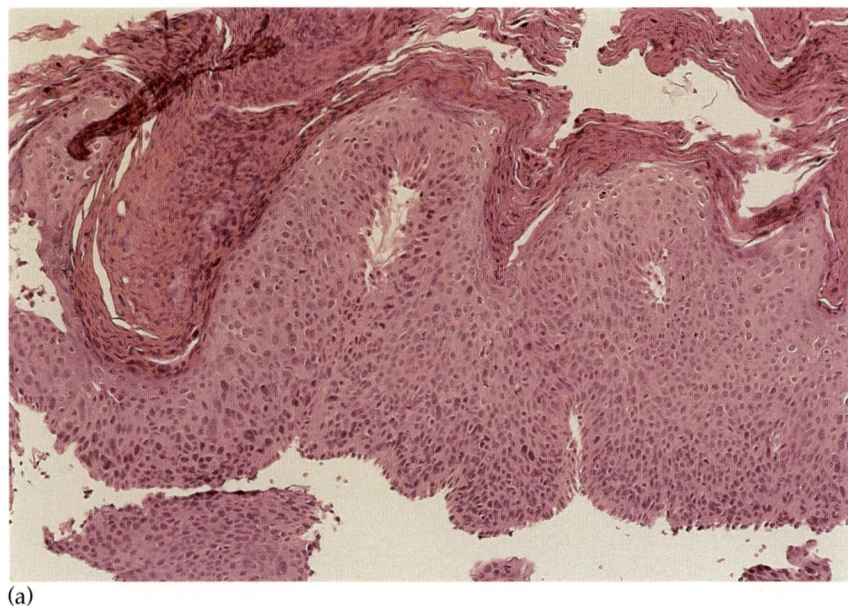

(a)

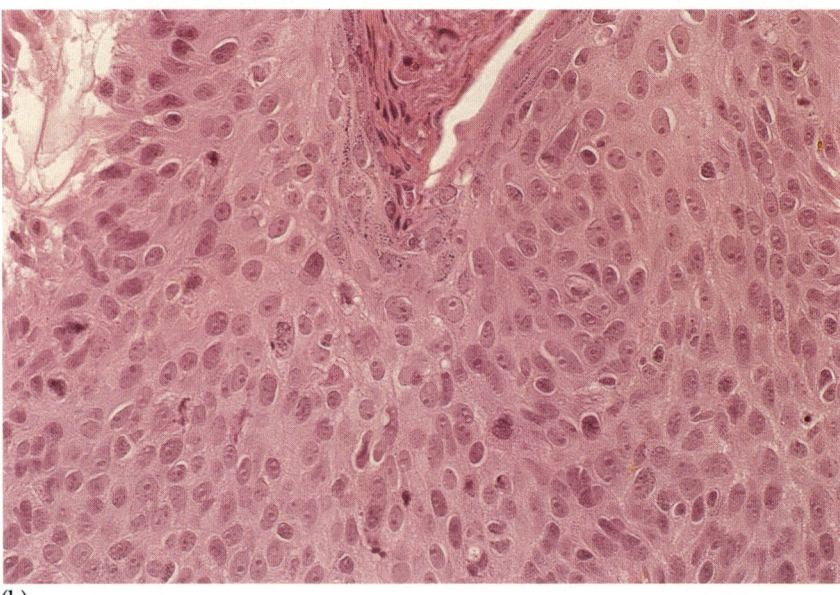

(b)

Plate 2   Bowenoid keratosis. (a) The epidermis is acanthotic with overlying hyperkeratosis and parakeratosis. (b) The keratinocytes show substantial atypia, but there is no dermal invasion.

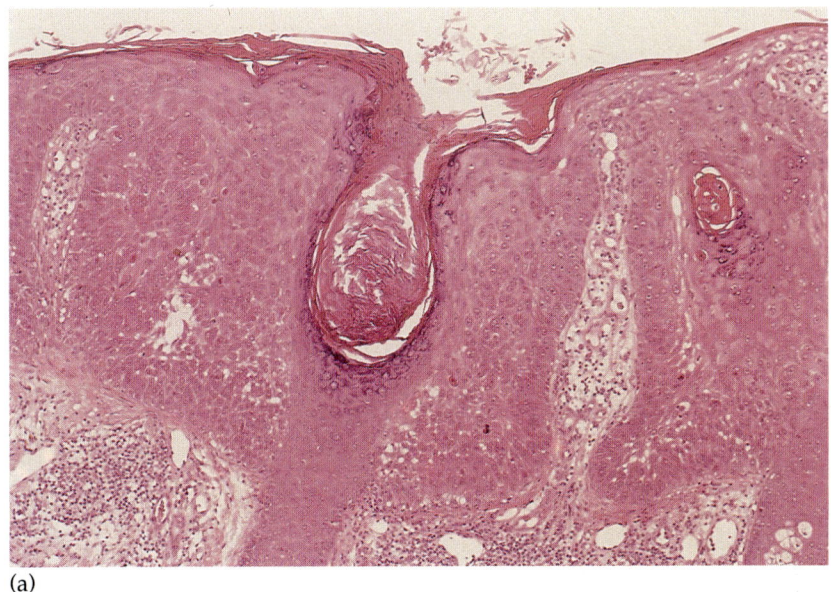

(a)

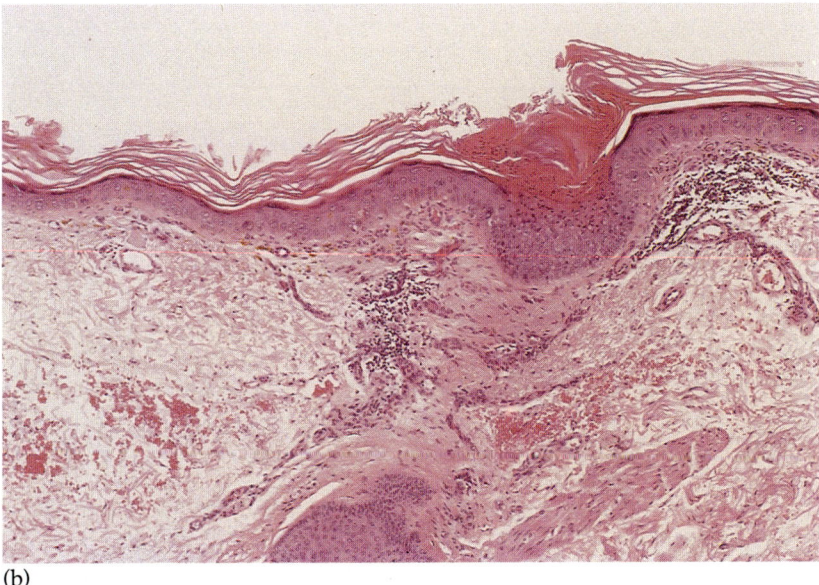

(b)

Plate 3   (a) Acantholytic keratosis. There is acantholysis in the lower portion of
the abnormal epidermis. The lesion involves hair follicle infundibulum.
(b) Disseminated superficial actinic porokeratosis. The cornoid lamella
arises on a base of moderately atypical keratinocytes.

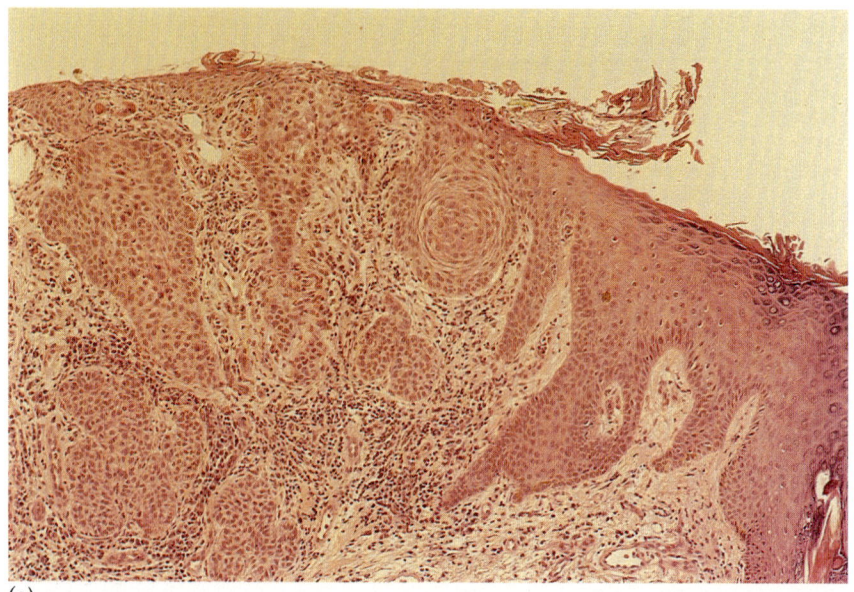

(a)

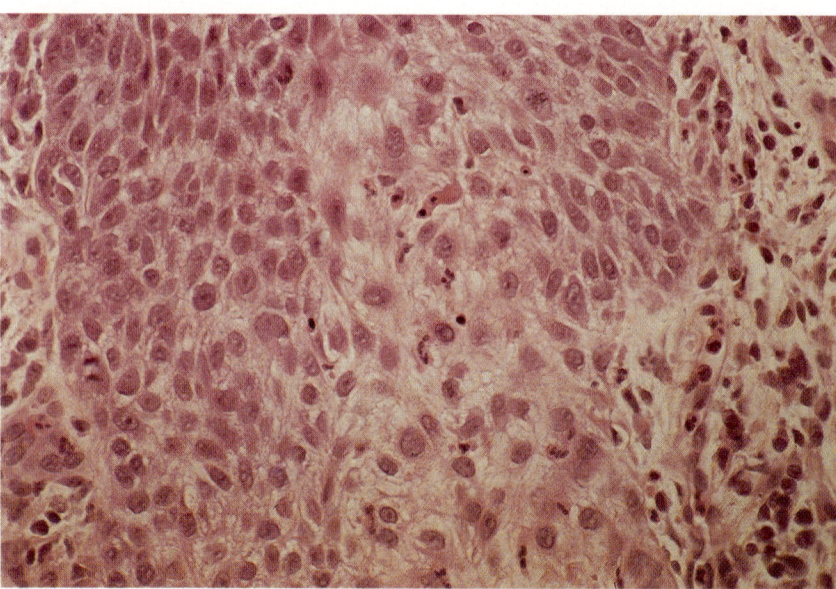

(b)

Plate 4   Clear cell acanthoma. (a) The acanthotic lesion is sharply demarcated from adjacent normal epidermis. (b) The lesional keratinocytes are enlarged with pale cytoplasm. Neutrophil granulocytes infiltrate between keratinocytes.

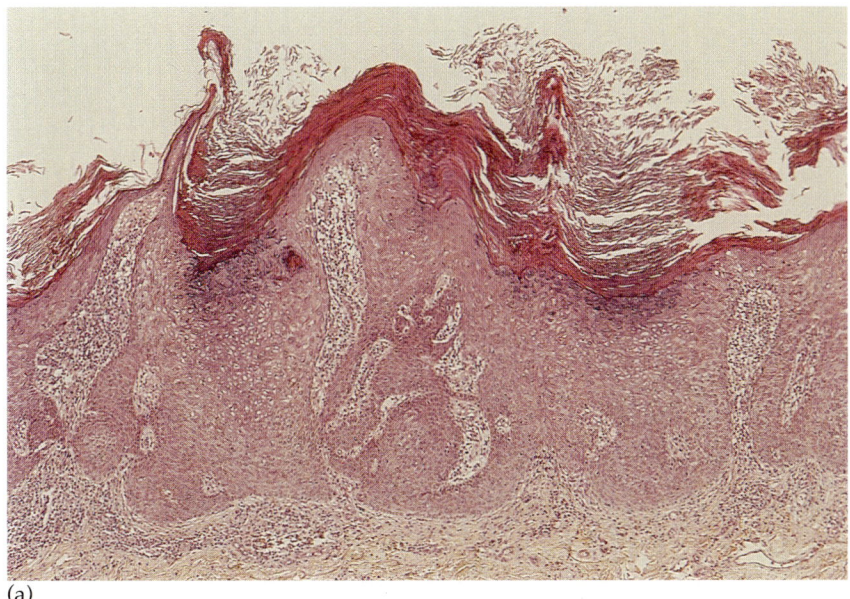

(a)

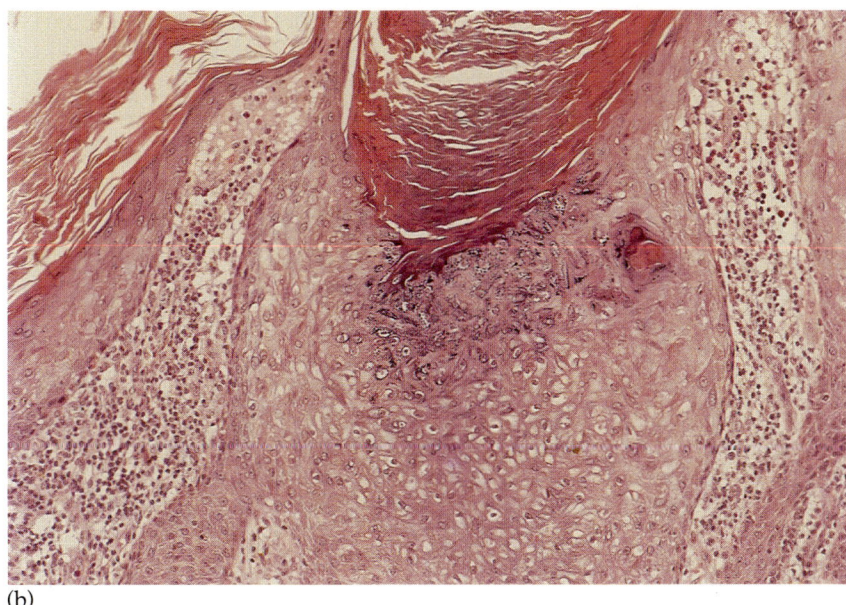

(b)

Plate 5   Viral wart. (a) The hyperkeratosis may be confused with an actinic
keratosis. (b) There is no keratinocyte atypia. Instead the keratinocytes
show perinuclear haloes and there is hypergranulosis.

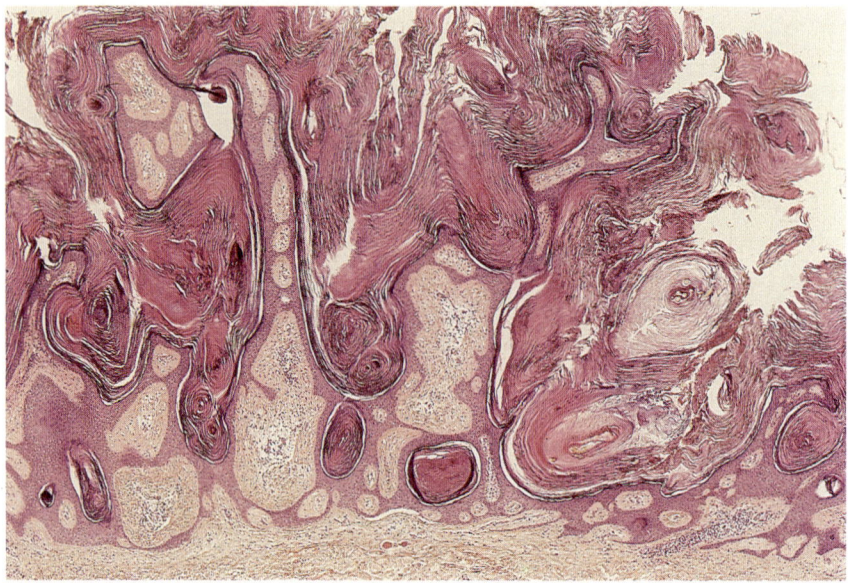

(a)

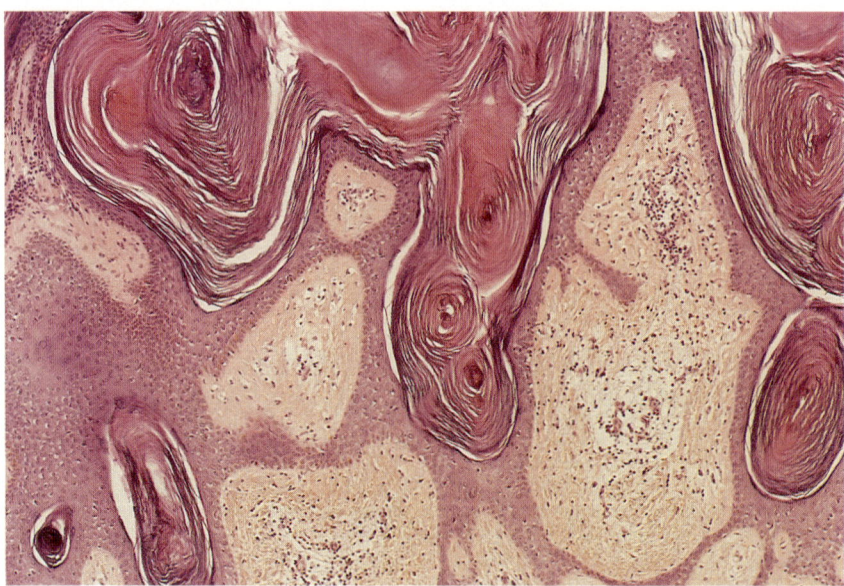

(b)

Plate 6   Seborrhoeic keratosis. (a) An exophytic papillary lesion that could be confused with a viral wart. (b) There is basal cell hyperplasia, without atypia, perinuclear haloes or hypergranulosis.

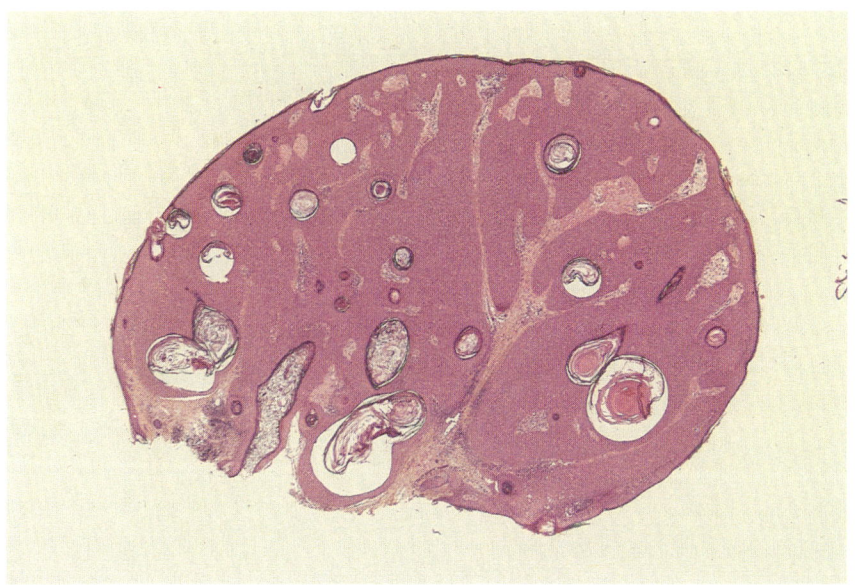

(a)

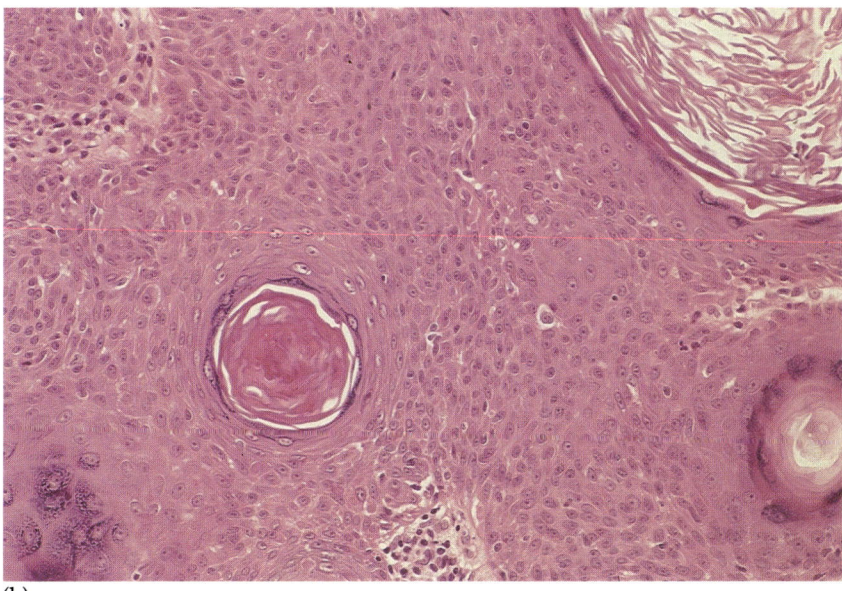

(b)

Plate 7   Seborrhoeic keratosis. (a) A rounded lesion difficult to distinguish clinically from a cellular naevus. (b) The lesion shows horn cysts and basal cell
hyperplasia but lacks cellular atypia.

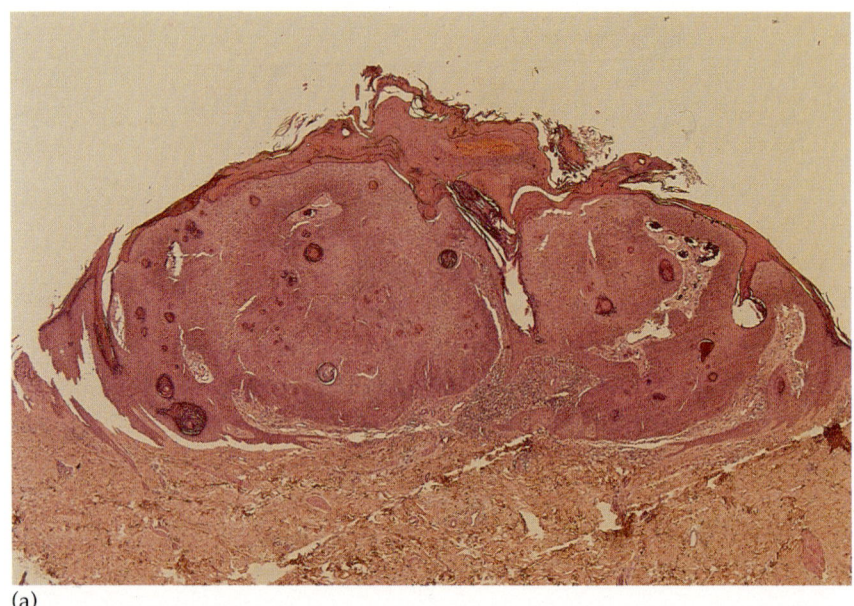

(a)

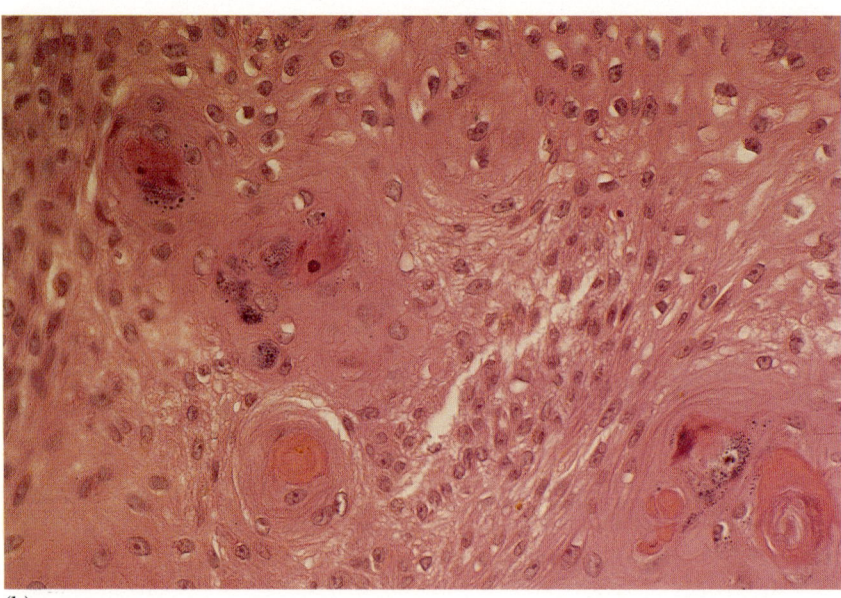

(b)

Plate 8 Inverted follicular keratosis. (a) The rounded lesion resembles a wart or seborrhoeic keratosis. (b) The characteristic feature is the presence of squamous eddies.

3.15   Warty dyskeratoma

Warty dyskeratomas present as solitary lesions on the sun exposed skin of the head and neck. They are usually curetted off and show a typical appearance of a large crypt at the base of which there are villi, usually covered by a single layer of basal cells. The upper part of the crypt contains keratinaceous debris. The lesions are entirely benign (Tanay and Mehregan, 1969).

3.16   Acanthosis nigricans

This condition is unfortunately named because neither acanthosis nor hyperpigmentation are features of the biopsy. Instead the epidermis is hyperkeratotic and shows a characteristic papillomatosis, with upward projection of the dermal papillae. Over the papillae the epidermis may be thin, whilst between them it is moderately acanthotic, with keratin filling the valleys. Its most prominent association is with gastro-intestinal malignancy, but it may occur as a simple naevoid lesion, as a secondary complication of obesity, of some drugs and as a manifestation of Bloom's syndrome, lipodystrophy, gigantism or insulin resistance (Hall *et al.*, 1988; Hernandez-Pérez, 1984).

References

Berger, B. W. and Hori, Y. (1978) Multicentric Bowen's disease of the genitalia. Spontaneous regression of lesions. *Arch. Dermatol.*, **114**, 1698–9.

Brownstein, M. H. (1985) The benign acanthomas. *J. Cut. Pathol.*, **12**, 172–88.

Burge, S. M., Fenton, D. A., Dawber, R. P. and Leigh, I. M. (1988) Darier's disease: an immunohistochemical study using monoclonal antibodies to human cytokeratins. *Br. J. Dermatol.*, **118**, 629–40.

Chernosky, M. E. and Freeman, R. G. (1967) Disseminated superficial actinic porokeratosis (DSAP). *Arch. Dermatol.*, **96**, 611–24.

Civatte, J. (1985) Pseudo-carcinomatous hyperplasia. *J. Cut. Pathol.*, **12**, 214–23.

Cohen, C. and DeRose, P. B. (1989) Histogenesis of extramammary and mammary Paget cells. An immunohistochemical study. *Am. J. Dermatopathol.*, **11**, 313–18.

Degos R. and Civatte J. (1970) Clear cell acanthoma. Experience of 8 years. *Br. J. Dermatol.*, **83**, 248–54.

Friedman, S. J., Herman, P. S., Pittelkow, M. R. and Su, W. P. (1988) Punctuate porokeratotic keratoderma. *Arch. Dermatol.*, **124**, 1678–82.

Grunwald, M. H., Lee, J. Y.-Y. and Ackerman, A. B. (1988) Pseudocarcinomatous hyperplasia. *Am. J. Dermatopathol.*, **10**, 95–103.

Hall, J. M., Moreland, A., Cox, G. J. and Wade, T. R. (1988) Oral acanthosis nigricans, report of a case and comparison of oral and cutaneous pathology. *Am. J. Dermatopathol.*, **10**, 68–73.

Hashimoto, T., Inamoto, N. and Nakamura, K. (1988) Two cases of clear cell acanthoma, an immunohistochemical study. *J. Cutan. Pathol.*, **15**, 27–30.

Hasebe, T., Yamamichi, N., Konishi, F. and Mukawa, A. (1988) [An immuno-histochemical analysis of extramammary Paget's disease compared with Paget's disease.] *Gan. No. Rinsho.*, **34**, 159–66.

Hernandez-Perez, E. (1984) On the classification of acanthosis nigricans. *Int. J. Dermatol.*, **23**, 605–6.

Himmelstein, R. and Lynnfield, Y. L. (1984) Punctate porokeratosis. *Arch. Dermatol.*, **120**, 263–4.

Hu, C.-H., Michel, B. and Farber, E. M. (1985) Transient acantholytic derma-tosis (Grover's disease). *Arch. Dermatol.*, **121**, 1439–41.

Kang, W. H. and Chun, S. I. (1988) Porokeratosis plantaris discreta. A case showing transepidermal elimination. *Am. J. Dermatopathol.*, **10**, 229–33.

Kao, G. F. and Sulica, V. I. (1989) Focal acantholytic dyskeratosis occurring in pityriasis rubra pilaris. *Am. J. Dermatopathol.*, **11**, 172–6.

Kirkham, N., Berry, N., Jones, D. B. and Taylor-Papadimitriou, J. (1985) Paget's disease of the nipple: immunohistochemical localisation of milk fat globule membrane antigens. *Cancer*, **55**, 1510–12.

Komorowski, R. A. and Clowry, L. J. (1989) Porokeratosis of Mibelli in trans-plant recipients. *Am. J. Clin. Pathol.*, **91**, 71–4.

Kyrle, J. (1916) Uber einen ungewohnlichen Fall von universeller follikularer und parafollikularer Hyperkeratose. *Ann. Derm. Syph.* (Berlin), **123**, 466–93.

Obalek, S., Jablonska, S., Beaudenon, S., Walczak, L. and Orth, G. (1986) Bowenoid papulosis of the male and female genitalia: risk of cervical neo-plasia. *J. Am. Acad. Dermatol.*, **14**, 433–44.

Pinkus, H. (1970) Epidermal mosaic in benign and precancerous neoplasia (with special reference to large-cell acanthoma). *Acta Dermatol.* (Kyoto), **65**, 75–81.

Price, M. L., Wilson Jones, E. and MacDonald, D. M. (1987) A clinicopatho-logical study of Flegel's disease (hyperkeratosis lenticularis perstans). *Br. J. Dermatol.*, **116**, 681–91.

Rabinowitz, A. D. (1983) Multiple large cell acanthomas. *J. Am. Acad. Der-matol.*, **8**, 840–5.

Raffle, E. J. and Rogers, J. (1969) Kyperkeratosis lenticularis perstans. *Arch. Dermatol.*, **100**, 423–8.

Rahbari, H., Cordero, A. A. and Mehregan, A. H. (1974) Linear porokeratosis. *Arch. Dermatol.*, **109**, 526–8.

Rahbari, H. and Pinkus, H. (1978) Large cell acanthomas. *Arch. Dermatol.*, **114**, 49–52.

Sanchez, Y. E., De Diego, V., and Urrutia, S. (1988) Large cell acanthoma. A cytologic variant of Bowen's disease? *Am. J. Dermatopathol.*, **10**, 197–208.

Schanne, R., Burg, G. and Braun-Falco, O. (1985) Zur nosologischen Beziehung der Dyskeratosis follicularis (Darier) und des Pemphigus benignus chronicus familiaris (Hailey-Hailey). *Hautarzt*, **36**, 504–8.

Scholl, W. (1982) Large cell acanthoma. *Z. Hautkr.*, **57**, 1002–5.

Steffen, C. and Ackerman, A. B. (1985) Intraepidermal epithelioma of Borst-Jadassohn. *Am. J. Dermatopathol.*, **7**, 5–24.

Steffen, C. (1988) Dyskeratosis and the dyskeratoses. *Am. J. Dermatopathol.*, **10**, 356–63.

Tanay, A. and Mehregan, A. H. (1969) Warty dyskeratoma (a review). *Derma-tologica*, **138**, 155–64.

Tappeiner, J., Wolff, K. and Schreiner, E. (1969) Morbus Kyrle. *Hautarzt*, **20**, 296–310.

Tazawa, T., Ito, M., Fujiwara, H., Shimizu, N. and Sato, Y. (1988) Immuno-logic characteristics of keratins in extramammary Paget's disease. *Arch. Dermatol.*, **124**, 1063–8.

Trau, H., Fisher, B. K. and Schewach-Millet, M. (1980) Multiple clear cell acan-thomas. *Arch. Dermatol.*, **116**, 433–4.

Wade, T. R., Kopf, A. W. and Ackerman, A. B. (1979) Bowenoid papulosis of the genitalia. *Arch. Dermatol.*, **115**, 306–8.

Wade, T. and Ackerman, A. B. (1980) Cornoid lamellation, a histologic reaction pattern. *Am. J. Dermatopathol.*, **2**, 5–15.

Wood, W. S. and Hegedus, C. (1988) Mammary Paget's disease and intraductal carcinoma. Histologic, histochemical and immunocytochemical comparison. *Am. J. Dermatopathol.*, **10**, 183–8.

4 Warts and viral dermatoses

After the keratoses, the warts are perhaps the commonest keratinocytic abnormality biopsied. Dermatologists often complain about the number of warts referred to them for treatment by family practitioners but, nevertheless, they are always worth examining histologically just to exclude the odd misdiagnosis and malignant lesion. Aligned with the common viral warts in this chapter are other warts and associated conditions of viral aetiology.

The differential diagnosis of warts is often difficult, especially if full clinical details do not accompany the biopsy. Of the warty lesions that may be curetted or excised, actinic keratosis, viral wart, seborrhoeic wart and squamous papilloma predominated as potential diagnoses. Whilst each of these conditions has typical features of its own, there can be considerable overlap. The presence of cellular atypia is very much in favour of a dysplastic process and probably indicates an actinic keratosis, especially if the biopsy is from a sun exposed site in an elderly person. Viral warts lack atypia and show varying degrees of papillary differentiation, hypergranulosis and hyperkeratosis and are commoner in younger people. Seborrhoeic warts typically show basal cell proliferation without atypia, and with associated horn cysts and often with pigmentation. Irritated variants may be more squamous and hyperkeratotic, overlapping in appearance with warts and keratoses, but lacking cellular atypia. These differences are illustrated in this chapter.

4.1 Viral warts

Many biopsies are submitted to the laboratory with an accompanying suggestion that the lesion is a wart. True viral warts show thick hyperkeratosis and a prominent granular cell layer in which the cells contain coarse haematoxophylic granules. Eosinophilic inclusions in these cells are rare. Beneath the granular cell layer acanthocytes may show foci in

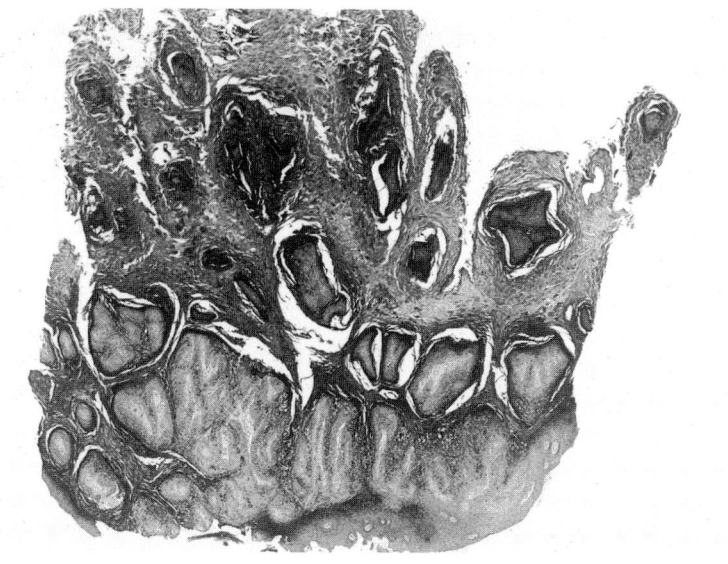

(a)

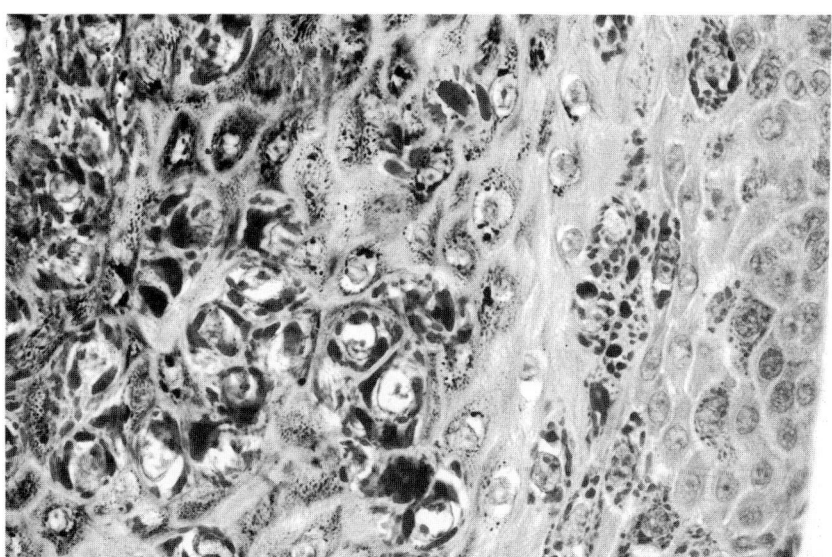

(b)

Figure 4.1 Curetted viral wart in active phase, showing (a) papillary hyperkeratotic lesion with well-defined base, and (b) hypergranulosis including both basophilic and eosinophilic granules.

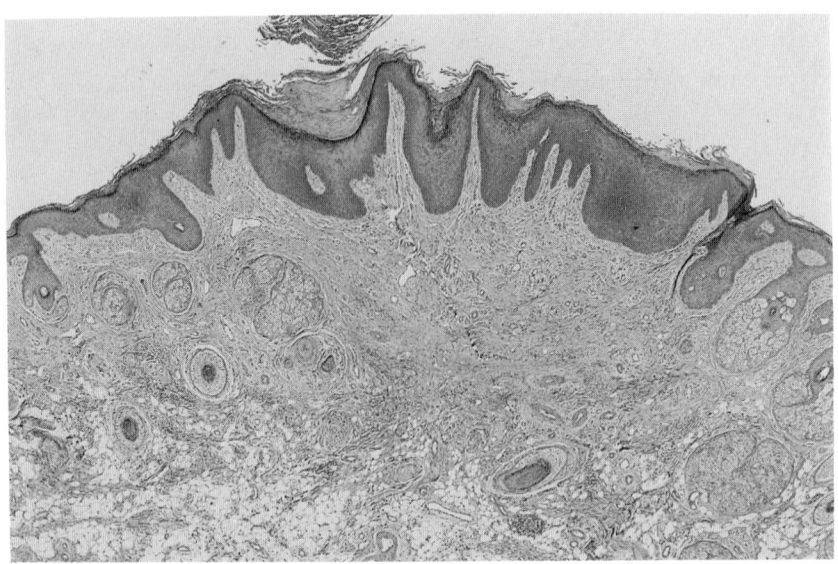

Figure 4.2 Excised viral wart showing irregular acanthosis, hypergranulosis and hyperkeratosis and architectural, but not cytological, similarity to an actinic keratosis.

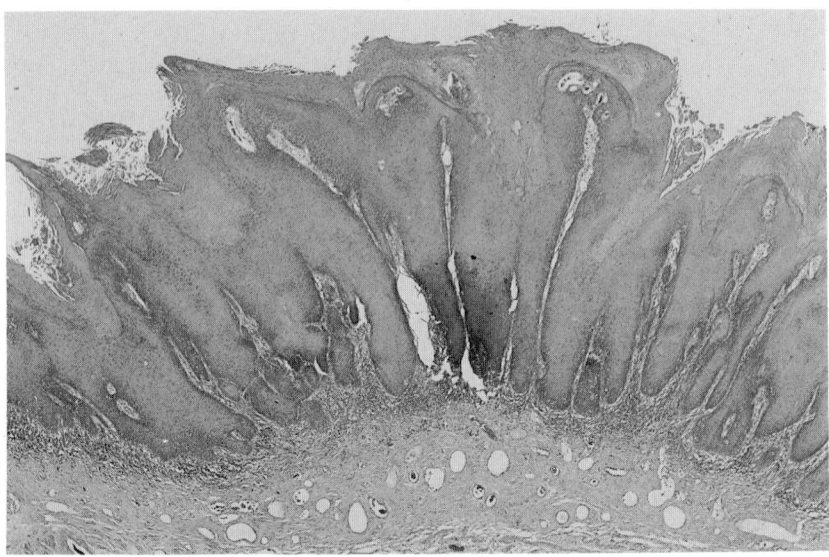

Figure 4.3 Papillary viral wart with elongated dermal papillae and pale eosinophilic keratinocyte cytoplasm.

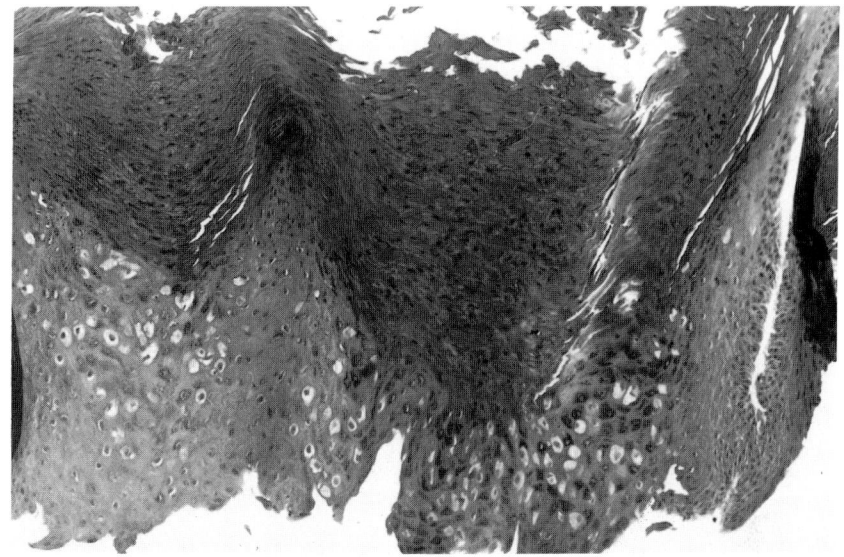

Figure 4.4 Curetting specimen of viral wart with prominent koilocytic change, typical of warts, and without cytological atypia.

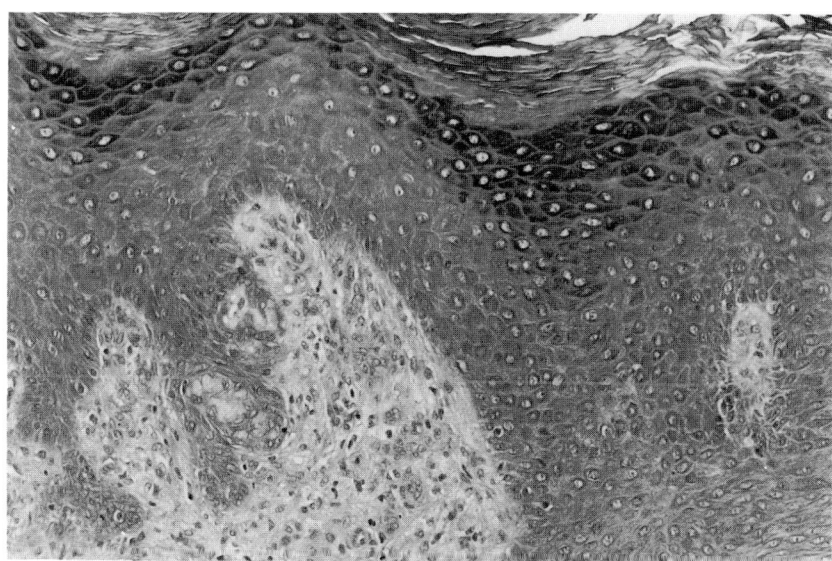

Figure 4.5 Viral wart with prominent hypergranulosis, but lacking koilocytic change, in an older lesion.

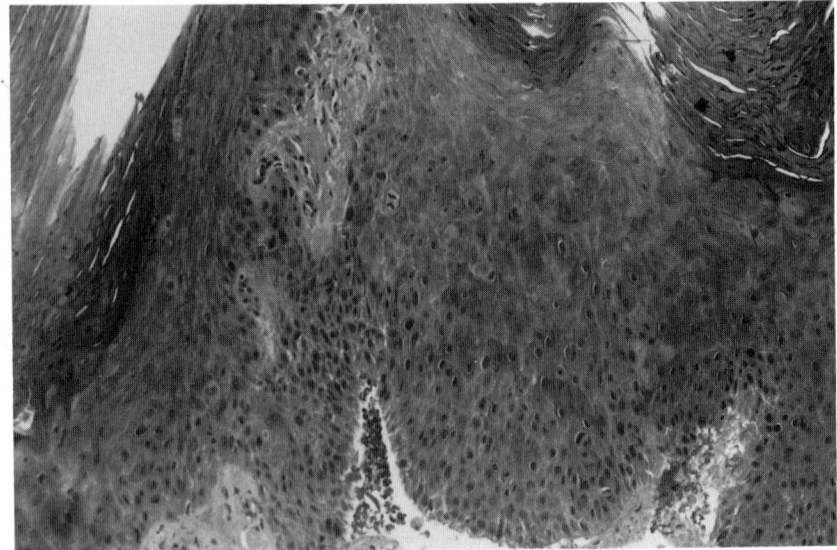

Figure 4.6   Viral wart from a renal transplant patient – occasional atypical cells are a feature.

which the perinuclear cytoplasm is clear – it does not stain with eosin. This is akin to the 'koilocytosis' associated with wart virus infection in the cervix.

Such lesions show no suggestion of nuclear or cellular atypia and have a well defined basal layer. There is no suggestion of dermal invasion. The warts may have been excised or curetted off, but the method of removal is unimportant as there is no suggestion of malignancy and local recurrence is unlikely.

In many cases the diagnosis is not so straightforward. Warts vary in appearance with age. As they get older, the features described above are less marked and the wart develops into a blander form showing little more than hyperkeratosis and irregular or papillary growth. However, in the absence of atypia a reasonably confident diagnosis can be made.

4.2   Renal allograft recipients

Allograft recipients and others who are receiving immunosuppressive therapy have an increased chance of developing viral warts, epidermal keratoses with cellular atypia and skin cancers, especially squamous cell carcinoma. Any of these lesions may show a greater than expected

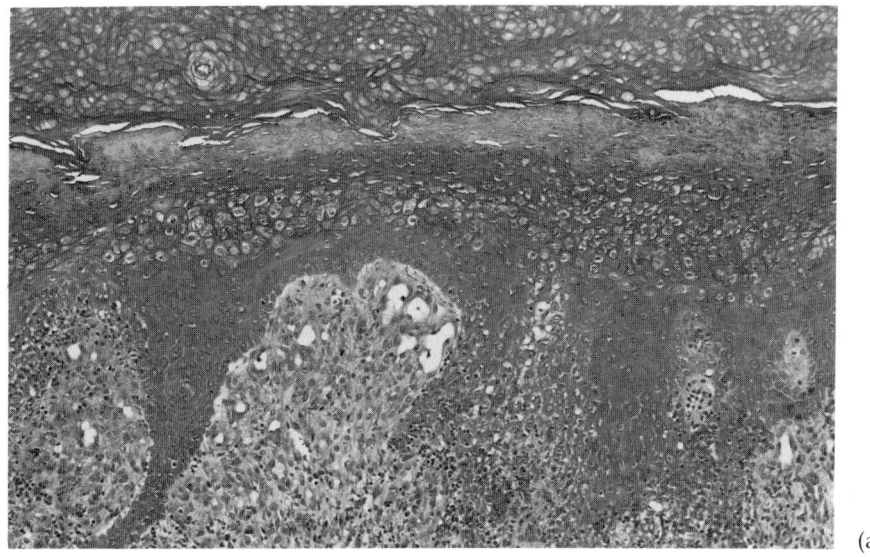

(a)

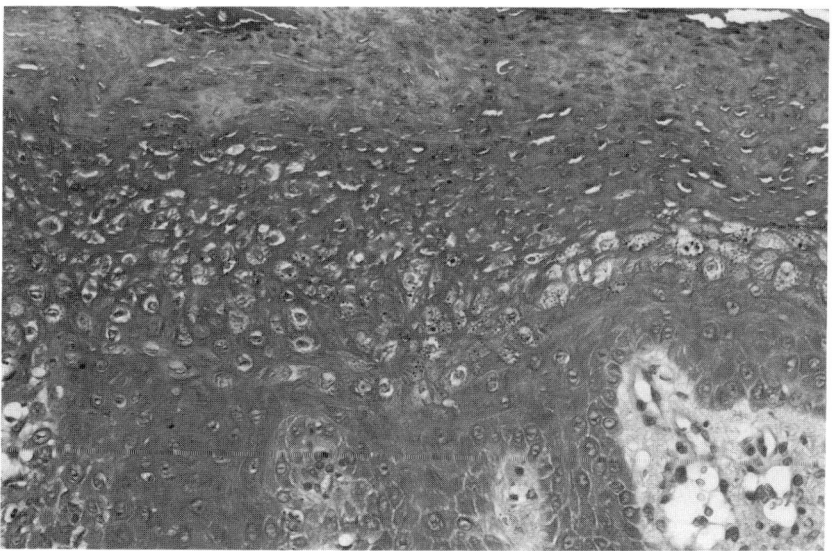

(b)

Figure 4.7 Milker's nodule. (a) Keratinocytes contain cytoplasmic inclusions, in a band (b) running through the suprabasal part of the lesion.

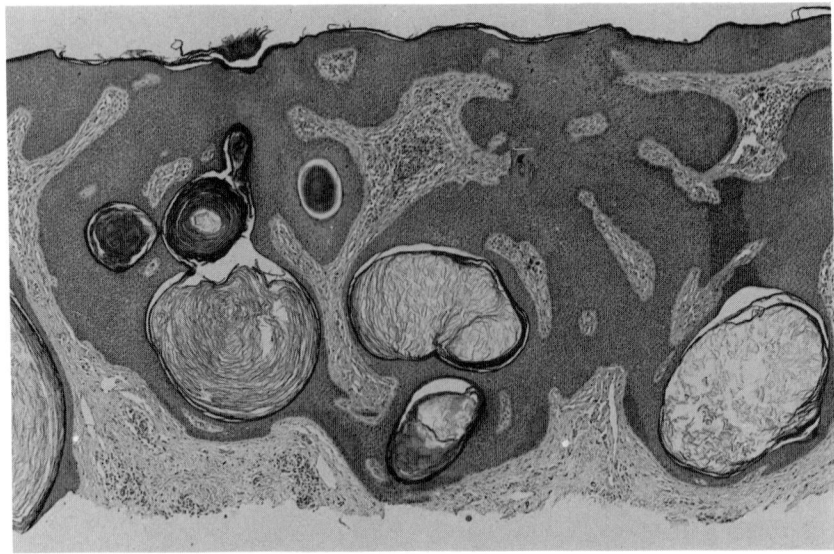

Figure 4.8   Seborrhoeic wart of typical type showing basal cell proliferation and horn cysts loosly filled with keratin.

degree of cellular atypia, out of proportion to the architectural change. Over 60% of invasive and in situ carcinomas contain HPV 5/8: these virus types have also been isolated from squamous carcinomas in patients with epidermodysplasia verruciformis (Blessing *et al.*, 1989).

4.3   Milker's nodule

Milker's nodules are caused by infection with a parapox virus acquired from cows' udders. The lesions develop quickly over just a few weeks, at which stage the biopsy shows a band of koilocytic keratinocytes in the upper epidermis, some of which may contain eosinophilic cyto-plasmic inclusions. Subsequently, the lesions break down and involute, with an associated inflammatory reaction in the dermis (Shelley and Shelley, 1983).

4.4   Seborrhoeic warts

'Seb warts' or basal cell papillomas are extremely common, usually occurring as well circumscribed brown-black lesions anywhere on the body except for the palms and soles, but usually on the trunk. Typically they have a greasy appearance with prominent keratotic plugs. Differ-

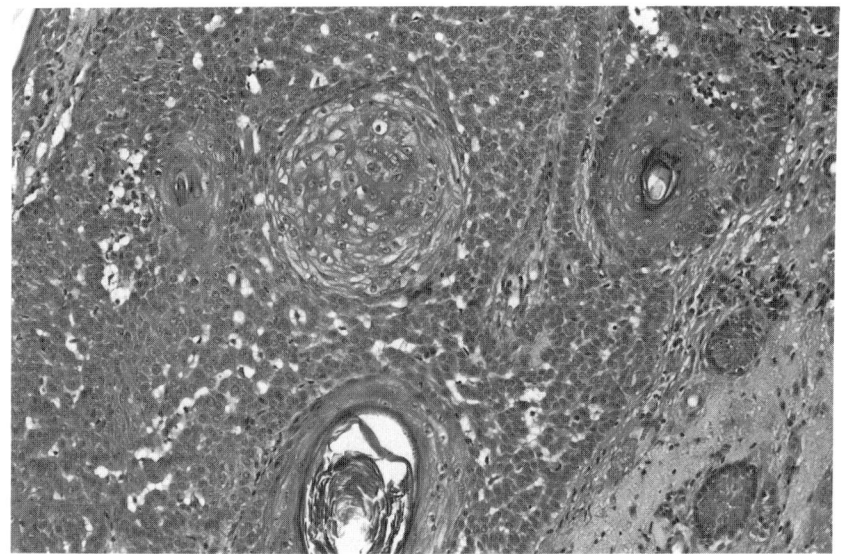

Figure 4.9 Seborrhoeic wart. A reticulated variant of basal cell proliferation.

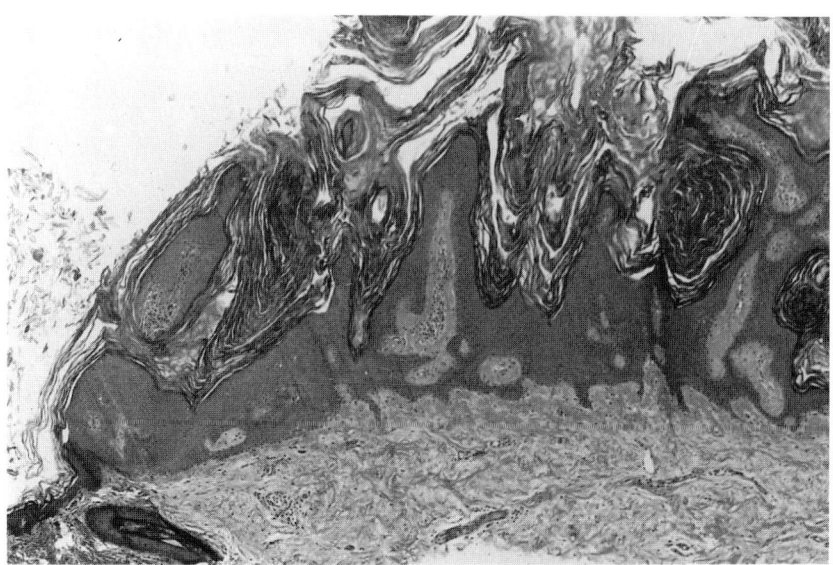

Figure 4.10 Irritated seborrhoeic wart showing marked hyperkeratosis, and architecture which may be confused with a viral wart.

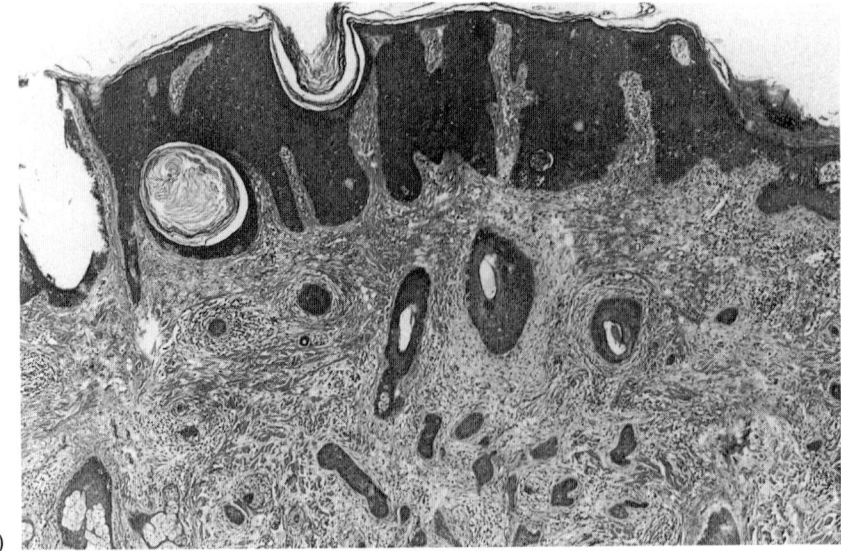

(a)

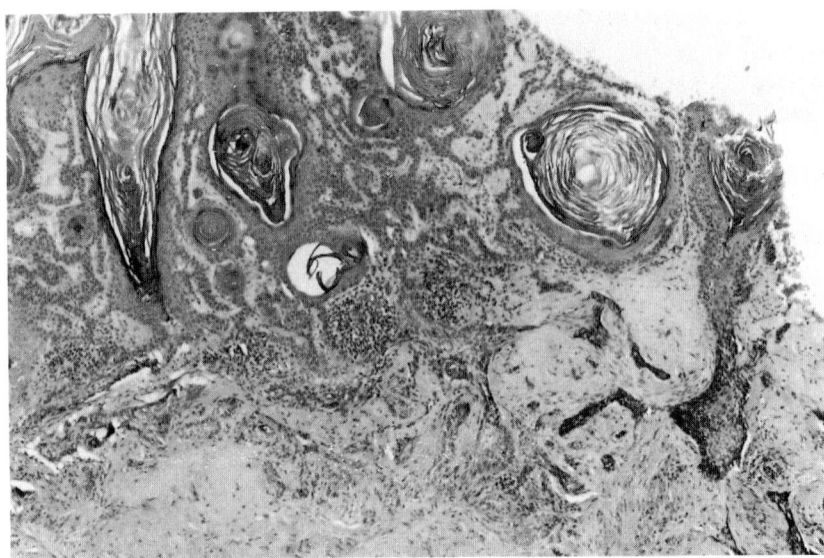

(b)

Figure 4.11 Combined warts (a and b). Two examples of basal cell carcinomas growing in the dermis beneath otherwise unremarkable seborrhoeic warts.

ential diagnosis from naevi and melanomas can be difficult clinically, because of the pigmentation. The melanin is produced by melanocytes, which are situated at the base of the epithelium, and is transported to the surface in keratinocytes (Mevorah and Mishima, 1965).

There are several subtypes which have in common an exophytic profile, with an essentially flat base, and an epithelial component showing hyperkeratosis, acanthosis and papillomatosis. The cells show a predominantly basaloid appearance. The commonest kind is the acanthotic, with thick bands of basaloid cells. The reticulated type shows cords of cells in a reticular pattern. The irritated type show squamous differentiation and hyperkeratosis. Sometimes a basal cell carcinoma can develop at the base of an otherwise unremarkable seborrhoeic wart (Mikhail and Mehregan, 1982; Goette, 1985).

4.5 Melanoacanthoma

Occasional seborrhoeic wart-like lesions contain melanocytes throughout the epithelial component, rather than just in the basal layer. These are the melanoacanthomas, which come in two varieties. The first shows dendritic melanocytes distributed diffusely through the lesion (Mishima and Pinkus, 1960). The second variety has circumscribed islands of basaloid cells within the lesion, with melanocytes concentrated within these islands (Prince et al., 1984).

4.6 Squamous cell papilloma

Sometimes a biopsy shows only a well differentiated papilloma with virtually normal epidermis and unremarkable dermis beneath. There are divergent views on the suitability of the description 'squamous cell papilloma' for this sort of lesion, and even of the legitimacy of the title at all. However, after lesions such as warts and keratosis have been excluded, there does remain a small group of 'benign squamous cell papillomas' for which no other description is appropriate. The squamous cell papilloma· the lesion dermatology forgot!

4.7 Molluscum contagiosum

The lesions of molluscum contagiosum are always striking. They are small and circumscribed with nests of eosinophilic keratinocytes containing characteristic inclusions. The lesions are caused by infection with a poxvirus. They are increased in HIV-positive patients and others who are immunosuppressed (Oriel, 1987).

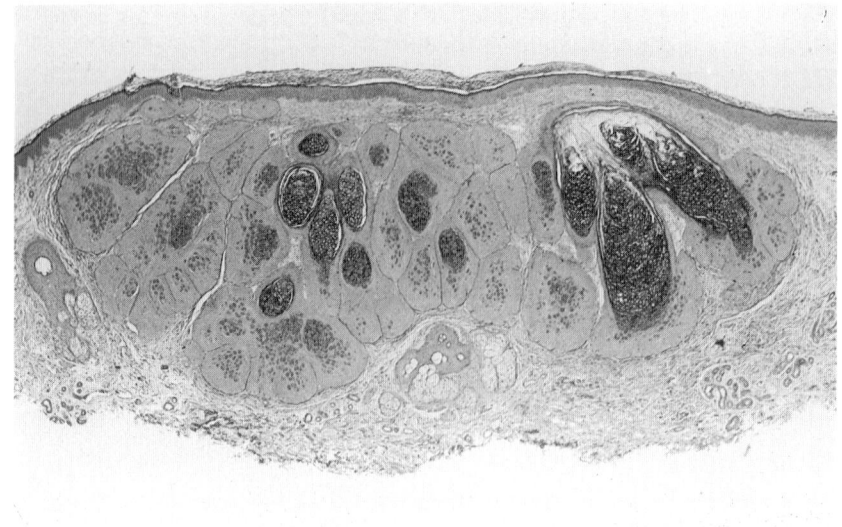

(a)

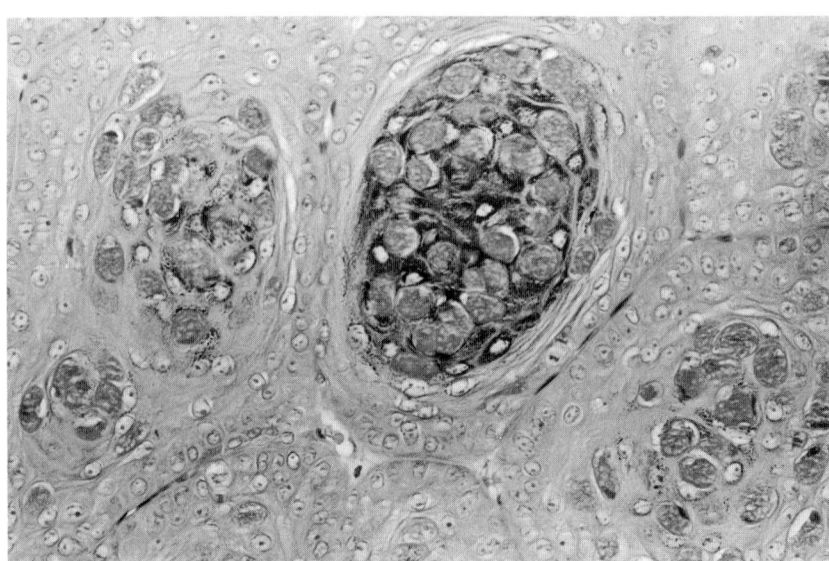

(b)

Figure 4.12 Molluscum contagiosum. (a) An unmistakable lobulated architecture, and (b) cytological pattern of cell nests with eosinophilic inclusions.

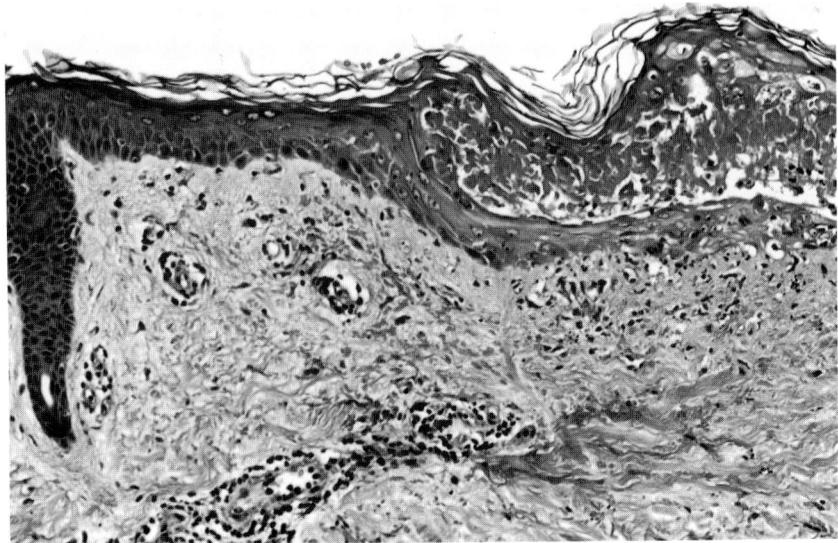

Figure 4.13 Acute herpetic lesion with blood-filled intraepidermal vescicle with associated epidermal necrosis.

4.8 Herpes

Infection with the herpes simplex and varicella-zoster viruses produce lesions which are indistinguishable and show varying degrees of epidermal vesicle formation, with ballooning degeneration of keratinocytes. Intranuclear eosinophilic inclusions may be seen, as may aggregated multinucleated epithelial cells (Chang, 1983).

For rapid diagnosis a smear can be made from a vesicle: the Tzanck smear, which can be stained with Giemsa, to show the acantholytic ballooned and multinucleated cells from the lesion.

References

Blessing, K., McLaren, K. M., Benton, E. C., Barr, B. B., Bunney, M H., Smith, I. W. and Beveridge, G. W. (1989) Histopathology of skin lesions in renal allograft recipients – an assessment of viral features and dysplasia. *Histopathol.*, **14**, 129–39.

Chang, T.-W. (1983) Herpes simplex virus infection. *Int. J. Dermatol.*, **22**, 1–7.

Goette, D. K. (1985) Basal cell carcinoma arising in seborrhoeic keratosis. *J. Dermatol. Surg. Oncol.*, **11**, 1014–16.

Mevorah, B. and Mishima, Y. (1965) Cellular response of seborrhoeic keratosis following croton oil and surgical trauma. *Dermatologica*, **131**, 452–62.

Mikhail, G. R. and Mehregan, A. H. (1982) Basal cell carcinoma in seborrhoeic keratosis. *Am. Acad. Dermatol.*, **6**, 500–6.

Mishima, Y. and Pinkus, H. (1960) Benign mixed tumour of melanocytes and malpighian cells. *Arch. Dermatol.*, **81**, 539–50.

Oriel, J. D. (1987) The increase in molloscum contagiosum. *Br. Med. J.*, **294**, 74.

Prince, C., Mehregan, A. H., Hashimoto, K. and Plotnick, H. (1984) Large melanoacanthomas, a report of five cases. *Cutan. Pathol.*, **11**, 309–17.

Shelley, W. B. and Shelley, E. D. (1983) Farmyard pox, parapox virus infection in man. *Br. J. Dermatol.*, **108**, 725–7.

5 Epidermal tumours

This chapter deals with the tumours of the epidermal basal cells and keratinocytes. The number of diagnoses is limited here but these are amongst the commonest, not just of skin tumours, but of all tumours and, indeed, are only less common than lung cancer in men and breast cancer in women (Harvey *et al.*, 1989). They are associated with sun damage, being especially common amongst whites in Australia. The impression has spread that these actinic squamous and basal cell carcinomas are unlikely to metastasize. This is not the case for squamous cell carcinomas, with reported rates of between 2.6% and 3.3% (Nixon *et al.*, 1986; Moller *et al.*, 1979). Basal cell carcinoma metastasis is more contentious (Domarus and Stevens, 1984), but reports suggest a rate of between 0.54% and 0.0028% (Beerman, 1969; Paver *et al.*, 1973).

As such the tumours need to be diagnosed accurately and treated appropriately (McGibbon, 1985). Treatment is either surgical or with cryotherapy or radiotherapy. Larger lesions will probably be excised in a skin ellipse. Smaller tumours may be treated by shave excision, possibly supplemented by curettage of the base (Harrison, 1987).

So whilst many biopsies will be attempts at excision and will contain all or most of the tumour, there are also those tumours which are not destined for surgical therapy. A small diagnostic biopsy is usually taken from these, in which case the specimen may be very small. It may need to be cut at several levels to find the tumour, or before finally concluding that there is no evidence of tumour in the tissue submitted.

There is a small debate about whether it is best to smear these small curettings onto a slide, in the clinic, and treat the sample as a cytology specimen, or whether to process them for sectioning. Both methods have their advantages. Although the smear is quick and easy to make, there are often large clumps of tissue which are too thick to examine in a smear and would be better analysed in a section. Other lesions may be excised completely, and in such biopsies it is important to look at the surgical margins to confirm complete excision.

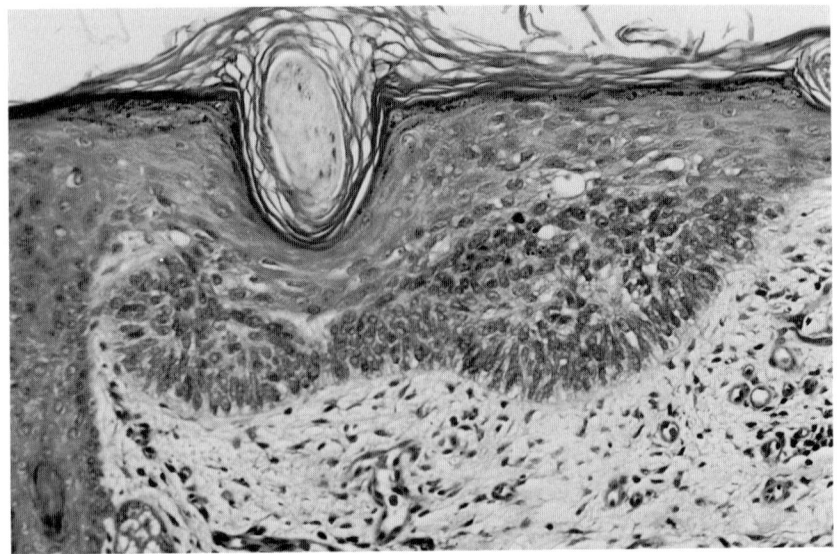

(a)

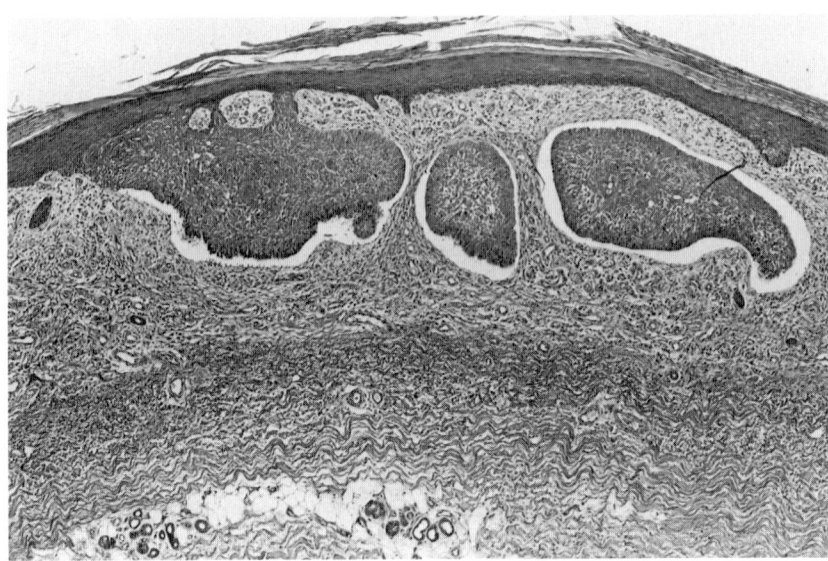

(b)

Figure 5.1 Superficial multicentric basal cell carcinoma showing (a) proliferation of tumour cells in continuity with the epidermis, and (b) retraction artefact between tumour and stroma.

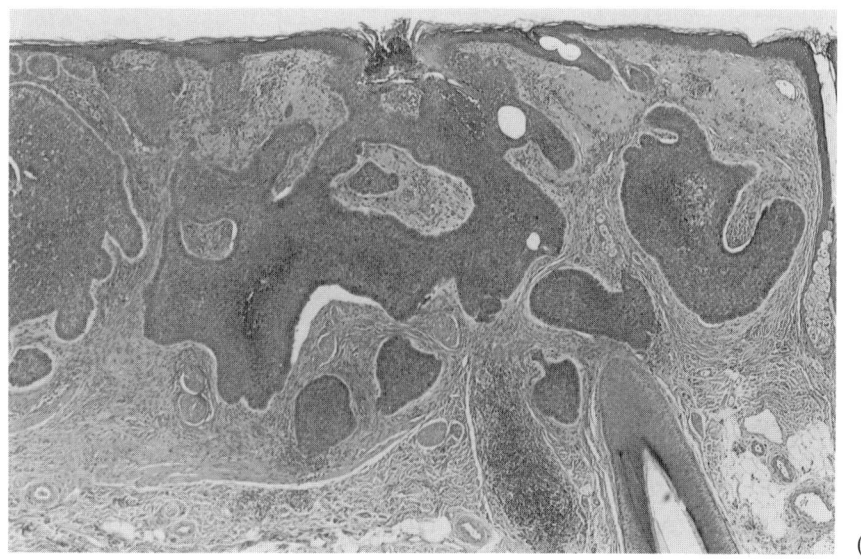

(a)

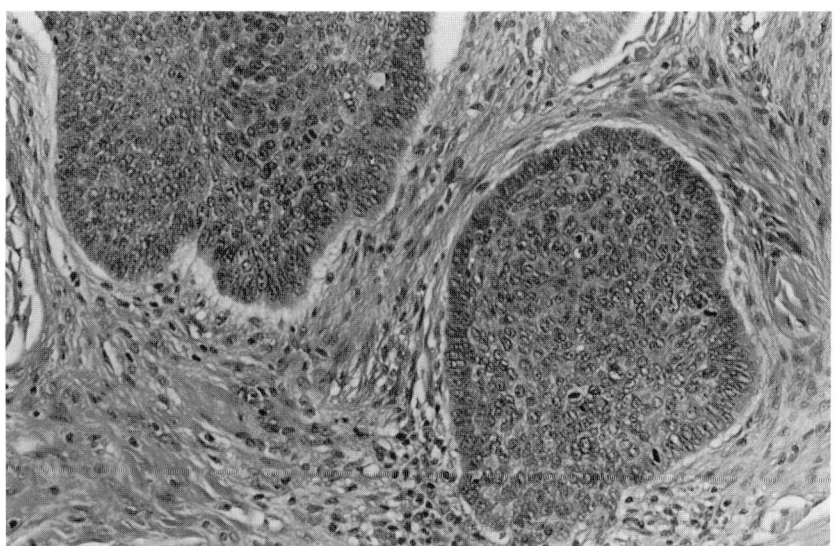

(b)

Figure 5.2 Nodular basal cell carcinoma, (a) with rounded nests of tumour cells extending into the reticular dermis, and (b) with well developed peripheral palisading of tumour cells.

5.1   Basal cell carcinoma

The archetype of basal cell carcinoma is a tumour composed of fairly regular cells with rounded haematoxophilic nuclei and little cytoplasm. The tumour cells are arranged in groups of varying size and shape, depending upon the sub-type concerned, but should show a regular palisade of cells around the margin of each group. The proliferating cell component of the tumour is found predominantly in these peripheral palisades at the edge of the tumour nodules, which corresponds to the way in which basal cell carcinomas grow by slow progressive, local invasion (Grimwood *et al.*, 1986).

Of the variants that are widely recognized, the superficial multicentric form is the smallest, being composed of small clusters of tumour cells budding off the basal layer of the epidermis. These tumours are often quite widely spread along the epidermis. The lateral margin can be difficult to define clinically, making complete excision an uncertain process. So there are two possible problems: early sections off the block of an excision biopsy may not show any lesion at all, and multiple sections may also have to be examined to confirm that the excision margins are clear. Very small examples can be difficult to see even in multiple sections. One clue to diagnosis is the presence of a constant artefact: the separation of the basal cells from the underlying stroma. This is possibly due to defective production of hemidesmosomes by the tumour (Jones *et al.*, 1989).

Perhaps the commonest form is the solid variant, characterized by well circumscribed clusters of cells, usually limited to the upper dermis. One of two variations may be present. Some tumours of this type may show a varying degree of adenoid differentiation progressing to actual cystic change. This is usually more prominent in the central tumour cell clusters of the lesion.

Tumours from the nose, nasolabial folds and adjacent cheeks often show small cysts or duct-like structures resembling hair follicles. This is often accompanied by dystrophic mineralization. These two features indicate that the tumours are trichoepitheliomas rather than basal cell carcinomas. The presence of hair follicle differentiation is a reassuring feature, suggesting a lower likelihood of local recurrence or aggressive behaviour.

Well-differentiated, nodular basal cell carcinomas with palisading of cells around the cell clusters and only a small stromal component do occur in young people. These lesions are essentially identical to similar lesions in older people, but present clinically as small naevi and are not associated with aggressive growth or ulceration (Rahbari and Mehregan, 1982). When multiple, naevoid basal cell carcinomas are present they

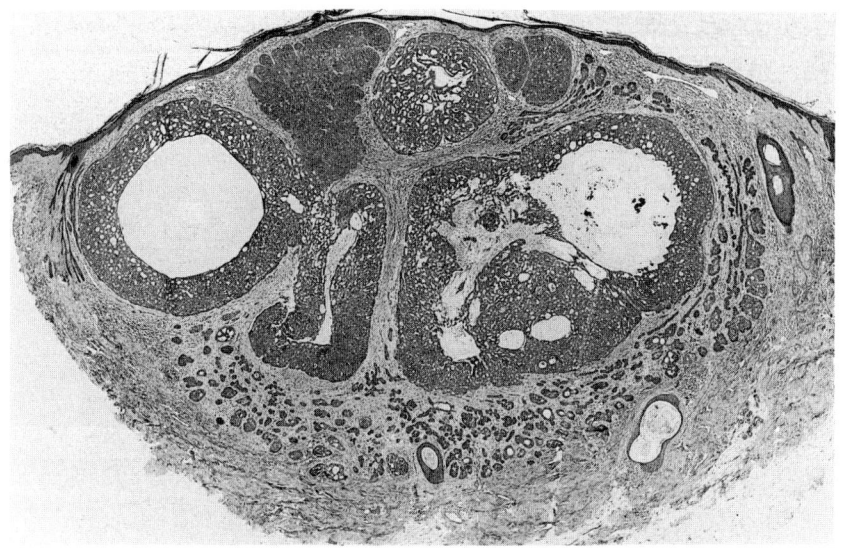

(a)

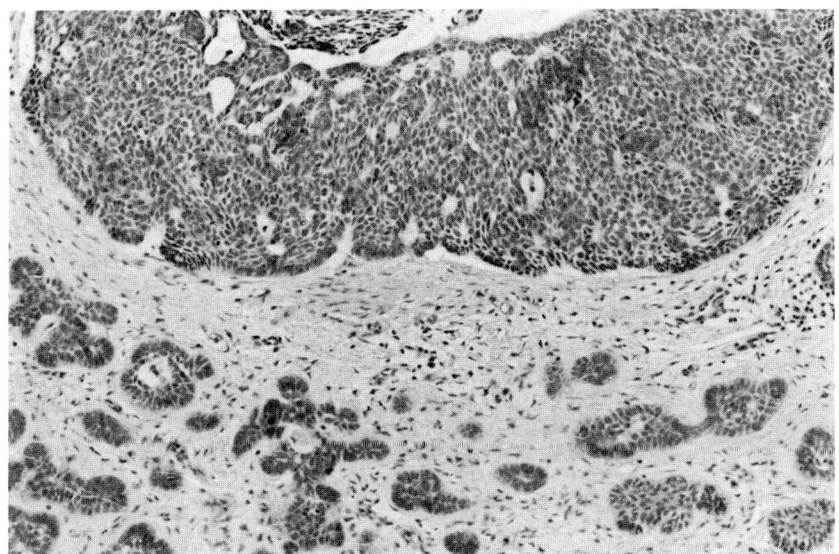

(b)

Figure 5.3 Adenoid basal cell carcinoma, with (a) central cystic change, and (b) non-infiltrative margins.

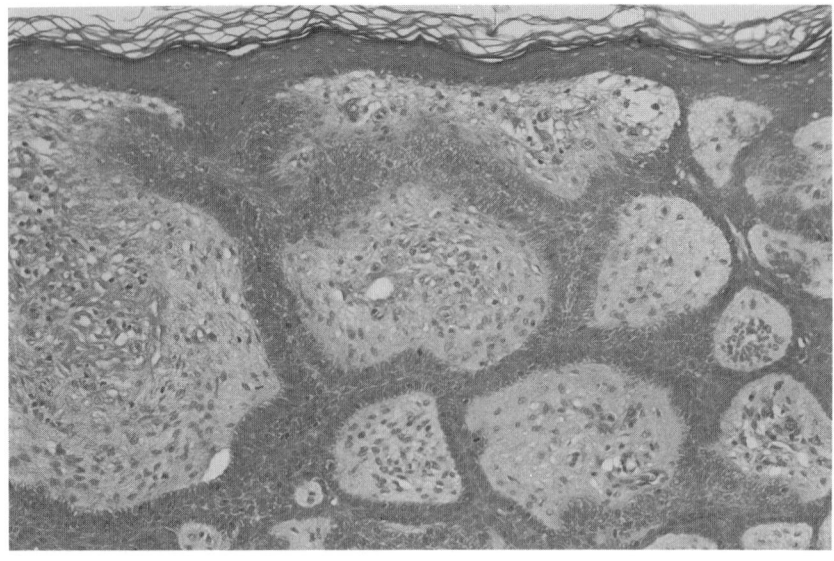

Figure 5.4   Fibroepithelioma of Pinkus showing strands of tumour cells compressed between an excess of stroma.

may be part of a Gorlin's syndrome, which is associated with jaw cysts, skeletal anomalies, medulloblastoma and hyporesponsiveness to parathormone (Gorlin *et al.*, 1965).

The final variant is the sclerosing or morphoea-like basal cell carcinoma, which is characterized clinically by lesions on the head and neck that resemble morphoea except for the frequent presence of telangiectasia and the possible eventual development of ulceration. The tumours grow slowly, have indistinct margins and frequently recur after attempted excision. They consist of small cords of tumour cells infiltrating within a larger amount of stroma (Caro and Howell, 1951).

Neuroendocrine differentiation has been described, but is uncommon, is rarely found by Grimelius' stain, needing immunohistochemical markers such as neurone specific enolase or chromogranin, and is probably of no clinical relevance (George *et al.*, 1989).

One of the interesting aspects of basal cell carcinoma is the close relationship that exists between the epithelial cell component and the specialized stroma, without which the epithelial cells cannot develop. This stroma is particularly abundant in sclerosing basal cell carcinoma and constitutes the major part of the tumour volume. The tumour stroma can be seen in H and E sections, but immunohistochemical staining with an antibody to type IV collagen is particularly good at

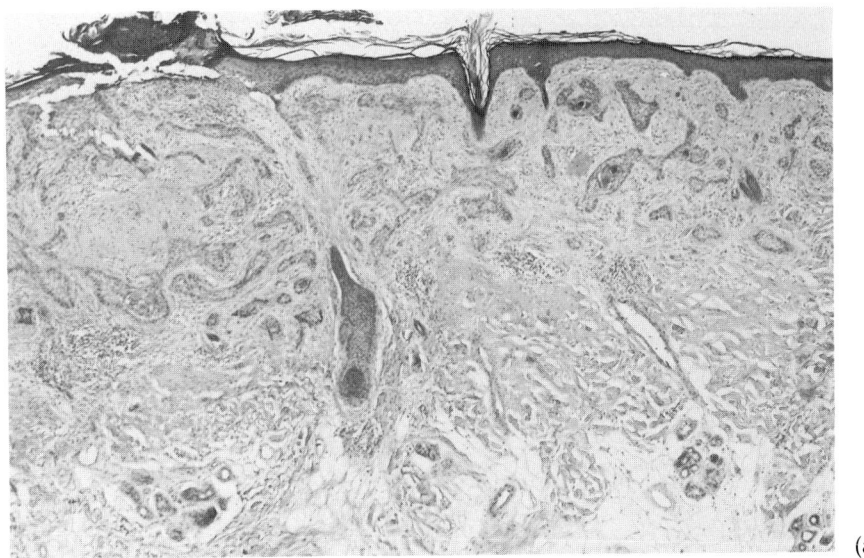

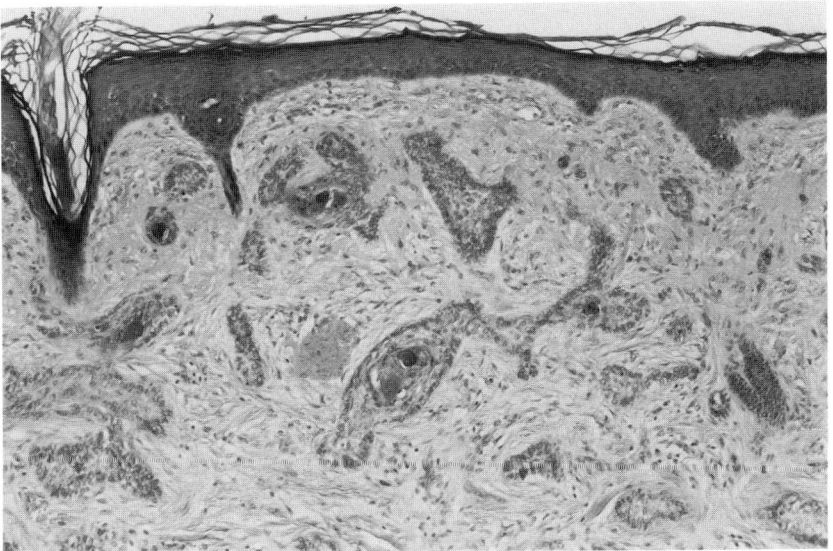

Figure 5.5 Recurrent basal cell carcinoma (for the second time), showing (a) diffuse infiltration of dermis, and (b) metatypical squamous differentiation and an aggressive growth pattern.

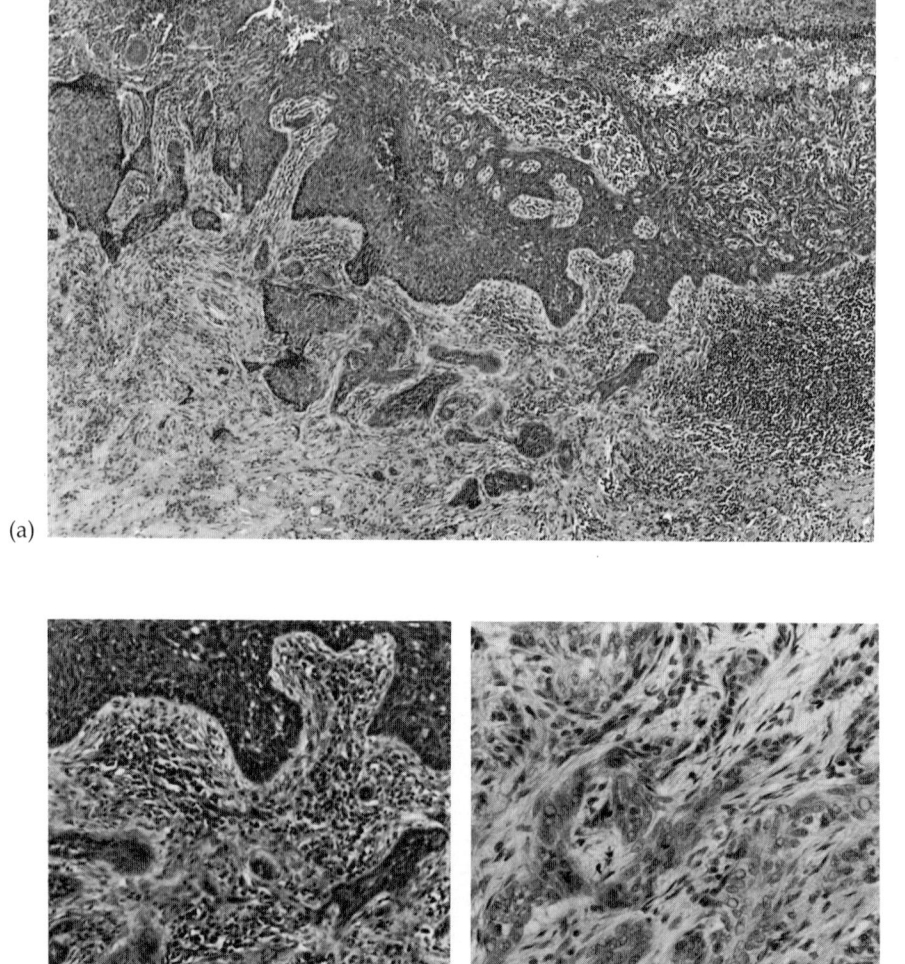

(a)

(b)

(c)

Figure 5.6 Basal cell carcinoma with (a) an aggressive growth pattern. Narrow cords of tumour cells are infiltrating deeply at the base of the tumour (b and c).

demonstrating the tumour stroma, which extends for some distance beyond the apparent limit of the epithelial component of the tumour. One should attempt, therefore, to decide whether or not the tumour stroma has been completely excised when assessing the surgical margins of an excision biopsy.

Sclerosing basal cell carcinoma tumour cells appear to elaborate factors that enhance collagen production by adjacent stroma fibroblasts. The reasons for the lack of such reaction in nodular basal cell carcinoma are not clear, but they may be due to a difference in the level of collagen synthesis within the tumours (Moy *et al.*, 1988). It is also possible that the tumours require contact with the epithelium of the epidermis or hair follicle in order to grow (Imayama *et al.*, 1987).

From a practical point of view, it is often difficult to decide whether a particular tumour is of a sclerosing type or not, because it may show a mixture of appearances. It is less of a problem, however, to look at the advancing margin to decide whether it is of the infiltrative, aggressive type seen in sclerosing basal cell carcinomas, or is of the well-circumscribed non-aggressive type seen in a typical nodular tumour. The aggressive tumours may be ulcerated and have thin cords of cells infiltrating through a hyalinized stroma, with loss of the peripheral

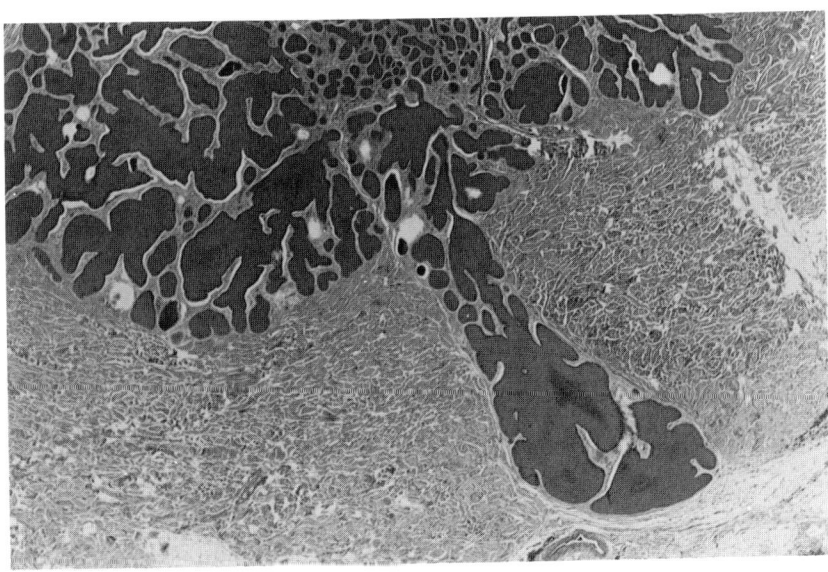

Figure 5.7   Nodular basal cell carcinoma, without an aggressive growth pattern, but with a deep penetrating component – another possible cause of local recurrence if incompletely excised.

palisading of nodular basal cell carcinomas. This seems to be a useful and important distinction, as the tumours with an aggressive pattern are more likely to recur if inadequately excised. So as well as reporting the variant type of tumour and commenting on the margins in an excision biopsy, it is also worth saying whether the tumour has an aggressive or non-aggressive growth pattern. This information may be of use in the follow-up of the patient, when looking for evidence of local recurrence. If tumour is present at the surgical margin of the biopsy, with a morphoeic basal cell carcinoma, there is a 90% chance of local recurrence (Jacobs et al., 1982; Dellon et al., 1985).

Dixon et al. (1989) have suggested that the likelihood of recurrence can be predicted by considering the following variables: 'inadequate surgical resection margins; an infiltrative, morphoea or superficial multicentric growth pattern; spiky shape of cell groups; infiltrating invading edge; poorly formed peripheral palisades; high degree of nuclear pleomorphism; and possibly marked fibrosis, absent cystic change, and markedly atypical squamous change'. They assert that a tumour containing several of these will have a high likelihood of recurrence and that tumour type is more important than the state of the surgical margins in predicting recurrence. They do point out, however, that despite this evidence there remain a small number of cases in which recurrence would have been difficult to predict.

The form of excision chosen depends to a large extent upon the size of the tumour. Simple shave excision is appropriate for small tumours and is an easy way of achieving a good cosmetic result (Harrison, 1987). Up to 93% of tumours less than 20 mm in diameter will be cured by local excision, with progressively worse results as the tumours increase in size (Petrovich et al., 1987).

Follow-up is also recommended because a patient who has had one basal cell carcinoma is likely to have another. Up to 20% of patients will have developed another basal cell carcinoma after 1 year and 36% after 5 years, the majority of which will be small and unsuspected by the patient (Epstein, 1973; Rahbari and Mehregan, 1982). Obviously the sooner the tumour is diagnosed and treated the better. The early lesion which can be cured in the dermatology clinic becomes much more of a problem if left to develop to the stage of the 'rodent ulcer', which was more familiar to our forebears (Robinson, 1987). Some cases of 'horrifying' basal cell carcinoma still occur. These are histological indistinguishable from regular basal cell carcinomas, but behave in a much more aggressive way. There does not seem to be an easy way of predicting which tumours will behave in this way (Jackson and Adams, 1973).

Basal cell carcinoma remains a slight semantic problem. In former times it was more commonly called epithelioma. This is not without reason, as it does seem to be a tumour which infiltrates locally but does not metastasize. There are very occasional reports in the literature of metastatic basal cell carcinoma but the reports are very sporadic, with one review suggesting a rate of <0.1% of all basal cell carcinomas (Wermuth and Fajardo, 1970). These reports suggest that the metastasizing tumours are histologically typical but large and long-standing, possibly from a primary which has been left to develop to a stage when it has invaded very deeply into the dermis or subcutaneous fat, with consequent greater likelihood of vascular invasion (Perrone *et al.*, 1987; Hoffman *et al.*, 1988). Alternatively, reports of metastasizing basal cell carcinoma raise doubts about true nature of the primary lesion (Lattes and Kesseler, 1951).

5.2 Squamous cell carcinoma

Unfortunately, patients still present with invasive, cutaneous squamous cell carcinomas, of varying extent, but often large. These often require formal excision by a plastic surgeon. Diagnosis is not usually a problem. The dermis will contain cords of malignant keratinized cells in a variety

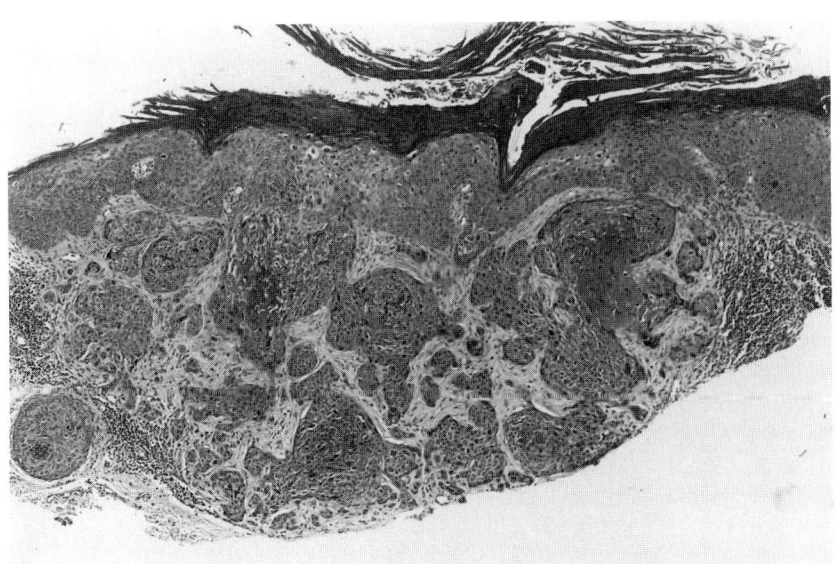

Figure 5.8 Squamous cell carcinoma arising in an actinic keratosis, and apparently incompletely excised. No tumour was found in the re-excision specimen.

of shapes, sizes and patterns, but having in common a squamous appearance, without the palisading outer layer of basal cells of the metatypical basal cell carcinoma.

It is, of course, important to examine the surgical margins to ensure that a complete excision has been performed. There does not seem to be any reliable way of predicting which squamous carcinomas are going to be cured by excision and which are going to metastasize, either to regional lymph nodes, or more widely. It may be useful to at least measure the size of the tumour accurately and record its thickness, as size does appear to be related to the possibility of metastasis (Dinehart and Pollack, 1989).

Squamous cell carcinoma has to be distinguished from pseudocarcinomatous hyperplasia, which is not a hyperplasia of the epidermal epithelium, but of the adnexal epithelium of follicular infundibulum and eccrine duct. Pseudocarcinomatous hyperplasia occurs as a response to an underlying inflammatory or neoplastic process. If the biopsy is deep enough the underlying process should be apparent (Grunwald et al., 1988). Even considering this way of attempting differential diagnosis, it can still be difficult to distinguish the two conditions. Further follow-up of the patient is perhaps offers the best chance of confirming that a diagnosis has been correct.

5.3   Keratoacanthoma

Keratoacanthomas are skin tumours that develop over a period of 6–8 weeks from a red papule to a domed nodule 2–3 cm in diameter and then gradually shrink, leaving a depressed, flat scar, if the lesion is not removed first. They occur mainly on sun exposed skin such as the face, hands and forearms. Men are three times more commonly affected than women. The lesions are commonest in the middle-aged and elderly. They also occur in association with defective cell mediated immunity, in association with immunosuppression after renal transplant, and in patients with xeroderma pigmentosum (Kern and McCray, 1980).

The aetiology of keratoacanthomas and the reasons for their rapid growth and resolution remain to be explained. They have been shown to have an increased number of S100 positive Langerhans cells when inflamed, as they usually are during the phase of resolution (Korenburg et al., 1988). Activation of the oncogene H-ras has been demonstrated, indicating that this change alone is not sufficient to maintain a malignant phenotype (Leon et al., 1988).

Histologically, there are similarities with squamous cell carcinoma. At either end of the spectrum differential diagnosis is possible, but there does exist a group of lesions in which it is difficult to make a

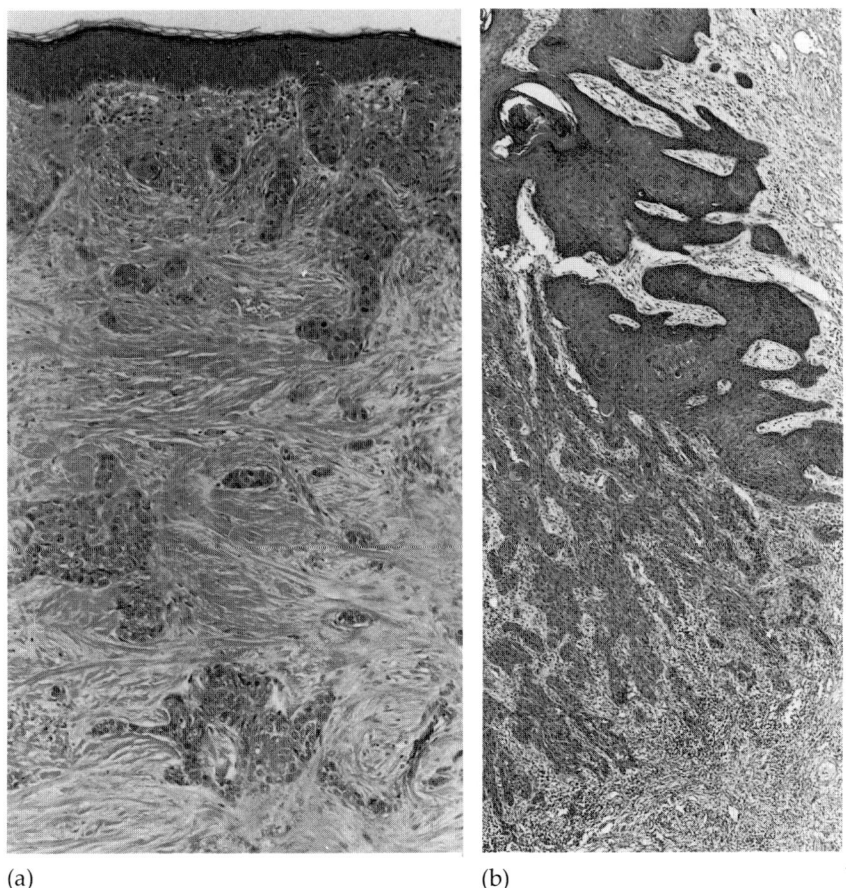

(a)   (b)

Figure 5.9   Squamous cell carcinomas showing (a) infiltration in a desmoplastic stroma, and (b) deep dermal invasion with associated inflammatory response.

confident distinction between keratoacanthoma and squamous cell carcinoma on morphological grounds. Indeed, examples of otherwise typical keratoacanthomas have been described showing perineural invasion and intravascular growth – features normally taken to indicate frank malignancy (Cooper and Wolfe, 1988). Furthermore a case has been made for examples of definite transition from keratoacanthoma to squamous cell carcinoma (Lawrence and Reed, 1990).

The classical description of keratoacanthoma as a symmetrical lesion

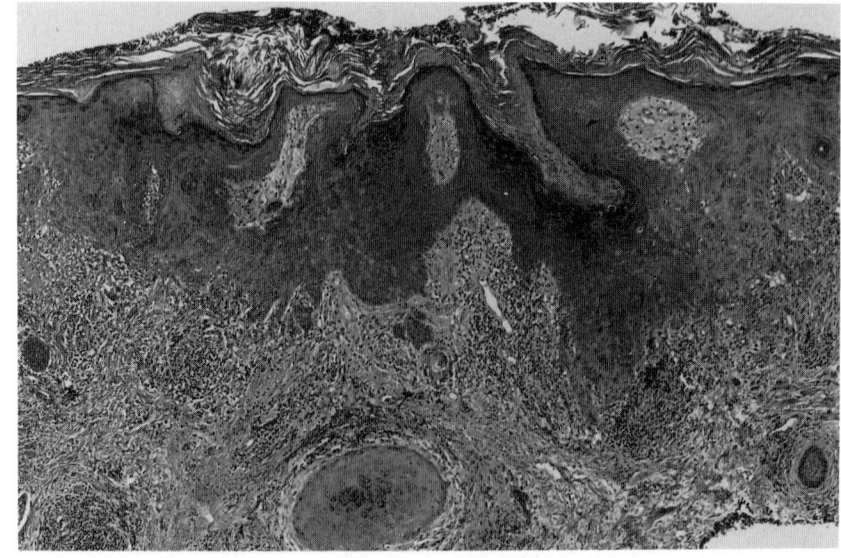

(a)

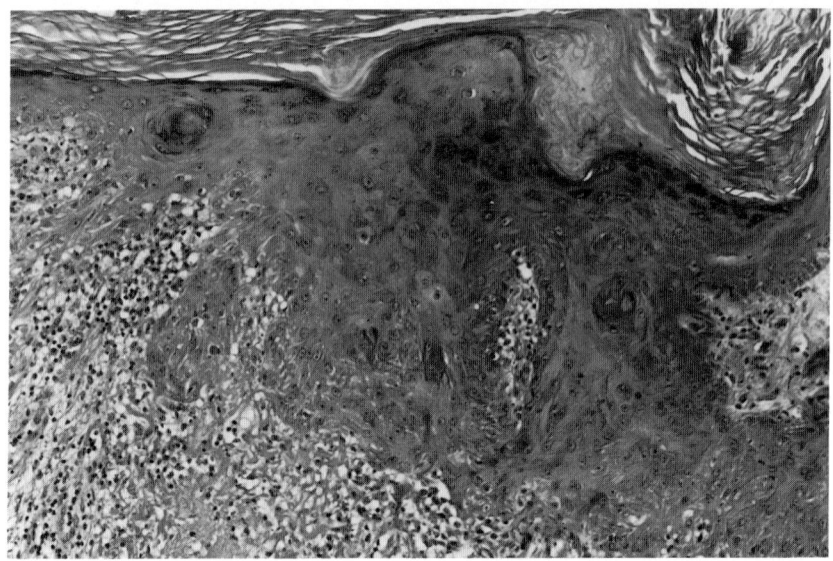

(b)

Figure 5.10   Pseudoepitheliomatous hyperplasia. The lesion shows (a) a close architectural resemblence to squamous cell carcinoma, but (b) lacks cytological atypia.

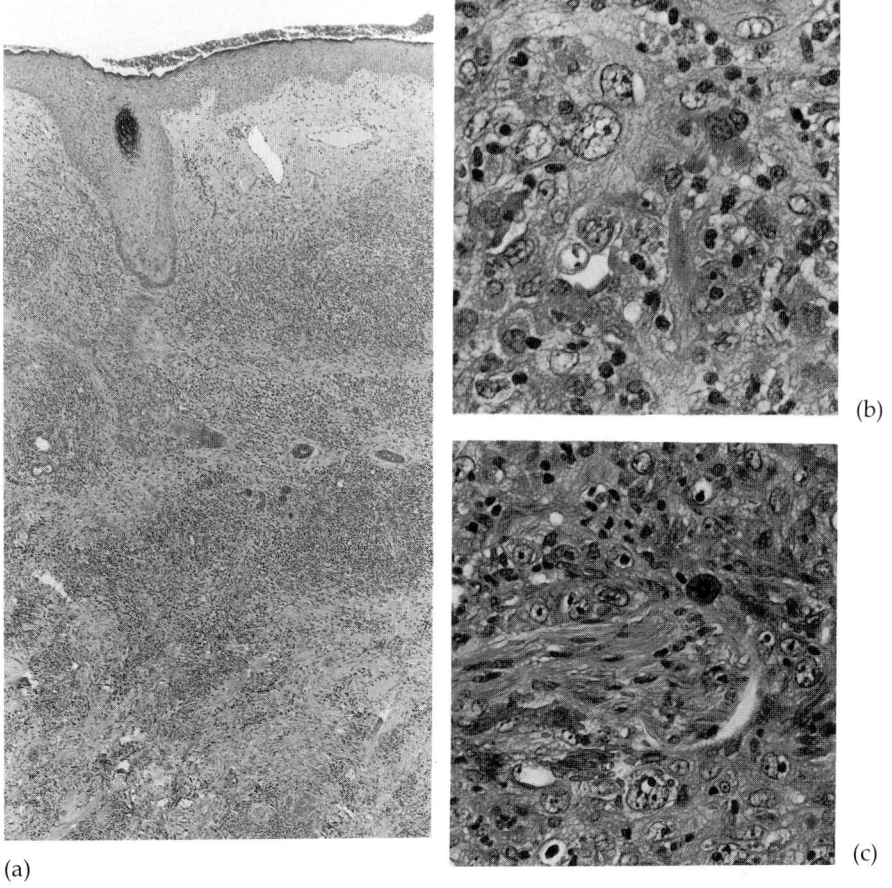

(a)

(b)

(c)

Figure 5.11 Inflammatory squamous cell carcinoma. At first sight (a) it is not obviously a tumour, but closer inspection (b) shows tumour cells, and (c) perineural infiltration.

with a central, keratin-filled cavity surrounded by tongues of proliferating epidermis at the sides and bottom remains valid (Seifert and Nasemann, 1989). One useful differential point is the larger size of cells in a keratoacanthoma and their hyaline eosinophilic cytoplasm. They do not show convincing cellular or nuclear atypia, mitoses are infrequent and atypical mitoses virtually unknown. Ultrastructural studies show abnormal keratinization and intracytoplasmic desmosome-like

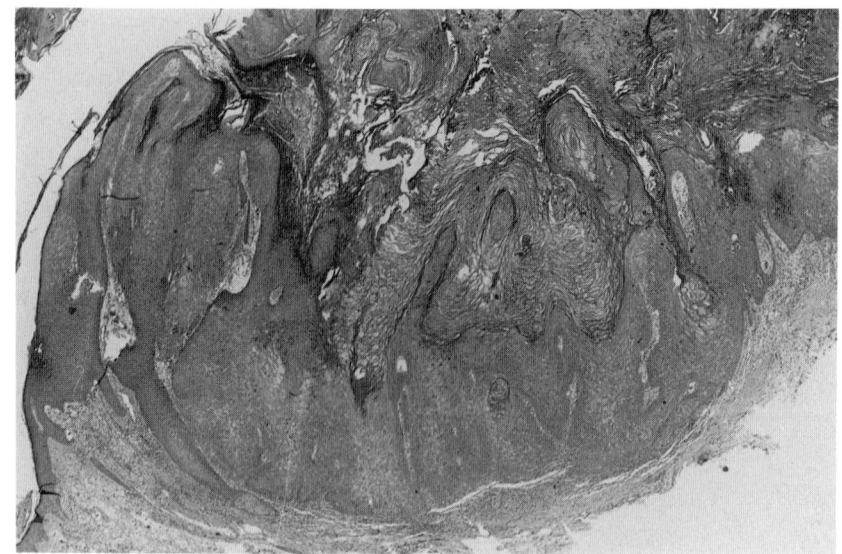

(a)

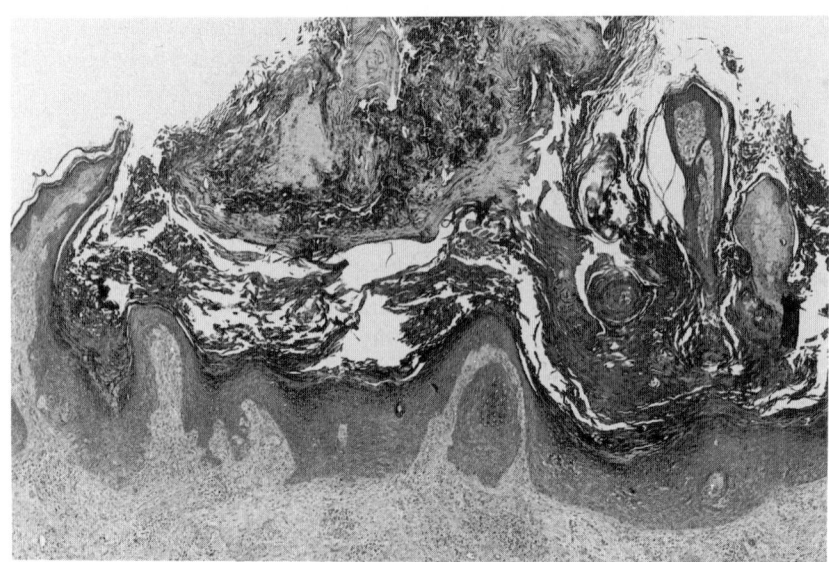

(b)

Figure 5.12 Keratoacanthoma (a and b). Two examples showing typical symmetrical architecture, circumscribed base and central accumulation of keratin.

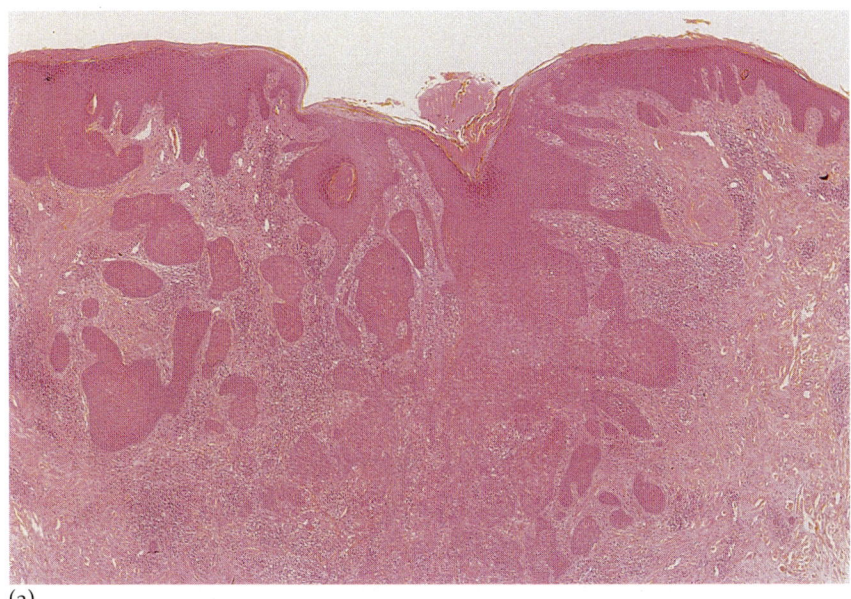
(a)

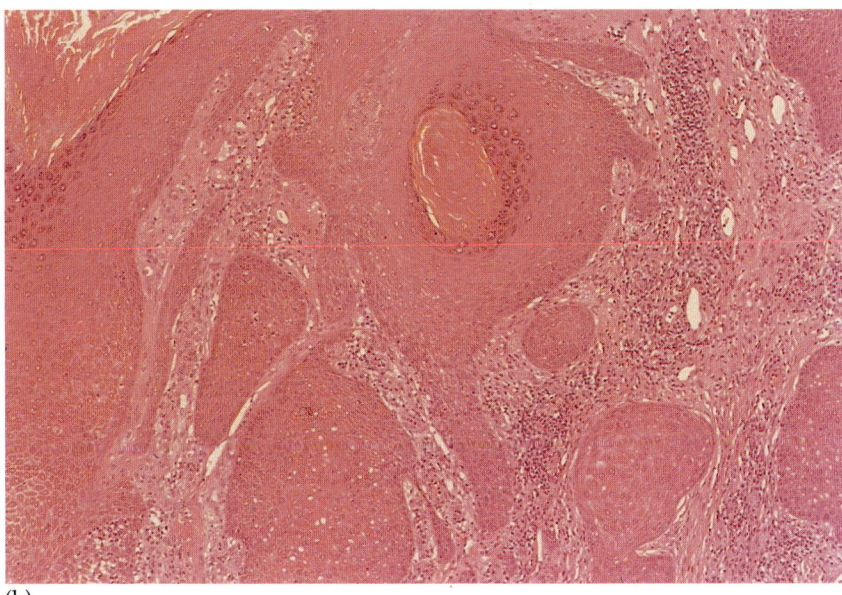
(b)

Plate 9 Pseudoepitheliomatous hyperplasia. (a) The lesion appears to be invading the dermis. (b) The dermal proliferation lacks atypia and represents hyperplasia of appendageal epithelium.

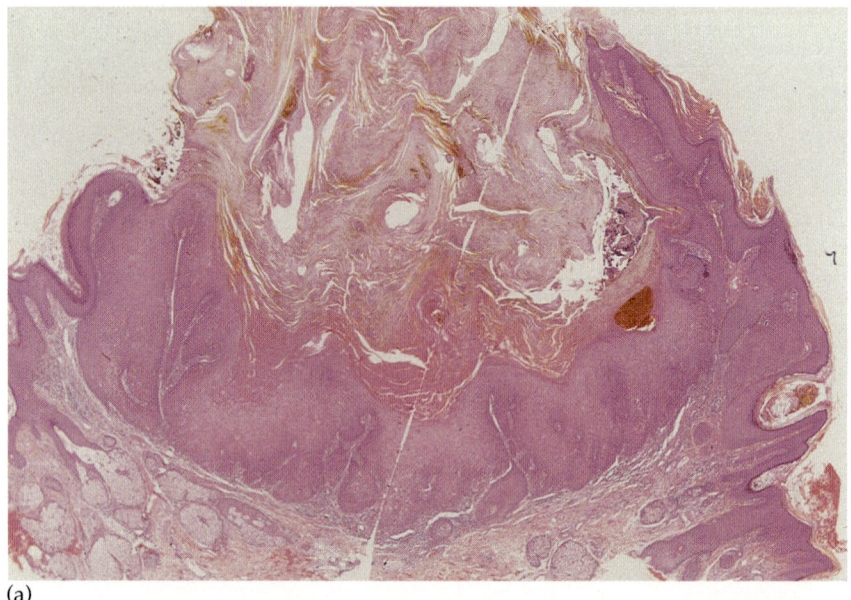

(a)

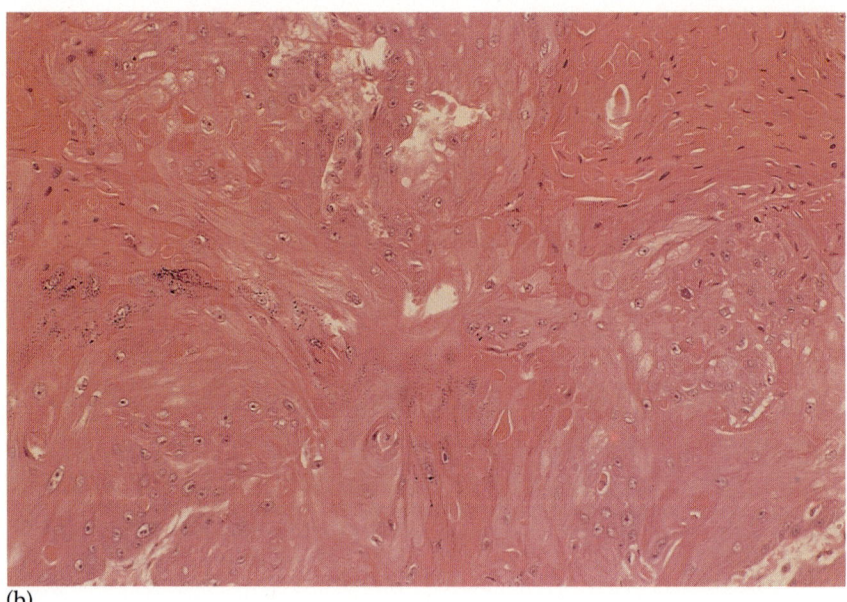

(b)

Plate 10 Keratoacanthoma. (a) This example shows typical radial symmetry and a central, keratin-filled cavity. (b) The keratinocytes are enlarged, with pale cytoplasm and without atypia.

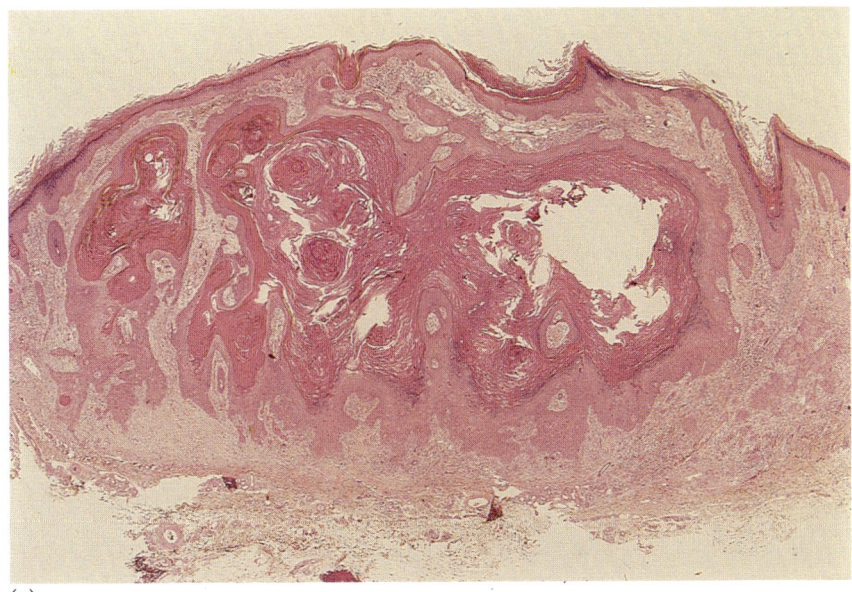

(a)

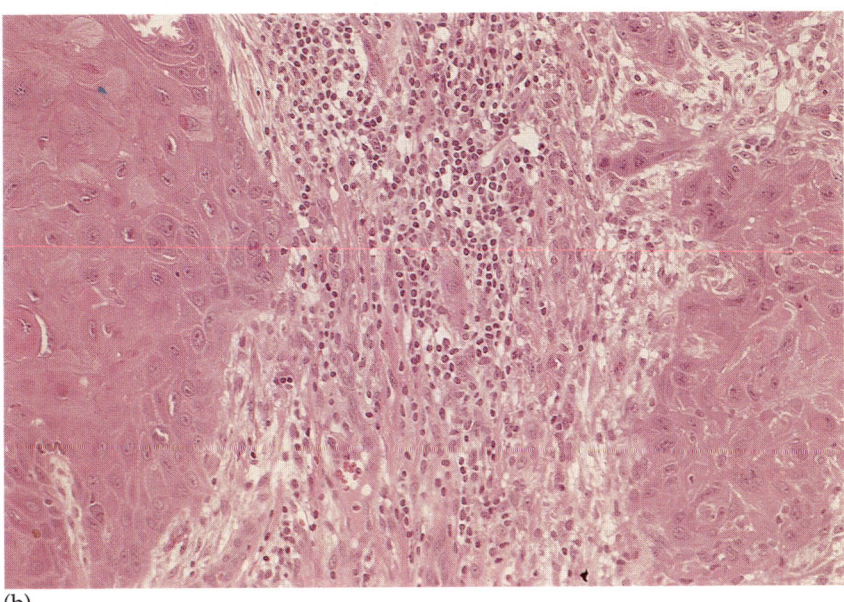

(b)

Plate 11   Keratoacanthoma. (a) This example shows typical architecture, but this is a biopsy of a recurrence after previous curettage. (b) There is evidence of an invasive component of squamous carcinoma to the side of the central lesion.

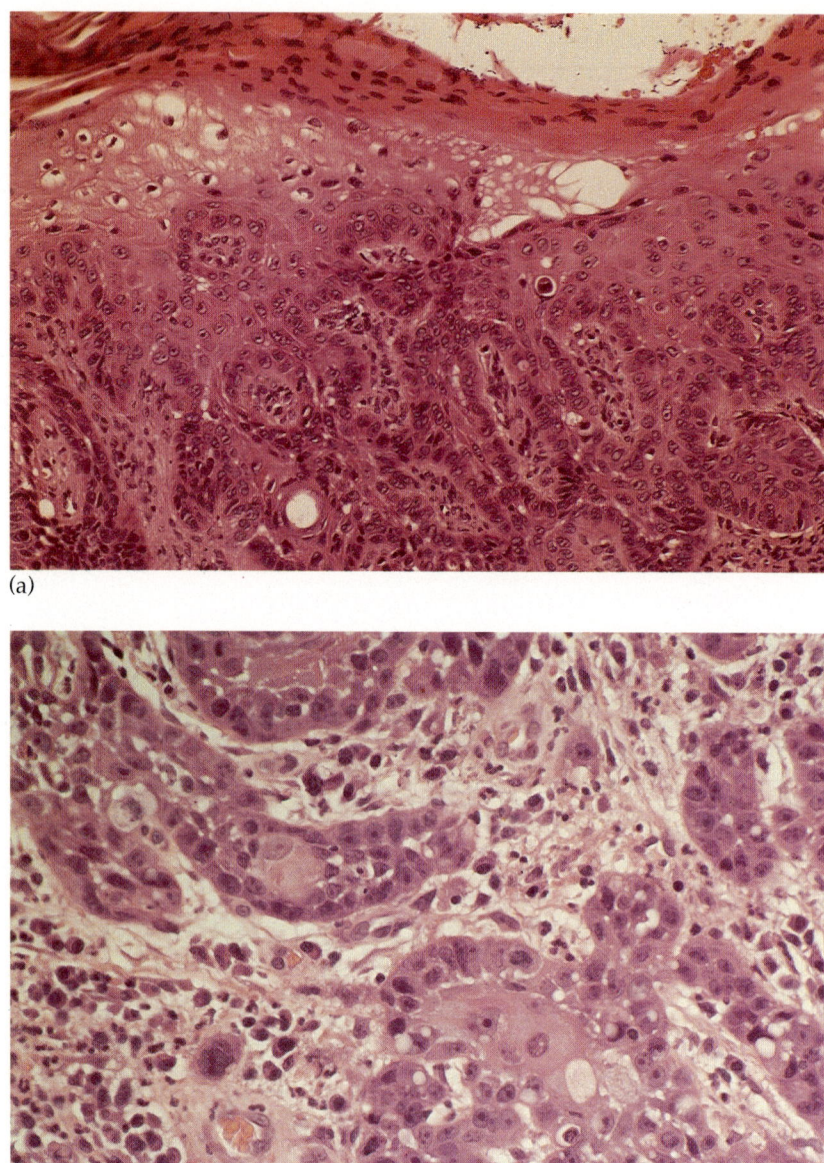

Plate 12 (a) Florid keratosis. There is prominent papillomatosis, but the basal layer remains intact, with no evidence of dermal invasion. (b) Squamous cell carcinoma. The tumour shows marked cellular pleomorphism, with definite dermal invasion.

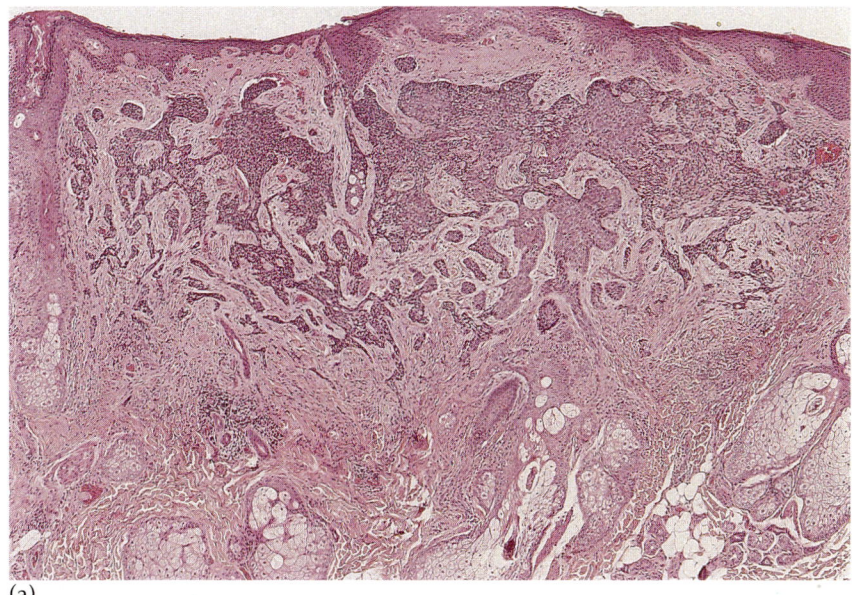
(a)

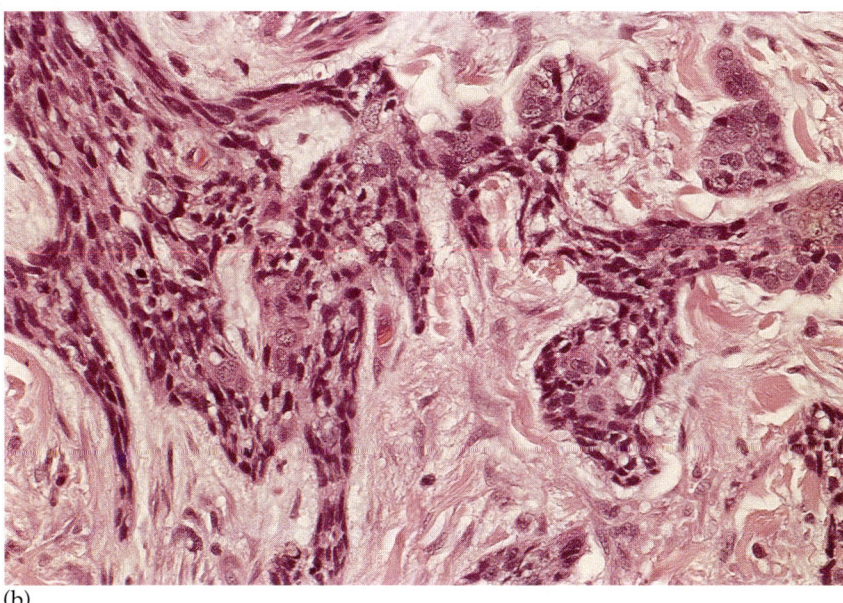
(b)

Plate 13 Basal cell carcinoma. (a) The cords of basaloid cells invade deeply into the dermis. (b) The advancing edge of the tumour shows an aggressive growth pattern, making local recurrence likely if excision is incomplete.

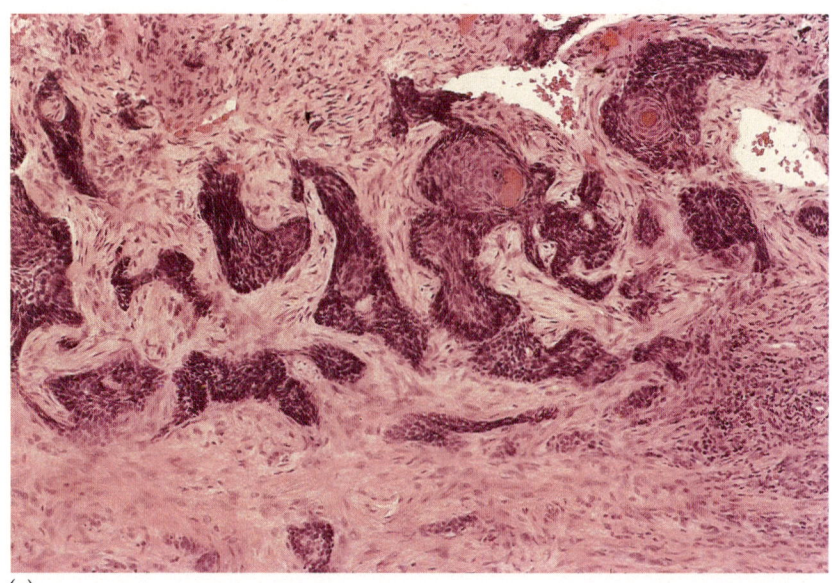

(a)

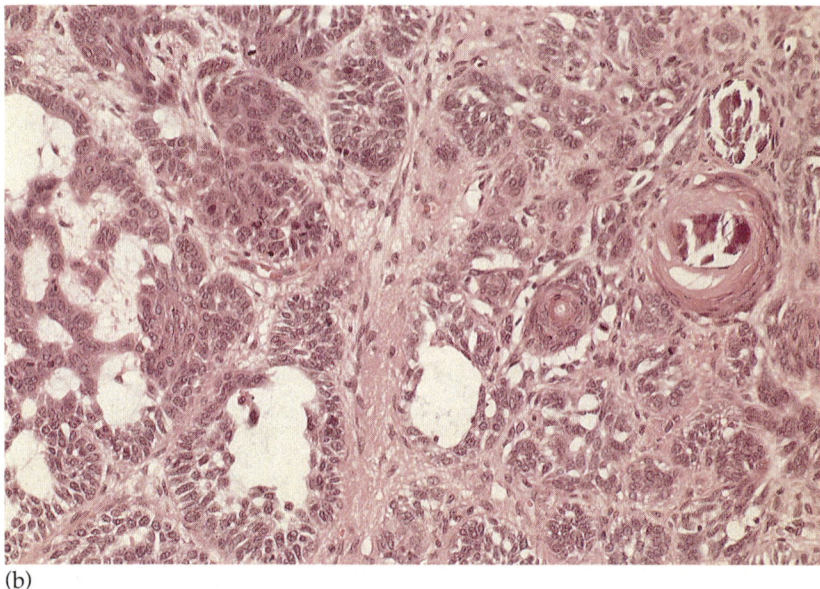

(b)

Plate 14 (a) Metatypical basal cell carcinoma. The advancing cords of tumour show squamous differentiation: a feature associated with frequent local recurrence. (b) Trichoepithelioma. This example shows focal calcification and an adenoid growth pattern.

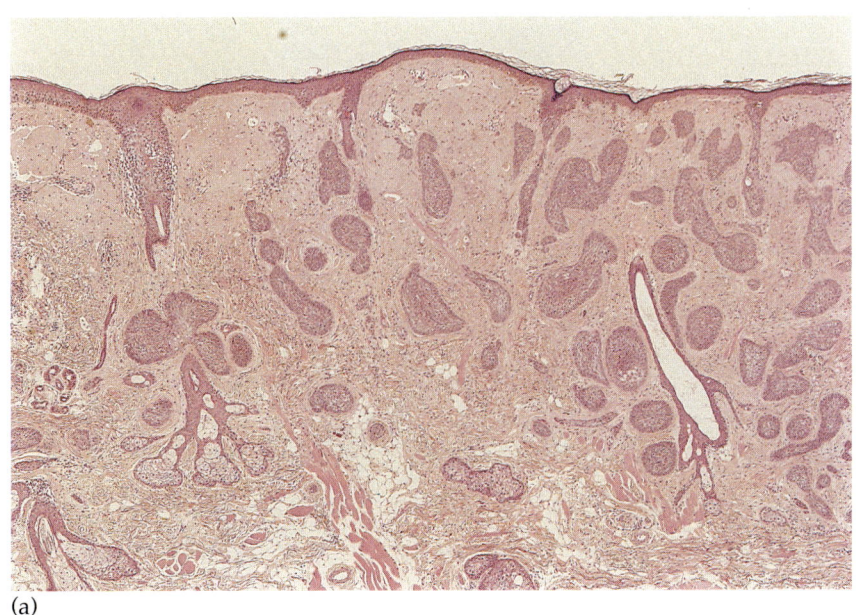

(a)

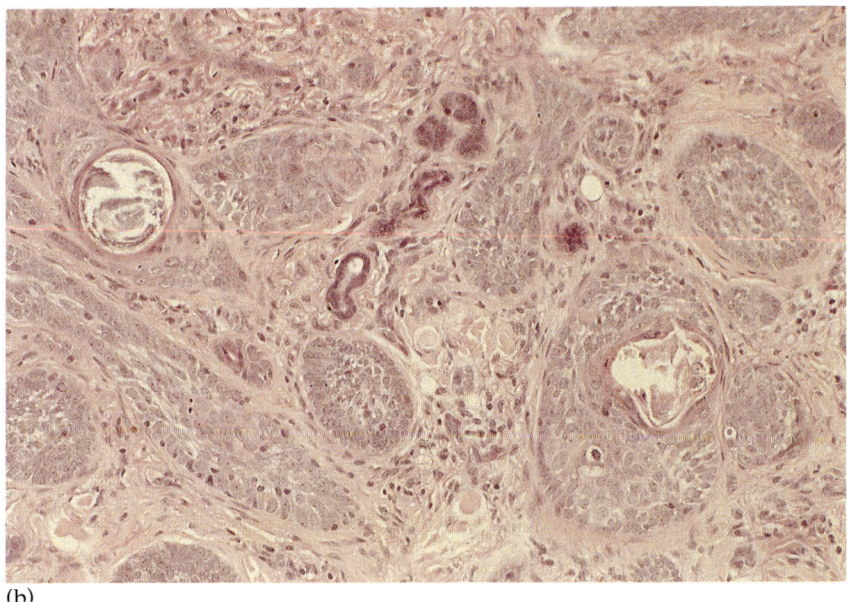

(b)

Plate 15   Trichoepithelioma. (a) Groups of tumour cells are seen arising from hair follicles. (b) The tumour shows calcification, rounded nests of tumour cells without an aggressive growth pattern and small horn cyst formation.

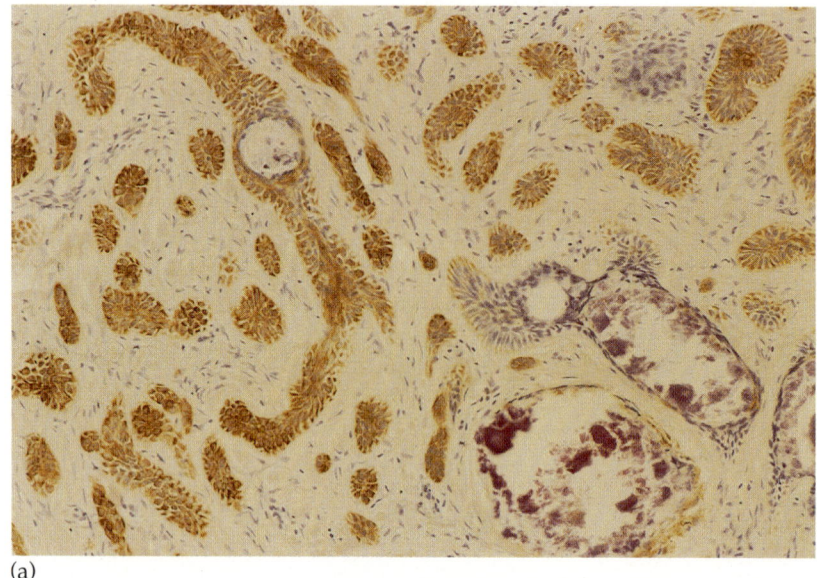

(a)

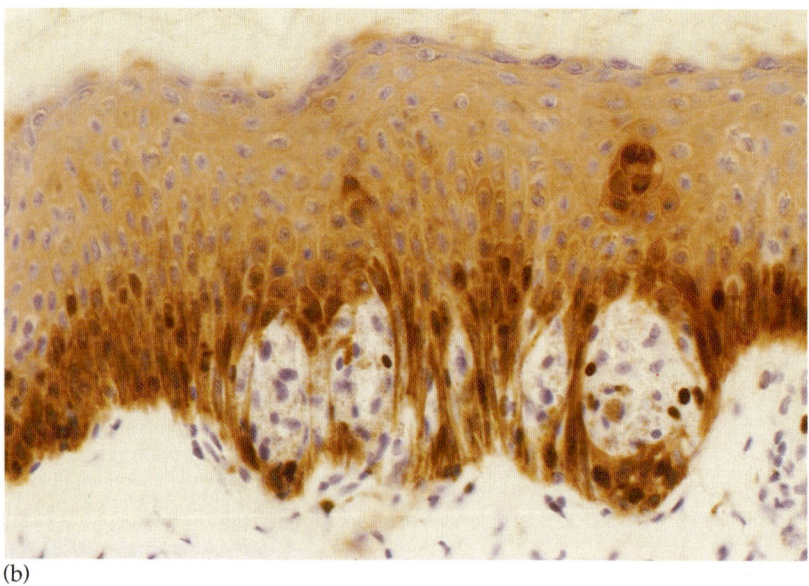

(b)

Plate 16 Immunoperoxidase staining (a) for high molecular weight cytokeratin (LP 34) shows positive immunoreactivity in tumour cells in a trichoepithelioma, and (b) the proliferation marker Ki-67 stains the nuclei of proliferating melanocytes in junctional nest. Basal cell cytoplasm staining is not related to cell proliferation.

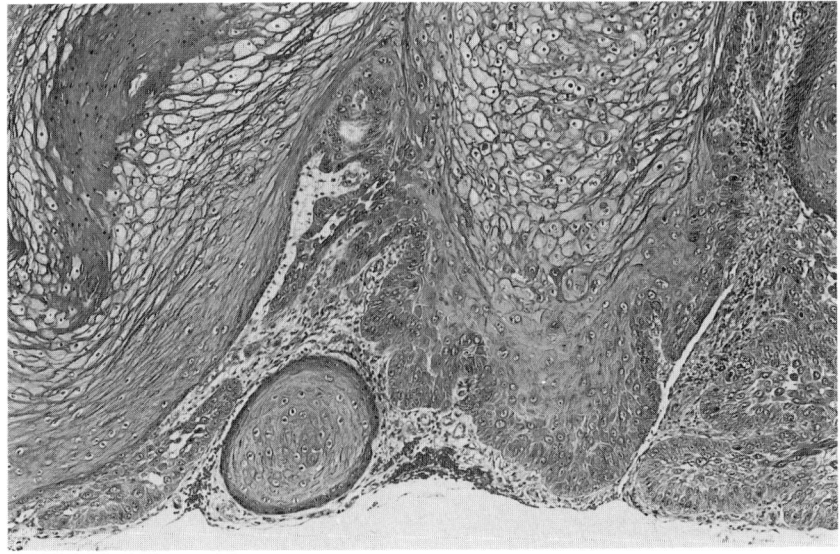

Figure 5.13   Keratoacanthoma. Well circumscribed base is seen in this curettage specimen.

structures (Takaki *et al.*, 1971). Squamous cell carcinomas are more likely to show cellular and nuclear atypia and mitotic activity.

Immunohistochemical staining has not offered much so far, although staining for involucrin may help. Keratoacanthomas show a relatively uniform staining pattern of all but the basal cells, whilst squamous cell carcinomas show considerable heterogeneity of immunoreactivity through the lesion (Smoller *et al.*, 1986).

There remains a small minority of biopsies with equivocal appearances in which it may not be possible to determine the correct diagnosis (Kern and McCray, 1980). These cases should be followed up to see whether the lesion recurs or has been cured.

The main problem in differential diagnosis is a consequence of the method of removal. Many of them are curetted off rather than excised. This produces a very friable specimen virtually devoid of surrounding normal skin. As a result, it is often difficult to produce a satisfactory, well-orientated section representative of the lesion and including its margins of excision. It is fruitless to spend time agonizing over the appearances of the base. If there is no cellular atypia or mitotic activity, then the lesion is unlikely to be a squamous cell carcinoma.

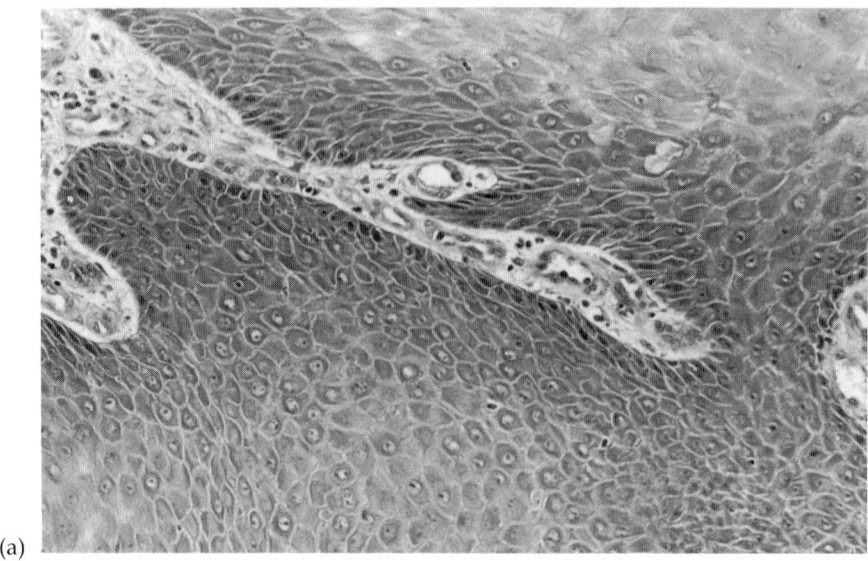

(a)

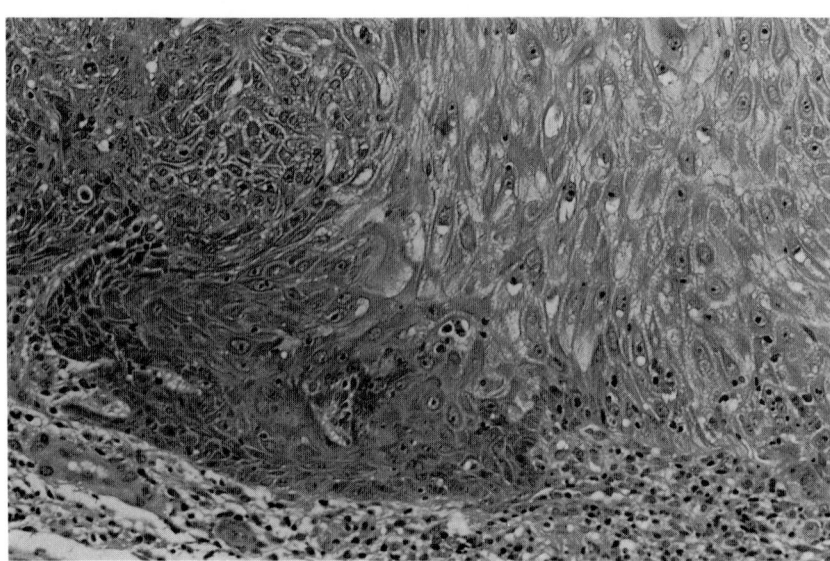

(b)

Figure 5.14 Keratoacanthoma (a and b). Proliferating squamous cells without atypia.

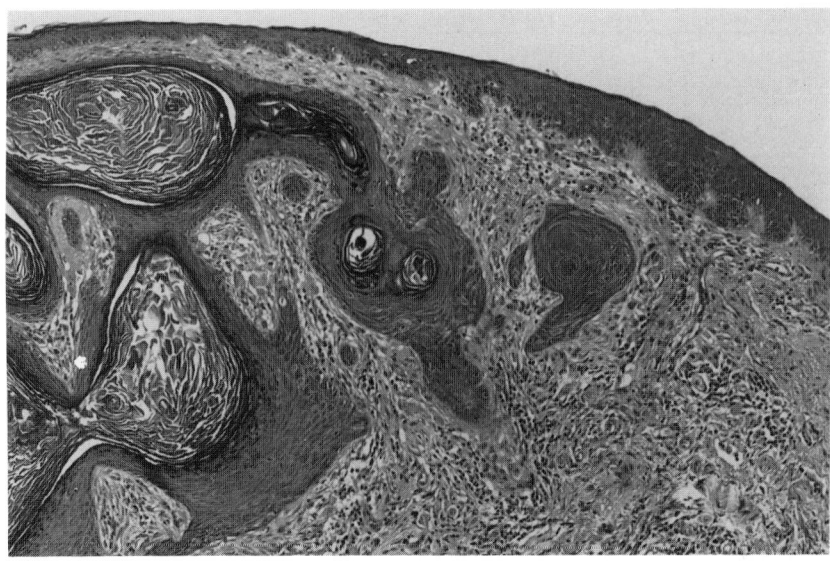

Figure 5.15   Keratoacanthoma. An involuting lesion with decreasing thickness of keratinocyte layer.

5.4   Spindle cell squamous cell carcinoma

A rare variant of squamous cell carcinoma is the spindle cell squamous cell carcinoma, which has to be distinguished from spindle cell melanoma and spindle cell sarcomas of various kinds. There is a close cytological resemblance to sarcoma (Sims and Kersch, 1948). If there is a clear attachment to the epidermis, intercellular prickles can be found and the tumour cells express high molecular weight cytokeratin and do not express vimentin, then a confident diagnosis can be made. These tumours are usually solitary, are sited on the head or an extremity and may present as a nodule, ulcer or fungating lesion. After adequate excision, they carry a favourable prognosis (Underwood *et al.*, 1951).

5.5   Basosquamous carcinoma

A small proportion of tumours show appearances in between basal and squamous cell carcinomas. The predominant impression is of a basal cell carcinoma with squamous differentiation taking place in the centre of larger groups of tumour cells. These tumours are unlikely to metastasize and should be regarded as variants of basal cell carcinoma from the point of view of clinical management. Differential staining for

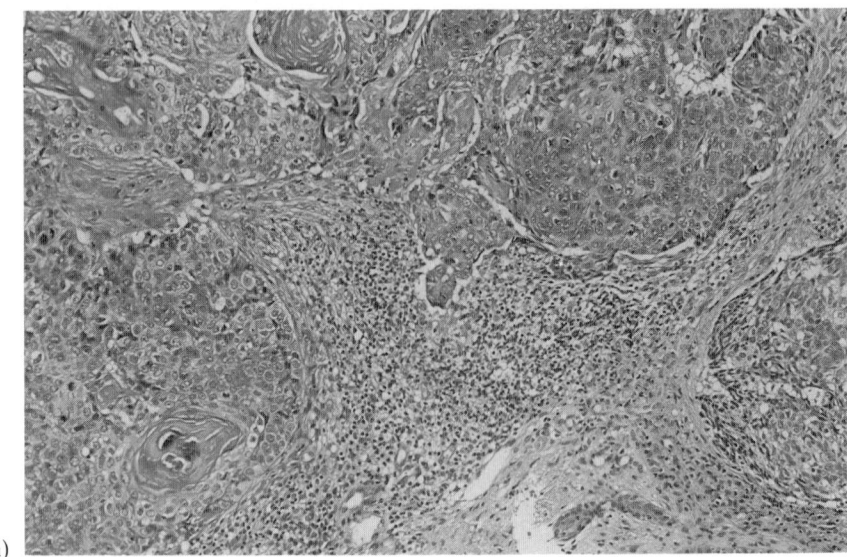

(a)

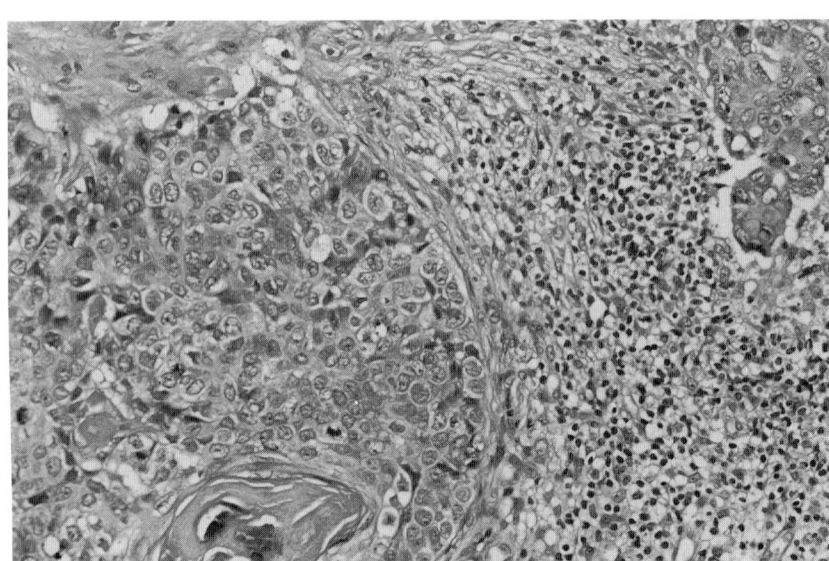

(b)

Figure 5.16 Basosquamous carcinoma (a and b). Basal cell carcinoma architecture with squamous cytological differentiation.

cytokeratins of low and high molecular weight may have a part to play in differential diagnosis (Thomas *et al.*, 1984).

Having said that, it should be borne in mind that the kind of basal cell carcinoma that they most resemble are those with an aggressive growth pattern and, as such, are more prone to local recurrence if not adequately excised. Furthermore occasional metastasizing cases have been recorded: cases which emphasized the need for an adequate biopsy when assessing these tumours. When metastasis occurs the prognosis is likely to be poor (Johnson *et al.*, 1989).

5.6 Adenosquamous carcinoma

Very occasional reports describe adenosquamous or mucoepidermoid carcinoma, which present in a fairly consistent way as moderately differentiated, deeply invasive, high-grade tumours with an aggressive clinical course including the possibility of local recurrence and distant metastasis (Underwood *et al.*, 1978). Well-differentiated low-grade tumours behave in a less aggressive way (Friedman, 1989). The tumours are probably derived from eccrine ducts.

References

Beerman, H. (1969) Some aspects of cutaneous malignancy. *Arch. Dermatol.*, **99**, 617–26.

Caro, M. R. and Howell, J. B. (1951) Morphoea-like epithelioma. *Arch. Derm. Syph.*, **63**, 53–7.

Cooper, P. H. and Wolfe, J. T. (1988) Perioral keratoacanthomas with extensive perineural invasion and intravenous growth. *Arch. Dermatol.*, **124**, 1397–1401.

Dellon, A. L., De Silva, S., Connolly, M. and Rees, A. (1985) Prediction of recurrence in incompletely excised basal cell carcinoma. *Plastic Reconstr. Surg.*, **75**, 860–71.

Dinehart, S. M. and Pollack, S. V. (1989) Metastases from squamous cell carcinoma of the skin and lip. An analysis of twenty-seven cases. *J. Am. Acad. Dermatol.*, **21**, 241–8.

Dixon, A. Y., Lee, S. H. and McGregor, D. H. (1989) Factors predictive of recurrence of basal cell carcinoma *Am. J. Dermatopathol.*, **11**, 222–32.

Domarus, H. V. and Stevens, P. J. (1984) Metastatic basal cell carcinoma. *J. Am. Acad. Dermatol.*, **10**, 1043–60.

Epstein, E. (1973) Value of follow-up after treatment of basal cell carcinoma. *Arch. Dermatol.*, **108**, 798–800.

Friedman, K. J. (1989) Low-grade primary cutaneous adenosquamous (mucoepidermoid) carcinoma. Report of a case and review of the literature. *Am. J. Dermatopathol.*, **11**, 43–50.

George, E., Swanson, P. E. and Wick, M. R. (1989) Neuroendocrine differentiation in basal cell carcinoma. An immunohistochemical study. *Am. J. Dermatopathol.*, **11**, 131–5.

Gorlin, R. J., Vickers, R. A., Kellen, E. and Williamson, J. J. (1965) The multiple basal-cell nevi syndrome. *Cancer*, **18**, 89–104.

Grimwood, R. E., Ferris, C. F., Mercill, D. B. and Huff, J. C. (1986) Proliferating cells of human basal cell carcinoma are located on the periphery of tumor nodules. *J. Invest. Dermatol.*, **86**, 191–4.

Grunwald, M. H., Lee, J. Y.-Y. and Ackerman, A. B. (1988) Pseudocarcinomatous hyperplasia. *Am. J. Dermatopathol.*, **10**, 95–103.

Harrison, P. V. (1987) Therapy of basal cell carcinoma – treatment in 1980–87 compared with 1985–86 and advantages of shave excision in smaller tumours. *Br. J. Dermatol.*, **117**, 349–57.

Harvey, I., Shalom, D., Marks, R. M. and Frankel, S. J. (1989) Non-melanotic skin cancer. Distribution and natural course are still open questions. *Br. Med. J.*, **299**, 1118–20.

Hoffman, M. S., Roberts, W. S. and Ruffolo, E. H. (1988) Basal cell carcinoma of the vulva with inguinal lymph node metastasis. *Gynecol. Oncol.*, **29**, 113–9.

Imayama, S., Yashima, Y., Higuchi, R. and Urabe, H. (1987) A new concept of basal cell epitheliomas based on the three-dimensional growth pattern of the superficial multicentric type. *Am. J. Pathol.*, **128**, 497–504.

Jackson, R. T. and Adams, R. H. (1973) Horrifying basal cell carcinoma, a study of 33 case and a comparison with 435 non-horror cases and a report on 5 metastatic cases. *J. Surg. Oncol.*, **5**, 431–63.

Jacobs, G. H., Reppey, J. J. and Allan (1982) Prediction of aggressive behaviour in basal bell carcinoma. *Cancer*, **49**, 533–7.

Johnson, B. F., Moore, P. J., Goepel, J. R. and Slater, D. N. (1989) Basosquamous carcinoma, a wolf in sheep's clothing? Report of 3 cases. *Postgrad. Med. J.*, **65**, 750–1.

Jones, J. C. R., Steinman, H. K. and Goldsmith, B. A. (1989) Hemidesmosomes, collagen VII, and intermediate filaments in basal cell carcinoma. *J. Invest. Dermatol.*, **93**, 662–71.

Kern, W. H. and McCray, M. K. (1980) The histopathologic differentiation of keratoacanthoma and squamous cell carcinoma of the skin. *J. Cut. Pathol.*, **7**, 318–25.

Korenberg, R., Penneys, N. S., Kowalczyk, A. and Nadji, M. (1988) Quantitation of S100 protein-positive cells in inflamed and non-inflamed keratoacanthoma and squamous cell carcinoma. *J. Cut. Pathol.*, **15**, 104–8.

Lattes, R. and Kesseler, R. W. (1951) Metastasizing basal cell epithelioma of the skin. *Cancer*, **4**, 466–78.

Lawrence, N. and Reed, R. J. (1990) Actinic keratoacanthoma. Speculations on the nature of the lesion and the role of cellular immunity in its evolution. *Am. J. Dermatopathol.*, **12**, 517–33.

Leon, J., Kamino, H., Steinberg, J. J. and Pellicer, A. (1988) H-*ras* activation in benign and self-regressing skin tumors (keratoacanthomas) in both human and an animal model system. *Mol. Cell. Biol.*, **8**, 786–93.

McGibbon, D. H. (1985) Malignant epidermal tumours. *J. Cut. Pathol.*, **12**, 224–38.

Moller, R., Reymann, F. and Hou-Jensen, K. (1979) Metastases in dermatological patients with squamous cell carcinoma. *Arch. Dermatol.*, **115**, 703–5.

Moy, R. L., Moy, L. S., Matsuoka, L. Y., Bennett, R. G. and Uitto, J. (1988) Selectively enhanced procollagen gene expression in sclerosing (morphoealike) basal cell carcinoma as reflected by elevated pro-alpha 1 (I) and pro-alpha 2 (III) procollagen messenger RNA steady-state levels. *J. Invest. Dermatol.*, **90**, 634–8.

Nixon, R. L., Dorevich, A. P. and Marks, R. (1986) Squamous cell carcinoma of the skin, accuracy of clinical diagnosis and outcome of follow-up in Australia. *Med. J. Aust.*, **144**, 235–9.

Paver, K., Poyzer, K., Burry, N. and Deakin, M. (1973) The incidence of basal carcinoma and their metastases in Australia and New Zealand. *Aust. J. Dermatol.*, **14**, 53.

Perrone, T., Twiggs, L. B., Adcock, L. L. and Dehner, L. P. (1987) Vulvar basal cell carcinoma, an infrequent metastasizing neoplasm. *Int. J. Gynaecol. Pathol.*, **6**, 152–65.

Petrovich, Z., Kuisk, H., Langholz, B., Astrahan, M., Luxton, G., Chak, L. and Rice, D. (1987) Treatment results and patterns of failure in 646 patients with carcinoma of the eyelids, pinna, and nose. *Am. J. Surg.*, **154**, 447–50.

Rahbari, H. and Mehregan, A. H. (1982) Basal cell epithelioma (carcinoma) in children and teenagers. *Cancer*, **49**, 350–3.

Robinson, J. K. (1987) Risk of developing another basal cell carcinoma. A 5 year prospective study. *Cancer*, **60**, 118–20.

Seifert, A. and Nasemann, T. (1989) Das Keratoakanthom und seine klinischen Varianten. Literaturubersicht und histopathologische Analyse von 90 Fallen. *Hautarzt*, **40**, 189–202.

Sims, C. F. and Kersch, N. (1948) Spindle cell epidermoid carcinoma simulating sarcoma in chronic radiodermatitis. *Arch. Dermatol. Syph.*, **57**, 63–8.

Smoller, B. R., Kwan, T. H., Said, J. W. and Banks-Schlegel, S. (1986) Keratoacanthoma and squamous cell carcinoma of the skin, immunohistochemical localization of involucrin and keratin proteins. *J. Am. Acad. Dermatol.*, **14**, 226–34.

Takaki, Y., Masutani, M, and Kawada, A. (1971) Electron microscopic study of keratoacanthoma. *Acta Dermatovener (Stockh.)*, **51**, 21–6.

Thomas, P., Said, J. W., Nash, G. and Banks-Schlegel, S. (1984) Profiles of keratin proteins in basal and squamous cell carcinomas of the skin. An immunohistochemical study. *J. Invest. Dermatol.*, **50**, 36–41.

Underwood, L. J., Montgomery, H. and Broders, A. C. (1951) Squamous-cell epithelioma that simulates sarcoma. *Arch. Derm. Syph.*, **64**, 149–58.

Underwood, J. W., Adcock, L. L. and Okagaki, T. (1978) Adenosquamous carcinomas of skin appendages of the vulva. A clinical and ultrastructural study. *Cancer*, **42**, 1851–8.

Wermuth, B. M. and Fajardo, L. F. (1970) Metastatic basal cell carcinoma. *Arch. Pathol.*, **90**, 458–62.

6 Melanocytic tumours

6.1 Naevi

Benign naevi are commonly excised, either completely or by shave biopsy, either for cosmetic reasons or because of concern about possible malignant change. The appearance depends to a certain extent upon the age of the patient. Naevi develop by proliferation of cells in the basal epidermis, which subsequently migrate down into the dermis; a process of progressive development which, in the context of minimal deviation melanoma, Reed has called 'accretive growth'.

Compound naevi, with both junctional and dermal naevus cells, are more common in young people. Claims have been made that congenital naevi can be differentiated from acquired naevi on histopathological features alone; this does not seem to be the case (Clemmensen and Kroon, 1988).

With age, the junctional component becomes less prominent and, indeed, if the junctional component is prominent in an older patient then one must look at the appearance of the cells and their distribution to exclude dysplastic naevus or melanoma. In the upper part of the dermal component, naevus giant cells may be present: when they are it is very reassuring as their presence is virtually pathognomonic of a benign naevus. Towards the base, the cells are usually smaller and may become more spindly or neuroid in appearance. This led Masson to suggest that whilst the upper naevoid cells were derived from epidermal melanocytes, the lower cells might be derived from Schwann cells (Masson, 1951).

Curran and McGann (1976) have described three types of naevus cells: type A is usually seen in the basal epidermis and forms nests, often containing melanin; type B is usually seen in the mid dermis and is arranged in clusters of three or four cells surrounded by collagen, and smaller in size; type C is present towards the base and consists of cells arranged singly, each surrounded by collagen, resembling fibroblasts or Schwann cells and rarely containing collagen. Other ultra-

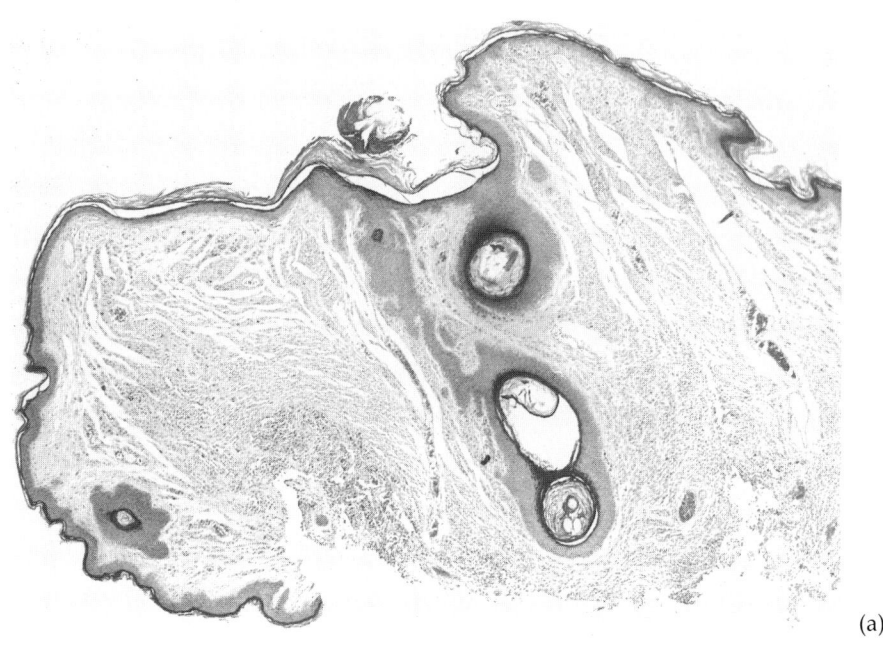

(a)

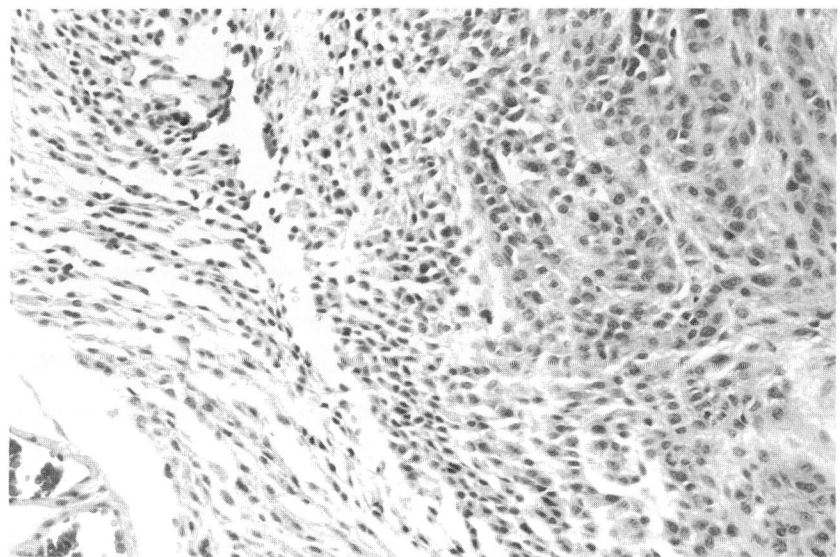

(b)

Figure 6.1 Unna's naevus. (a) A soft exophytic naevus with (b) naevus cells filling an expanded papillary dermis.

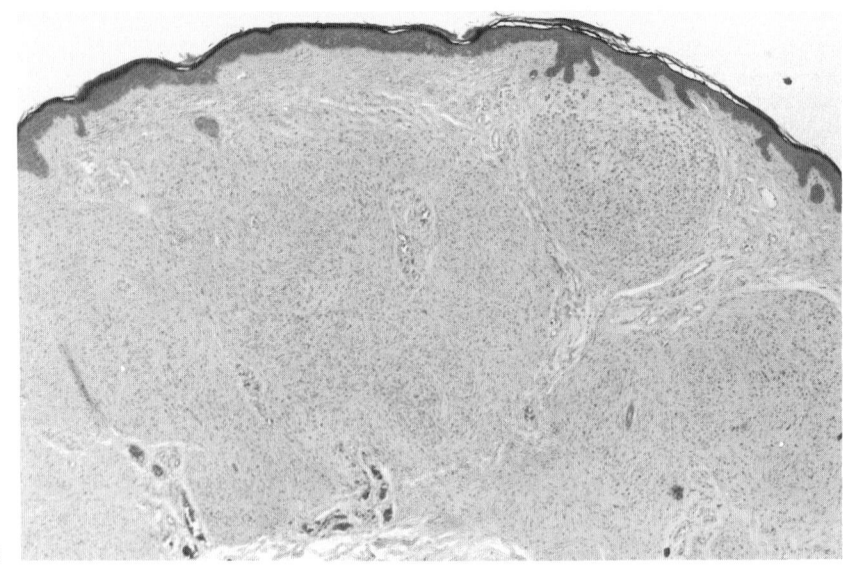

(a)

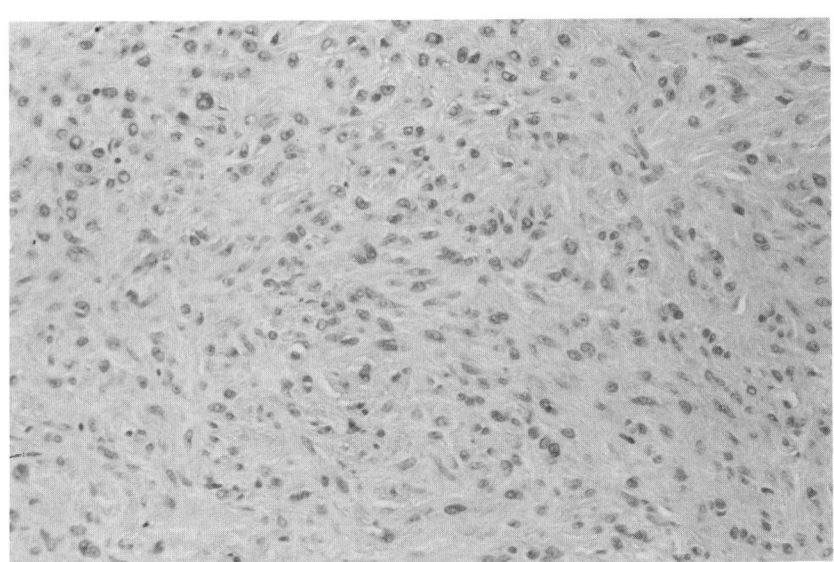

(b)

Figure 6.2 Meischer's naevus. (a) A domed naevus with (b) the whole dermis filled with naevus cells.

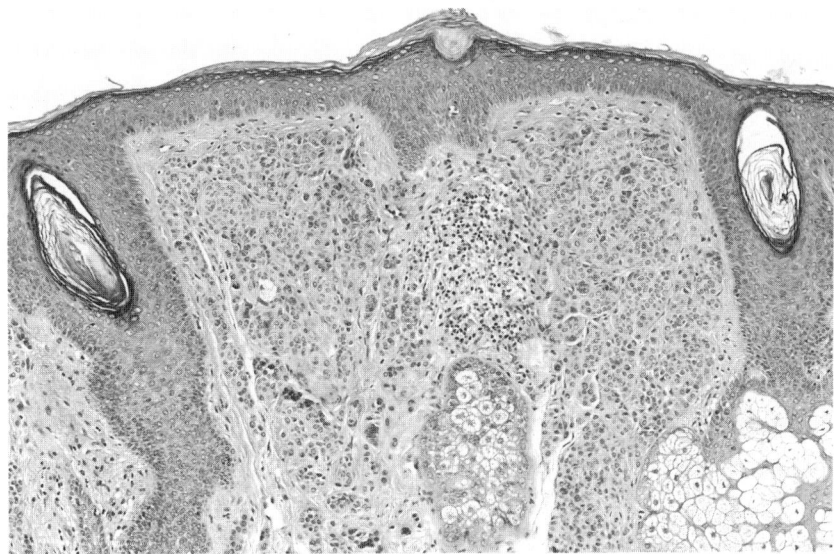

Figure 6.3 Meischer's naevus. The more superficial naevus cells are larger than those below them. Occasional multinucleated cells are also present in the upper part.

structural studies have shown that as naevus cells migrate into the dermis the numbers of cytoplasmic mitochondria and microfilaments decrease, implying that the changes seen are more attributable to a process of atrophy rather than maturation (Goovaerts and Buyssens, 1988).

Many naevi are shaved off rather than excised. Whilst this offends the pathologist's desire to examine the whole lesion, it does lead to a better cosmetic result. Malignant changes develop in the basal epidermis or upper epidermis, and so if there are no atypical features in the tissue present in the shave specimen, it is most unlikely that there will be anything worrying in what remains of the lesion in the patient. It does tend to shroud the differences between congenital and acquired naevi – congenital naevi being characterized by naevus cells spreading down into the deeper dermis and surrounding appendages.

The acquired cellular intradermal naevi fall into two main categories. Unna's naevus is a soft, exophytic polypoidal lesion which has naevus cells filling an expanded papillary dermis, with the reticular dermis uninvolved. Miescher's naevus is the commonest form seen, with naevus cells filling the dermis of a tightly confined mole, without any exophytic tendency (Ackerman and Magana-Garcia, 1990).

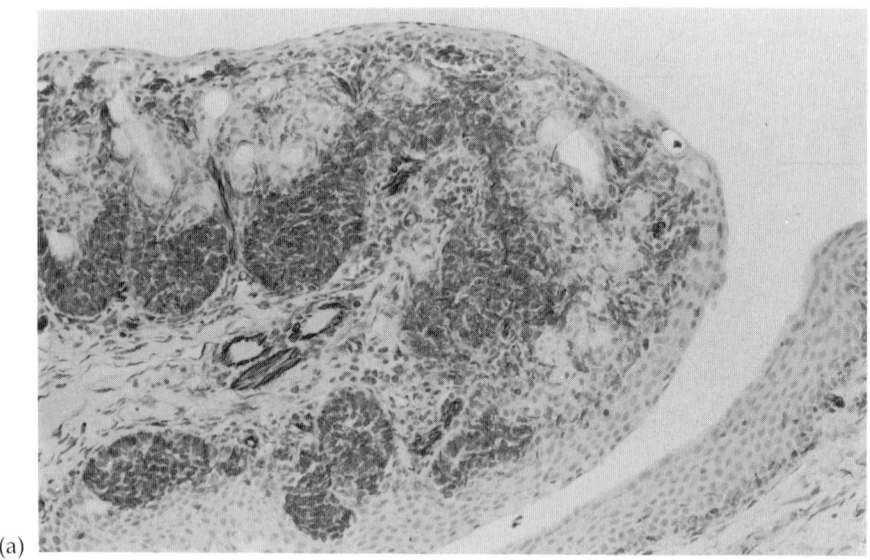

(a)

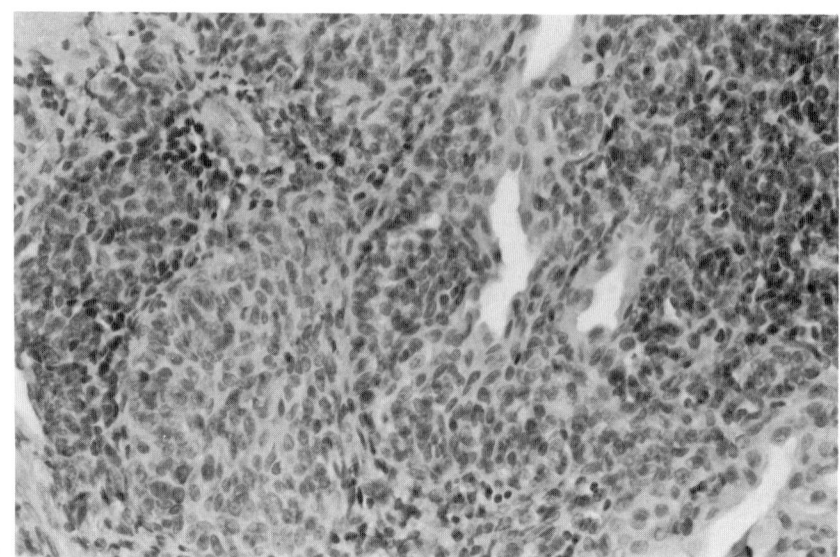

(b)

Figure 6.4 Naevus of conjunctiva. (a) S100 staining differentiates the naevus cells from epithelial cells and lymphocytes, (b) a differentiation which is more difficult on H and E.

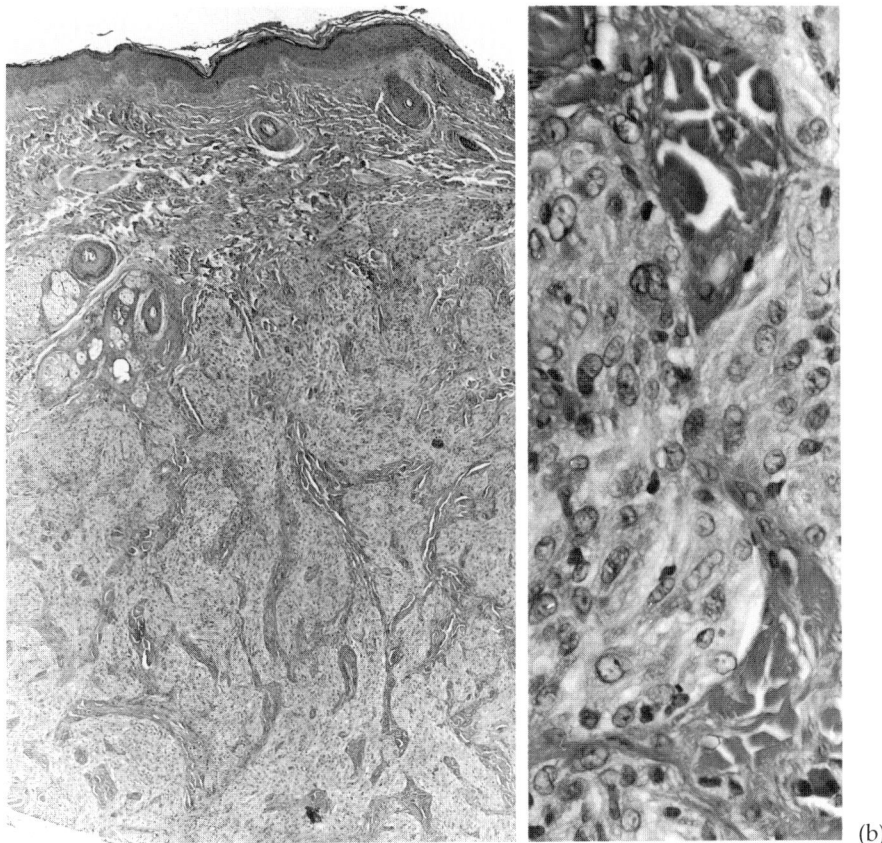

(a)

(b)

Figure 6.5 Deep penetrating naevus with (a) fasciculated pattern of dermal infiltration, and (b) benign cytological appearance. The cells have small nuclei and indistinct nuclei.

6.2 Deep penetrating naevus

Some naevi, called 'deep penetrating naevi', may be misinterpreted as melanoma, because of the presence of nuclear pleomorphism and extension into the deep dermis and subcutaneous fat. However, the appearance of these naevi is characteristic. Almost all examples are solitary and occur typically on the face of teenagers or young adults. They are pigmented and dome shaped with a smooth margin, and range in diameter from 2 to 9 mm. Recurrence after local excision has not been described.

The biopsy will show naevus cells with pleomorphic vacuolated nuclei, usually with rather smudged chromatin and without prominent nucleoli. Pigment is present both in the naevus cells and in scattered melanophages. Extension into reticular dermis is usual and naevus cells may extend into subcutaneous fat. Occasional mitoses may be present but are uncommon.

Other lesions to consider in differential diagnosis include Spitz naevus, which is usually seen in younger patients and shows junctional nests of naevus cells, epidermal acanthosis and dermal vascular telangiectasia. Considerably less melanin pigment is also present than in deep penetrating naevus. Knowledge of the clinical features of the lesion is therefore of prime importance (Seab et al., 1989).

6.3   Spitz naevus

Juvenile melanomas should not be diagnosed any more: the description Spitz naevus is far more appropriate. It avoids any possible implication of malignancy in what is a benign lesion, and it also recognizes the contribution of Sophie Spitz in characterizing this entity. The Spitz naevi are a variant of compound naevi, which are mainly found in juveniles, but can also present in young adults.

These naevi typically show radial symmetry. The epidermal component is similar to that found in a compound naevus of usual type. There is no tendency to the individual cell 'buckshot pattern' spread in the epidermis, which is a common feature of malignant melanoma. Occasional eosinophilic Kamino bodies may be present (Kamino et al., 1979).

The junctional component is often not prominent, but a constant feature is the gradual maturation in appearance of the cells at deeper levels of the dermis. In the upper dermis, the naevus cells can have a most worrisome appearance, with quite large nuclei and single nucleoli and abundant eosinophilic cytoplasm. They may be more spindled in shape and appear to 'rain down', as they become aligned around appendages (Paniago-Pereira et al., 1978). Mitoses may be present but should not look atypical. In the deeper part, the naevus cells appear smaller and more typical. Crucially, the lesions are not heavily pigmented and have a rounded, symmetrical profile, with no tendency to intralesional variation. Dilated, thin-walled blood vessels are present in the upper dermis.

When this constellation of clinical and morphological features is taken into account, there should be little occasion for confusing Spitz naevus with malignant melanoma. If a lesion shows definite asymmetry, intralesional variation, atypical mitoses, or mitoses in the lower part of the lesion, then it is likely to be a melanoma.

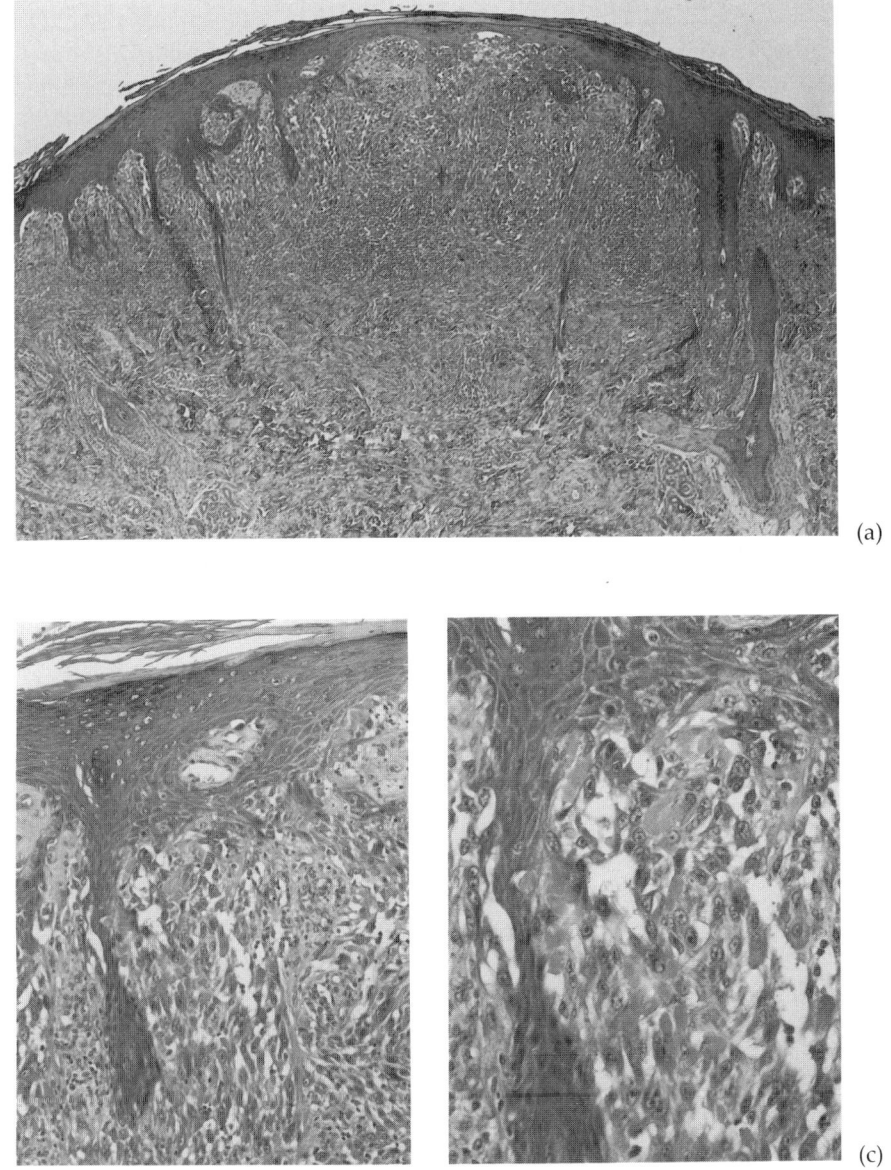

Figure 6.6 Spitz naevus. (a) A radially symmetrical lesion, with (b) vertically orientated spindle cells, and (c) small junctional component.

6.4   Pigmented spindle cell naevus of Reed

These lesions present typically as small, round, symmetrical, domed lesions on the legs of young women and are darkly pigmented. Essentially, they represent a pigmented variant of Spitz naevus. Whereas Spitz naevi are red and without significant amounts of melanin, these lesions are heavily pigmented. They are benign and must, therefore, be recognized and not confused with melanoma (Sagebiel *et al.*, 1984; Smith, 1987)

6.5   Blue naevus

These lesions are so called because they have their melanin in dendritic cells in the reticular dermis, beneath a relatively normal papillary dermis and epidermis. The collagen between the pigment and the overlying epidermis changes the appearance of the melanin from brown to blue. Typically the lesions are small and have heavy, coarse pigmentation in individual cells, separated by bundles of collagen. Mitoses are absent and nuclei are essentially unremarkable (Leopold and Richards, 1968).

The cells of blue naevi can be stained with the melanoma marker HMB-45, which does not mark adult melanocytes or naevus cells. This finding has been taken as evidence to support the proposition that the cells are not purely melanocytic or Schwannian, but are possibly derived from some precursor with features in common with both types of cell (Sun *et al.*, 1990).

6.6   Cellular blue naevus

An uncommon variant of the common blue naevus is the cellular blue naevus, which shows a variety of appearances that may lead to confusion with malignant melanoma (Leopold and Richards, 1967; Rodriguez and Ackerman, 1968). There are two main types, the biphasic and alveolar forms, both of which can protrude downwards into subcutaneous fat in the 'dumb-bell' fashion also seen with deep penetrating naevi.

A particularly difficult feature of benign blue naevi is that they may present as 'benign metastases' in lymph nodes. This is reported quite widely in contrast to the paucity of reports of truly malignant cellular blue naevi. It is important to differentiate these from true metastatic malignant melanoma so that unnecessary further surgery can be avoided (Lambert and Brodkin, 1984). The phenomenon of benign naevus cells in lymph nodes is relatively well recognized (Ridolfi *et al.*, 1977). Levene has suggested that their presence in lymph nodes may not be a mani-

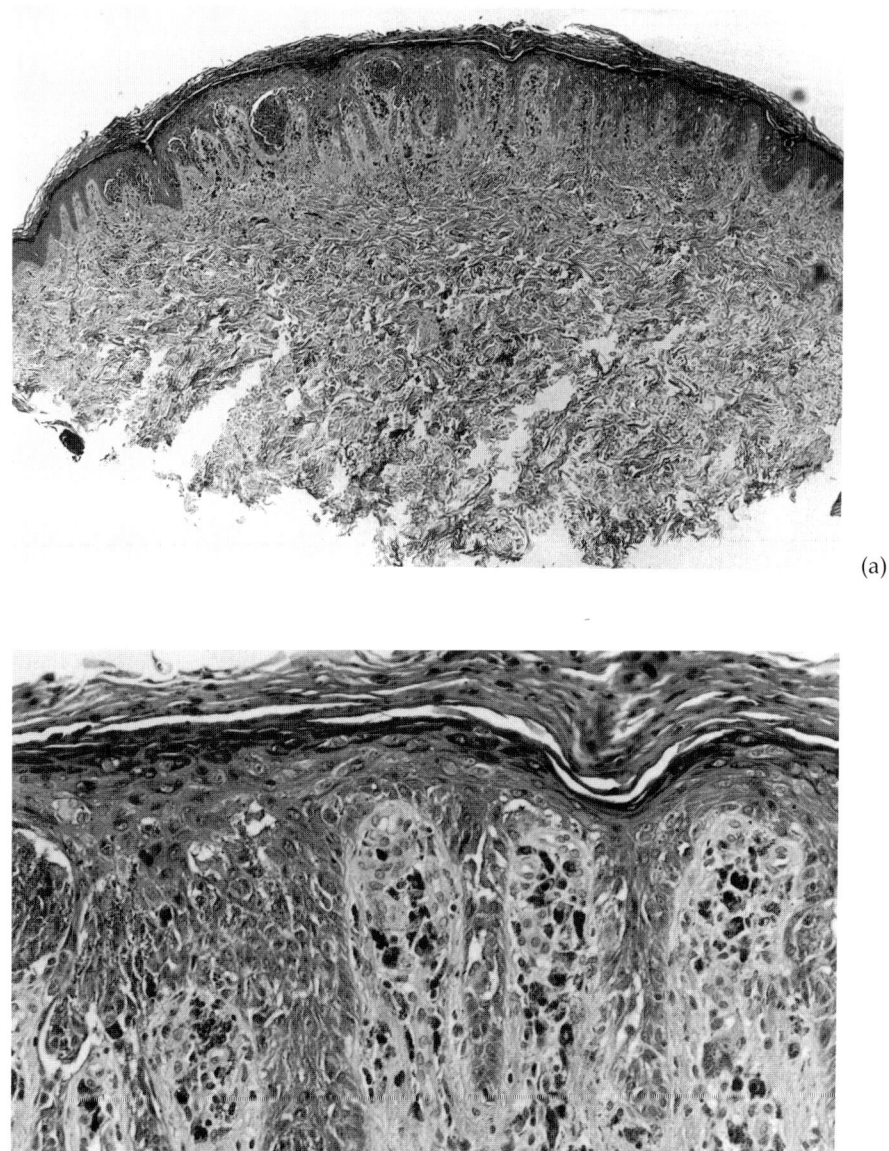

(a)

(b)

Figure 6.7 Pigmented spindle cell naevus. (a) A radially symmetrical naevus with (b) prominent transepidermal elimination of melanin.

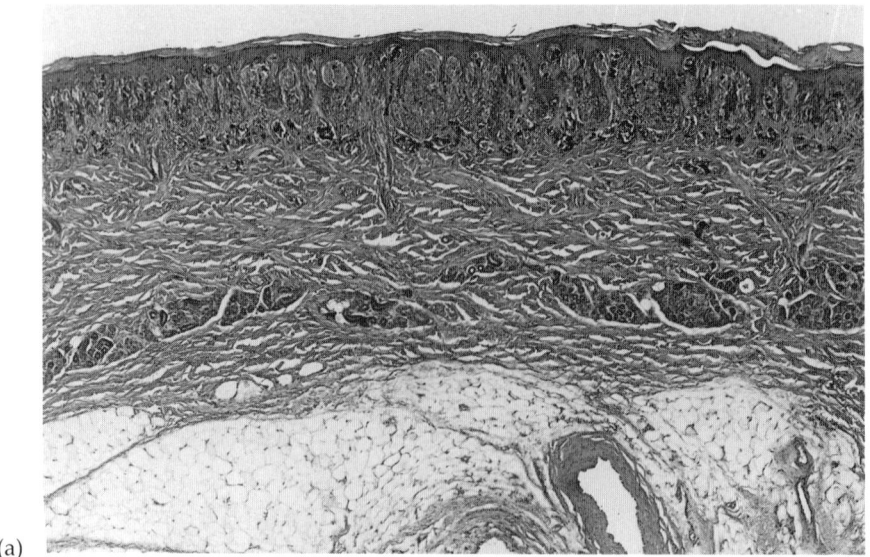

(a)

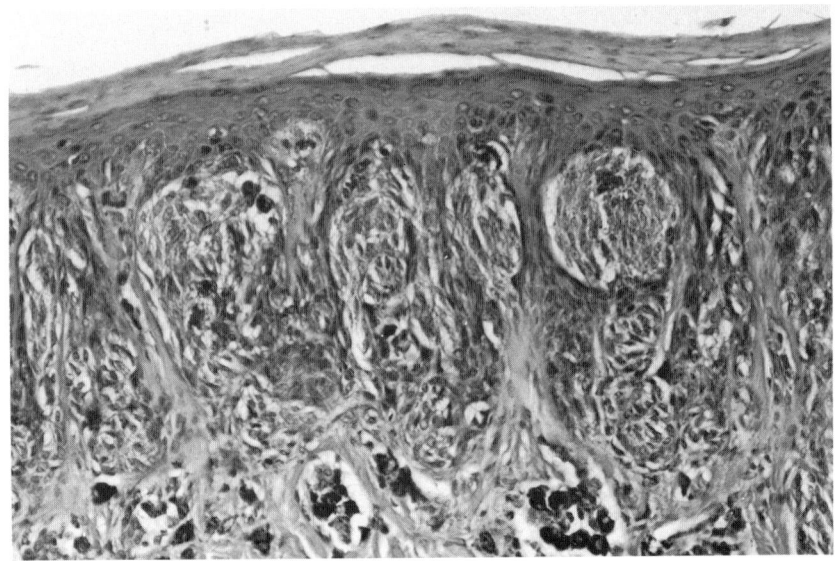

(b)

Figure 6.8 Blue naevus. (a) A loosely circumscribed lesion in the dermis with (b) pigment containing dendritic cells.

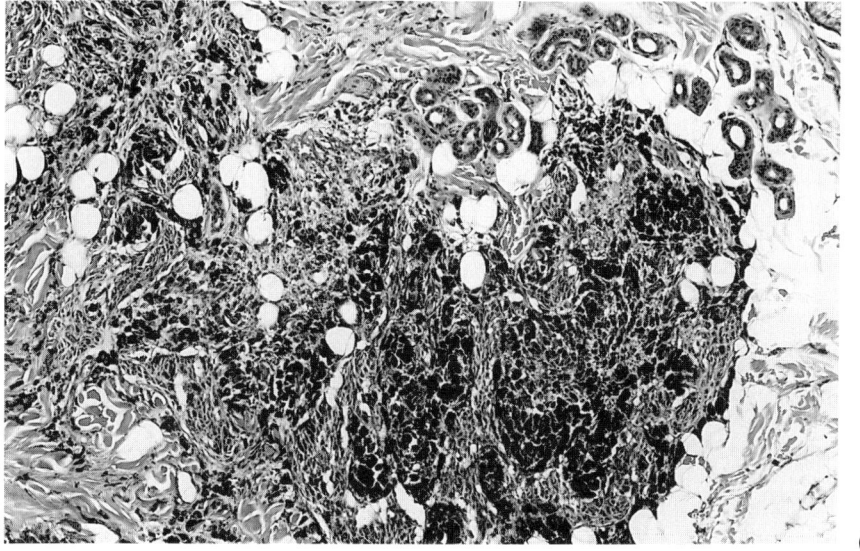

(a)

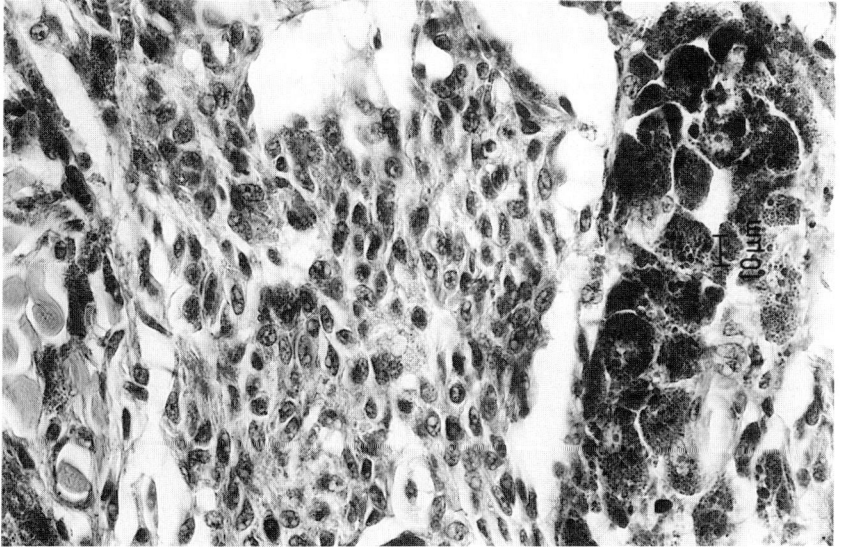

(b)

Figure 6.9 Cellular Blue naevus. (a) Cellular and pigmented nests of cells extend to the subcutis. (b) The naevus cells have oval nuclei, with single nucleoli and varying amounts of melanin.

festation of metastasis, but may instead represent a disorder of neural crest development (Levene, 1980). The presence of cellular blue naevus cells within a node is merely an extension of the phenomenon, but should be borne in mind, especially when considering a diagnosis of metastatic melanoma on a fine needle aspiration specimen.

Malignant cellular blue naevi are difficult to characterize with confidence. They usually present as progressively enlarging or multinodular, blue-black tumours. The presence of widespread necrosis does seem to be a common feature of the few malignant lesions that have been reported, but has also been seen in benign lesions. Other features, such as a high mitotic rate, vascular invasion and marked cytological atypia, with vascular invasion, are also in favour of malignancy (Temple-Camp *et al.*, 1988). There may be quite marked intralesional variation of the cytological appearances within the tumour, so an adequate biopsy is essential. Metastasis to regional lymph nodes is relatively common (Goldenhersh *et al.*, 1988).

6.7   Dysplastic naevus

It is worth describing some of the background to this name (Elder, 1985). Wallace Clark first drew attention to a syndrome of familial

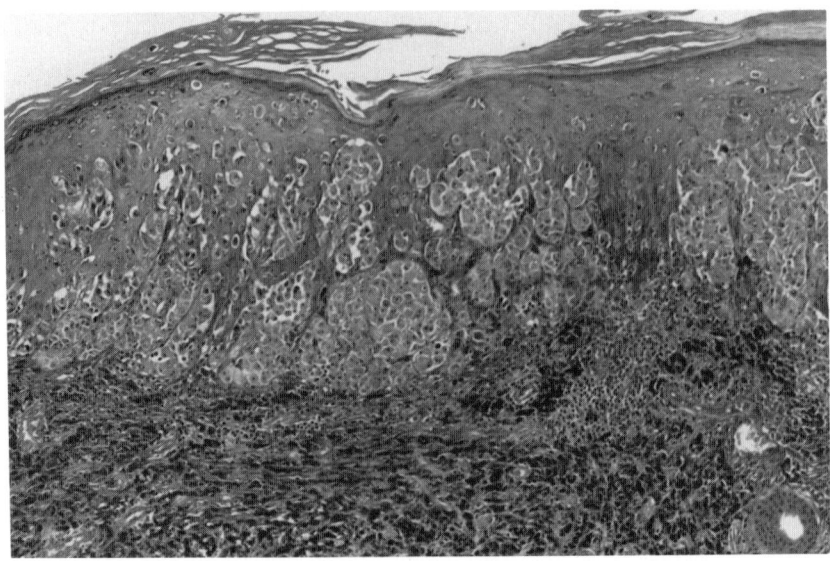

Figure 6.10   Combined naevus. Blue naevus beneath a compound cellular naevus.

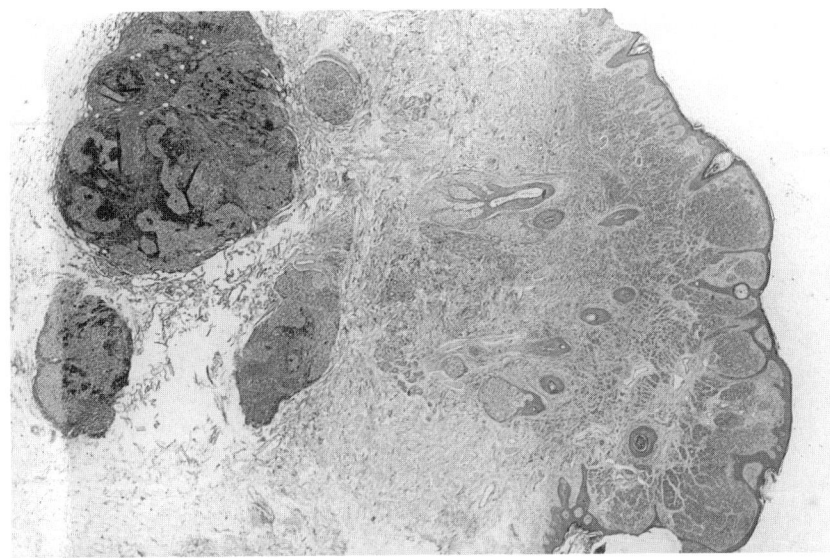

Figure 6.11 Combined naevus with a superficial cellular naevus and a deep nodular component of cellular blue naevus.

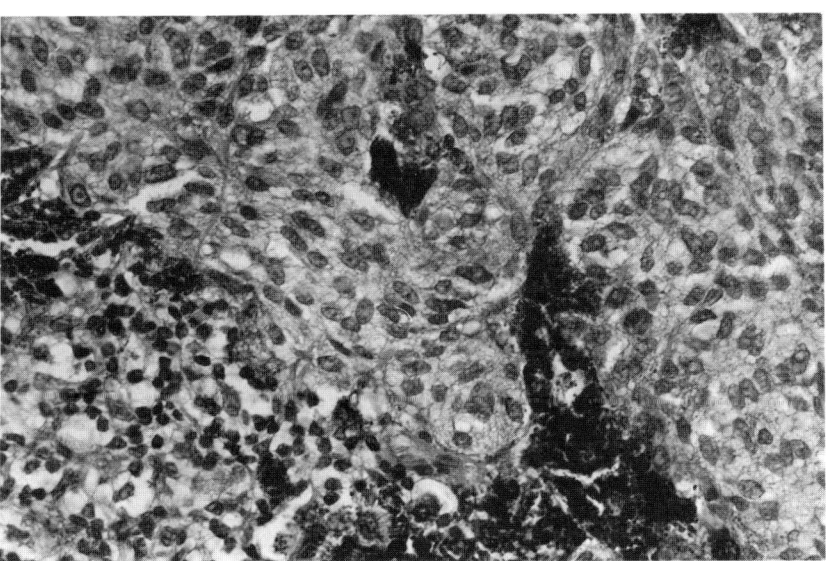

Figure 6.12 Combined naevus. Appearance of the deep cellular blue naevus component seen in Figure 6.11.

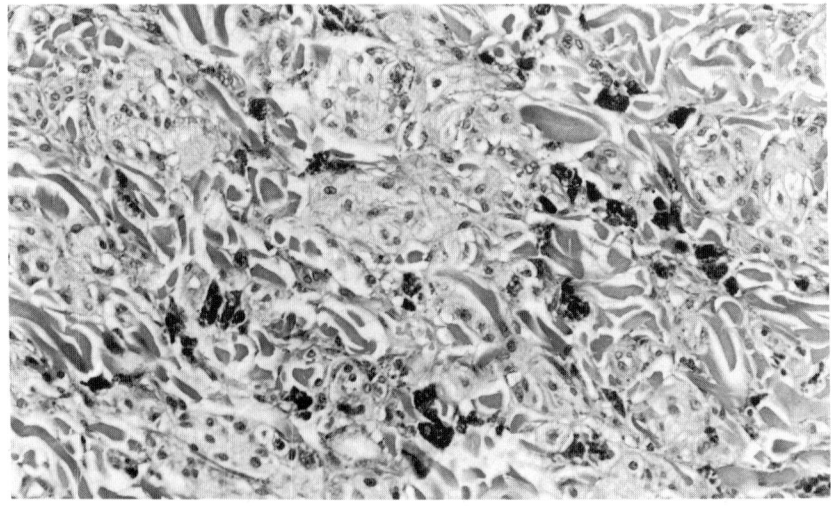

Figure 6.13 Balloon cell naevus. (a) Ballooned naevus cells infiltrated between dermal collagen bundles and (b) are associated with moderate numbers of stromal melanophages.

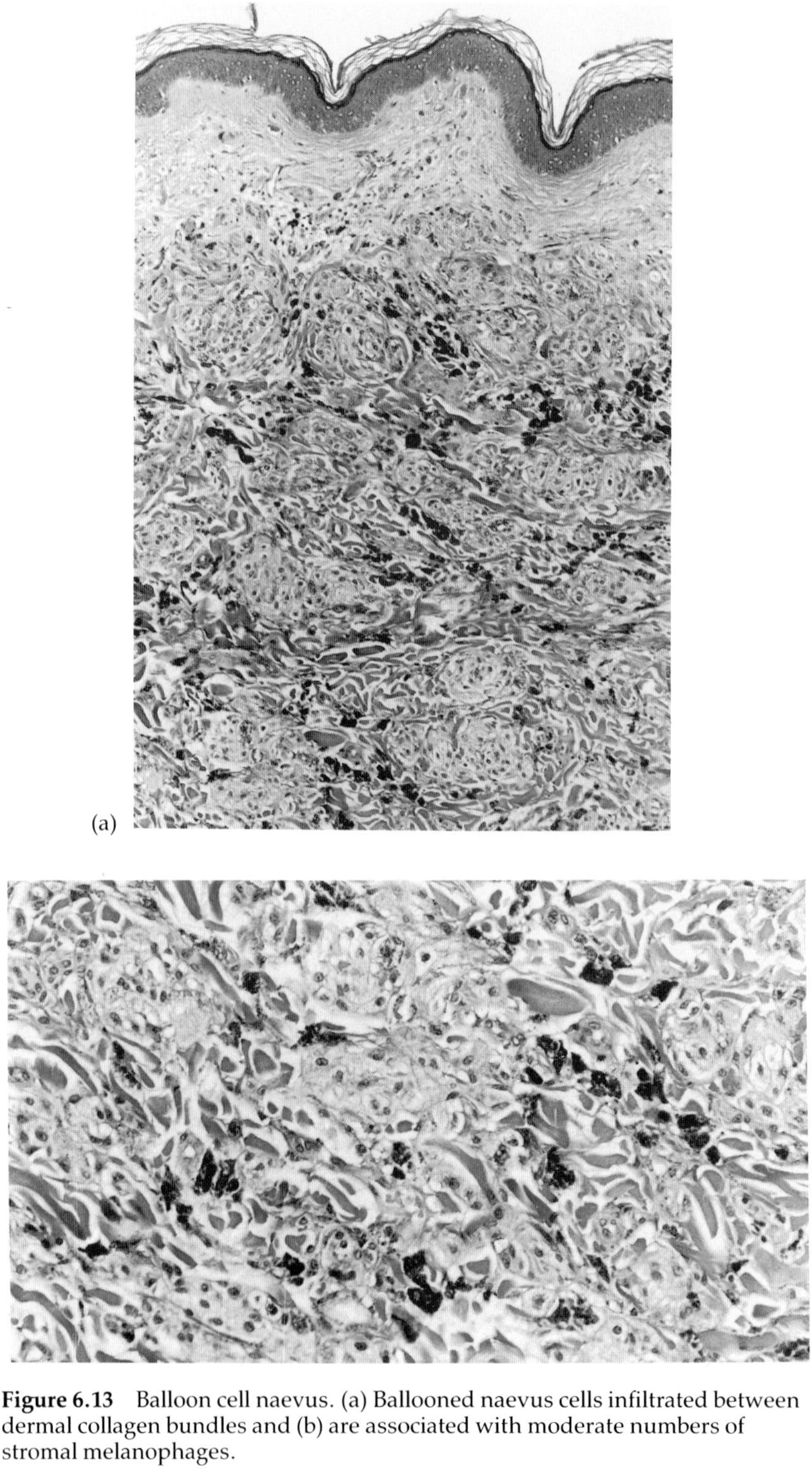

melanoma in which the affected individuals developed lesions that looked as though they might be precursors of melanoma. Because he did not claim to understand these lesions in any detail, the phenomenon was originally described as the 'B-K mole syndrome', using the initials of the two families studied (Clark *et al.*, 1978). This non-committal approach to nomenclature has much to recommend it, but there is always a demand for names. Clark therefore drew up a short list of possible alternatives which was shown around to colleagues. The pathologists involved chose 'dysplastic naevus', giving as a reason the reassurance that dysplasia was a familiar, widely understood and un-contentious concept (Elder *et al.*, 1980). The irony is obvious when we consider how successful the use of CIN concept in the cervix has been in providing a framework for biopsy classification and clinicopatho-logical communication, without using the word 'dysplasia', which can be readily applied to both neoplastic and non-neoplastic conditions (Fox, 1990). It has been suggested that we should adopt a similar classification for melanocytic intraepidermal neoplasia (Sagebiel, 1985; Frankel, 1987). In the meantime, it has been said that 'more people have died of boredom, listening to lectures on the dysplastic naevus syndrome, than have died of the syndrome itself' (Cotton, personal communication).

Moles similar to those seen in the B-K mole syndrome were sub-sequently described in sporadic cases (Elder *et al.*, 1980). 'Dysplastic naevus' is in danger of becoming a diagnostic dustbin for all sorts of dubious pigmented lesions. There are those who decry the whole concept (Ackerman, 1988). It is clear, however, that there are a group of lesions which have appearances in between benign naevi and malig-nant melanomas, and that even if these lesions are not in themselves malignant, they do indicate an increased risk of developing melanoma in the affected individual (Cook and Fallowfield, 1990). This view is further supported by the way in which a spectrum of immunohisto-chemical reactivity is seen with a number of melanocytic markers. For instance, the melanocyte specific antibody HMB-45 shows weak or negative staining of naevus cells, moderate staining of cells in dysplastic naevi and strong staining in melanomas (Smoller *et al.*, 1989). Similar results can be obtained in frozen sections with the progression marker PAL-M1.

Thus dysplastic naevi have a similar relationship to melanoma as colorectal adenomas have to adenocarcinoma: there are cytological and architectural similarities that are easily apparent and one is a marker for an increased risk of the other. Adenomas are of course much more commonly seen than carcinomas and do not necessarily progress to the stage of metastasizing malignancy in the majority of cases.

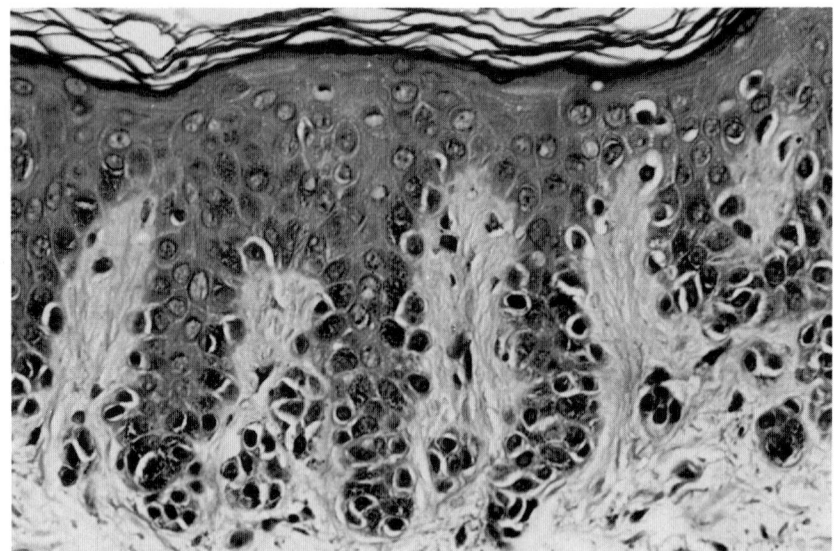

(a)

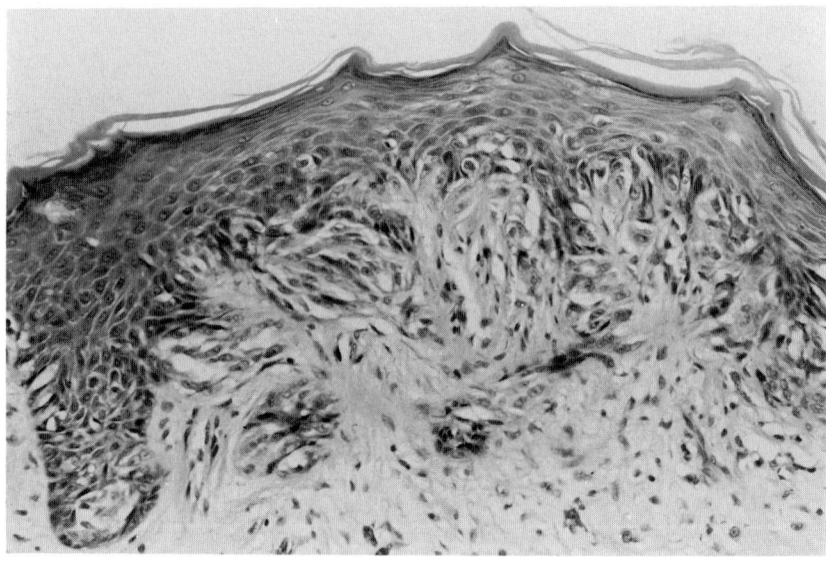

(b)

Figure 6.14 The spectrum of melanocytic abnormalities – 1. (a) A junctional naevus showing minimal abnormality, and (b) a mildly dysplastic naevus with horizontally orientated spindle shaped melanocytes.

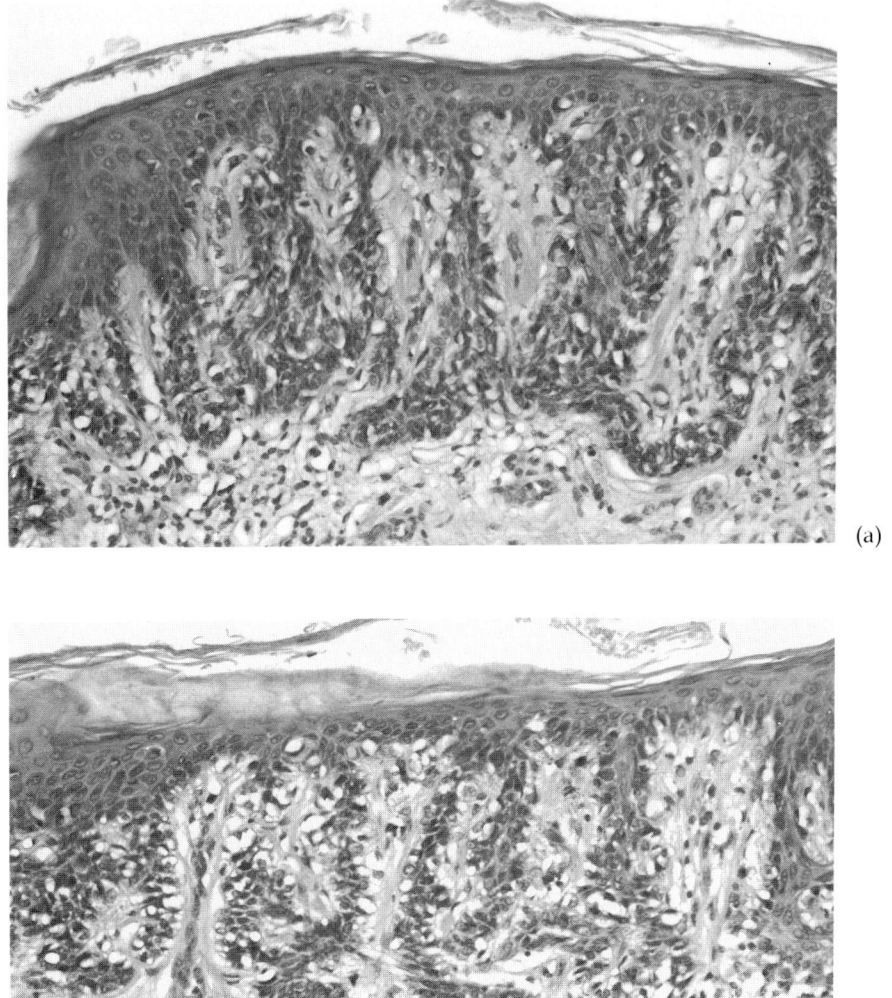

(a)

(b)

Figure 6.15 The spectrum of melanocytic abnormalities – 2. (a and b) A dysplastic naevus with lamellar fibroplasia of collagen in the dermal papillae and extension of melanocytes all around the rete ridges.

Clinically dysplastic naevi show an irregular margin and irregular pigmentation, but the pigmentation will usually be differing shades of brown rather than black. The microscopic appearances include a varying degree of junctional melanocytic proliferation and atypia, but with little evidence of spread into the upper epidermis by single pigmented cells. Some of the lesions look as though they have arisen in compound naevi, but the dermal naevus cell component will usually show little atypia; the proliferation takes place in the junctional component. A common finding is the presence of spindle-shaped, junctional cells bridging across the rete. Another constant feature is that these lesions are always thin; usually of the order of 0.5 mm thick or less.

Dysplastic naevi are markers of an increased risk of patients developing melanoma. The patients must be advised against excessive sun exposure and of the advantages of regular examination of their skin lesions. They will then have the opportunity of having potential melanomas excised at a time when they are still curable by excision. This risk must be put into perspective. The risk of a person with two atypical moles developing a melanoma is the same as the risk associated with having red hair or freckles: that is a very low risk. The full syndrome of familial atypical moles and malignant melanoma (FAMMM) is associated with a more substantial risk.

We have yet to develop a satisfactory way of labelling these lesions. It is the author's practice to assess the degree of change present and describe it as being mild, moderate or severe, measure the Breslow thickness and satisfy myself that the abnormalities are intraepidermal. The lesion is then described as a 'dysplastic naevus', qualified by a statement about the degree of atypia and the thickness, and a recommendation that no further wide excision is indicated. Even this must be done with caution given the likelihood that such a diagnosis may affect the patient's chances of buying life insurance and also carries the implication that follow-up should continue for the rest of the person's life. Ackerman and Magana-Garcia's suggestion (1990) that these lesions could be called 'Clark's naevi' is a possible solution to the tired argument of nomenclature.

6.8   Malignant melanoma

Melanoma is such a potentially lethal condition that it is particularly important to diagnose it accurately and provide adequate information to the surgeon to ensure appropriate and adequate treatment. In the past there have been various attempts to subclassify melanoma of which the Sydney classification is the most successful (McGovern *et al.*, 1986). It does, however, appear to be the case that cutaneous melano-

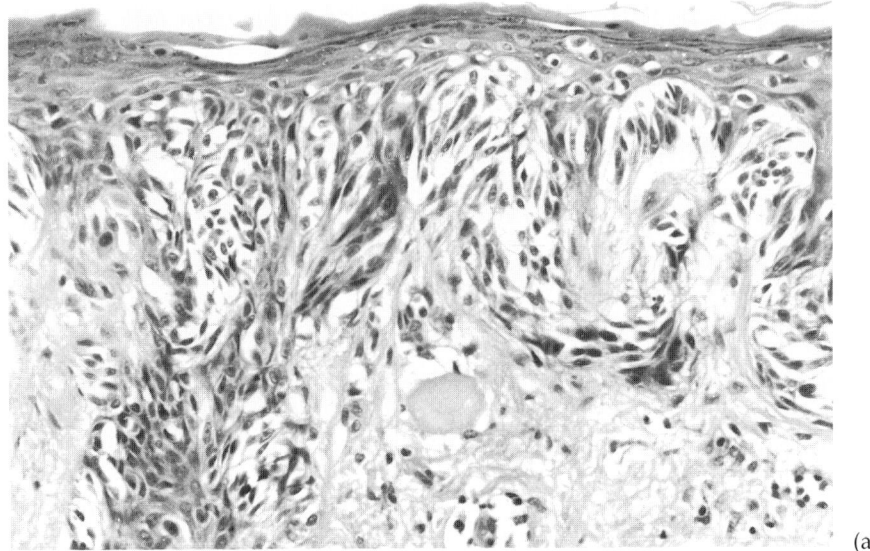

(a)

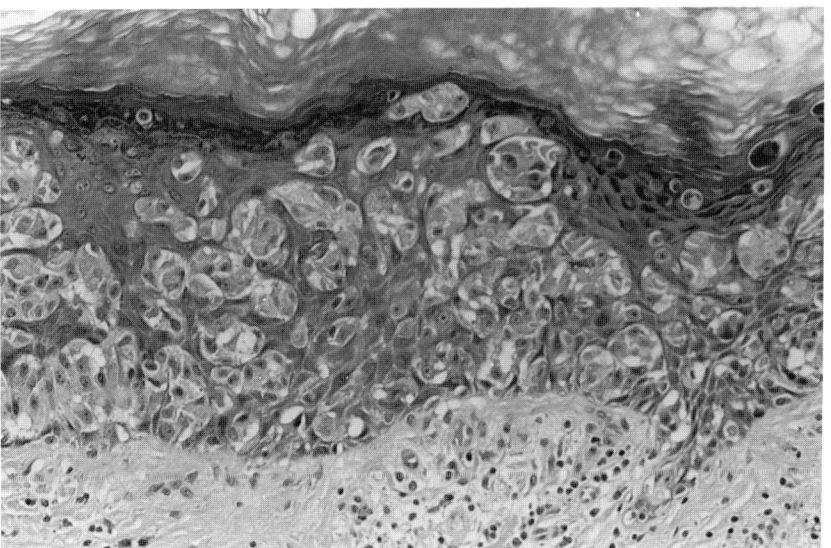

(b)

Figure 6.16 The spectrum of melanocytic abnormalities – 3. (a) Dysplastic naevus showing extension of atypical melanocytes into the upper epidermis, and (b) Pagetoid spread of malignant melanoma, Clark's level 1.

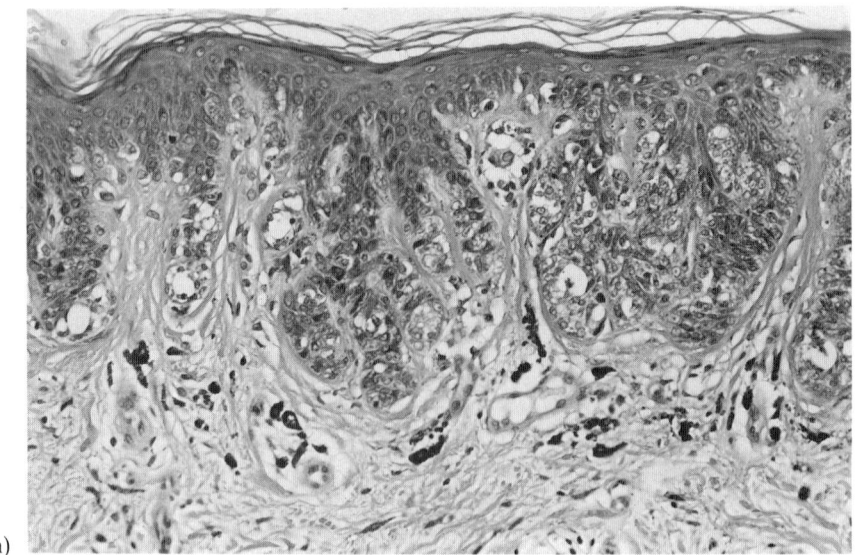

(a)

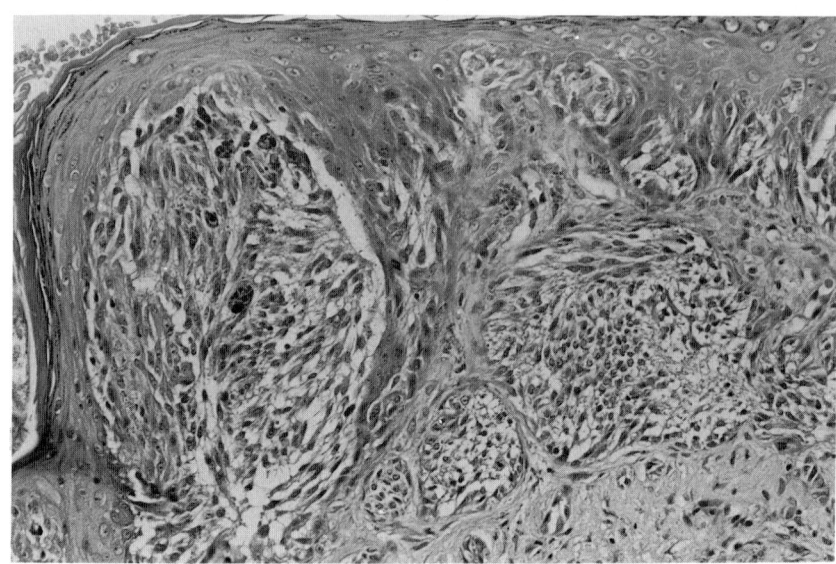

(b)

Figure 6.17 The spectrum of melanocytic abnormalities – 4. (a) Dysplastic naevus without evidence of dermal invasion, and (b) melanoma with prominent junctional component and with definite dermal invasive component.

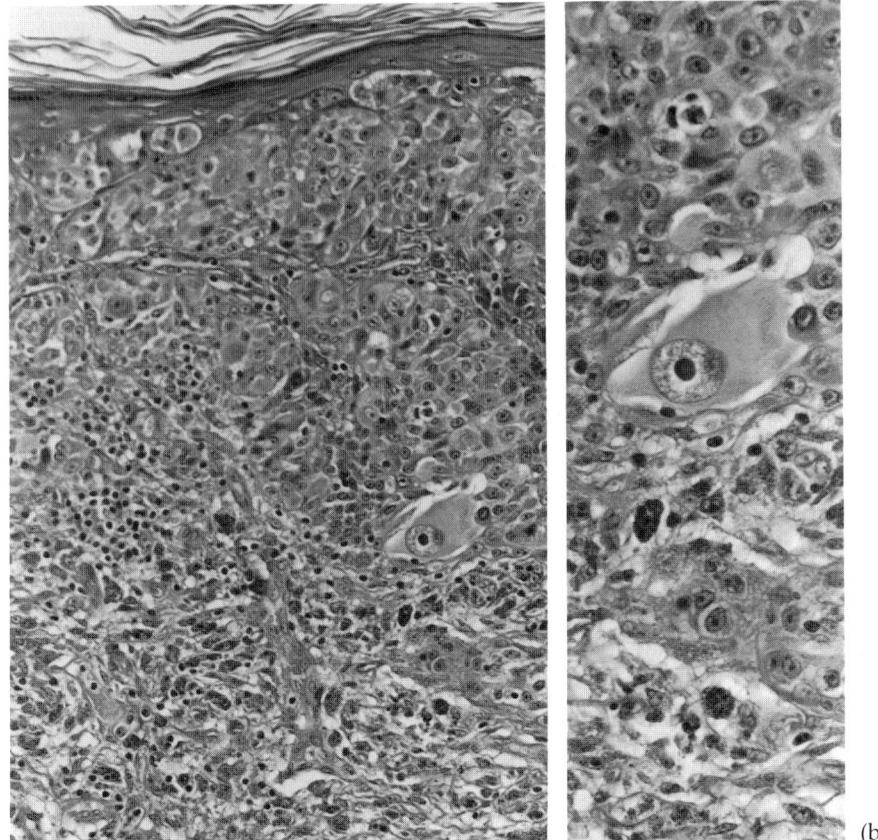

Figure 6.18   Melanoma (a) in vertical growth phase, with (b) marked cellular pleomorphism and giant epithelioid tumour cells with prominent single nucleoli.

mas should be regarded as a single group of tumours, whose behaviour is best determined by measuring the thickness of the tumour, from the top of the granular layer of the epidermis to the bottom of the deepest tumour cell in the dermis (Breslow, 1970). The classification based upon levels of invasion proposed by Clark *et al.* has been a useful way of analysing tumours, but does not provide as reliable prognostic information. Clark's levels are: I, intraepidermal tumour only; II, invasion into the papillary dermis; III, extension to the papillary-reticular boundary; IV, invasion of the reticular dermis; and V, invasion of subcutis (Clark *et al.*, 1969).

The principal distinction to make is that between melanomas in the

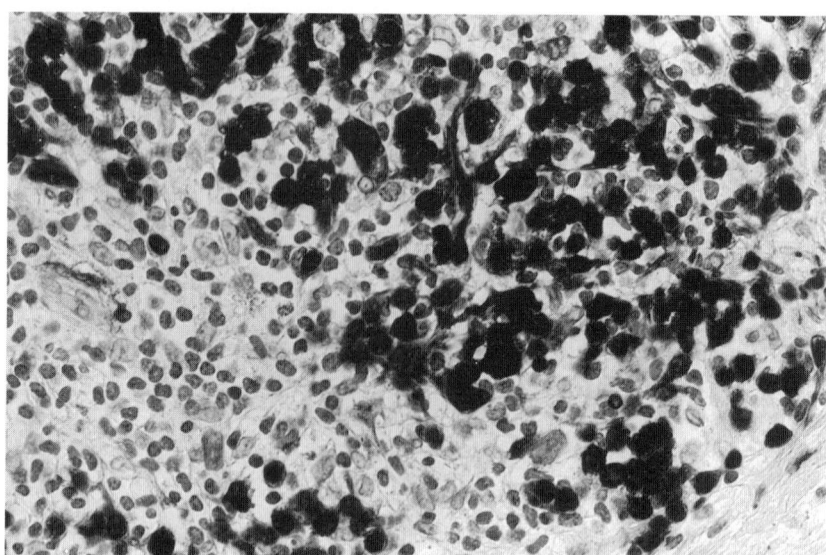

Figure 6.19   Melanoma. S100 staining of melanoma as a way of identifying the extent of the tumour, especially within the inflammatory reaction at the base of the tumour.

horizontal and vertical growth phases (Clark *et al.*, 1984). Those in the horizontal growth phase have an excellent chance of survival (Elder *et al.*, 1984; Clark *et al.*, 1989). This may be because they are still mainly intraepidermal, invasion through the basement membrane being difficult to identify with confidence in all routine H and E sections (Kirkham *et al.*, 1989). The vertical growth phase describes a tumour which is unequivocally invasive. It is these tumours which kill. When the tumour has reached a thickness of 0.9 mm it starts to acquire its own new blood supply (Srivastava *et al.*, 1988). This is of particular importance because it seems clear that melanomas metastasize through blood vessels rather than lymphatics (Fallowfield and Cook, 1990).

Having dispensed with subclassification, the next problem is to decide which lesions are malignant and which are benign mimics of melanoma. The malignant lesions are best characterized by considering a combination of cytological and architectural factors. The cells of melanoma have large nuclei with prominent, usually single, nucleoli and a variable amount of cytoplasm. Mitoses are variable in number. Atypical forms are often seen.

Most melanomas start as proliferations of atypical melanocytes at the base of the epidermis. It is important, therefore, to start by looking at the biopsy at low power, or scanning magnification. This will show the overall nature of the lesion and emphasize its asymmetrical nature and highlight variations in cell type and pigmentation from place to place.

As the tumour develops, the cells move in all directions. One of the most helpful features is the presence of individual melanocytes in the upper layers of the epidermis. It is virtually unknown for benign melanocytic lesions to show individual cell spread above the basal layer. Therefore when one sees this pattern of spread, sometimes called 'buckshot spread', it is a good indication that the lesion is likely to be malignant. Special stains for Langerhans cells show a diminution in their numbers as the tumours increase in size (Stone et al., 1988).

It is also crucial to examine the cells in the dermis. The cytological features of malignancy are usually obvious, as is the presence of mitoses. The variant known as minimal deviation melanoma may cause difficulty, but is an uncommon problem in the author's experience. Melanoma will also usually show marked variation within the lesion. This 'intralesional variation' may be manifested by variations in the cells themselves or in the degree of pigmentation. The variation suggests a polyclonal type of tumour development. There is unlikely to be much difference between the tumour cells at the top and the bottom dermal component.

There are two variants of which one should be aware. Many thin lesions look as though they have grown from the junctional component of a compound naevus. The cells in the upper part of the dermis appear more atypical than those beneath. At the time of writing there is no clear answer to this sort of tumour. We cannot be sure whether the Breslow thickness should be taken to the bottom of the upper component or to the bottom of the whole lesion. For the time being it is probably best to measure the thickness of the whole lesion when deciding on appropriate further treatment.

In difficult cases it may be helpful to undertake immunohistochemical staining to confirm the melanocytic nature of the tumour in hand. Of the intermediate filaments only vimentin is found in melanomas (Caselitz et al., 1983). S100 is useful, as it is positive in almost all melanomas, but although highly sensitive it is not specific, being positive in other structures such as nerve and cartilage (Springall et al., 1983). The newer antibody HMB-45 is more specific and, like the other two, can be used in paraffin sections (Colombari et al., 1988).

There is no clear evidence to decide upon the best form of excision, but it is now clear that the very extensive excisions practised in the past have no advantage over more modest excisions (Heenan et al., 1985; Milton, 1985a). The author's practice is to recommend a 1 cm radius of excision for melanomas less than 0.7 mm thick, 2 cm from 0.8 to 1.7 mm

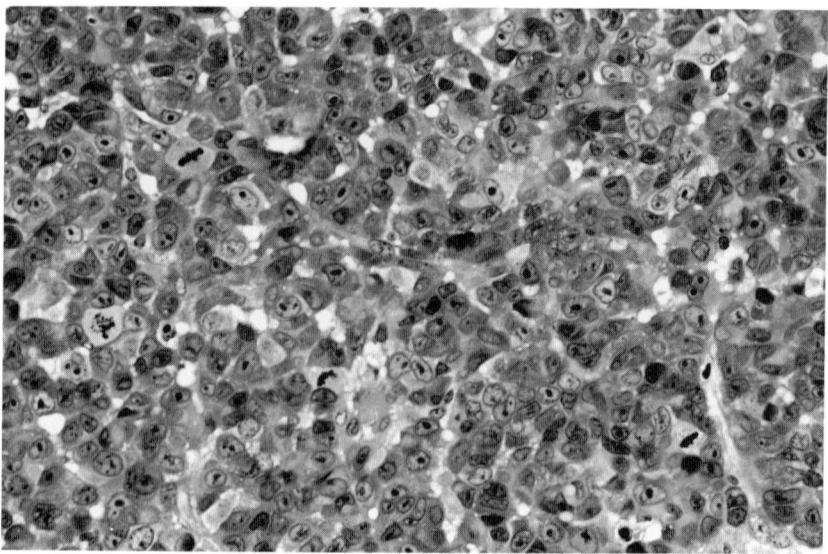

Figure 6.20   Melanoma. Plastic-embedded section allows cellular features to be seen in detail.

and no more than 3 cm thereafter. There is reasonably good evidence that this approach leads to good control of local recurrence (Veronesi *et al.*, 1988). Failures are usually seen in sites such as the head and neck, where it may be difficult to achieve the necessary margin within local anatomical limitations. The form of local treatment does of course only affect the chances of local recurrence. The likelihood of metastasis is a function of the size and character of the tumour at the time that it is excised. More information is needed to understand the heterogeneity of behaviour which exists within tumours of the same thickness. The degree of tumour vascularity appears to be one variable of some importance in predicting the chances of tumour recurrence in intermediate thickness melanomas (Srivastava *et al.*, 1988).

Furthermore, in deciding upon the appropriate surgery it is perfectly safe to undertake a diagnostic excisional biopsy of a malignant melanoma followed by delayed wide excision. The delay to the second procedure can be 21 days or more without any effect on survival (Landthaler *et al.*, 1989). Indeed, the long-standing taboo against incisional biopsy has been disproven: there is no difference in long-term survival of stage I melanoma whether the diagnostic biopsy is incisional or excisional (Lee, 1985; Lederman and Sober, 1985).

Clark and his colleagues have recently proposed a prognostic index

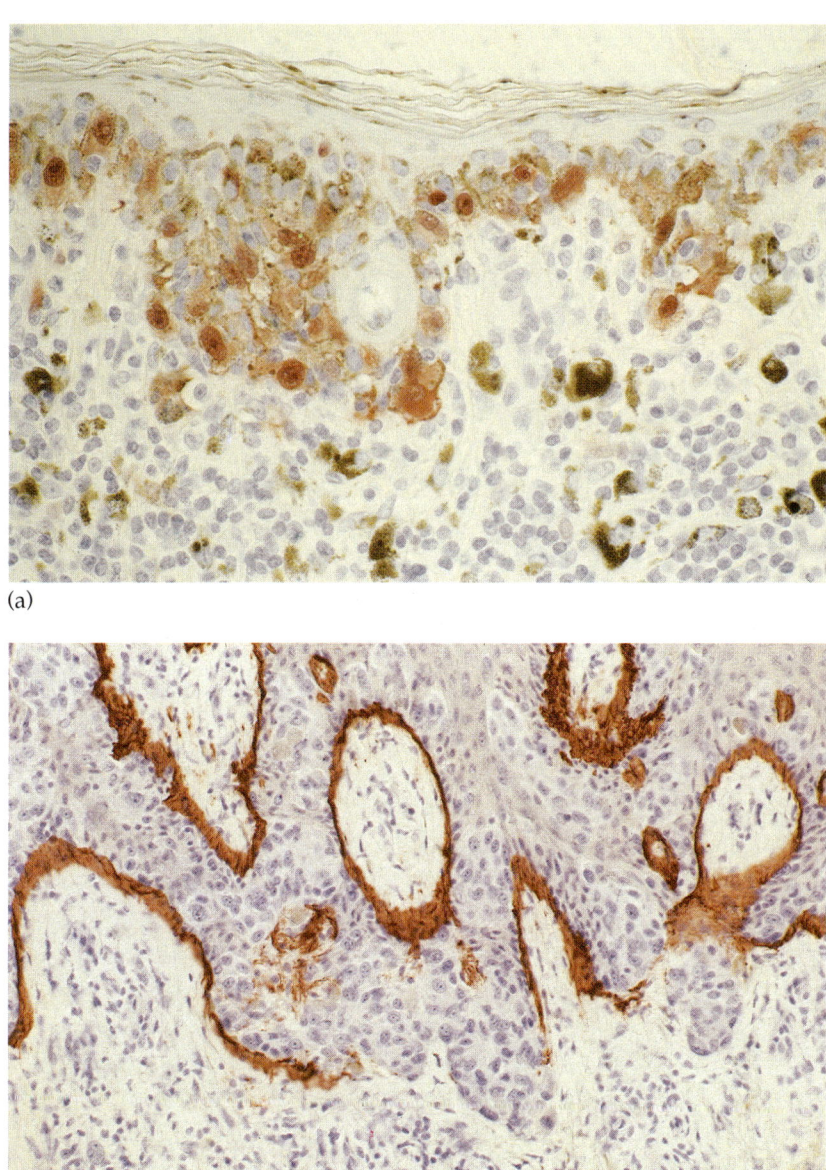

(a)

(b)

Plate 17 Melanoma (a) Immunoperoxidase staining for S100 protein using aminocarbazole allows the red colour reaction to be distinguished from brown
melanin in the lesion. (b) Immunoperoxidase staining of a frozen section,
using the antibody LH 7.2, shows epidermal basement membrane that
is breached by invasive tumour.

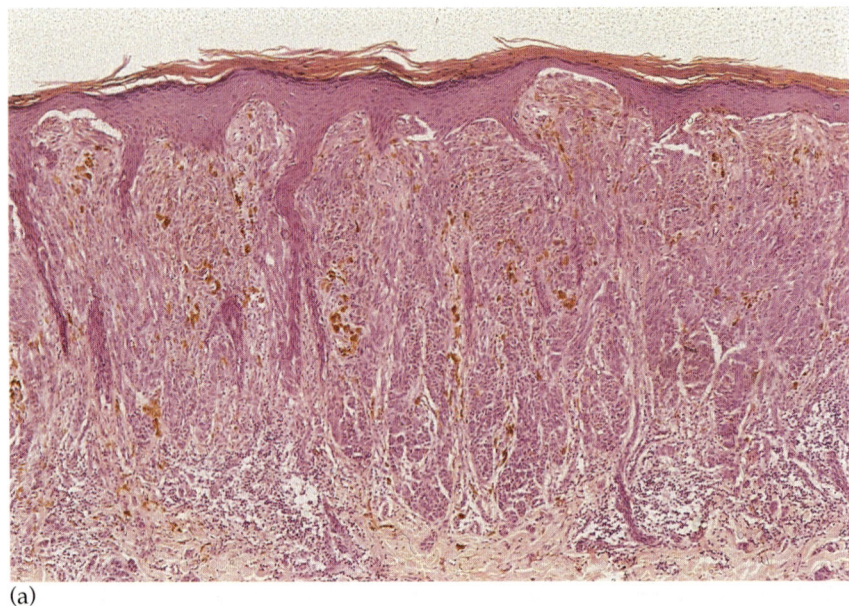

(a)

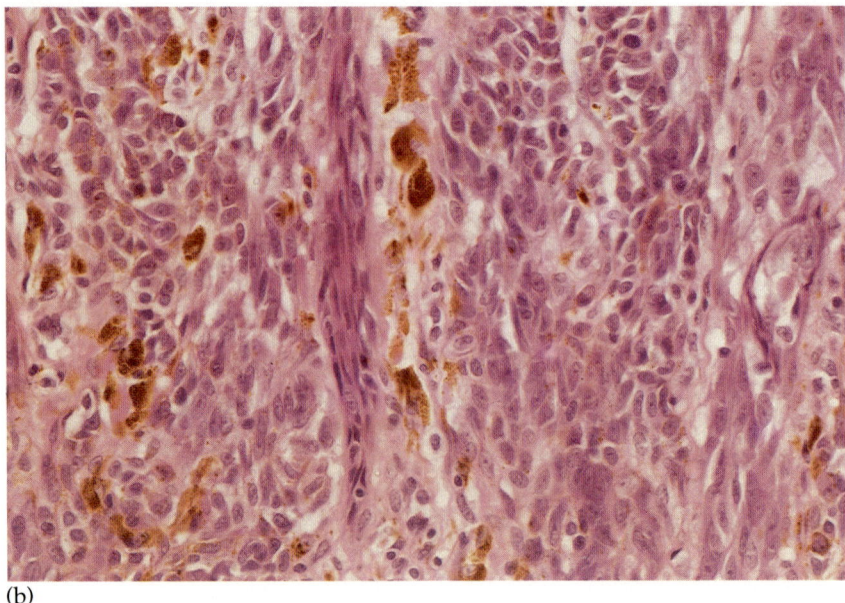

(b)

Plate 18   Pigmented spindle cell naevus of Reed. (a) The vertically-orientated spindle cells are cytologically benign and (b) show no tendency to epidermal invasion.

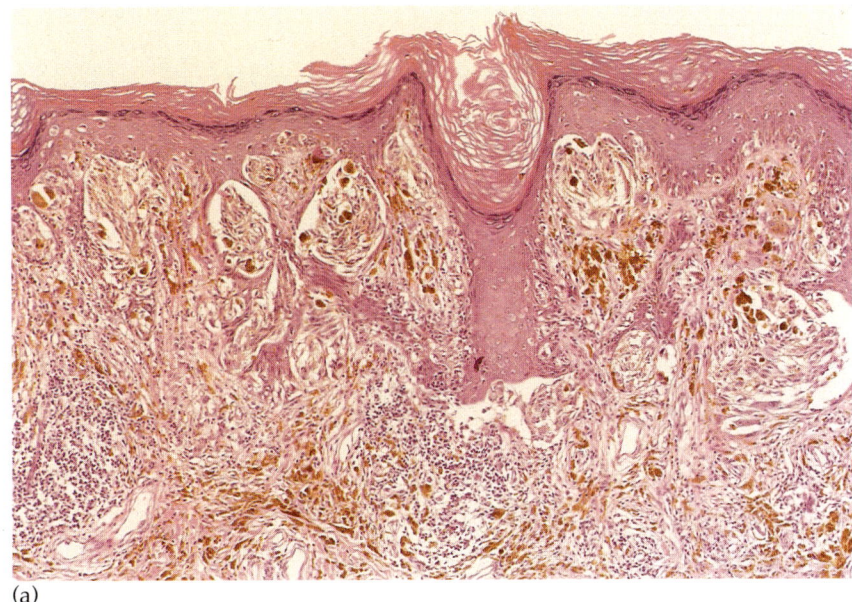
(a)

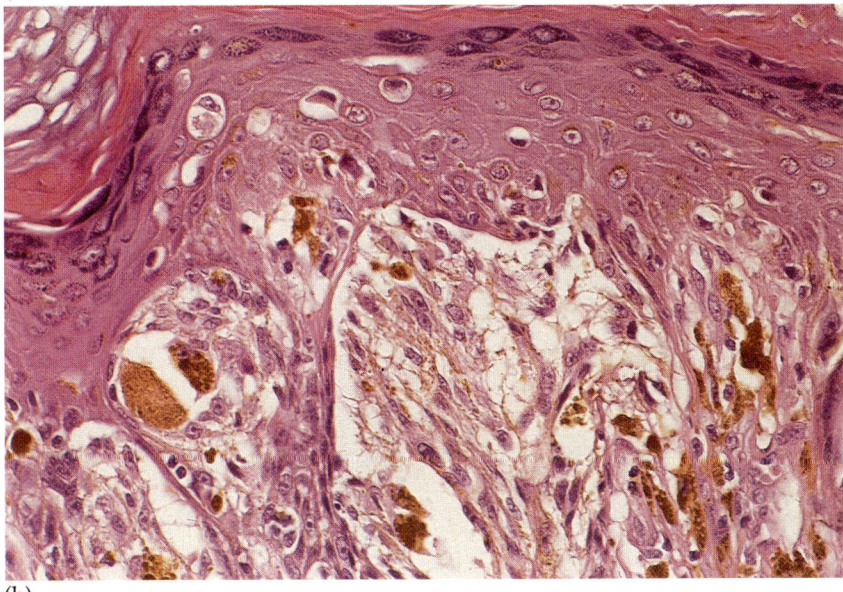
(b)

Plate 19 Malignant melanoma. (a) The tumour is pigmented and with a tendency to spindle cell morphology. (b) The tumour cells are cytologically malignant and invade the epidermis.

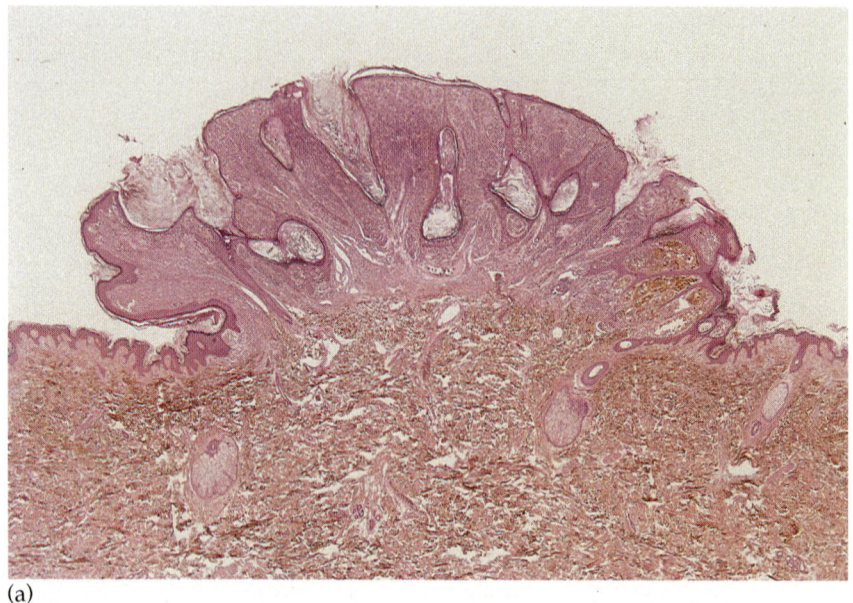

(a)

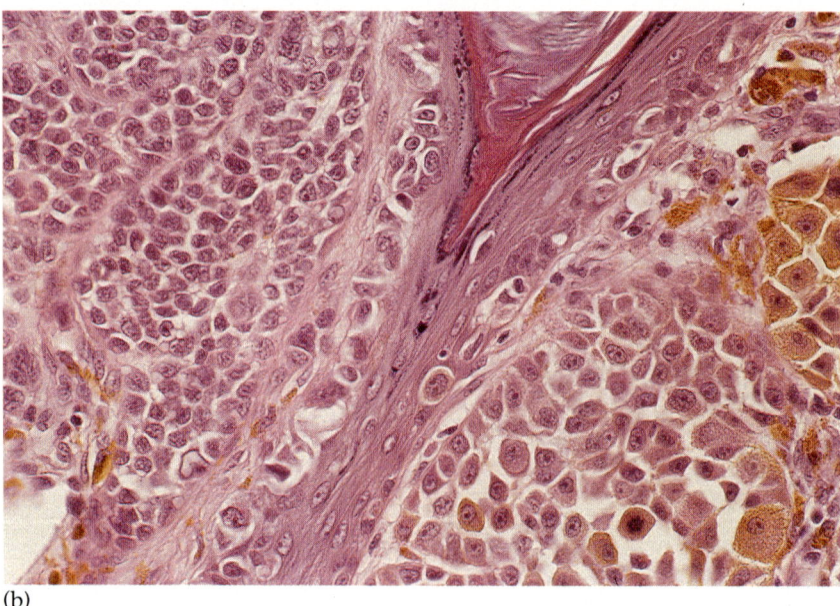

(b)

Plate 20 Naevoid melanoma. (a) The scanning view resembles a naevus. (b) There is cytological malignancy, with intralesional variation in the appearance of the cells and the degree of pigmentation.

for stage I melanoma. The results of a detailed multi-variate analysis of 23 variables showed that six had independent predictive value. These were:

i.   mitotic count per square millimetre
ii. tumour-infiltrating lymphocytes
iii. Breslow thickness
iv. anatomic site of the primary tumour
v.   sex of the patient
vi. histological evidence of regression.

Tumour thickness remains the strongest predictor of 8-year survival, but the other five are also independent predictors (Clark *et al.*, 1989).

6.9   Regression and halo naevi

Halo naevi show a clinical appearance in which there is a zone of depigmentation around a naevus, which corresponds to an underlying inflammatory reaction, which may be so prominent as to obscure the naevus cell component (Langer and Konrad, 1990). Staining with a melanocyte marker will show up the cells within the infiltrate.

Spontaneous regression of a primary melanoma is sometimes cited as the cause of an apparently absent primary in the presence of metastases. The presence of regression certainly does not seem to mean that an anti-tumour reaction has taken place, and that the tumour is likely to behave in a benign fashion as a consequence, as evidenced by the high rate (6 out of 9 cases) of metastases seen in one report (Smith and Stehlin, 1965). If regression is incomplete, it can also cause a problem, because the primary may have a thickness which is less than its true potential; the original maximum thickness of the unregressed lesion probably represents the true potential of the lesion and so the tumour may behave more aggressively than anticipated. Indeed, Shaw *et al.* (1989) found regression in all 28 of their cases who presented with stage II disease (metastasis to regional lymph nodes) in a series of primary melanomas <0.76 mm thick.

In a completely regressed lesion the epidermis may be flat, relatively atrophic and depigmented, with absent melanocytes in the basal layer. There may be a variable degree of pigmentary incontinence in the underlying dermis, which in the absence of other pointers may be mistaken as a tattoo. Alternatively, there may be a residual junctional lesion, of relatively innocuous appearance, but which may give the clue to the diagnosis, especially if the biopsy is being viewed with the retrospectoscope, after the discovery of metastases.

The main problem is that regression is poorly described and defined

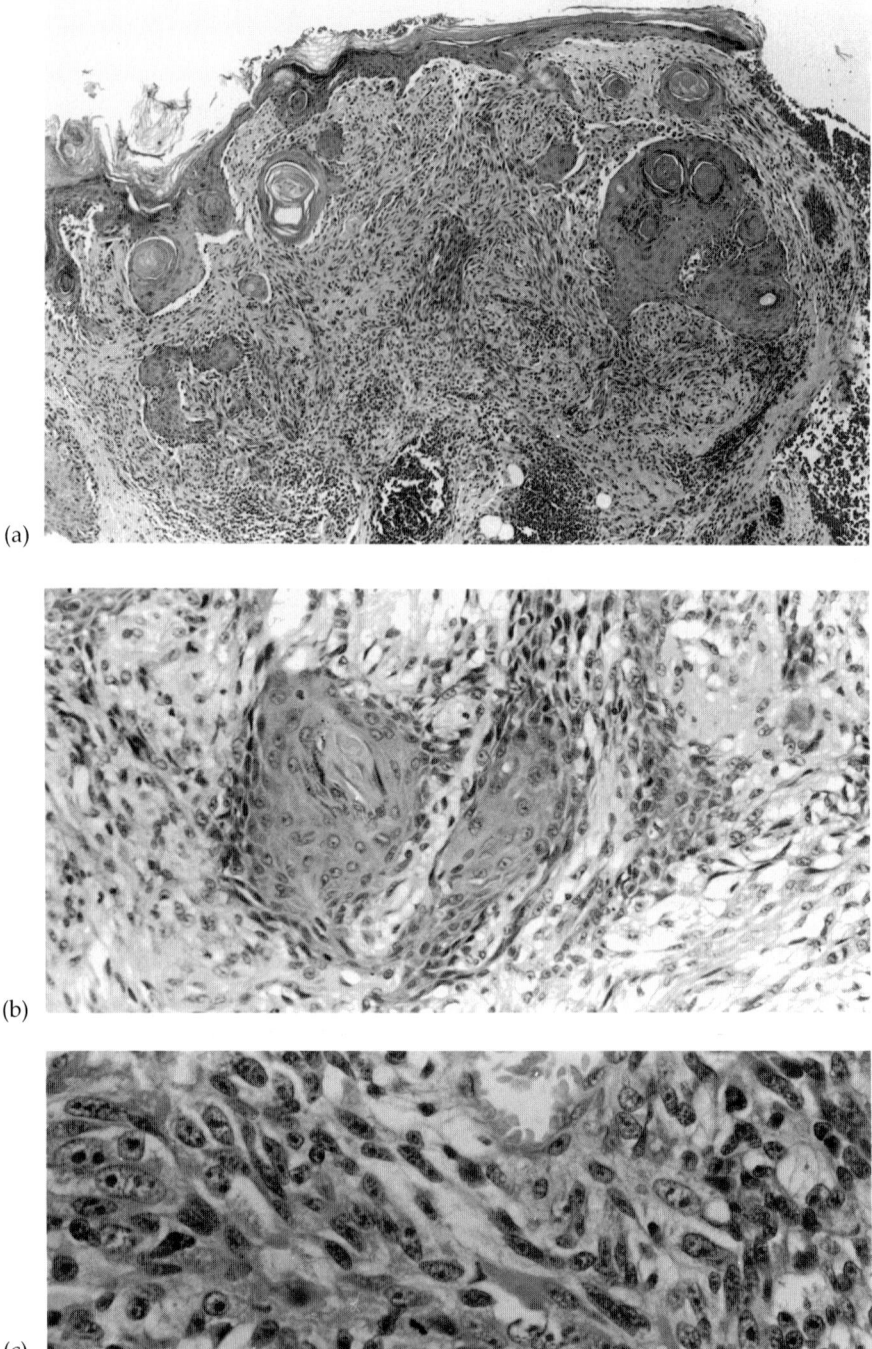

Figure 6.21 A curetting specimen showing (a) squamous proliferation which was originally diagnosed as squamous carcinoma. Review of the first (b) and second (c) recurrences revealed the true nature of the lesion: a spindle cell malignant melanoma.

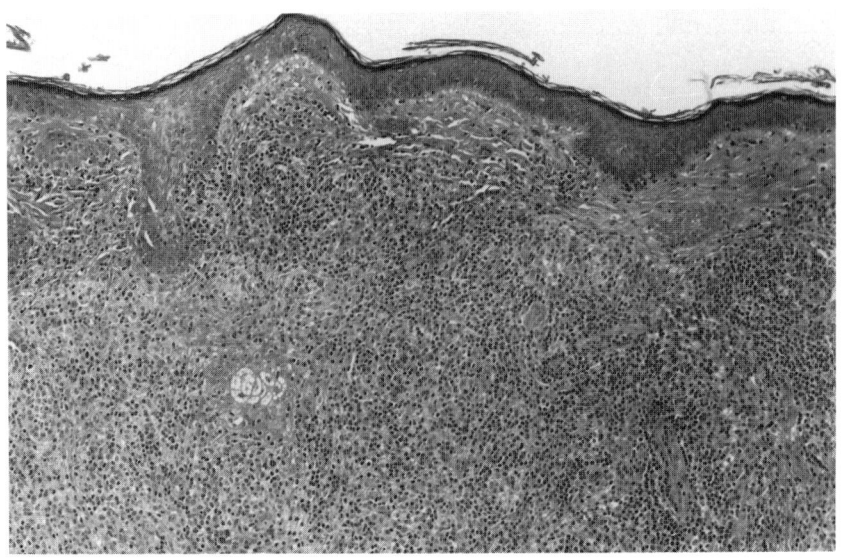

(a)

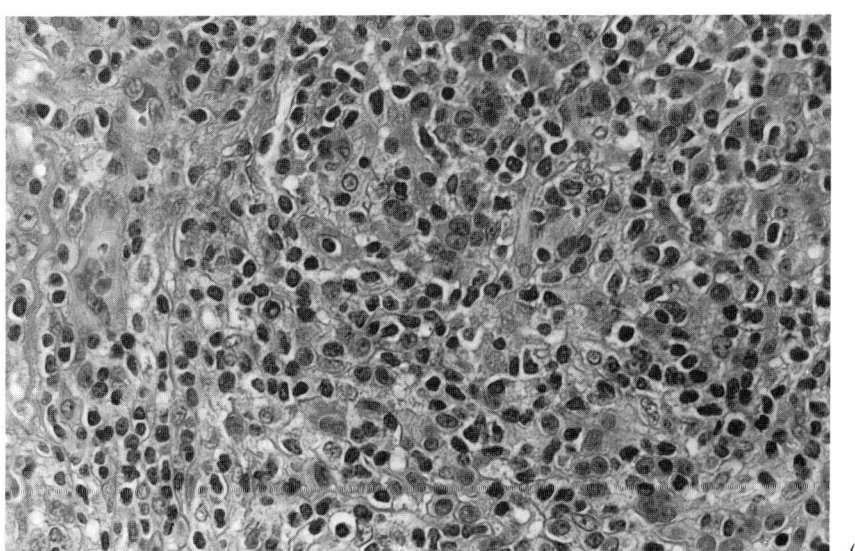

(b)

Figure 6.22   Halo naevus (a) with heavy inflammatory cell infiltration, in which (b) it is difficult to see the naevus cell component.

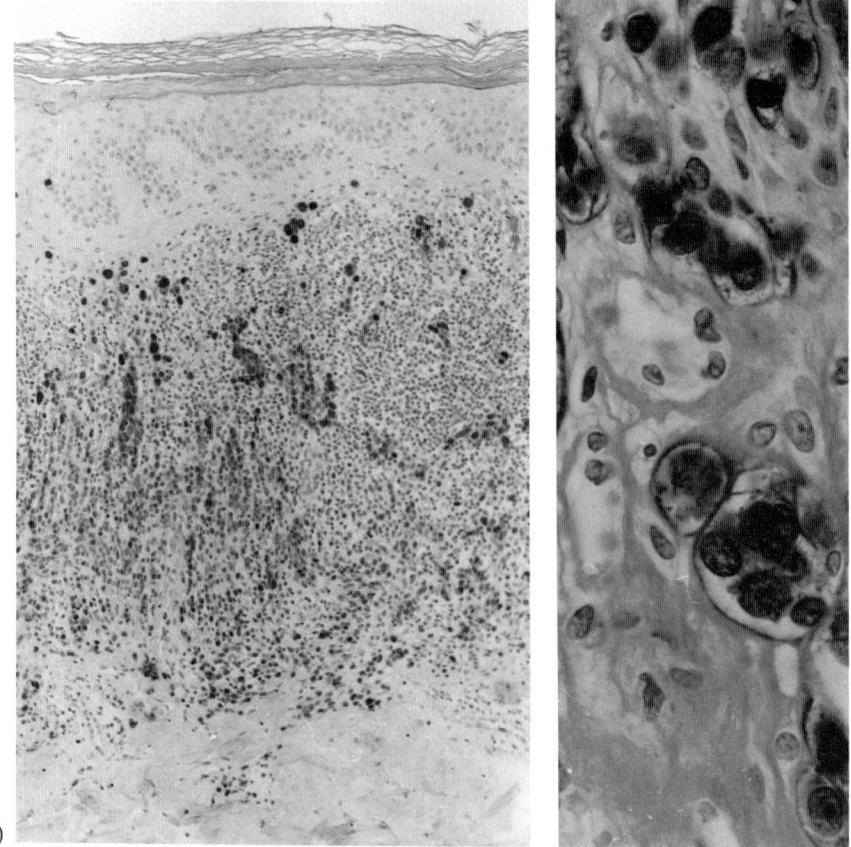

(a)
(b)

Figure 6.23   S100 staining of (a) a halo naevus and (b) a melanoma, showing nuclear and cytoplasmic immunoreactivity.

in the literature, so how are we to define it and diagnose it in a consistent fashion? It is not easy. Regression is probably best character-ized by the presence of scarring or abnormal dermal collagen, a change emphasized by viewing in polarized light, together with an increase in dermal vascularity, in the absence of tumour. It usually starts towards the central and upper part of the tumour. Staining with a marker such as type IV collagen may help to accentuate these often subtle changes.

   Related to regression is the phenomenon of the halo naevus. Some naevi may undergo an inflammatory involution. Clinically, this is manifested by a depigmented halo around the lesion. In the biopsy the lymphocytic reaction may be so vigorous as to mask the naevus cells. Staining with a melanocyte marker, such as S100, will reveal the nature of the process. This reaction is not confined to benign naevi, but can also be seen in some melanomas, especially the minimal deviation type.

6.10   Lentigo maligna

Lentigo maligna, the melanotic freckle, was the first kind of premalignant melanocytic lesion to be recognized, and was described as a pigmented macular lesion, showing a variegated black-brown colour and irregular outline, which enlarged slowly and was most commonly found on the face (Hutchinson 1894; Dubreuilh, 1894, 1912). It is a premalignant, intraepidermal lesion in a similar way to senile keratosis and Bowen's disease (Wayte and Helwig, 1968).

If the lesion progresses beyond the macular stage and develops a nodule or plaque and definite histological evidence of dermal invasion by atypical melanocytes, then the description 'lentigo maligna melanoma' applies. True lentigo maligna melanoma is rare. The impression has grown up that it is different from melanoma elsewhere and carries a better prognosis (McGovern *et al.*, 1980). This is almost certainly wrong. Koh *et al.* (1984) have shown quite conclusively that when Breslow thickness is taken into account, in stage I disease, there is no

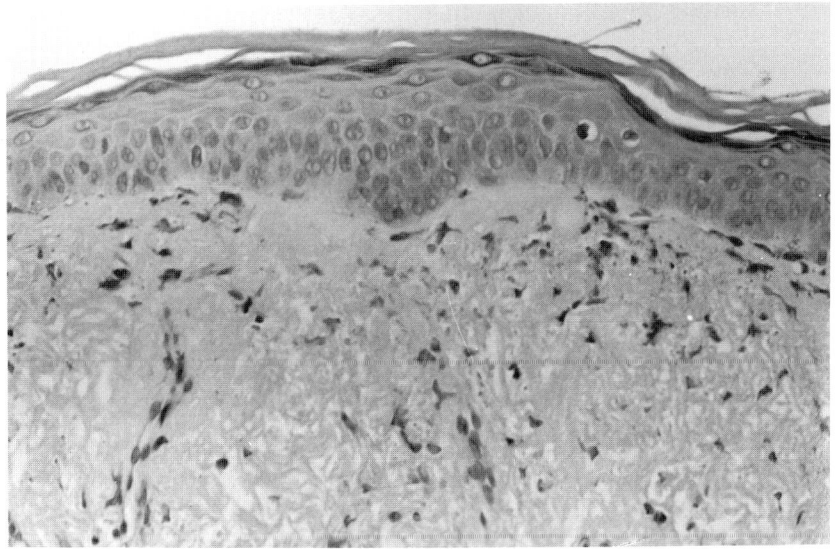

Figure 6.24   Senile lentigo of face. Clinically quite markedly pigmented, but shows only dermal elastosis and pigmentary incontinence.

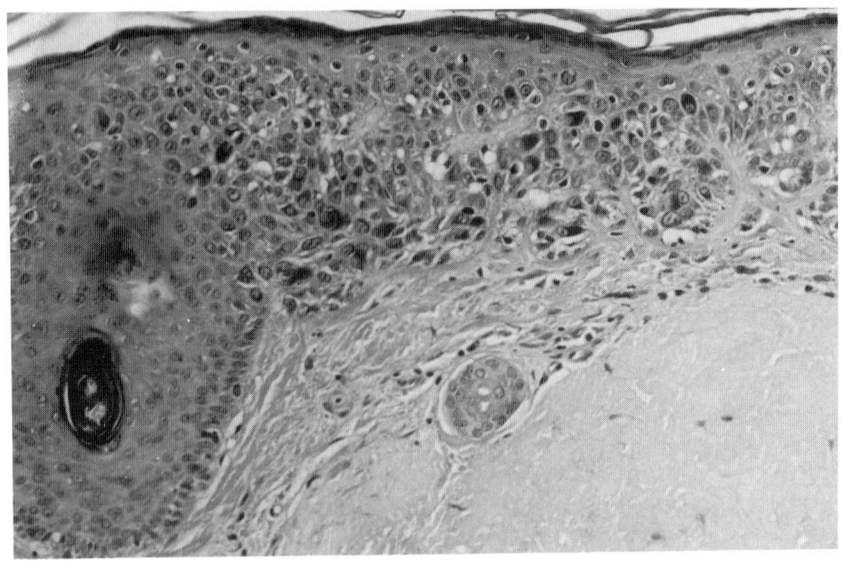

Figure 6.25 Lentigo maligna. Proliferation of melanocytes in the lower epidermis and with associated dermal elastosis.

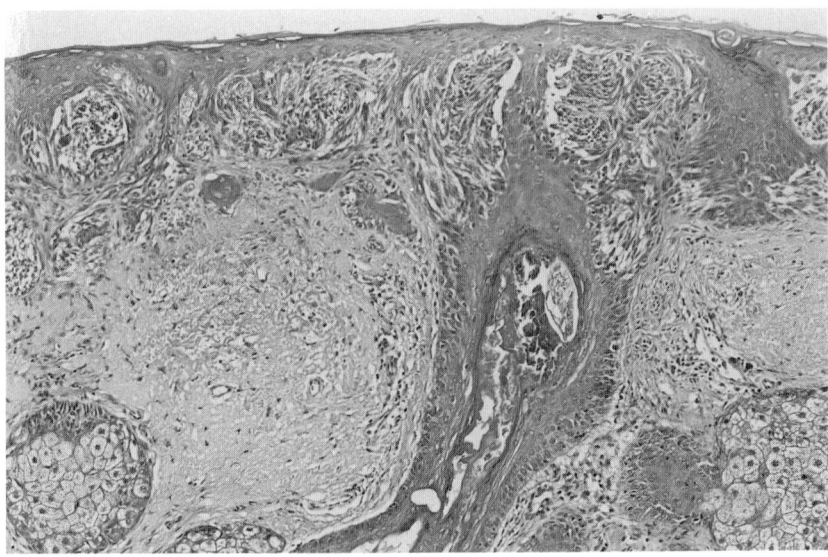

Figure 6.26 Lentigo maligna. Marked proliferation of melanocytes in the lower epidermis, but without dermal invasion.

difference in behaviour between tumours classified as lentigo maligna melanoma and those merely called melanoma. If there is a difference it is at the earlier stage of development of the macular lentigo maligna: which is an usually indolent lesion when compared to other melanomas which may be more rapidly progressive.

The histological criteria for diagnosis have been stated as:

i.   an atrophic epidermis with an almost continuous layer of atypical melanocytes in the basal layer and with little or no spread of atypical melanocytes into the upper epidermal layers,
ii. infiltration down into the epithelium of appendages by atypical melanocytes,
iii. solar elastosis, with or without inflammation in the dermis,
iv. definite evidence of dermal invasion by atypical melanocytes.

The main differential point to separate this condition from superficial spreading melanoma is the way in which the atypical melanocytes tend to be restricted to the basal epidermis, in contrast to the upward spread of atypical melanocytes which is more characteristic of melanomas of usual type (Clark and Mihm, 1969; Green et al., 1983).

6.11   Minimal deviation melanoma

Reed has spent some time pursuing the problem of thin, malignant melanomas that show a low degree of cellular atypia. He has used this term to describe thin melanomas that are, nevertheless, in the vertical growth phase. However, it is probably not useful to distinguish these lesions from melanoma of usual type because the two behave in a similar way, thickness for thickness. Reed has extended the concept to include some other problematic features of melanomas. The basic minimal deviation melanoma shows a gradation of abnormality, with the most abnormal cells in the upper part of the lesion and more benign looking naevoid cells towards the base. Other variants may show features of Spitz naevus or of halo naevus (Reed et al., 1990). It is not known whether these variants are associated with different prognoses, thickness for thickness, than melanoma, NOS.

6.12   Spindle cell melanoma

When considering the differential diagnosis of spindle cell tumours in the dermis it is always important to consider the possibility of melanoma: a distinction of some clinical importance because of the greater likelihood of metastasis when compared to spindle cell tumours of keratinocyte or fibrohistiocyte origin. As well as looking carefully at the

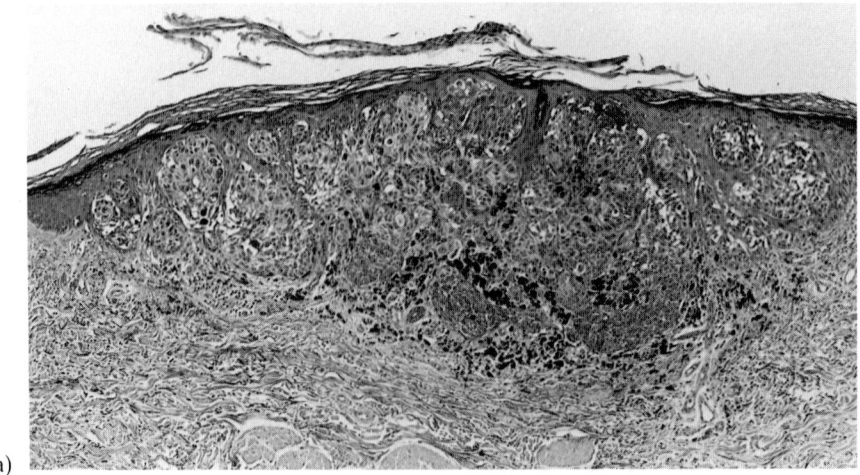

(a)

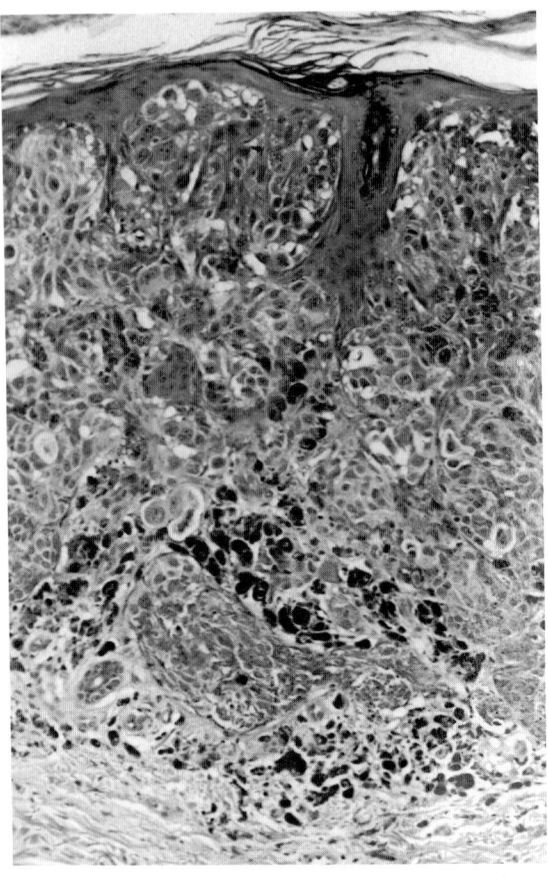

(b)

Figure 6.27 Minimal deviation melanoma (a and b). A melanoma with apparent maturation of cells towards the base of the tumour.

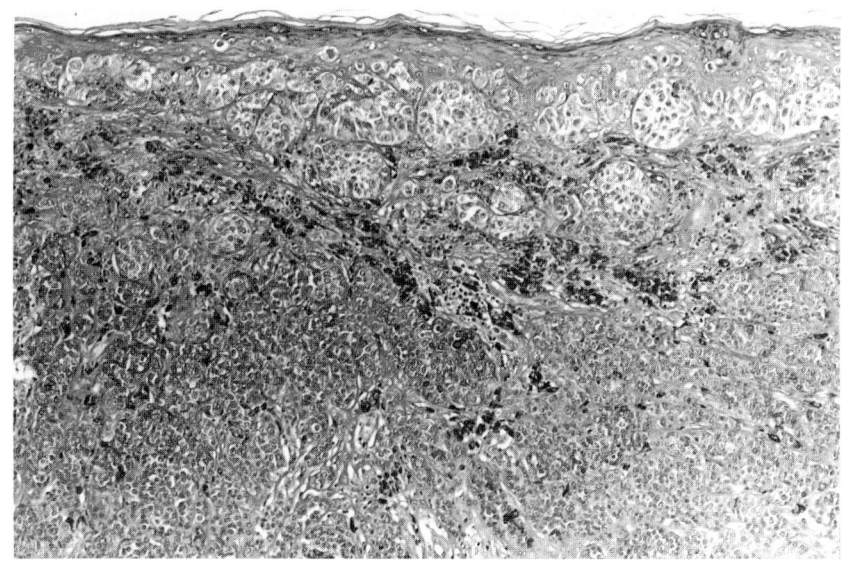

(a)

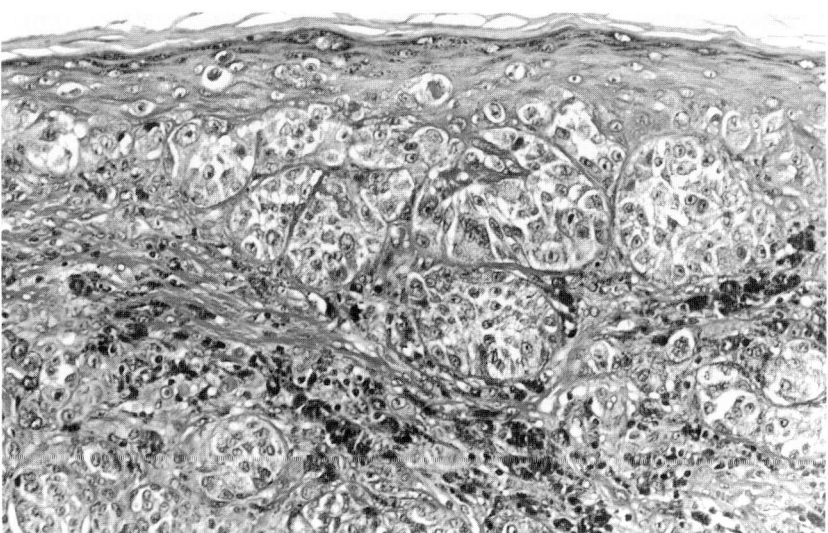

(b)

Figure 6.28 Minimal deviation melanoma (a and b). Large pleomorphic tumour cells in the upper component and naevoid cells at the base.

nuclei to find large, single nucleoli one can also use a panel of markers. The differential diagnosis of spindle cell and pleomorphic tumours includes spindle cell carcinoma, atypical fibroxanthoma, leiomyosarcoma, and angiosarcoma. Using a panel of antibodies, including vimentin, cytokeratin, S100 protein, desmin, and factor-VIII-related antigen can provide information for the appropriate classification of malignant, cutaneous spindle cell tumours (Walker and Morton, 1988). The typical spindle cell melanoma will be positive for S100, vimentin and NKI/C3 and negative for cytokeratins. Fibrohistiocytic tumours will express vimentin but not the other melanoma markers. The antibody HMB-45, which is otherwise a very sensitive marker of melanoma, does not appear to react with most spindle cell melanomas (Wick *et al.*, 1988).

6.13   Desmoplastic melanoma

There is an important group of melanomas, usually arising in sun-damaged skin of fair individuals, which are often misdiagnosed. These were first described by Conley, Lattes and Orr (1971) when they described seven non-pigmented, subcutaneous, fibrosarcoma-like tumours in which there was a minimal degree of melanocytic atypia in the overlying epidermis. Further cases were described which showed prominent neurotropism of tumour cells, for which the title 'neurotropic melanoma' was proposed (Reed and Leonard, 1979). More recently the subject has been reviewed and the proposal made that these are aspects of the same tumour and that in addition reports of malignant epithelioid schwannomas of superficial soft tissues (Enzinger and Weiss, 1983) and many malignant schwannomas of sun-exposed skin are also examples of desmoplastic melanoma (Jain and Allen,1989).

The main problem in diagnosis is to recognize that there is a malignant tumour present in the biopsy. The epidermis may show little or even no melanocytic atypia and the dermis is only sparsely infiltrated by tumour cells. Mitoses are almost always present, however, amongst the cells which are arranged singly or in small bundles or fascicles within the dermis. A useful clue is that the spindle-shaped cells have quite large epithelioid nuclei and are arranged perpendicular to the epidermis. When neurotropism is present, nerves are expanded by the tumour cell infiltrate. The tumour cells are usually S100 positive (Egbert *et al.*, 1988). Antibodies to S100 protein have been used widely as markers for melanoma, despite abundant evidence that they react with a whole variety of other structures. The antibody HMB-45 offers an alternative. Positive immunoreactivity is 100% specific and 93% sensitive for the diagnosis of malignant melanoma in paraffin sections. Only spindle cell melanomas are not stained reliably (Wick *et al.*, 1988).

The prognosis is poor, with overall survival rates quoted from 36% (Jain and Allen, 1989) to 67% (Reiman *et al.*, 1987). Those cases with head and neck primary tumours have a mortality rate of approaching 100%. Widespread distant metastasis is relatively common and perhaps more so than regional lymph node spread. In the head and neck neurotropism may be particularly evident. Surgery should therefore attempt to include the involved cranial nerve and associated skin within the resection field. Recurrence is a common consequence of inadequate initial resection (Egbert *et al.*, 1988).

6.14   Balloon cell melanoma

Both naevi, halo naevi and melanomas can show balloon cell change, which when present usually affects the large part of the lesion. The balloon cell appearance does not seem to affect the nature or behaviour of the underlying lesion, which behaves the same way as a non-ballooned analogue. The cells in a balloon cell melanoma should be S100 positive, which will help in distinguishing it from metastatic clear cell carcinoma or renal carcinoma (Akslen and Myking, 1989; Aloi *et al.*, 1988; Cote *et al.*, 1986; Napoli, 1988).

6.15   Signet-ring cell melanoma

A further variant of melanoma has been described recently, in which the tumour cells contain cytoplasmic inclusions, which lead to a signet-ring cell appearance. The inclusions stain for vimentin, but their nature and function remains obscure. Few cases have been reported. Those that have so far have been associated with lymph node metastasis (Sheibani and Battifora, 1988; Al-Talib and Theaker, 1991).

References

Ackerman, A. B. (1988) What naevus is dysplastic, a syndrome and the commonest precursor of malignant melanoma? A riddle and an answer. *Histopathology*, **13**, 241–56.

Ackerman, A. B. and Magana-Garcia, M. (1990) Naming acquired melanocytic nevi. Unna's, Miescher's, Spitz's, Clark's. *Am. J. Dermatopathol.*, **12**, 193–209.

Akslen, L. A. and Myking, A. O. (1989) Balloon cell melanoma mimicking clear cell carcinoma. *Pathol. Res. Pract.*, **184**, 548–53.

Aloi, F. G., Coverlizza, S. and Pippione, M. (1988) Balloon cell melanoma: a report of two cases. *J. Cutan. Pathol.*, **15**, 230–3.

Al-Talib, R. K. and Theaker, J. M. (1991) Signet-ring cell melanoma; light microscopic, immunohistochemical and ultrastructural features. *Histopathology*, **18**, 572–5.

Breslow, A. (1970) Thickness, cross-sectional areas and depth of invasion in the prognosis of cutaneous melanoma. *Ann. Surg.*, **172**, 902–8.

Caselitz, J., Janner, M., Brutbach, E., Weber, K. and Osborn, M. (1983) Malignant melanomas contain only the vimentin type of intermediate filaments. *Virchows Arch. (A)*, **400**, 43–51.

Clark, W. H., From, L., Bernardino, E. A. and Mihm, M. C. (1969) The histogenesis and biologic behaviour of primary malignant human melanomas of the skin. *Cancer Res.*, **29**, 705–26.

Clark, W. H. and Mihm, M. C. (1969) Lentigo maligna and lentigo maligna melanoma. *Am. J. Pathol.*, **55**, 39–67.

Clark, W. H., Reimer, R. R., Greene, M., Ainsworth, A. M. and Mastrangelo, M. J. (1978) Origin of familial malignant melanomas from heritable melanocytic lesions. 'The B-K mole syndrome'. *Arch. Dermatol.*, **114**, 732–8.

Clark, W. H., Elder, D. E., Guerry, D., Epstein, M. E., Greene, M. H. and Van Horn, M. (1984) A study of tumour progression: the precursor lesions of superficial spreading and nodular melanoma. *Hum. Pathol.*, **15**, 1147–65.

Clark, W. H., Elder, D. E., Guerry, D., Braitman, L. E., Trock, B. J., Schultz, D., Synnestvedt, M. and Halpern, A. C. (1989) Model predicting survival in stage I melanoma based on tumor progression. *J. Natl Cancer. Inst.*, **81**, 1893–1904.

Clemmensen, O. J. and Kroon, S. (1988) The histology of "congenital features" in early acquired melanocytic nevi. *J. Am. Acad. Dermatol.*, **19**, 742–6.

Colombari, R., Bonetti, F., Zamboni, G., Scarpa, A., Marino, F., Tomezzoli, A., Capelli, P., Menestrina, F., Chilosi, M. and Fiore-Donati, L. (1988) Distribution of melanoma specific antibody (HMB-45) in benign and malignant melanocytic tumours. An immunohistochemical study on paraffin sections. Virchows Archiv. A. *Pathol. Anat.*, **413**, 17–24.

Conley, J., Lattes, R. and Orr, W. (1971) Desmoplastic malignant melanoma: a rare variant of spindle cell melanoma. *Cancer*, **28**, 914–36.

Cook, M. G. and Fallowfield, M. E. (1990) Dysplastic naevi – an alternative view. *Histopathology*, **16**, 29–35.

Cote, J., Watters, A. K. and O'Brien, E. A. (1986) Halo balloon cell nevus. *J. Cutan. Pathol.*, **13**, 123–7.

Curran, R. C. and McGann, B. G. (1976) The ultrastructure of benign pigmented naevi and melano-carcinomas in man. *J. Pathol.*, **119**, 135–45.

Dubreuilh, M. W. (1894) Lentigo malin des vieillards. *Ann. Derm. Syph. (Paris)*, **5**, 1092–9.

Dubreuilh, M. W. (1912) De la melanose circonscrite precancereuse. *Ann. Derm. Syph. (Paris)*, **5**, 129–51.

Egbert, B., Kempson, R. and Sagebiel, R. (1988) Desmoplastic malignant melanoma. A clinicohistopathologic study of 25 cases. *Cancer*, **62**, 2033–41.

Elder, D. E., Goldman, L. I., Goldman, S. C., Greene, M. H. and Clark, W. H. (1980) Dysplastic nevus syndrome: a phenotypic association of sporadic cutaneous melanoma. *Cancer*, **46**, 1787–94.

Elder, D. E., Guerry, D., Epstein, M. N., Zehngebot, C., Lusk, E., Van Horn, M. and Clark, W. H. (1984) Invasive malignant melanomas lacking competence for metastasis. *Am. J. Dermatopathol.*, **6** (suppl. 1), 55–62.

Elder, D. E. (1985) The dysplastic nevus. *Pathology*, **17**, 291–7.

Enzinger, F. M. and Weiss, S. W. (1983) *Soft Tissue Tumours* (1st edn) Mosby, St Louis, pp. 644–8.

Fallowfield, M. E. and Cook, M. G. (1990) Lymphatics in primary cutaneous melanoma. *Am. J. Surg. Pathol.*, **14**, 370–4.

Fox, H. (1990) Dysplastic naevi. Histopathology, **16**, 105–6.

Frankel, K. A. (1987) Intraepithelial melanocytic neoplasia: a classification by pattern analysis of proliferations of atypical melanocytes. *Am. J. Dermatopathol.*, **9**, 80–1.

Goldenhersh, M. A., Savin, R. C., Barnhill, R. L. and Stenn, K. S. (1988) Malignant blue nevus. Case report and literature review. *J. Am. Acad. Dermatol.*, **19**, 712–22.

Green, A., Little, J. H. and Weedon, D. (1983) The diagnosis of Hutchinson's melanotic freckle (lentigo maligna) in Queensland. *Pathology*, **15**, 33–5.

Goovaerts, G. and Buyssens, N. (1988) Nevus cell maturation or atrophy? *Am. J. Dermatopathol.*, **10**, 20–7.

Heenan, P. J., Weeramanthri, T., Holman, C. D. J. and Armstrong, B. K. (1985) Surgical treatment and survival from cutaneous malignant melanoma. *Aust. NZ J. Med.*, **55**, 229–34.

Hutchinson, J. (1894) Lentigo melanosis. *Arch. Surg.*, **5**, 252–6.

Jain, S. and Allen, P. W. (1989) Desmoplastic malignant melanoma and its variants. A study of 45 cases. *Am. J. Surg. Pathol.*, **13**, 358–73.

Kamino, H., Misheloff, E., Ackerman, A. B., Flotte, T. J. and Greco, M. A. (1979) Eosinophilic globules in Spitz's naevi. *Am. J. Dermatopathol.*, **1**, 319–24.

Kirkham, N., Price, M. L., Gibson, B., Leigh, I. M., Coburn, P. and Darley, C. R. (1989) Type VII collagen antibody LH 7.2 identifies basement membrane characteristics of thin malignant melanomas. *J. Pathol.*, **157**, 243–8.

Koh, H. K., Michalik, E., Sober, A. J., Lew, R. A., Day, C. L., Clark, W., Mihm, M. C., Kopf, A. W., Blois, M. J. and Fitzpatrick, T. B. (1984) Lentigo maligna melanoma has no better prognosis than other types of melanoma. *J. Clin. Oncol.*, **2**, 994–1001.

Lambert, W. C. and Brodkin, R. H. (1984) Nodal and subcutaneous cellular blue nevi. A pseudometastasizing pseudomelanoma. *Arch. Dermatol.*, **120**, 367–70.

Landthaler, M., Braun-Falco, O., Leitl, A., Konz, B. and Holzel, D. (1989) Excisional biopsy as the first therapeutic procedure versus primary wide excision of malignant melanoma. *Cancer*, **64**, 1612–6.

Langer, K. and Konrad, K. (1990) Congenital melanocytic naevi with halo phenomenon, report of two cases and a review of the literature. *J. Derm. Surg. Oncol.*, **16**, 377–83.

Lederman, J. S. and Sober, A. J. (1985) Does biopsy type influence survival in clinical stage I cutaneous melanoma. *J. Am. Acad. Dermatol.*, **13**, 983–97.

Lee, Y. N. (1985) Diagnosis treatment and prognosis of early melanoma: the importance of depth of microinvasion. *Ann. Surg.*, **191**, 87–96.

Leopold, J. G. and Richards, D. B. (1967) Cellular blue naevi. *J. Path. Bact.*, **94**, 247–55.

Leopold, J. G. and Richards, D. B. (1968) The interrelationship of blue and common naevi. *J. Pathol.*, **95**, 37–43.

Levene, A. (1980) On the natural history and comparative pathology of the blue naevus. *Ann. R. Coll. Surg. Engl.*, **62**, 327–34.

Masson, P. (1951) My conception of cellular naevi. *Cancer*, **4**, 9–38.

McGovern, V. J., Shaw, H. M., Milton, G. W. and Farago, G. A. (1980) Is malignant melanoma arising in a Hutchinson's melanotic freckle a separate disease entity? *Histopathol.*, **4**, 235–42.

McGovern, V. J., Cochran, A. J., Van der Esch, E. P., Little, J. H. and MacLennan, R. (1986) The classification of malignant melanoma, its histological reporting and registration: a revision of the 1972 Sydney classification. *Pathologica*, **18**, 12–21.

Milton, G. W., Shaw, H. and McCarthy, W. H. (1985) Resection margins for melanoma. *Aust. NZ J. Med.*, **55**, 225–6.

Milton, G. W., Balch, C. M. and Shaw, H. M. (1985) Clinical characteristics. In *Cutaneous Melanoma. Clinical Management and Treatment Results Worldwide*, eds Balch, C. M. and Milton, G. W. JB Lippincott, Philadelphia, pp. 13–28.

Napoli, P. (1988) [Balloon cell malignant melanoma]. *Pathologica*, **80**, 379–85.

Paniago-Pereira, C., Maize, J. C. and Ackerman, A. B. (1978) Nevus of large spindle and/or epithelioid cells (Spitz's nevus). *Arch. Dermatol.*, **114**, 1811–23.

Reed, R. J. and Leonard, D. D. (1979) Neurotropic melanoma: a variant of desmoplastic melanoma. *Am. J. Surg. Pathol.*, **3**, 301–11.

Reed, R. J., Webb, S. V. and Clark, W. H. Jr. (1990) Minimal deviation melanoma (halo nevus variant). *Am. J. Surg. Pathol.*, **14**, 53–68.

Reiman, H. M., Goellner, J. R., Woods, J. E. and Mixter, R. C. (1987) Desmoplastic melanoma of the head and neck. *Cancer*, **60**, 2269–74.

Ridolfi, R. L., Rosen, P. P. and Thaler, H. (1977) Nevus cell aggregates associated with lymph nodes: estimated frequency and clinical significance. *Cancer*, **39**, 164–71.

Rodriguez, H. A. and Ackerman, L. V. (1968) Cellular blue nevus. Clinico-pathologic study of forty-five cases. *Cancer*, **21**, 393–405.

Sagebiel, R. W., Chinn, E. K. and Egbert, B. M. (1984) Pigmented spindle cell nevus. *Am. J. Surg. Pathol.*, **8**, 645–53.

Sagebiel, R. W. (1985) Histopathology of precursor melanocytic lesions. *Am. J. Surg. Pathol.*, **9** (suppl.), 41–52.

Seab, J. A., Graham, J. H. and Helwig, E. B. (1989) Deep penetrating neavus. *Am. J. Surg. Pathol.*, **13**, 39–44.

Shaw, H. M., McCarthy, S. W., McCarthy, W. H., Thompson, J. F. and Milton, G. W. (1989) Thin regressing malignant melanoma: significance of concurrent regional lymph node metastases. *Histopathology*, **15**, 257–65.

Sheibani, K. and Battifora, H. (1988) Signet-ring cell melanoma. A rare morphologic variant of malignant melanoma. *Am. J. Surg. Pathol.*, **12**, 28–34.

Smith, J. L. and Stehlin, J. S. (1965) Spontaneous regression of primary malignant melanomas with regional metastases. *Cancer*, **18**, 1399–415.

Smith, N. P. (1987) The pigmented spindle cell tumor of Reed, an underdiagnosed lesion. *Semin. Diagn. Pathol.*, **4**, 75–87.

Smoller, B. R., McNutt, N. S. and Hsu, A. (1989) HMB-45 staining in dysplastic naevi. Support for a spectrum of progression toward melanoma. *Am. J. Surg. Pathol.*, **13**, 680–4.

Springall, D. R., Cun, J., Cocchia, D., Michetti, F., Levene, A., Levene, M. M., Marangos, P. J., Bloom, S. R. and Polak, J. M. (1983) The value of S100 immunostaining as a diagnostic tool in human malignant melanomas. *Virchows Arch. [A]*, **400**, 331–44.

Srivastava, A., Laidler, P., Davies, R. P., Horgan, K. and Hughes, L. E. (1988) The prognostic significance of tumor vascularity in intermediate-thickness (0.76–4.0 mm thick) skin melanoma. A quantitative histologic study. *Am. J. Pathol.*, **133**, 419–23.

Stone, M. A., Balajanians, M., Bhuta, S. and Cochran, A. J. (1988) Quantative alterations in cutaneous Langerhans cells during the evolution of malignant melanoma of the skin. *J. Invest. Dermatol.*, **91**, 125–8.

Sun, J., Morton, T. H. and Gown, A. M. (1990) Antibody HMB-45 identifies the cells of blue nevi. *Am. J. Dermatopathol.*, **14**, 748–51.

Temple-Camp, C. R. E., Saxe, N. and King, H. (1988) Benign and malignant cellular blue nevus. A clinicopathological study of 30 cases. *Am. J. Dermatopathol.*, **10**, 289–96.

Veronesi, U., Cascinelli, N., Adamus, J., Balch, C., Bandiera, D., Barchuk, A., Bufalino, R., Craig, P., De Marsillac, J., Durand, J. C. *et al.* (1988) Thin stage 1 primary cutaneous malignant melanoma. Comparison of excision with margins of 1 or 3 cm. *N. Engl. J. Med.*, **318**, 1159–62.

Wayte, D. M. and Helwig, E. B. (1968) Melanotic freckle of Hutchinson. *Cancer*, **21**, 893–911.

Walker, A. N. and Morton, B. D. (1988) Immunohistochemistry: a useful adjunct in the evaluation of malignant cutaneous spindle cell tumors. *South. Med. J.*, **81**, 1505–8.

Wick, M. R., Swanson, P. E. and Rocamora, A. (1988) Recognition of malignant melanoma by monoclonal antibody HMB-45. An immunohistochemical study of 200 paraffin-embedded cutaneous tumors. *J. Cutan. Pathol.*, **15**, 201–7.

7 Adnexal tumours

Before embarking on an attempt to list and describe many of the more readily identifiable adnexal tumours, a few words of introduction are in order. The identification and subclassification of adnexal skin tumours is a subject which often worries the histopathologist. Many entities have emerged over the years in a continuing campaign of 'splitting'; over ten varieties of hair follicle tumour alone have been described. On the other hand the majority of these tumours are essentially benign in behaviour. So although it is a great source of satisfaction to achieve a definitive subclassification, it is usually largely irrelevant from a clinical point of view; if the tumour has been adequately excised the patient will have been cured and need not be seen again once the stitches have been removed. The archetypes probably also represent the best differentiated examples: less well differentiated tumours causing more problems in classification.

The even rarer tumours that show histological features of malignancy are also best treated by surgical excision. There is no evidence that radiotherapy or chemotherapy has any part to play in their management. However, because of their rarity the patients should be followed-up carefully (Wick, 1985).

Nevertheless, these lesions have been described and subclassified and their clinical and pathological features delineated, so it is the duty of the pathologist to attempt a definitive diagnosis, rather than merely to 'lump' a lesion into some convenient diagnostic garbage can.

The classifications have been based on the morphological and phenotypic resemblances to be drawn between the tumours and parallel, normal, adnexal components. Some tumours are markers of internal malignancy, such as epidermal and pilar cysts in Gardner's syndrome, tricholemmomas in Cowden's syndrome and cutaneous myxomas in Carney's complex, so these lesions must be recognized so that the possible underlying tumours can be recognized and treated at an early stage.

Table 7.1 Markers used in phenotyping eccrine tumours

Marker	Specificity
LP34	high molecular weight cytokeratin all keratinocytes
PKK1	epidermal basal cells
CEA	duct luminal lining cells
CAM 5.2	low molecular weight cytokeratin most secretory coil lining cells
S100	some secretory coil cells
HMFG1	secretory canaliculi
EMA	secretory canaliculi

It should also be borne in mind that whilst convention dictates that there are four kinds of adnexal skin tumours, classified into those showing eccrine, apocrine, sebaceous or hair follicle differentiation, there is, in addition, a fifth group not commonly mentioned which shows features of two or more of these four categories. Many adnexal tumours encountered in clinical practice fall into this fifth category. Unfortunately, this is not sufficient grounds for complacency, because some of the combined tumours have now started to be described in the literature (Nakhleh et al., 1990).

Furthermore, the classification of sweat gland tumours has been complicated by the description of the hybrid apoeccrine glands, which represent 45% of axillary glands and are also found in the pubes, face, scalp and breast. These develop at puberty from eccrine precursors, show features of both eccrine and apocrine secretion, and are especially common in naevus sebaceous (Sato and Sato, 1987; Sato et al., 1987).

7.1 Eccrine sweat gland tumours

The subclassification of benign eccrine sweat gland tumours has been well reviewed by Cotton (1987, 1991). Using a combination of conventional morphology and immunohistochemistry, he has simplified the diagnostic possibilities into four categories based on the apparent relationships between the four regions of the sweat gland (intraepidermal duct, intradermal straight duct, intradermal coiled duct and secretory coil), and the tumours which correspond to each region.

The basis of this classification is the use of antibodies to high and low molecular weight cytokeratins, CEA, S100 and epithelial membrane antigen allows the direction of differentiation of an individual tumour to be analysed (Tables 7.1, 7.2). High molecular weight cytokeratin

Table 7.2 Immunophenotype of eccrine tumours

Tumour type	HMWCK	CEA	LMWCK	S100	EMA
Intraepidermal duct	+	+	–	–	–
Dermal straight duct	–	+	+	–	–
Dermal coiled duct	–	–	+	–	–
Secretory coil	–	–	+	+	+

(HMWCK) is found in epidermal keratinocytes. CEA is found in the lining of eccrine ducts (Penneys *et al.*, 1982a, b). The majority of cells in the secretory epithelium and lower duct contain low molecular weight cytokeratin (LMWCK) in their cytoplasm. A minority of cells in the secretory coil are LMWCK negative and S100 protein positive. Differential staining for the alpha and beta subunits of S100 protein shows that the epithelial cells in the secretory coil stain for the alpha subunit and the luminal surface of cells in the coil and in the duct may show granular staining for the beta subunit (Noda *et al.*, 1988). The secretory canaliculi between secretory coil cells stain with HMFG1 or epithelial membrane antigen (EMA). Corresponding patterns of expression can be found in tumours and by establishing the tumour phenotype the tumour can be classified correctly. This approach may also help to identify the metastatic clear cell carcinoma of the kidney which may occasionally present with a cutaneous metastasis.

True squamous differentiation may be seen occasionally in both benign and malignant eccrine tumours. The presence of squamous islands within these tumours may represent entrapment of hair follicle or epidermal epithelium, squamous metaplasia or true malignant transformation (Kohda *et al.*, 1990).

7.1.1 Tumours of the intraepidermal duct

Three entities have been described, which all represent variations on a theme and these are *hidroacanthoma simplex*, *poroma* and *dermal duct tumour*. Of these three, *eccrine poroma* is the most widely recognized (Pinkus *et al.*, 1956; Hyman and Brownstein, 1969; Penneys *et al.*, 1970; Pylyser *et al.*, 1983). It is usually a solitary lesion on the sole of the foot, although rare cases occur on the palms and 'poromatosis' have been described, with hundreds of lesions on both palms and soles. The tumour is usually painful and consists of a central, raised nodule with a surrounding depression: the so-called 'moat and hillock' appearance.

The tumour is usually attached to the lower epidermis and has a well

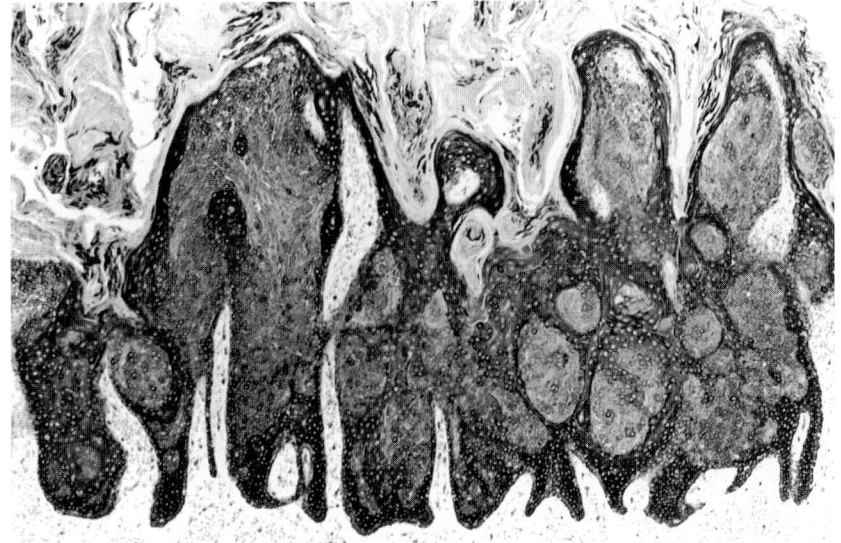

Figure 7.1   Hidroacanthoma simplex. Immunoperoxidase staining for high molecular weight cytokeratin (LP34) accentuates the boundaries between the nests of palely stained lesional cells and the surrounding darkly stained keratinocytes of the epidermis.

circumscribed margin with sharp demarcation from the surrounding epidermis. The tumour cells have a basaloid appearance, but with intercellular prickles. Staining for CEA will demonstrate the attempts at sweat duct differentiation within the tumour. This feature will not be seen in basal cell carcinomas, which never develops from sweat gland epithelium. Differentiation from seborrhoeic wart is sometimes a problem, but if the tumour contains horn cysts or duct-like structures filled with keratin and there is no evidence of CEA lined ducts, then it is not a poroma.

This description is of a circumscribed nodular tumour attached to the epidermis, which probably sits at the centre of a spectrum. At one end there is a form of poroma which is entirely intraepidermal, but is similar cytologically; this has been called 'hidroacanthoma simplex' (Smith and Coburn, 1956; Warner *et al.*, 1982). This is probably an unnecessary distinction, as is the description of a variant which is cytologically identical but lacks a direct connection with the epidermis: the so-called 'dermal duct tumour' (Hu *et al.*, 1978) which is entirely similar to poroma except for the lack of an epidermal connection.

Although the majority of these lesions are benign, occasional malig-

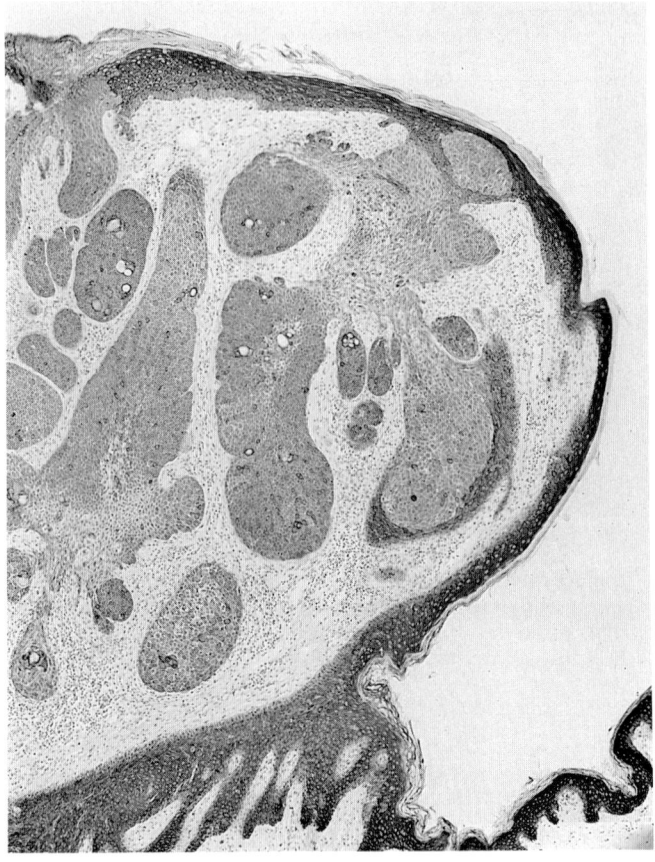

(a)

Figure 7.2 Hidradenoma. (a) In this apparently solid lesion staining for high molecular weight cytokeratin (LP 34) is weaker in the tumour than in the epidermis.

Normal skin. (b) Sweat gland acrosyringium with CEA positivity of duct lining cells, whilst (c) in the secretory coil the lumen and secretory canaliculi are demonstrated by membrane staining (HMFG 1).

Hidradenoma. (d) Low molecular weight cytokeratin (CAM 5.2) immunoreactivity is similar in tumour cells and in the epithelial cells of an adjacent sweat gland duct. (e) CEA staining shows foci of duct lumen differentiation within the tumour (Immunoperoxidase).

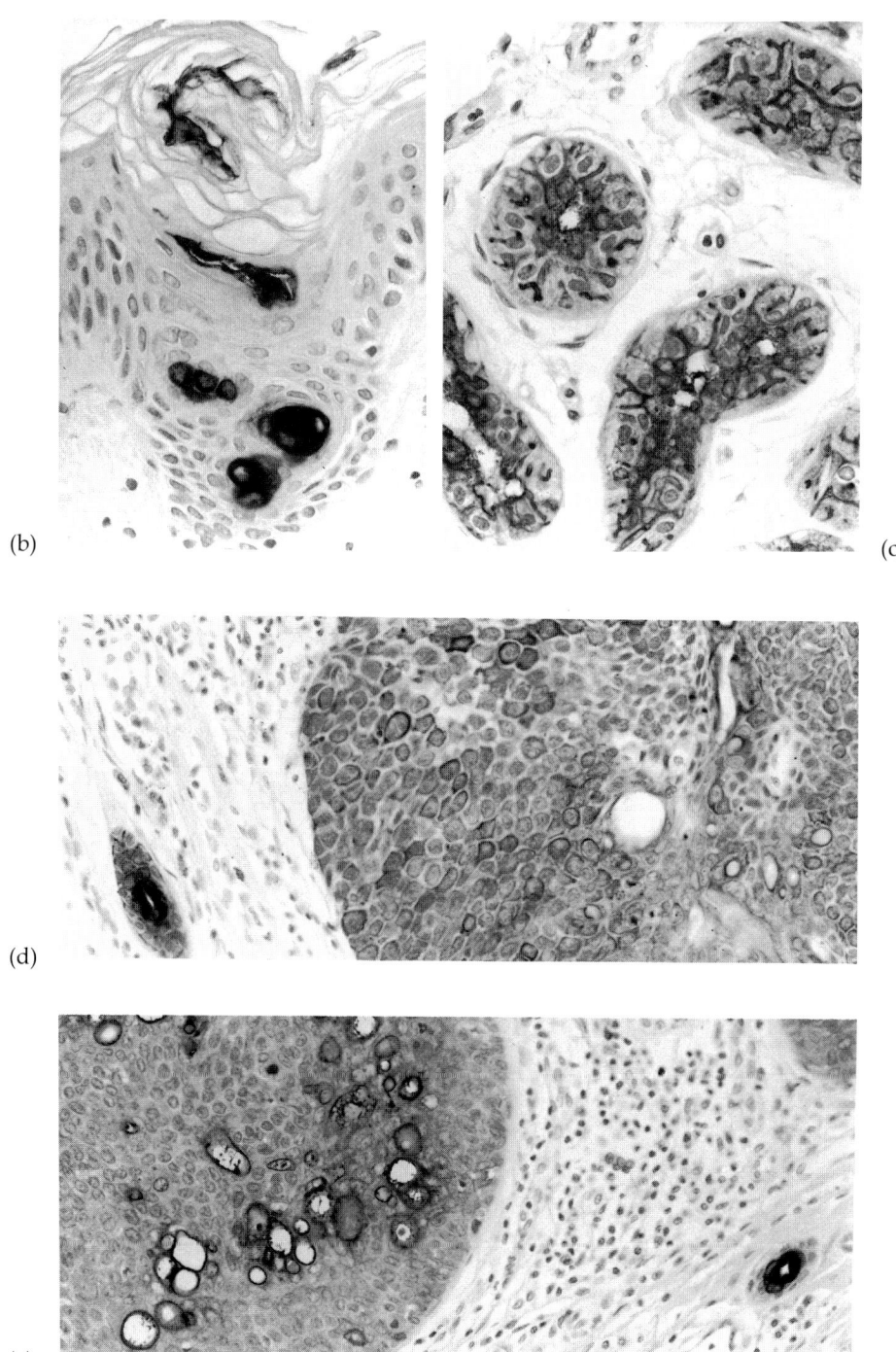

(b)

(c)

(d)

(e)

nant examples have been reported, usually on the lower limb (Darley *et al.*, 1983; Puttick *et al.*, 1986; Ryan *et al.*, 1986; Walsh, 1990).

Other lesions which appear to fall within this group include the syringoacanthoma, which resembles a seborrhoeic wart, Bowen's disease or squamous carcinoma clinically. The biopsy shows an acanthotic, papillomatous and hyperkeratotic lesion with well circumscribed nests of basaloid syringeal cells, with small, oval nuclei and moderate eosinophilic cytoplasm, surrounded by keratinocytes. Within the lesion there are small duct spaces containing mucin which is PAS and Alcian blue positive (Rahbari, 1984). The syringofibroadenoma also shows features suggesting an acrosyryngial origin: it consists of thin, anastamosing strands of epithelium attached to the underside of the epidermis and forming a lattice within which there are PAS positive acrosyryngeal formations (Kanitakis *et al.*, 1987). A similar lesion has been called acrosyryngeal naevus (Weedon and Lewis, 1977).

7.1.2   *Tumours of the intradermal straight duct*

In this category Cotton (1987) placed four groups of tumours: syringoma, spiradenoma, hidradenoma and mixed dermal tumour.

7.1.3   *Syringoma*

These occur as multiple small macules or papules on the lower eyelids and cheeks of women. They may erupt quite suddenly. They can also occur at other sites, such as the vulva, penis, abdomen, upper chest and neck.

The biopsy shows tiny ductal structures lined by a two-cell thick eccrine epithelium, often tapering off into comma- or tadpole-shaped tails. The ducts contain PAS-positive secretion and also contain CEA. They are surrounded by a dense, sclerotic and sparsely cellular stroma, which contains variable numbers of cells which are sometimes called myoepithelial cells, although they could probably be derived from any cell type within the sweat gland (Argenyi *et al.*, 1989). The differential diagnosis is from desmoplastic trichepithelioma, which is a lesion characterized by trichoepithelial duct-like structures in a desmoplastic stroma.

7.1.4   *Spiradenoma*

These tumours occur as single nodules, or groups of nodules, in the dermis and without any epidermal connection (Revis *et al.*, 1988). There are two types of cells present: peripheral cells with small, dark

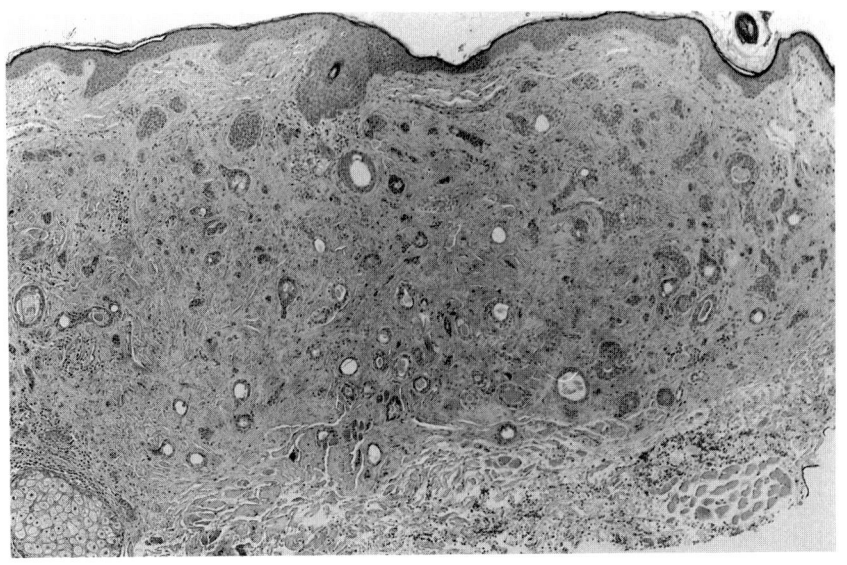

(a)

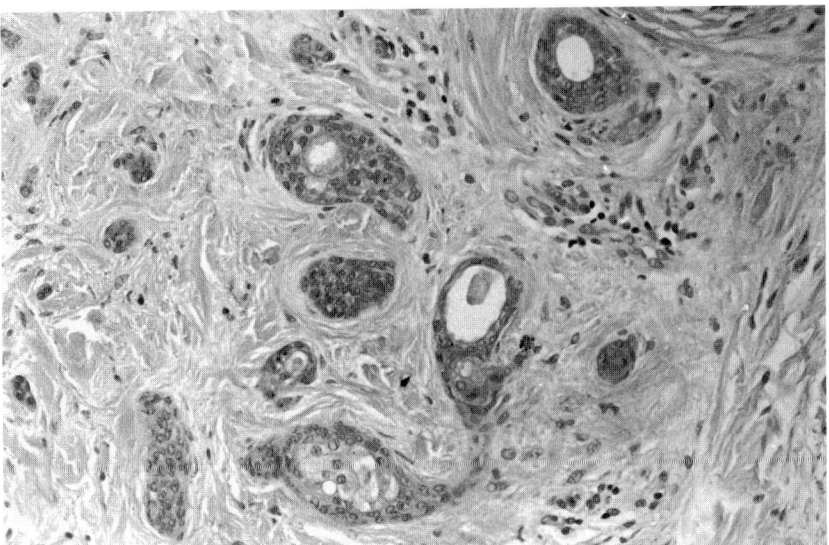

(b)

Figure 7.4 Syringoma. (a) A moderately well circumscribed tumour filling the dermis, and (b) containing epithelial elements differentiated to small ducts and 'tadpoles'.

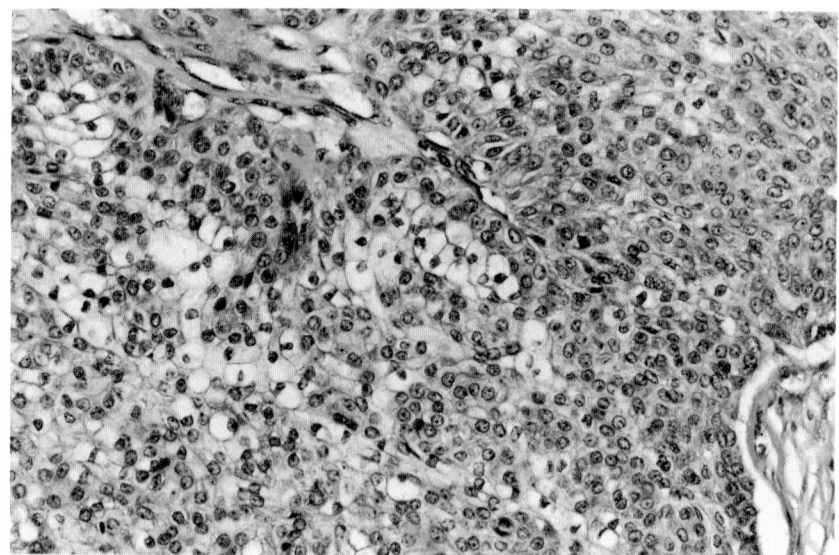

Figure 7.5 Clear cell hidradenoma. A solid sheet of relatively uniform cells with clear cytoplasm.

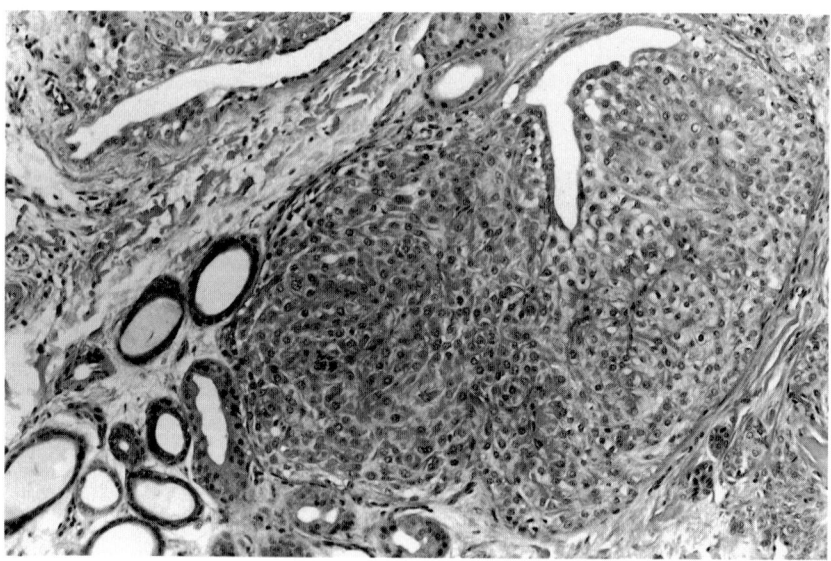

Figure 7.6 Hidradenoma showing close relationship with residual normal ducts.

nuclei and little cytoplasm, and larger, more centrally placed cells with larger, paler nuclei and moderate amounts of pale cytoplasm. Often, these pale cells form cords which appear to spiral within the tumour and may contain small ducts. Mitoses are rare. The ducts may contain CEA (Penneys, 1982), but do not contain HMFG1 or EMA-like antigens (Kariniemi, 1984).

On this basis, it seems most likely that spiradenomas are derived from the dermal straight duct, with predominant features of duct supporting cells rather than duct luminal cells: a proposal that is supported by electron microscopy, which also shows features of ductal rather than secretory coil cells (Jitsukawa *et al.*, 1987).

Malignant transformation has been described in spiradenoma (Cooper *et al.*, 1985a; Wick *et al.*, 1987), as has an associated malignant stromal component giving rise to an appearance of carcinosarcoma (McKee *et al.*, 1990).

7.1.5   Giant vascular eccrine spiradenoma

This rare variant of spiradenoma is characterized by its large size (up to 50 mm) and high vascularity. The tumours occur in elderly patients and usually have a relatively short history. The cellular component is similar to the usual type of spiradenoma, but the vascular component, consisting of cavernous, thin-walled vessels is very prominent (Cotton *et al.*, 1986).

7.1.6   Hidradenoma

There is great variation within this category. Many different names have been given to variants of hidradenoma, with consequent grounds for confusion and misdiagnosis. Cotton (1987) found that hidradenomas fell into two overlapping groups. One group showed predominant features of secretory coil differentiation, whilst the other showed features more in favour of an origin from intradermal straight duct.

Individual tumours are likely to be predominantly solid, multilobular and possibly with cystic areas. The presence or absence of slits, lumina and cysts corresponds to whether the lesion is of predominantly secretory coil or predominantly ductal type.

7.1.7   Mixed dermal tumour

Otherwise known as chondroid syringomas, these tumours present as firm, solitary intradermal or subcutaneous nodules on the face and occasionally on the eyelid (Jordan *et al.*, 1989). They are the cutaneous

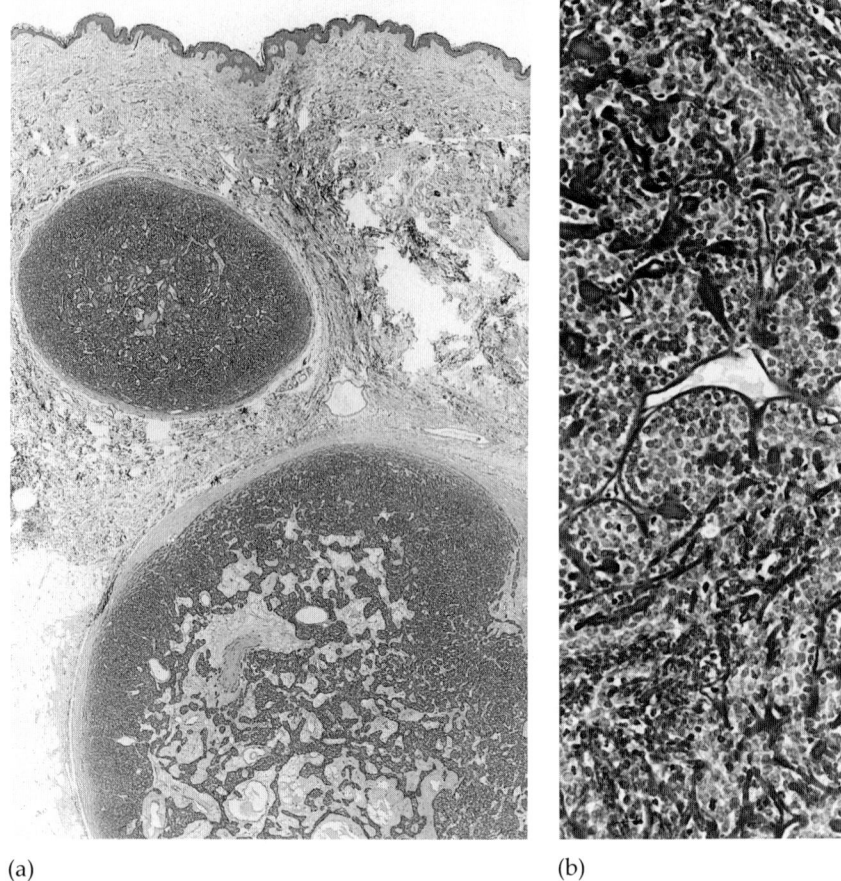

(a)   (b)

Figure 7.7   Spiradenoma. (a) A nodular tumour showing straight duct differentiation with two cell types, and with (b) PAS-positive basement membrane material between cords of cells.

analogue of pleomorphic adenomas of salivary gland and consist of well circumscribed dermal nodules containing a mixture of epithelial and stromal components (Noda *et al.*, 1986). The inner layers of epithelial cells stain for CEA and EMA, consistent with a ductal origin, whilst the outer layers and stroma do not show any evidence of a myoepithelial phenotype (Argenyi *et al.*, 1988). The stroma appears 'chondroid' and although true cartilage is not formed, stromal cells may be S100 positive in the same way as true chondrocytes may be. In essence, these tumours appear to be a form of hidradenoma in which an unusual stroma is secreted, probably by the S100 positive cells (Dominguez

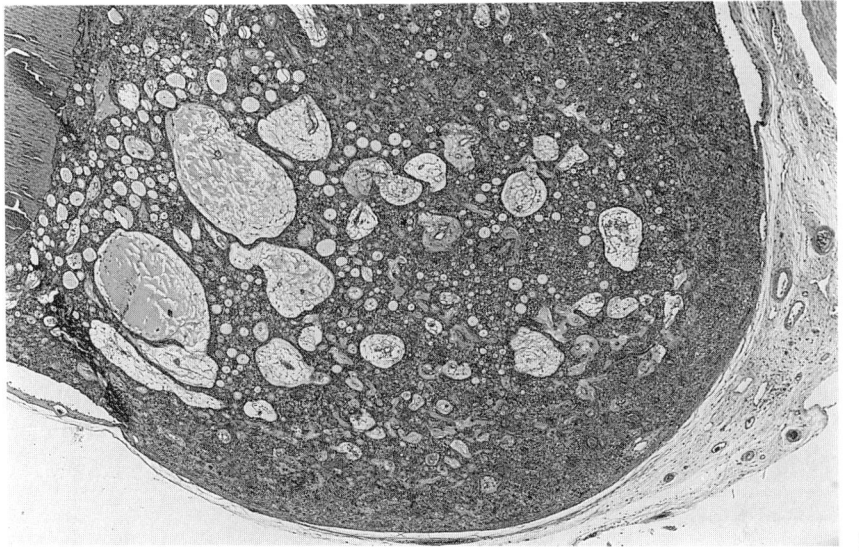

(a)

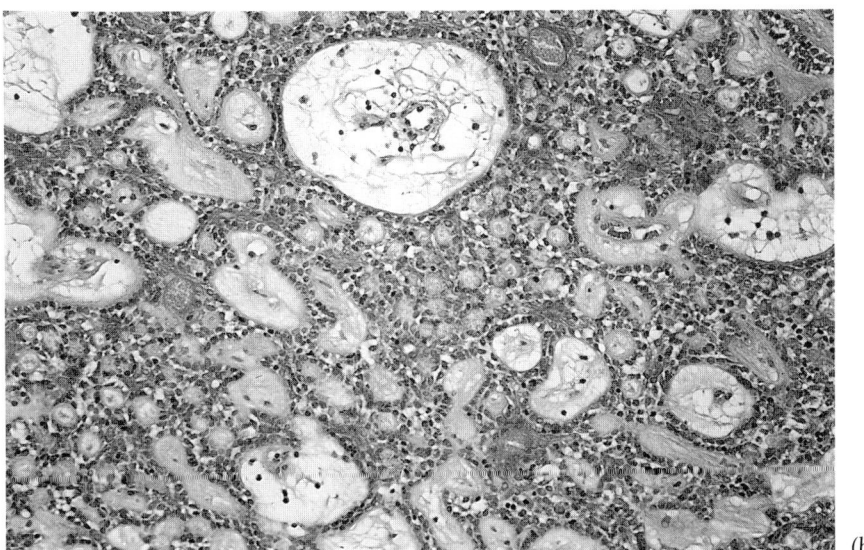

(b)

Figure 7.8 Spiradenoma (a and b). A multi-nodular tumour showing straight duct differentiation with two cell types present.

Inglesias *et al.*, 1990). Having said that two variants have been described, showing either apocrine or eccrine differentiation, only one of which may be seen in any one tumour. Either variant can contain elements showing follicular or sebaceous differentiation (Hassab-El-Naby *et al.*, 1989). Malignant change can occur (Shvili and Rotham, 1986). Similar tumours may occur in the salivary glands, especially the parotid gland, usually in association with multiple dermal tumours (Batsakis and Brannon, 1981; Herbst and Utz, 1984).

7.1.8   *Tumours of the intradermal coiled duct*

Only one tumour falls into this category; the cylindroma (Cotton and Braye, 1984). This occurs sporadically as a tumour of the scalp or forehead, and classically, but rarely, as an autosomal dominantly inherited condition, with the development of multiple tumours on the scalp and forehead, which can spread to cover the scalp, forming a 'turban' tumour.

The cylindroma consists of well circumscribed groups of surrounded by PAS-positive-diastase resistant hyalin. These groups of cells form a 'jigsaw-puzzle-like' appearance, in keeping with their suggested origin from a coiled duct. Within the cellular lobules there are two sorts of rounded spaces: one contains hyalin whilst the other takes the form of small ducts lined by clear, cuboidal epithelial cells secreting mucin.

As might be expected from a tumour which shows appearances consistent with an origin in the coiled duct, individual tumours may show overlapping appearances of hidradenoma, either of secretory coil or straight duct type.

7.1.9   *Tumours of the secretory coil*

The broad spread of lesions described as hidradenoma includes tumours of apparent secretory coil origin, as described above.

7.2   Apocrine gland tumours

Apocrine gland tumours are rare but are fairly easy to diagnose if the typical features of apocrine differentiation are found. Apocrine glands have an essentially similar structure to eccrine glands but a different form of secretion. Tumours can be divided into those showing features of ductal or of secretory differentiation. In a typical gland, the epithelial cells are columnar, with parabasal nuclei, prominent supranuclear cytoplasmic palor, corresponding to the Golgi zone, and with decapitation secretion taking place at the luminal pole of the cell.

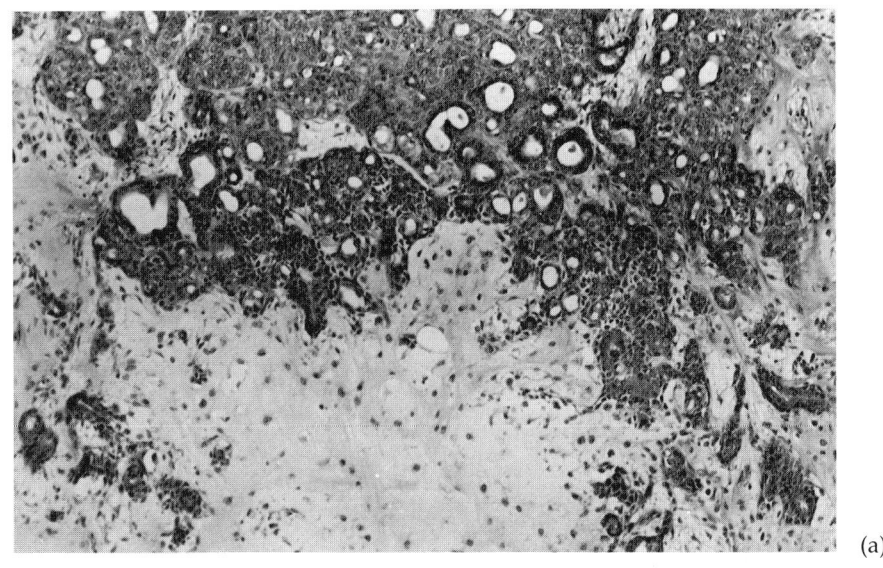

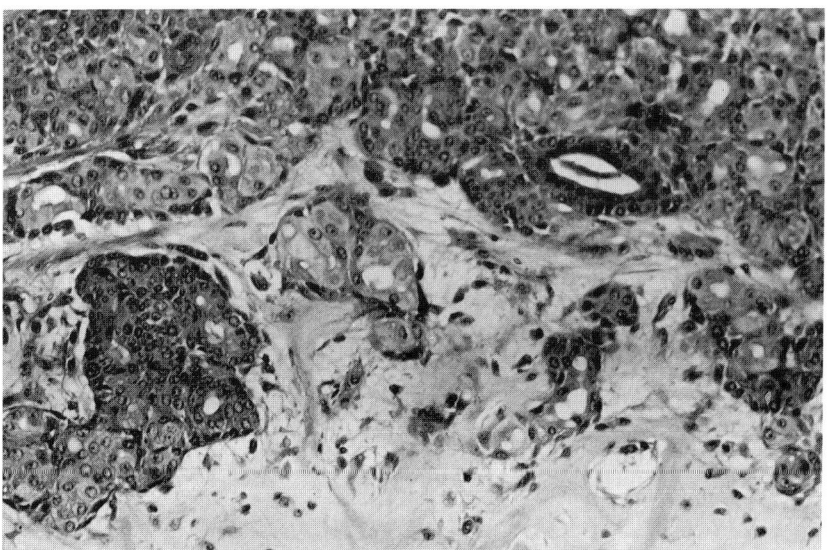

Figure 7.9 Mixed dermal tumour (a and b). Well-differentiated epithelial component with duct differentiation and a chondroid stroma.

They are found particularly in the axilla, but also occur around the face, scalp and genitalia, as well as in association with the specialized apocrine glands of the eyelids (Moll's glands) and the ceruminous glands of the external auditory canal (Sacks *et al.*, 1987; Ahmed and Nath, 1988).

7.2.1   Papillary syringadenoma

Most of these adenomas occur on the head and neck, most commonly as part of an organoid naevus. They usually have a verrucous surface with numerous ductal structures leading to glands, which often have apoeccrine rather than simply apocrine features.

7.2.2   Papillary hidradenoma

These tumours resemble intraduct papillomas of breast and occur almost always in women, arising mainly in the skin of the vulva and sometimes at other sites in the milk line. They probably arise from ectopic breast tissue.

7.2.3   Fibroadenoma

Occasional reports of apocrine fibroadenoma of the perineum describe tumours which are similar to fibroadenomas of the breast.

7.2.4   Apocrine carcinoma

Apocrine carcinoma is extremely rare and of those cases reported the majority have arisen in the axilla, where the problem is to differentiate them from carcinomas of the breast. They also occur in the eyelid, but reports are too few to draw conclusions about likely behaviour (Thomson and Tanner, 1989).

7.3   Microcystic adnexal carcinoma

This entity is rare and is distinguished by benign histological features and locally aggressive behaviour. The lesions typically occur as a single, flesh-coloured papule on the upper lip of a woman, aged about 44, but have also been seen in the axilla and on the buttock. This tumour is an example of the fifth category of adnexal tumour, showing a variety of forms of differentiation.

The biopsy shows a lesion containing nests of basal cells, some of which form horn cysts and abortive follicles lying in a desmoplastic

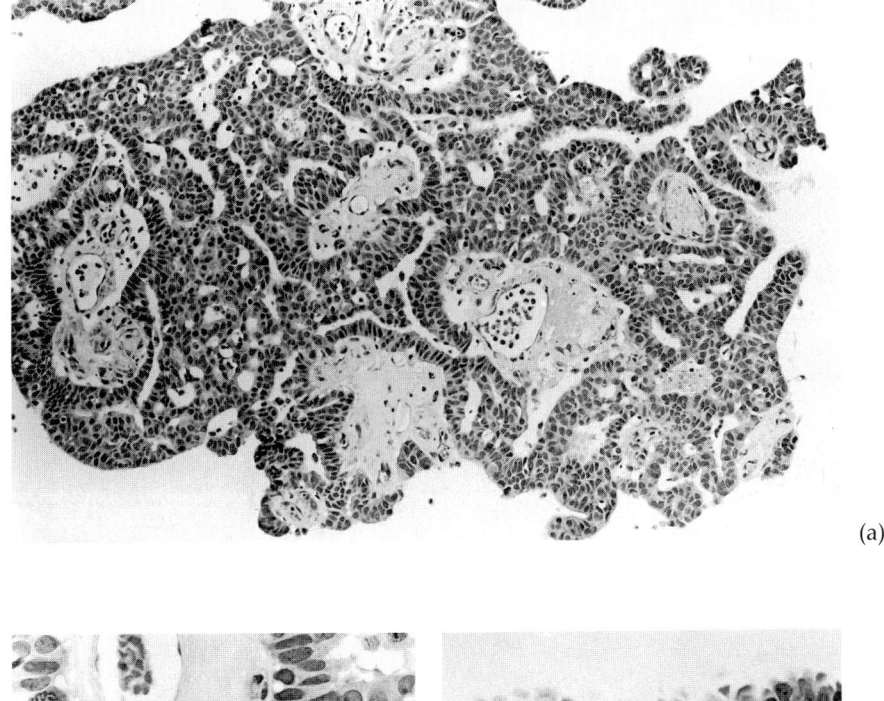

(a)

(b)

(c)

Figure 7.10 Papillary hidradenoma (a, b and c). The tumour has a moderate amount of stroma within papillae and shows apocrine differentiation of the epithelial cells.

stroma. Elsewhere there are eccrine structures; ducts and glands lined by a two cell thick epithelium. Stromal amyloid may also be present (Kato *et al.*, 1989). At the base, strands and individual cells dissect between collagen bundles and skeletal muscle and there may also be perineural invasion. Cytological atypia and mitotic figures are, however, rare and excision with clear margins is sufficient treatment. Local recurrence has been reported in about 40% of cases including one after 30 years (Lupton and McMarlin, 1986). One case of lymph node involvement, probably due to direct perineural spread, has also been recorded (Cooper *et al.*, 1985b). Immunohistochemical studies have shown reactivity for CEA within the ducts but not the horn cysts (Nickoloff, 1986).

Origin from a pluripotential adnexal keratinocyte, capable of both follicular and sweat gland differentiation has been suggested (Goldstein *et al.*, 1982). Previous radiotherapy has also been suggested as an aetiological factor (Nickoloff, 1986). There has been some debate about the most appropriate name. The alternative title of sclerosing sweat duct carcinoma has been proposed by Cooper (1985b, 1986), and similar lesions were reported under the title of sclerosing epithelial hamartoma (Macdonald *et al.*, 1977). Irrespective of the name used, it is an important tumour to recognize because of the high likelihood of local recurrence (Chow *et al.*, 1989).

7.4 Hair follicle tumours

Tumours of the hair follicle can also be classified according to the differentiation that they show (Massa and Medenica, 1985; Mehregan, 1985a). As with sweat gland tumours, there are tumours which show features of the intraepidermal follicle, the external hair sheath, the hair matrix and the hair germ, as well as tumours of the perifollicular mesenchyme. There are also a group of tumours which appear to be of hair follicle type but do not show specific features of one part of the structure.

One clue to the hair follicle nature of a lesion is the presence of calcification. If a putative adnexal tumour shows areas of calcification, it is almost certainly going to be a hair follicle tumour. The calcification is related to the production of a parathyroid hormone-related protein, which has been demonstrated in hair follicles and epidermis but is not found in sweat glands (Kukreja *et al.*, 1988; Danks *et al.*; 1989; Hayman *et al.*, 1989).

Malignant hair follicle tumours are exceedingly rare, to such an extent that the differential diagnosis between basal cell carcinoma and trichoepithelioma sorts tumours into those that may or may not recur. A review of extensive experience of such tumours in the eyelid showed very few recurrences in trichoepithelioma, which allows a more conservative approach to be made to the removal of the tumour (Simpson *et al.*, 1989).

7.4.1 *Tumours of intraepidermal follicle and infundibulum*

Examples of tumours which fall into this classification are difficult to come by but a case of an intraepidermal nesting epithelial tumour

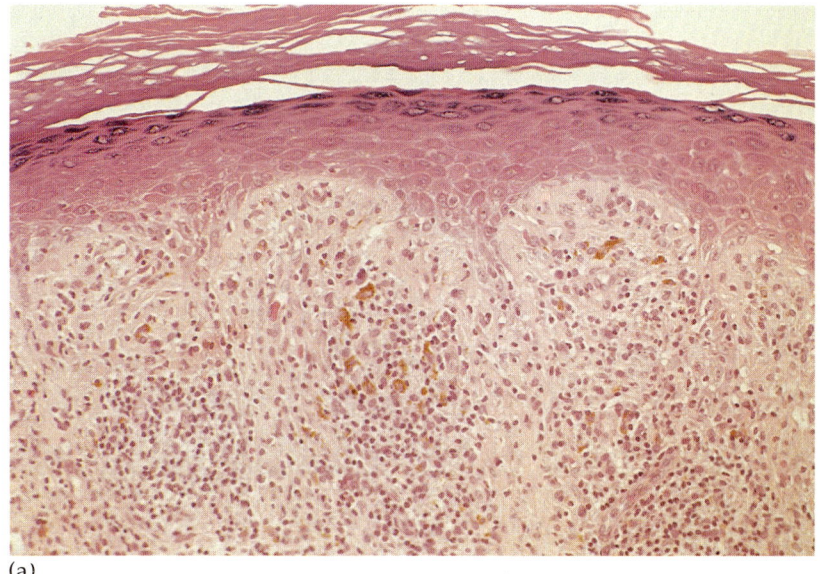

(a)

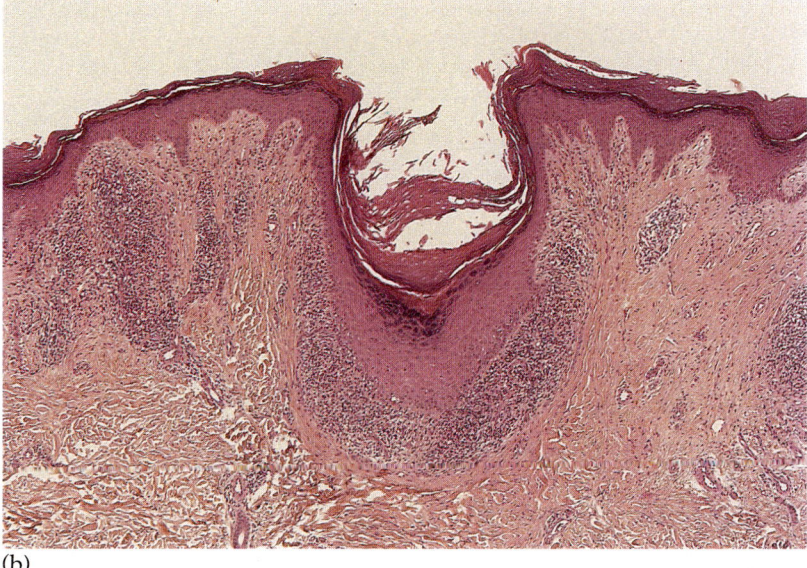

(b)

Plate 21 (a) Lichen planus. The lesion shows orthokeratotic hyperkeratosis, with a band of lymphocytes infiltrating the papillary dermis and basal epidermis, which shows a saw tooth profile. (b) Lichen planopilaris. The lichenoid infiltrate of lymphocytes surrounds the hair follicle and spares the intervening epidermis.

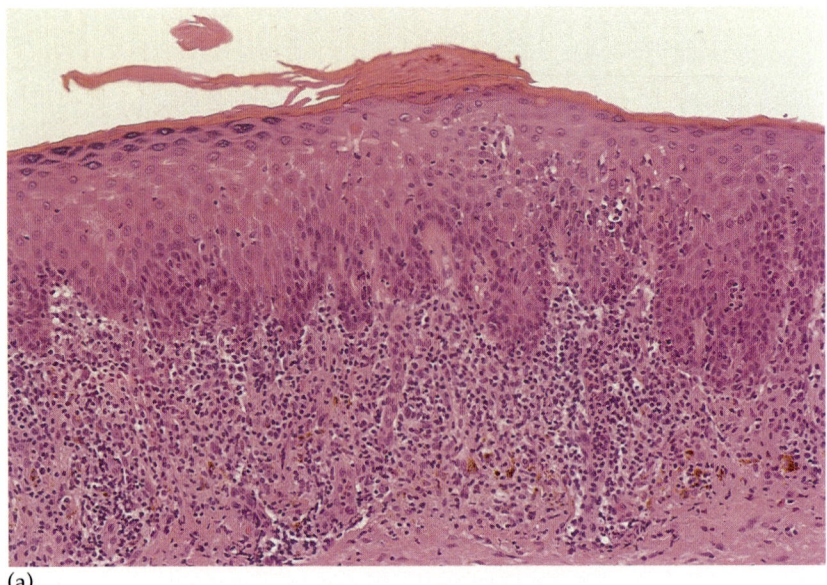

(a)

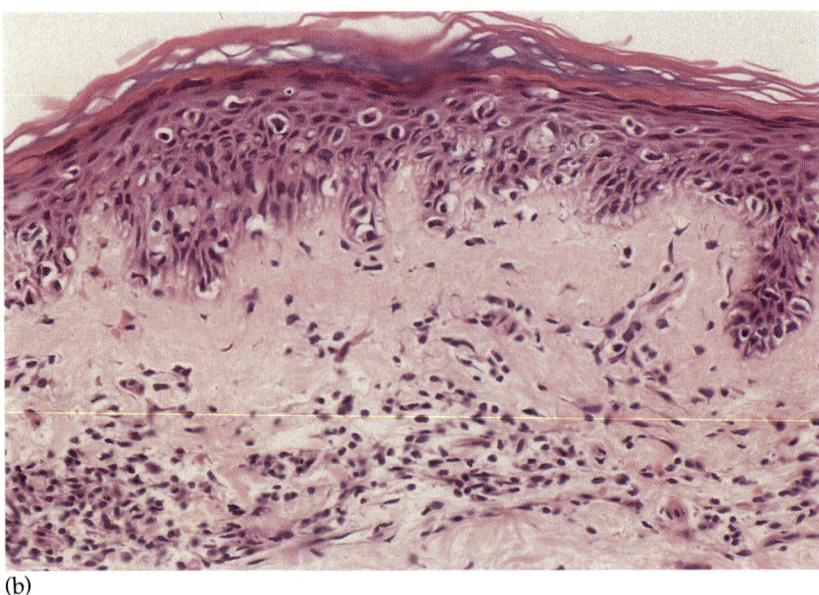

(b)

Plate 22 (a) Psoriasis. The epidermis is acanthotic, with overlying hyperkeratotic scale and with a dermal lymphocytic infiltrate showing little epidermotropism. (b) Cutaneous T-cell lymphoma. The epidermotropic infiltrate has a pagetoid appearance, but T-cell markers were positive.

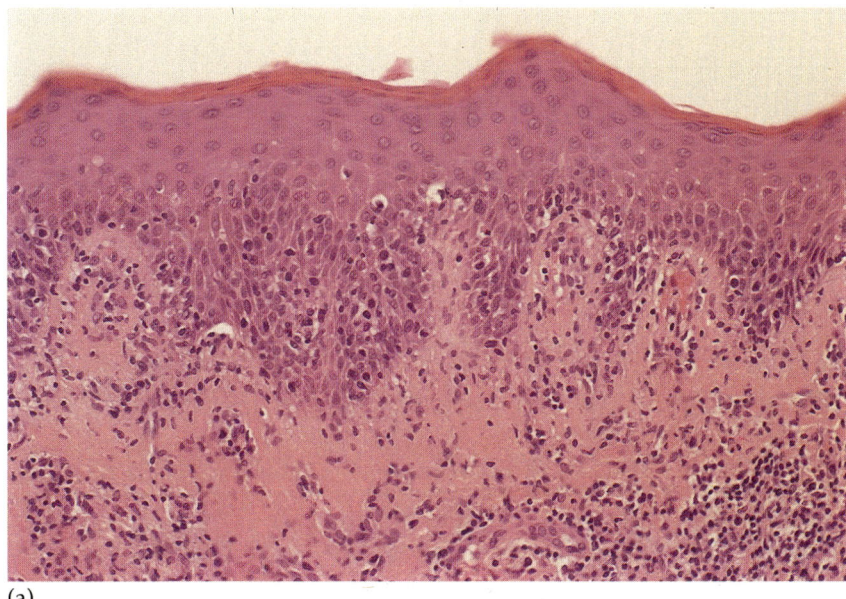

(a)

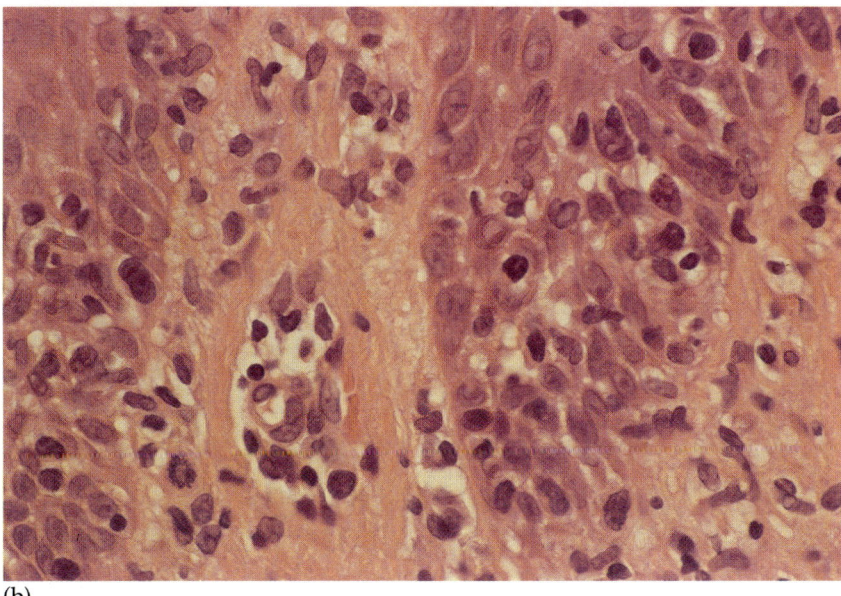

(b)

Plate 23 Cutaneous T-cell lymphoma. (a) A biopsy from the erythematous stage, with a moderately cellular, epidermotrophic infiltrate. (b) The infiltrating lymphocytes are medium-sized with a few showing cerebriform nuclei.

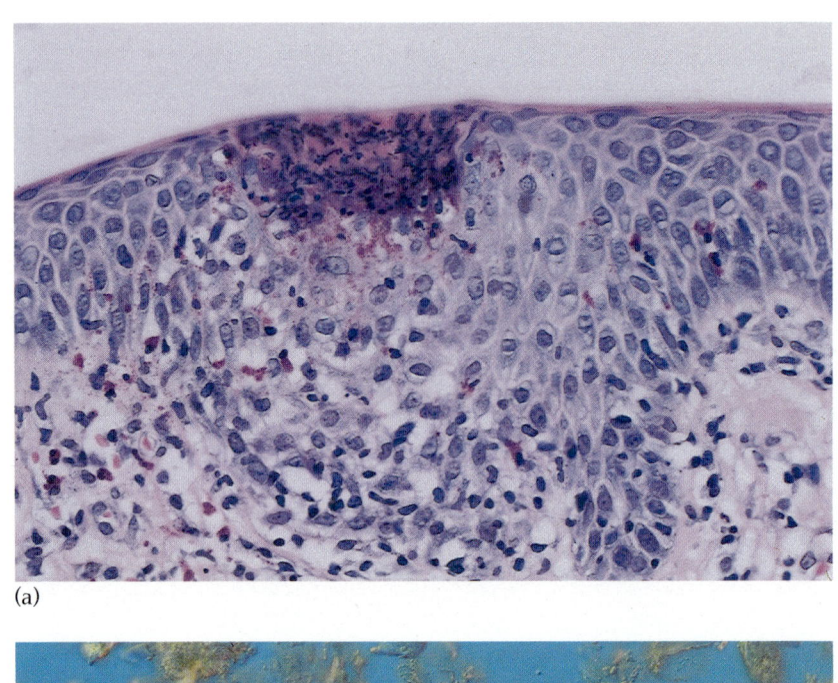

(a)

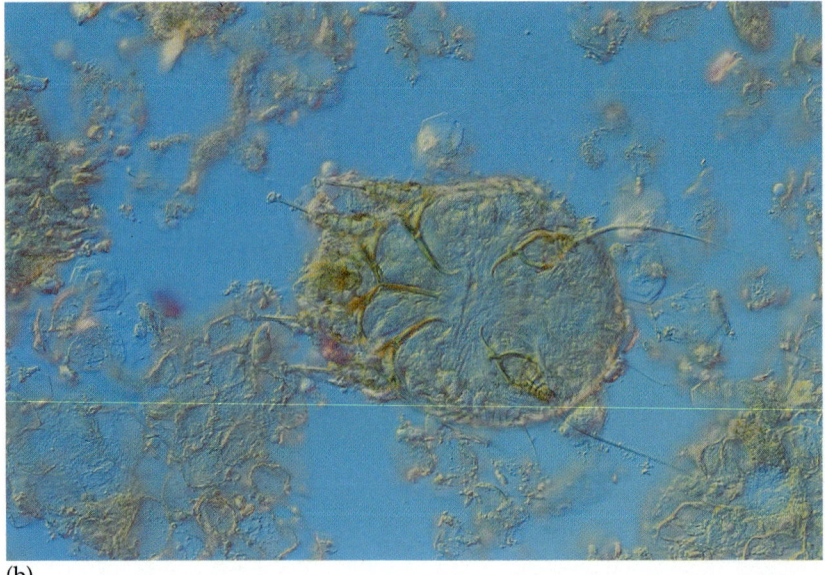

(b)

Plate 24   Scabies. (a) The epidermis shows a spongiotic lesion with occasional eosinophils, together with a superficial microabscess (Acid orcein Giemsa). (b) The *Sarcoptes scabei* mite can be found in scrapings from active lesions (Nomarski interference contrast).

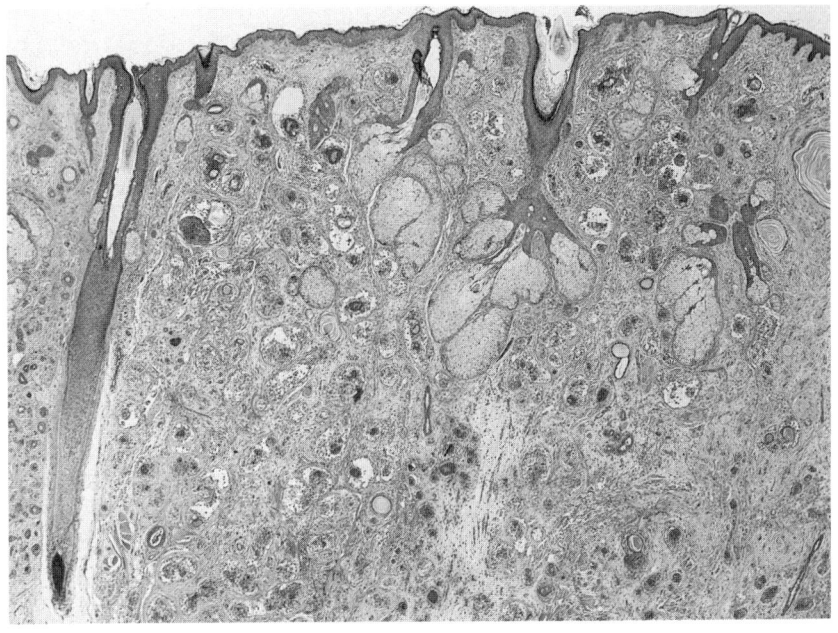

(a)

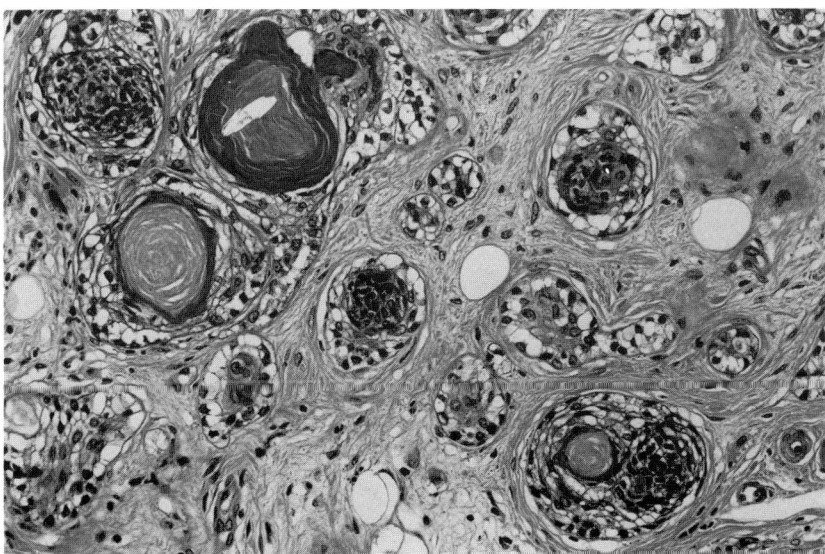

(b)

Figure 7.11 Microcystic adnexal carcinoma. (a) The tumour infiltrates deeply into the dermis and around appendages, with (b) nests of clear cell with central keratin-filled spaces.

showing cytological similarity to hair follicle cortical cells and with histo-chemical and immunohistochemical features of hair follicle differentia-tion has been described. As well as containing hair follicle cytokeratins the tumour was PAS and CEA negative. The term intraepidermal pilar epithelioma was proposed as a name for this tumour (Ito *et al.*, 1988).

7.4.2   Inverted follicular keratosis

Most of these nodular lesions occur on the head and neck and show a variety of morphologies resembling warts, keratoacanthomas and cysts. The lesions have in common a proliferation of outer root sheath epithe-lium with basaloid cells at the periphery and larger keratinizing cells towards the centre, producing the characteristic feature: the squamous eddy (Mehregan, 1985a).

7.4.3   Dilated pore of Winer

This is a relatively common lesion and presents as an enlarged follicle plugged with keratin. The biopsy shows a pit lined by outer root, sheath-type epithelium, filled with keratin in the manner of a large follicle infundibulum and with a varying degree of budding of epithe-lial projections into the surrounding stroma (Winer, 1954).

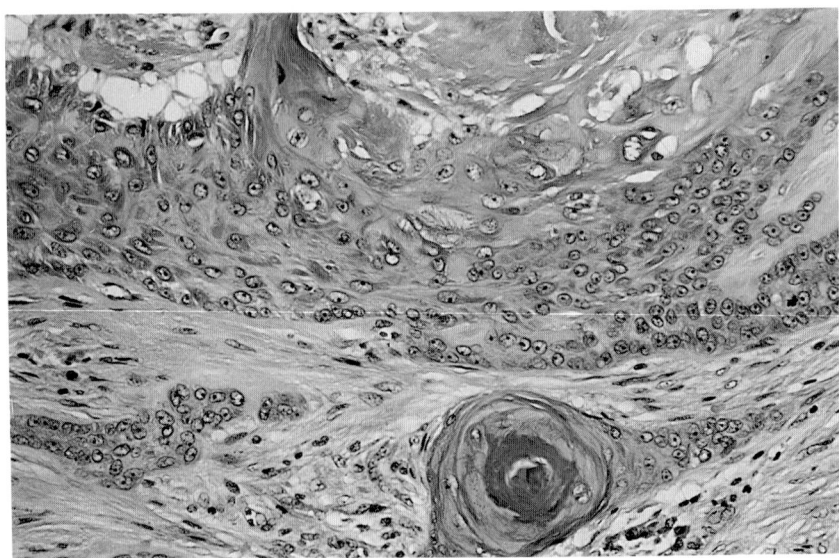

Figure 7.12 Proliferating pilar tumour. Tricholemmal cells form interconnecting lobules, with mild cytological atypia and occasional mitoses.

7.4.4   Trichofolliculoma

These lesions present as small, single, flesh-coloured nodules on the face, with a tuft of white hairs protruding from the centre. They consist of a central, dilated primary follicle, filled with hair and keratin, with many small, complete or incomplete secondary follicles arranged around it (Pinkus and Sutton, 1965).

7.4.5   Tumours of external hair sheath

Pilar or tricholemmal cyst

One of the two kinds of cyst beloved to general surgeons as sebaceous cysts, they occur mainly on the scalp, but also at other sites. The cyst is lined by outer root, sheath-type epithelium and shows tricholemmal keratinization. There is no granular cell layer in the epithelium. The cyst contents may calcify, in keeping with other hair follicle tumours.

Proliferating pilar or tricholemmal tumour

These tumours are usually exophytic and can achieve a quite large size and show marked cytological atypia. The appearance is one of inter-connecting lobules of keratinocytes, showing predominantly tricholem-mal differentiation, in an otherwise well circumscribed tumour. Clear cell change may occur and mimic other clear cell adnexal tumours. There may be keratin formation at the periphery of the tumour, which may also be present in the surrounding tumour-associated stroma. There may also be a locally aggressive growth pattern, which together with associated cytological atypia and abnormal mitoses, raises the possibility of true malignant behaviour (Jawarski, 1988). The overwhel-ming majority of these tumours do not metastasize, irrespective of their cytological appearance.

Tricholemmoma

The tricholemmoma is often in continuity with the epidermis and has a rounded, smooth lobular pattern. The basal layer of cells is palisaded and there is usually a prominent basement membrane. There may be keratotic elements within the epithelium and the stroma may be quite sclerotic (Headington, 1980).

Tricholemmoma may be solitary but also forms part of Cowden's syndrome, in which multiple small papules appear on the face, repre-

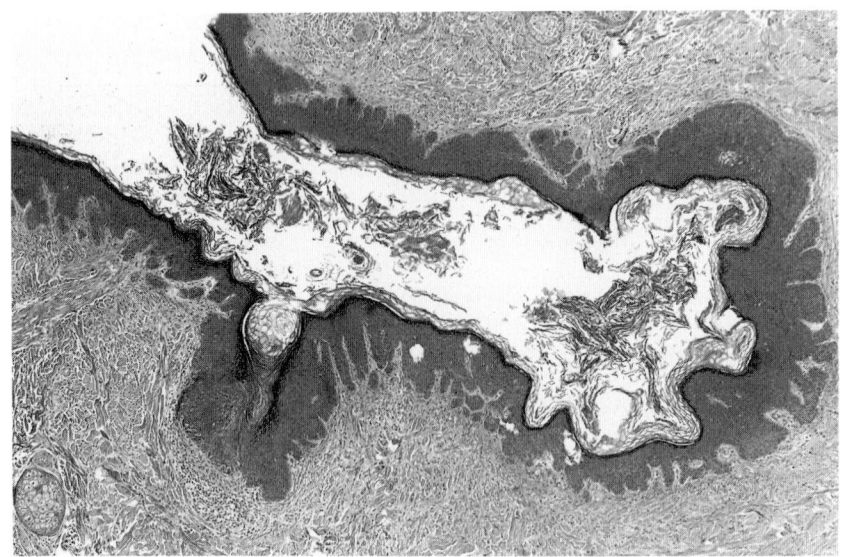

(a)

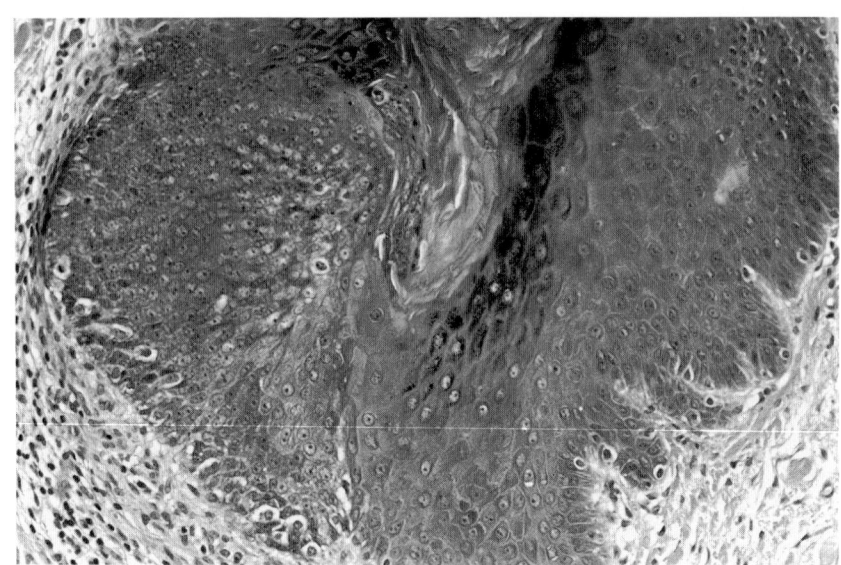

(b)

Figure 7.13 Pore of Winer. (a) A deep pit, with (b) attempts at hair follicle differentiation in parts of the wall.

senting fibromas, neuromas and verrucous keratoses as well as tricholemmomas. Sometimes combined lesions may be present, with a
verrucous surface and tricholemmal base. The importance of this condition is its association with an increased risk of breast cancer (Brownstein *et al.*, 1979; Thyresson and Doyle, 1981).

Tricholemmal carcinoma

Low grade tricholemmal carcinomas are likely to grow in continuity
with the epidermis, or with the outer root sheath of the follicle, with a
lobular growth pattern, with clear cell change and malignant cytological
features. Such tumours are likely to behave no more aggressively than
a nodular basal cell carcinoma.

Less well differentiated tumours are more difficult to define and to
differentiate from other poorly characterized tumours such as a clear
cell type of proliferating tricholemmal tumour, clear cell acrospiroma
and so-called clear cell squamous cell carcinoma. High grade tumours
are probably indistinguishable from squamous cell carcinoma.

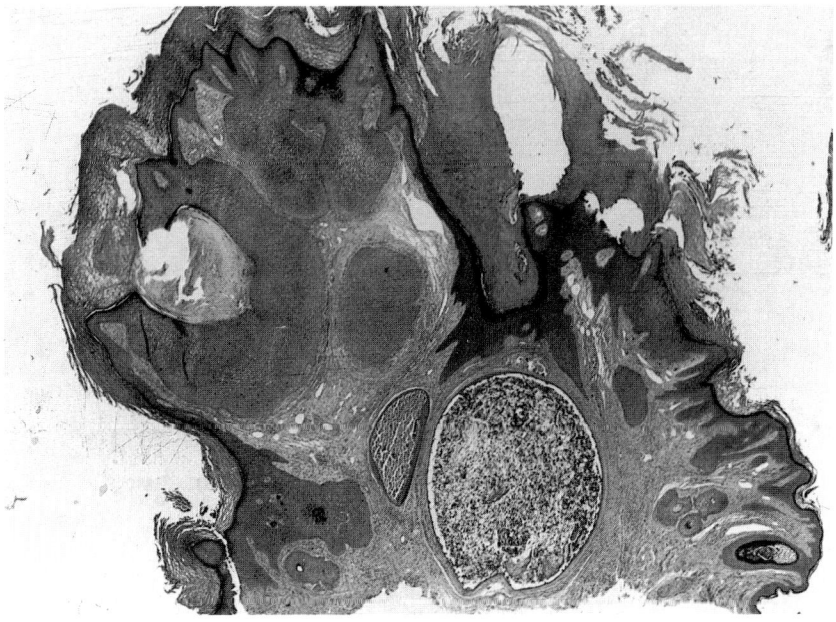

(a)

Figure 7.14   Tricholemmoma. (a) A warty lesion, with (b) pale acanthotic
epithelium resembling outer root sheath. (Cont.)

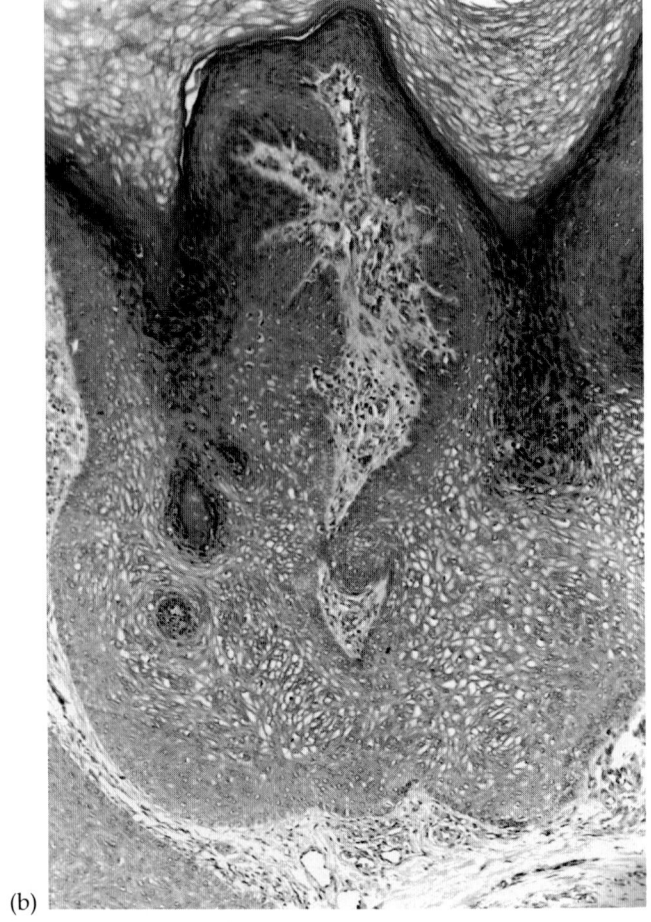

(b)

Figure 7.14 (Cont.)

7.4.6 Tumours of hair matrix

Pilomatrixoma

Also known as the calcifying epithelioma of Malherbe, these lesions present as firm dermal nodules, usually on the limb of a child (Malherbe and Chenantais, 1880; Moehlenbeck, 1973). They show a characteristic, scrambled-up appearance, with epithelium merging into ghost cells and with stromal calcification, often associated with giant cell granulomatous reaction, sometimes progressing to ossification.

Analysis of the keratins present showed that the predominant pattern

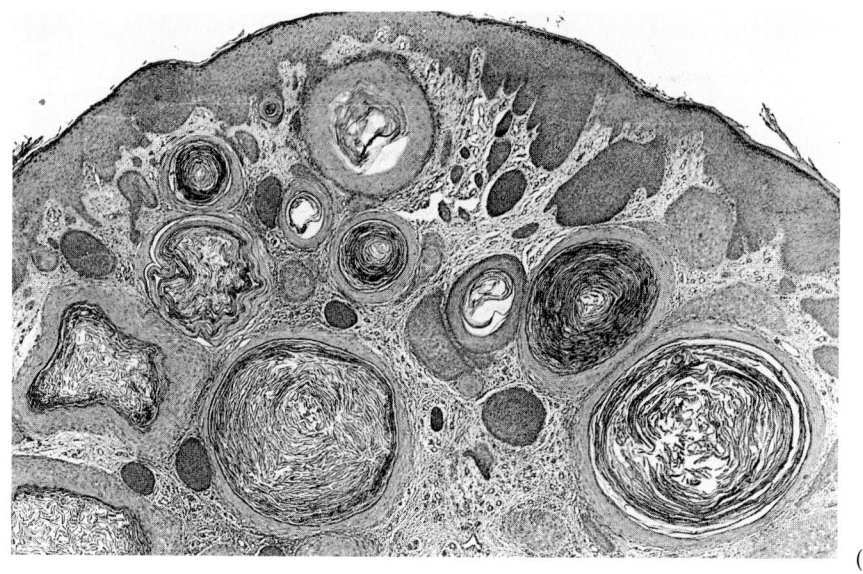

(a)

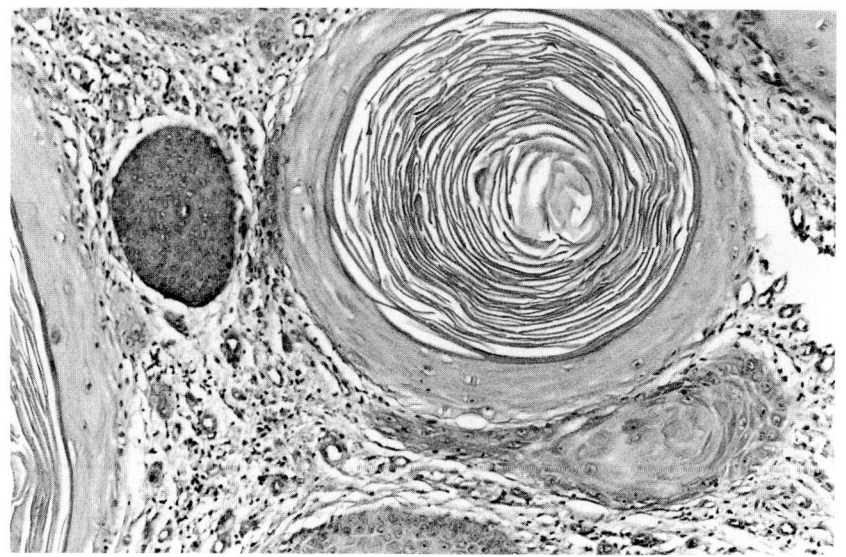

(b)

Figure 7.15 Trichoadenoma. (a) A circumscribed tumour; (b) with many horn cysts.

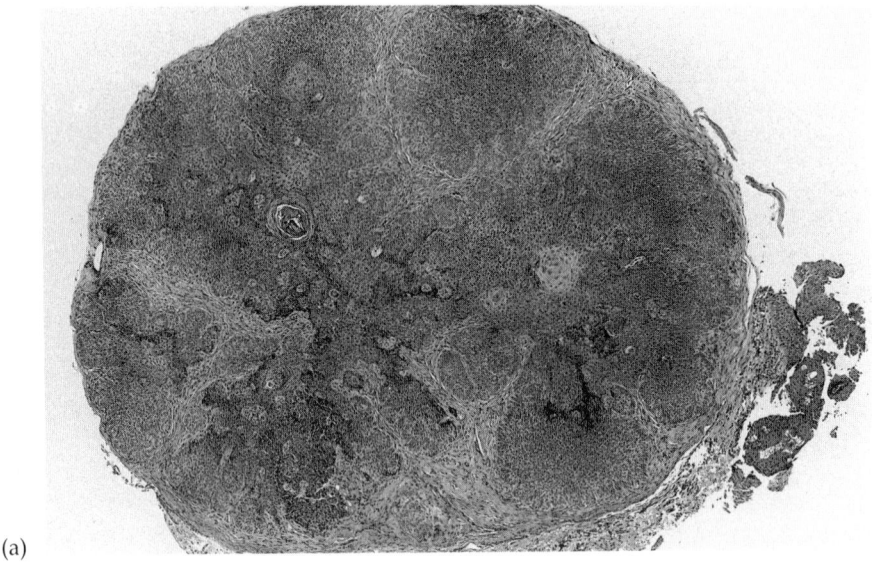

(a)

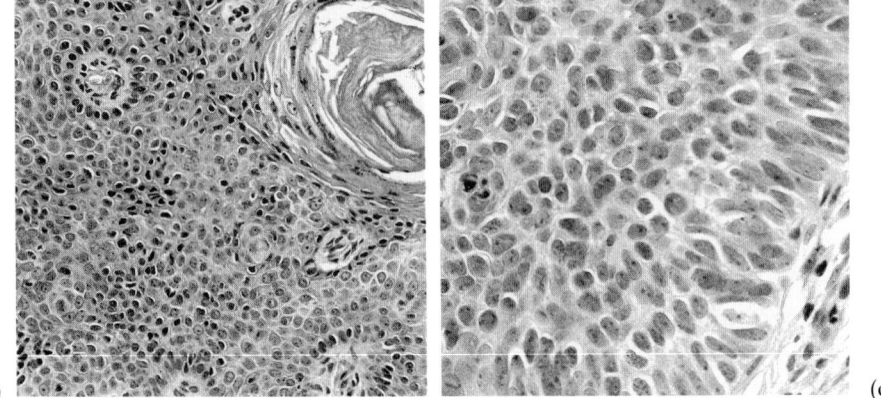

(b)

(c)

Figure 7.16 Trichoadenoma. (a) A solid nodular tumour removed by curettage, with (b) horn cyst formation and (c) pale outer root sheath type epithelium.

was one of hair cortex lineage, but with a proportion showing an epidermal phenotype (Moll *et al.*, 1988).

Giant calcifying epithelioma, or matrical carcinoma

Sometimes these tumours of the head and neck may be large and show an increased cellularity, cytological atypia and a high mitotic rate. They may have an infiltrative margin, erosion of the overlying epidermis, local recurrence and vascular invasion suggestive of malignant change (Gromiko, 1927; Prandetsky and Iuzuinkevich, 1969; Reed and Lamar, 1966; Rothman *et al.*, 1976; Lopansri and Mihm, 1989, Sasaki *et al.*, 1976; Van der Walt and Rohlova, 1984; Weedon *et al.*, 1980), although only one definite example of distant metastasis has been reported (Gould *et al.*, 1984).

   These large lesions can, therefore, be treated by simple excision in the majority of cases, although there may be a bias in that, paradoxically, the poorly-differentiated examples of matrical carcinoma may not be recognized, because they lack a well differentiated matrix component.

7.4.7   Tumours of hair germ

These are very rare tumours and fall into three groups depending on whether they show absent (trichoblastoma), partial (trichoblastic fibroma), or complete (trichogenic trichoblastoma) induction of hair follicle differentiation by the associated stroma (Headington, 1976). Differential diagnosis is mainly from basal cell carcinoma.

(*a*)   *Trichoblastomas*   These do not show fibroblastic stroma, but consist of small uniform lobules of basaloid cells (Headington, 1976).

(*b*)   *Trichoblastic fibromas*   These are occur as solitary nodules of about 1 cm in size on hairy sites, such as the scalp and vulva, and have no familial associations. Microscopically, there are well differentiated and well circumscribed nests and strands of basaloid cells in a cellular fibroblastic stroma forming a circumscribed dermal nodule, with no epidermal connection. Small keratinizing microcysts may be present, occasionally with follicular-like structures budding from the cysts. Frequent mitoses may be present. All of the cases reported have been benign (Headington, 1976; Slater, 1987; Gilks *et al.*, 1989).

(*c*)   *Trichogenic trichoblastomas*   These show the features of trichoblastic fibroma but, in addition, contain hair follicles in various stages of

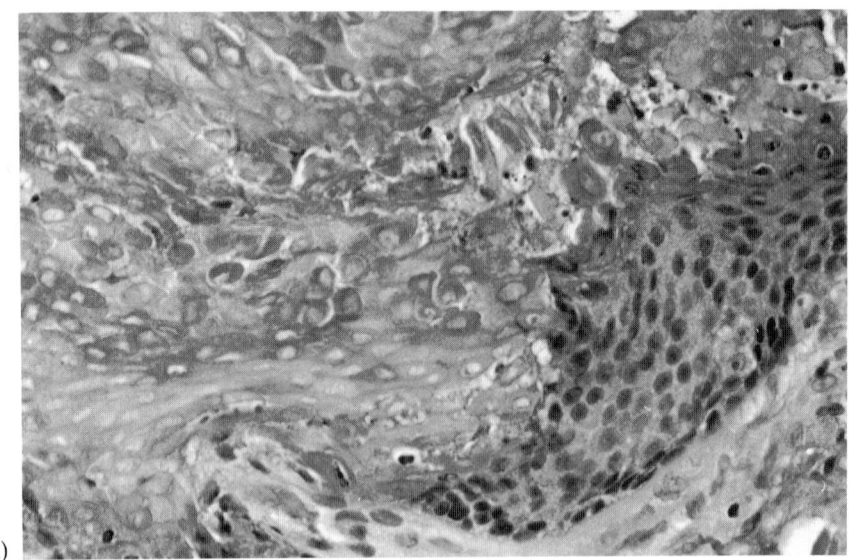

(a)

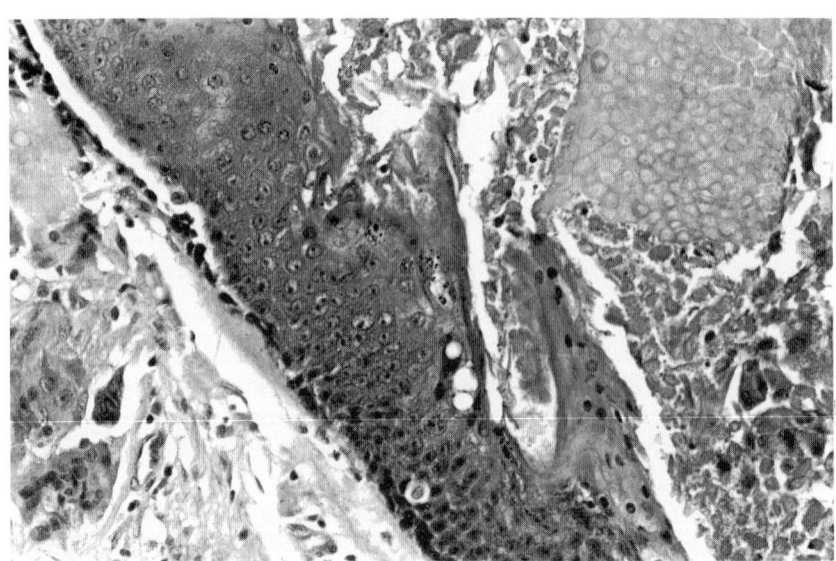

(b)

Figure 7.17 Pilomatrixoma. (a) A complex mix of epithelium with development of ghost cells, and (b) giant cell stromal reaction.

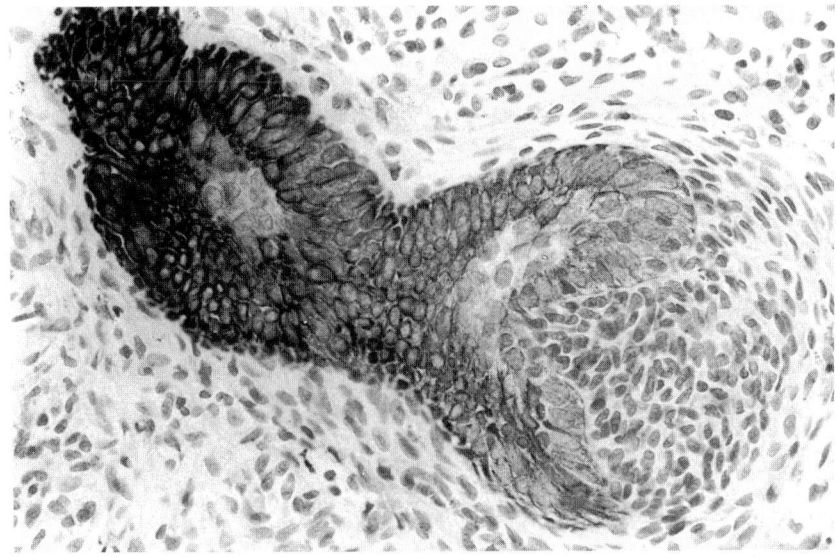

Figure 7.18   Hair follicle stained for cytokeratin, showing the hair germ (immunoperoxidase).

development, lying in continuity with the epithelial cords (Headington, 1976; Requena *et al.*, 1990).

7.4.8   Tumours of perifollicular mesenchyme

Perifollicular fibroma

A lesion has been described in which there is a marked perifollicular arrangement of collagen fibres. It is not certain whether this represents a true tumour, or whether it is a scarring response to previous follicular inflammation (Zackheim and Pinkus, 1960). A related description of perifollicular elastolysis refers to the loss of perifollicular elastic fibres, but without active inflammation. This may be due to the effects of elastase produced by *Staphylococcus epidermidis* in the affected follicles (Varadi and Saqueton, 1970).

7.4.9   Trichoepithelioma

The most typical feature of trichoepithelioma is the presence of multiple solid islands of basaloid tumour cells in a mosaic or lace-like pattern with multiple, small horn cysts, in which the centre is fully

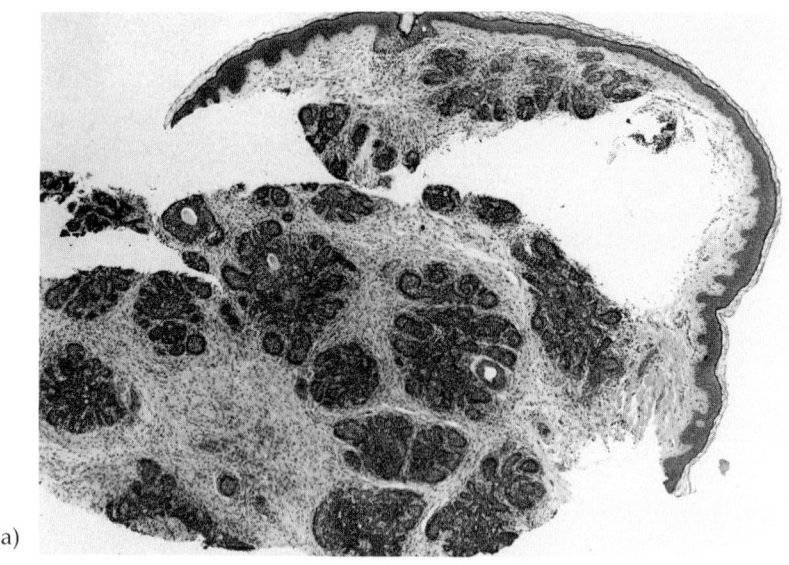

(a)

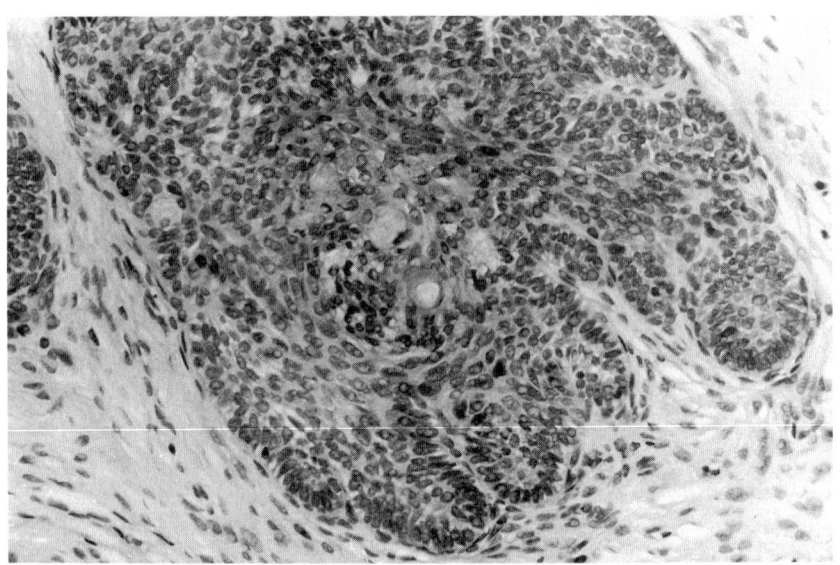

(b)

Figure 7.19 Trichoepithelioma adenoides sebaceum. (a) One of many small lesions on a child's face showing basaloid nests, with (b) foci of hair germ differentiation.

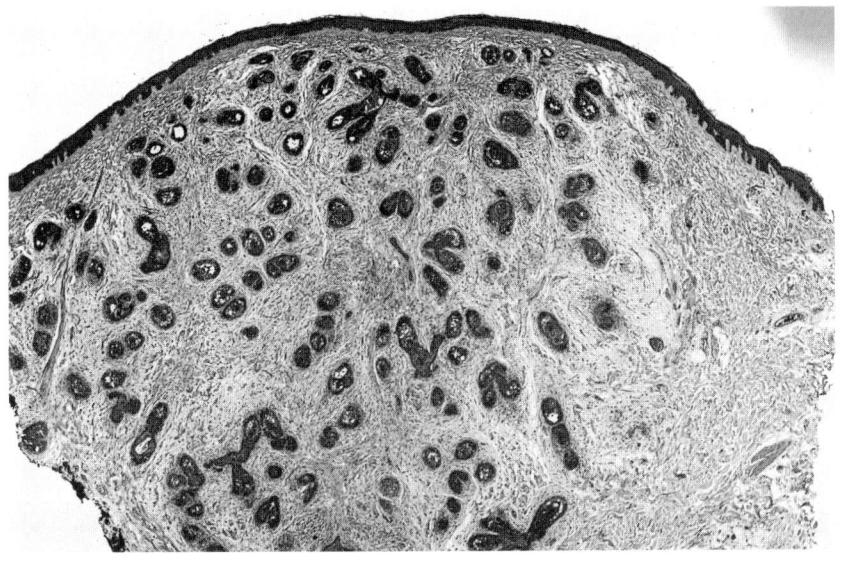

(a)

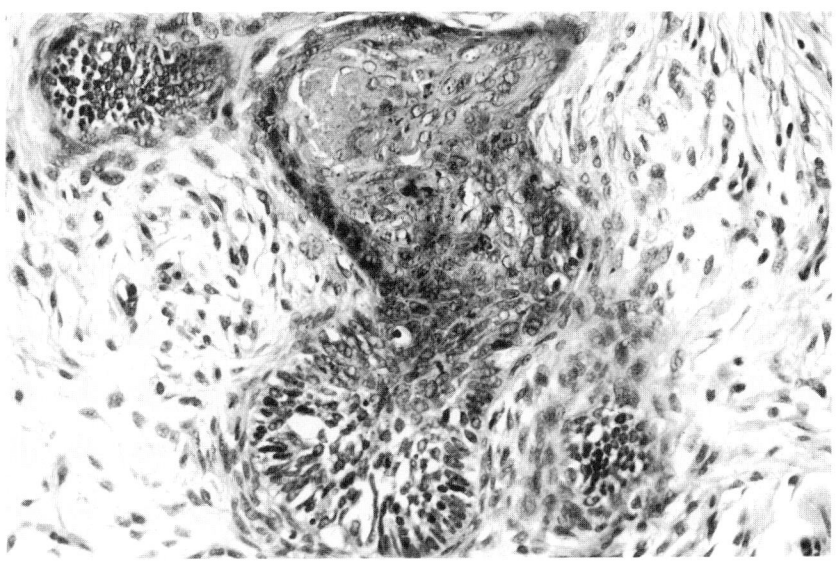

(b)

Figure 7.20 Trichoblastic fibroma. (a) A well differentiated and well circumscribed nodular tumour, with (b) follicle-like structures budding from microcystic structures. Immunohistochemical staining for (c) high molecular weight cytokeratin (LP34), (d) type IV collagen, and (e) vimentin show both epithelial and stromal features of hair follicle differentiation. (Cont.)

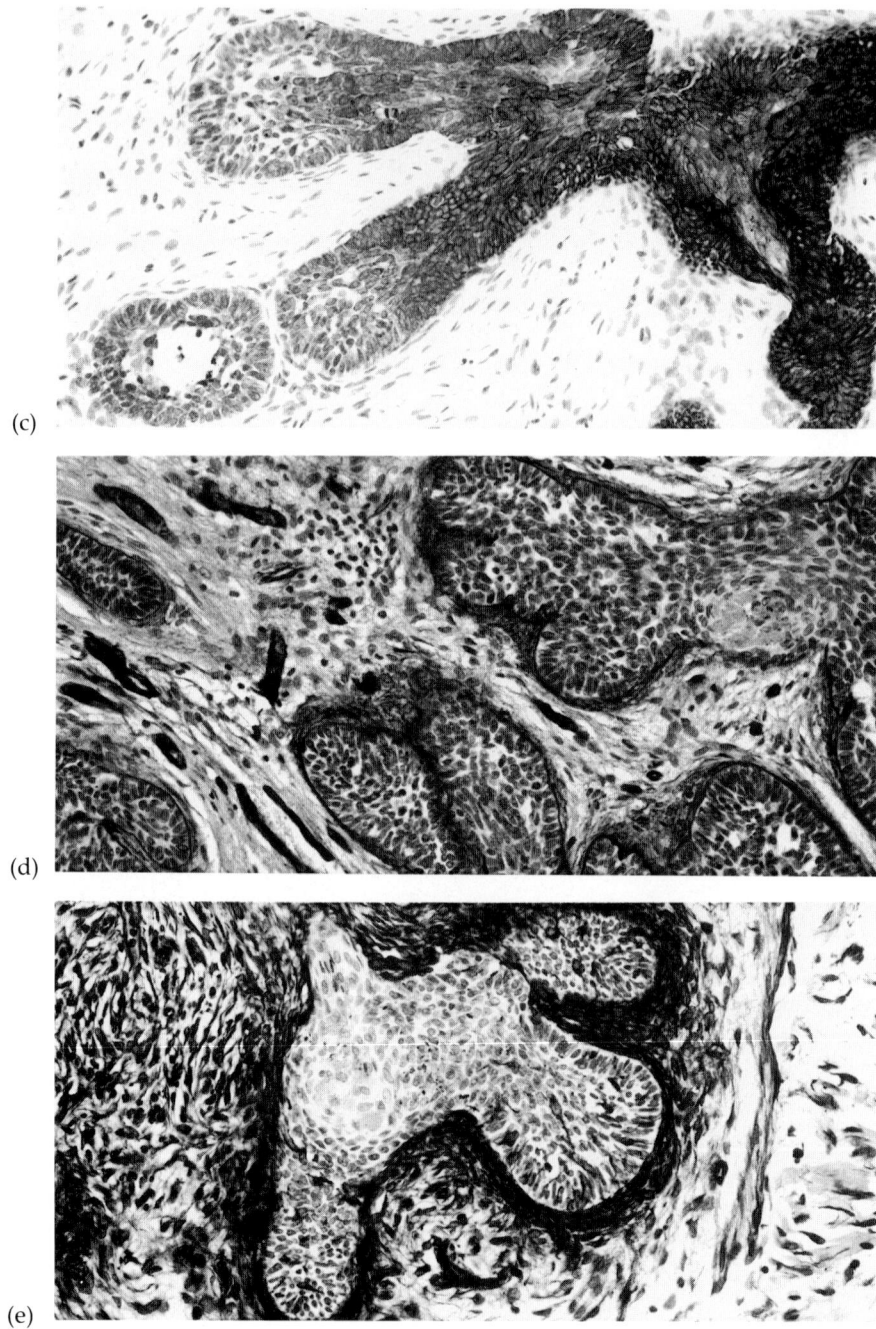

(c)

(d)

(e)

Figure 7.20 (Cont.)

keratinized. The basaloid cells show peripheral palisading in the manner of basal cell carcinoma.

Trichoepithelioma is found especially in the snout area of the face. Curettings from putative basal cell carcinomas around the region of the nose, nasolabial folds and cheeks commonly show a tumour with many features of a basal cell carcinoma, but including small cysts filled with eosinophilic keratinized cells. If this feature is present and if calcification is also seen then the diagnosis can be made with confidence. Conversely, when such changes are seen in a specimen which has been submitted innocent of clinical information, one can reasonably speculate about the likely site of the lesion on the patient, and most times be correct.

Trichepithelioma is less likely to recur than a basal cell carcinoma (Simpson *et al.*, 1989), although a giant variant has been reported which did recur (Beck and Cotton, 1988).

7.5   Sebaceous tumours

The variety of sebaceous tumours is fairly limited, but does cover examples from the whole spectrum from hyperplasia to frank malignancy, and like many other adnexal tumours they do have associations

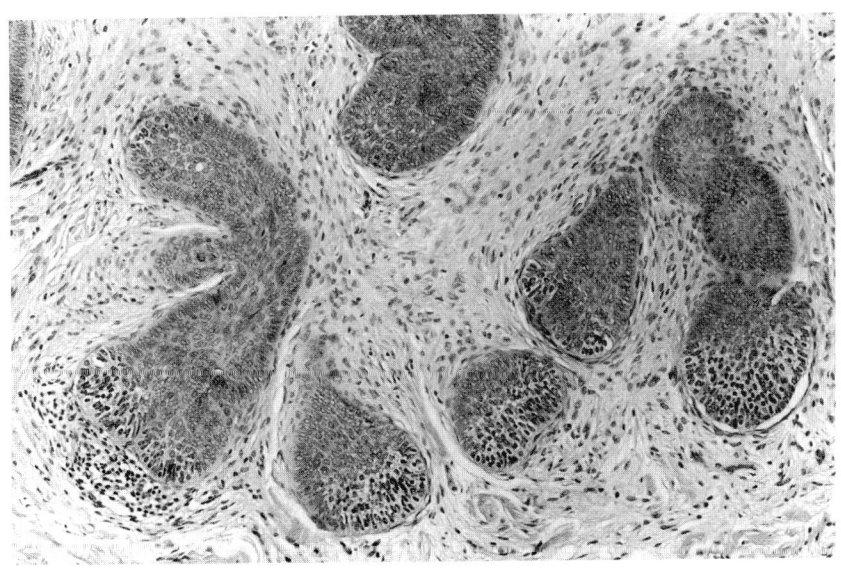

Figure 7.21   Trichogenic trichoblastoma. Hair germ and more differentiated elements of hair follicle, in a fibroblastic stroma.

with internal malignancy (Mehregan, 1985b; Massa and Medenica, 1985).

7.5.1   Organoid naevus

Also known as naevus sebaceous, these lesions occur almost exclusively as hairless plaques on the scalp and are present in childhood. They combine several elements of which a papillary acanthotic epidermis and enlarged sebaceous glands predominate. There are also increased numbers of apoeccrine glands present. The importance of organoid naevus is the increasing risk with age of the development of true neoplasms albeit locally infiltrating and non-metastasizing ones. The tumours that develop are usually basal cell carcinoma-like, but with apocrine features: probably derived from the apoeccrine glands (Morioka, 1985; Alessi et al., 1988).

7.5.2   Sebaceous hyperplasia

Sebaceous hyperplasia is a relatively common lesion, presenting as small, yellow papules on the face of the middle aged and elderly. Biopsy shows large sebaceous lobules branching from a central duct which is, in turn, connected to the surface epidermis.

7.5.3   Sebaceous adenoma

Adenomas of sebaceous glands are usually clinically undiagnostic nodules up to 1 cm in diameter. Biopsy shows irregular groups of sebaceous lobules with multiple layers of undifferentiated cells at the periphery of the lobules.

7.5.4   Sebaceous epithelioma

Sebaceous epithelioma presents as either a solitary nodule on the head and neck, or as a nodule developing within a naevus sebaceous. The tumour contains irregular lobules of basophilic cells with multiple small foci of squamous differentiation.

There is an association between sebaceous adenoma, epithelioma and carcinoma with underlying visceral carcinoma, which is known as Torre's syndrome (Lynch et al., 1981). When combined with multiple keratoacanthomas this is known as Muir-Torre's syndrome (Fahmy et al., 1982).

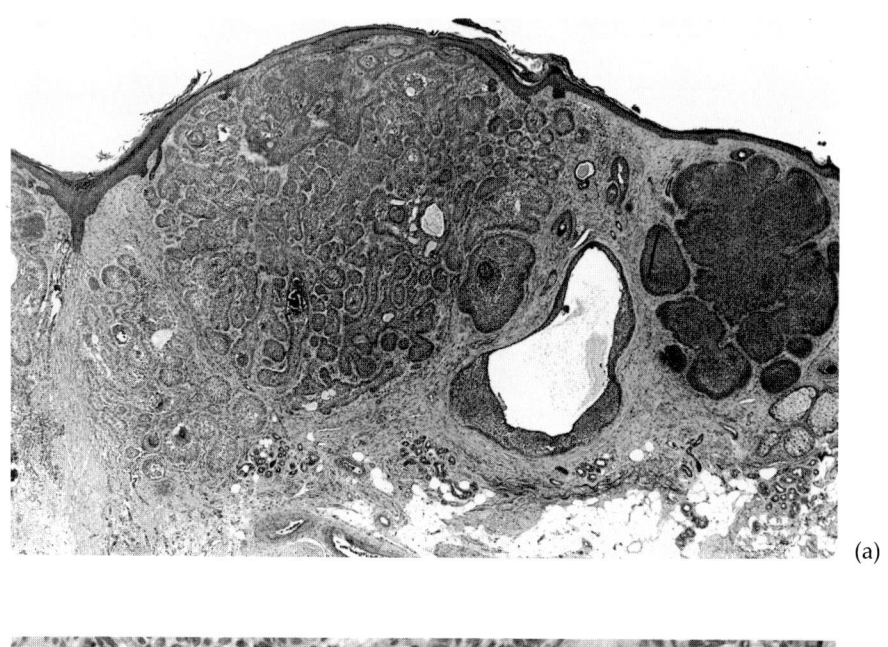

(a)

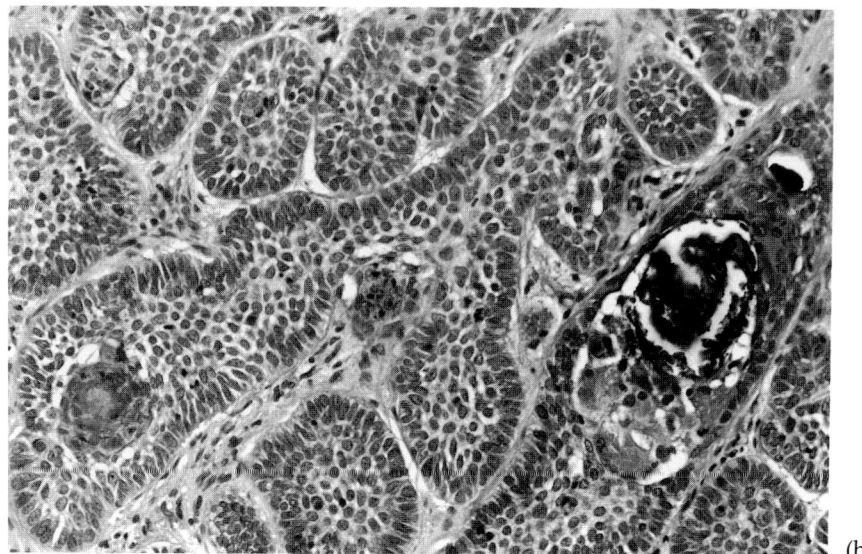

(b)

Figure 7.22 Trichoepithelioma. (a) This is not a nodular basal cell carcinoma, but (b) a tumour with focal calcification.

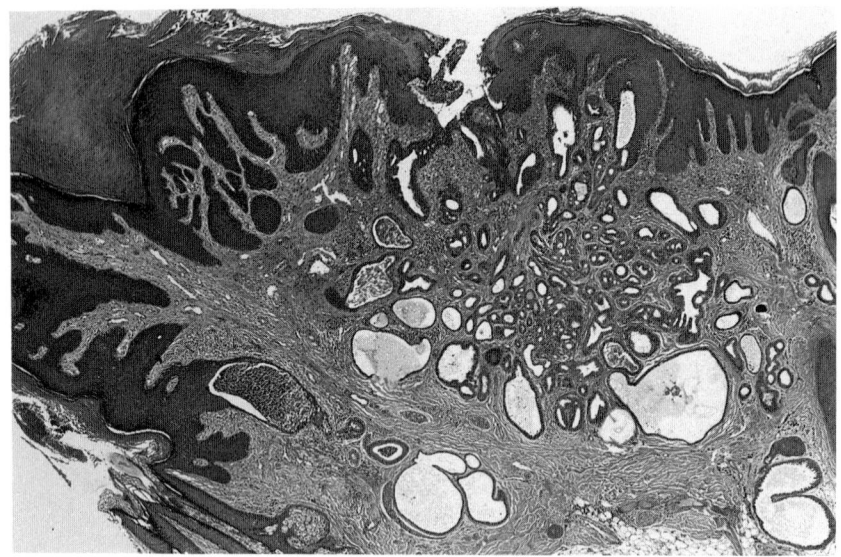

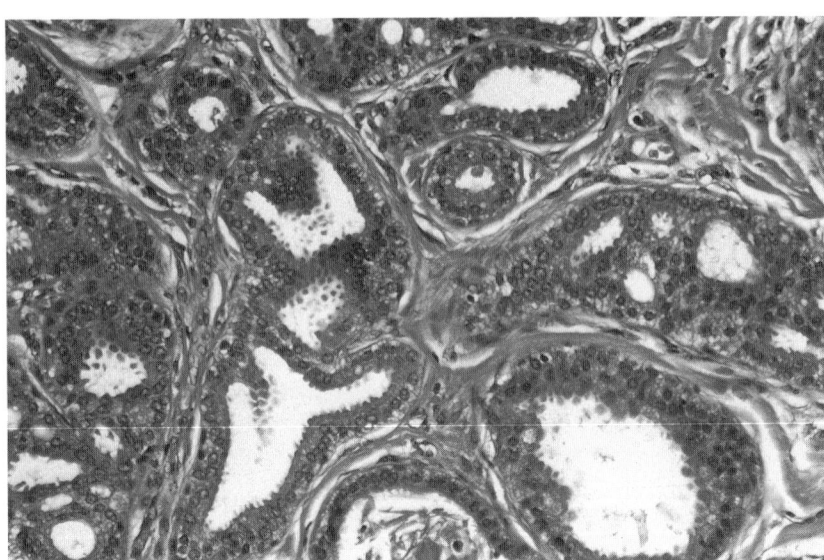

Figure 7.23 Organoid naevus. (a) The epidermis is warty and hyperkeratotic and the naevus shows (b) development of papillary syringadenoma at its base.

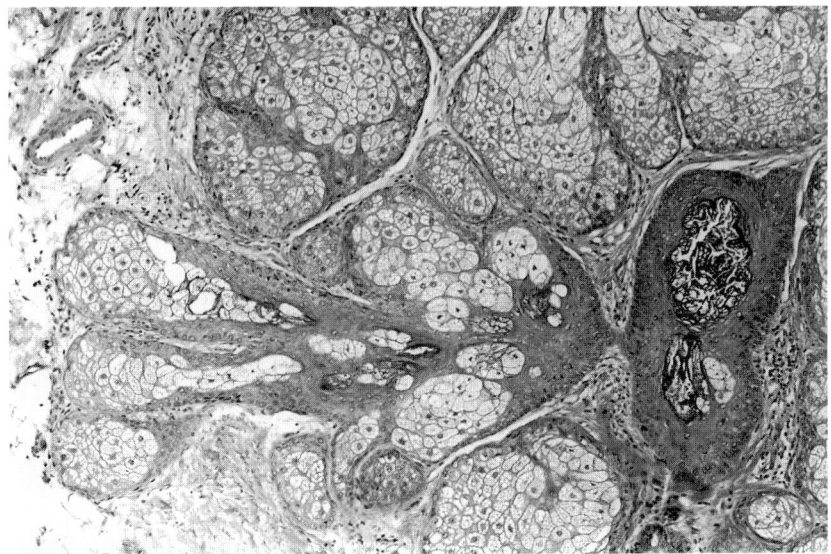

Figure 7.24 Sebaceous hyperplasia. Enlarged sebaceous glands connecting with a keratin-filled follicle.

7.5.5 *Sebaceous carcinoma*

Sebaceous carcinoma is one of the few adnexal carcinomas with a definite propensity for regional, but not usually distant, metastasis. They are particularly common around the eye. The tumours resemble sebaceous epitheliomas but with more marked cytological atypia. They may show Pagetoid spread into the overlying epidermis. This feature together with a size of more than 1 cm and the presence of a highly infiltrative growth pattern are adverse prognostic features (Rao *et al.*, 1982).

7.6 Cysts

Finally, a word about cysts. It seems impossible to get across to general surgeons that 'sebaceous cysts' do not exist. Most of such surgical specimens are either epidermal cysts with an epidermal type lining, or pilar or tricholemmal cysts, showing tricholemmal keratinization, without a granular layer. In either case the cyst is filled with keratin. The two types can be differentially labelled using appropriate keratin antibodies (Cotton *et al.*, 1984). When the cysts rupture, a granulomatous reaction to keratin ensues, with keratin flakes visible within the giant

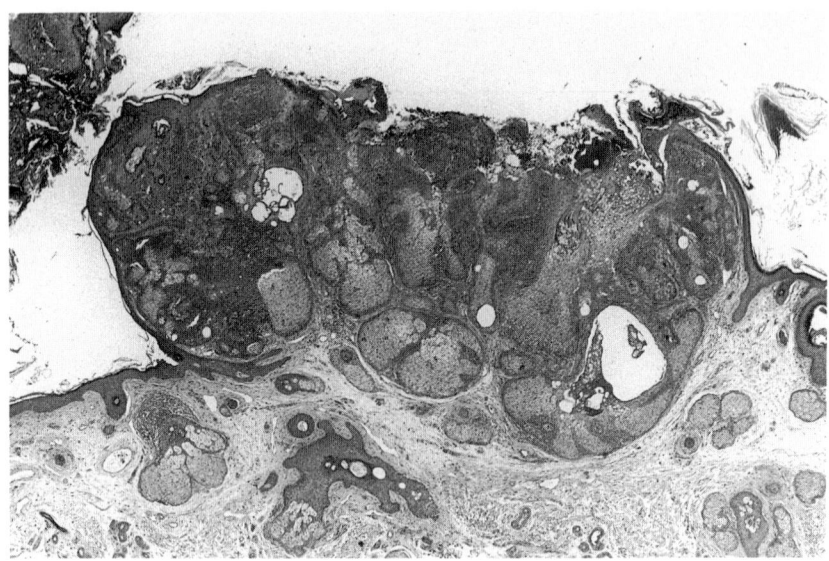

(a)

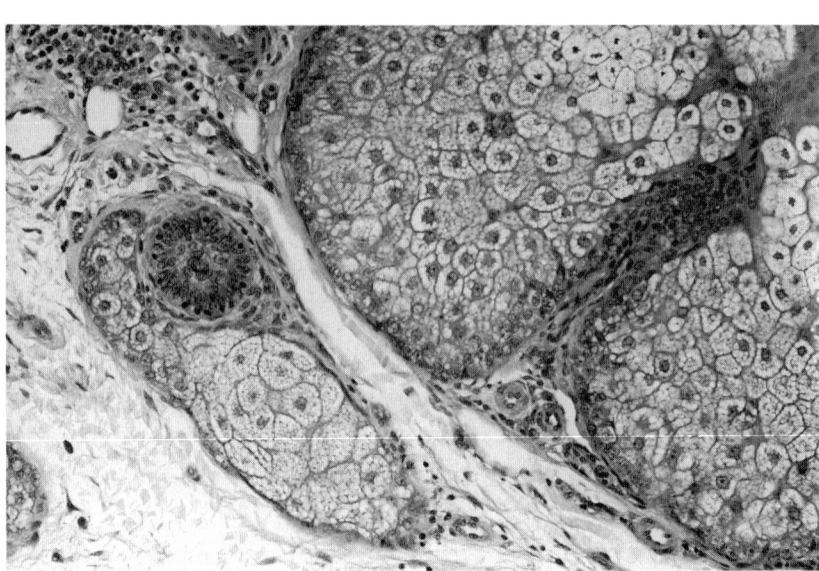

(b)

Figure 7.25 Sebaceous adenoma. (a) An ulcerated exophytic nodule with (b) sebaceous differentiation at the base.

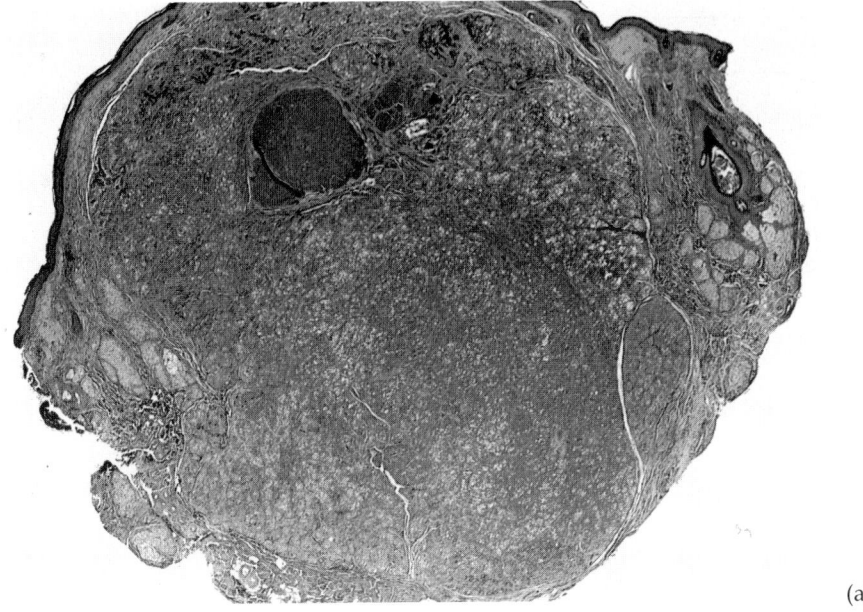

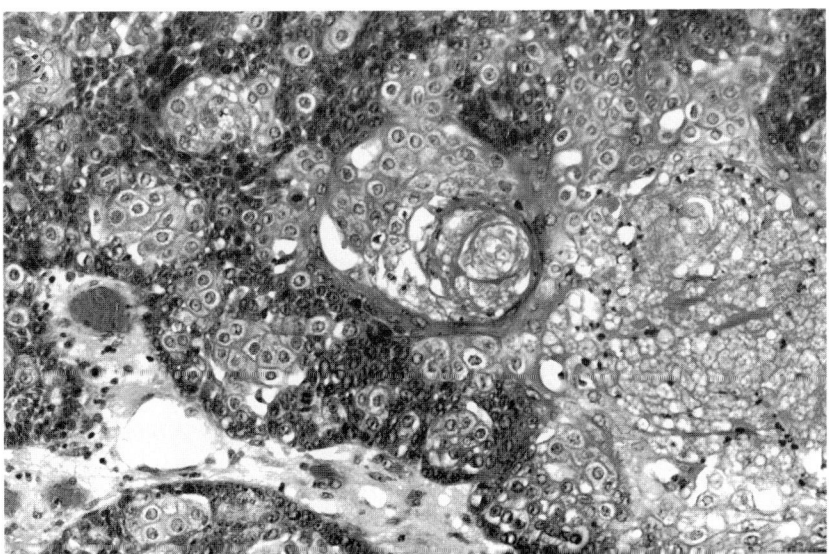

Figure 7.26 Sebaceous epithelioma. (a) A curetted nodule, showing (b) sebaceous cells surrounded by basaloid cells.

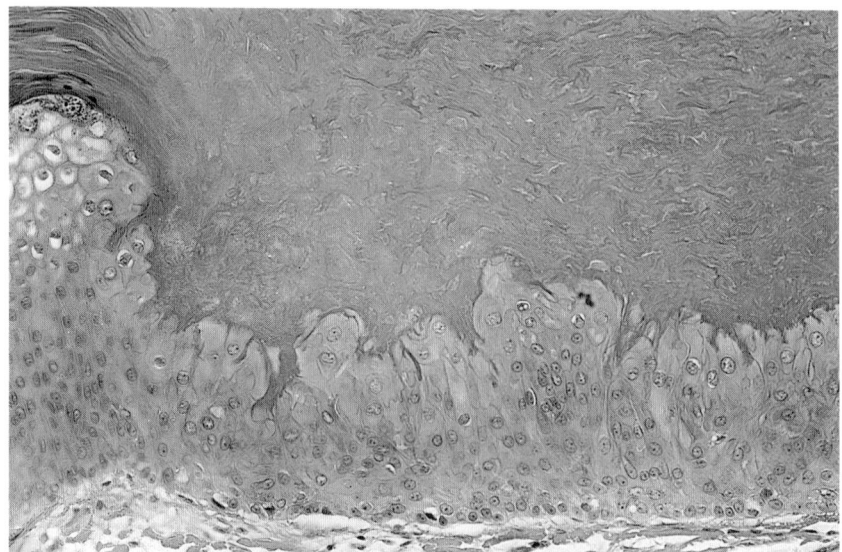

Figure 7.27 Pilar cyst. The lining epithelium shows trichilemmal keratinization, without a granular layer.

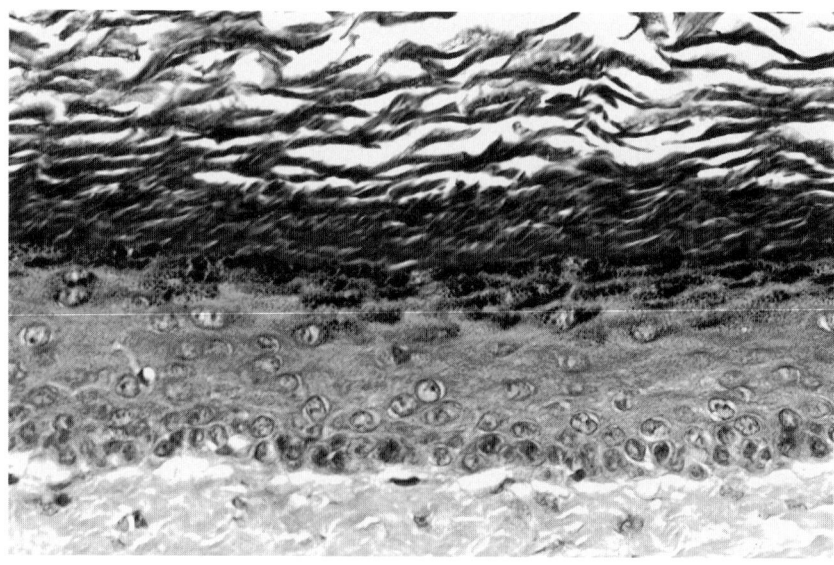

Figure 7.28 Epidermal cyst. The lining epithelium has a prominent granular layer and the cyst is filled with keratin flakes rather than surgical sebum.

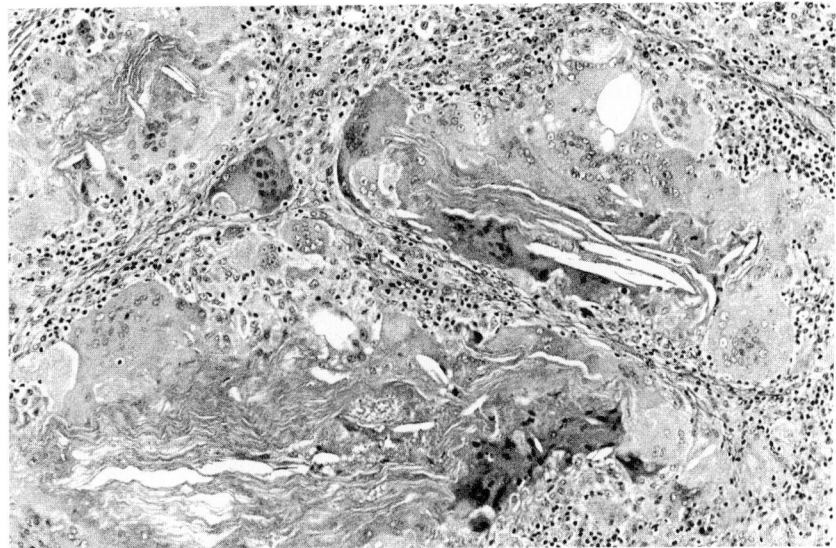

Figure 7.29 Keratin granuloma. These granulomas are common associations following partial or complete rupture of a keratin-filled epidermal or pilar cyst. Giant cells surround keratin flakes in the granuloma.

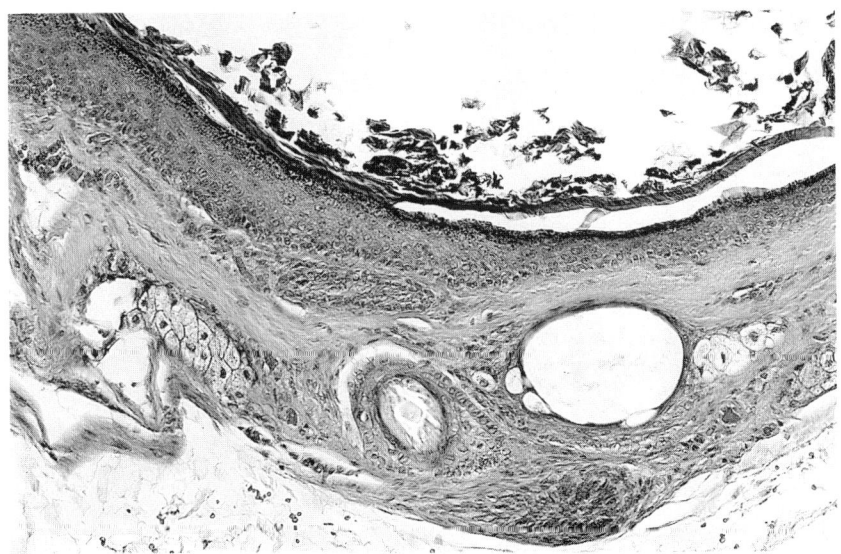

Figure 7.30 External angular dermoid, with hair follicle and sebaceous gland rudiments in the wall.

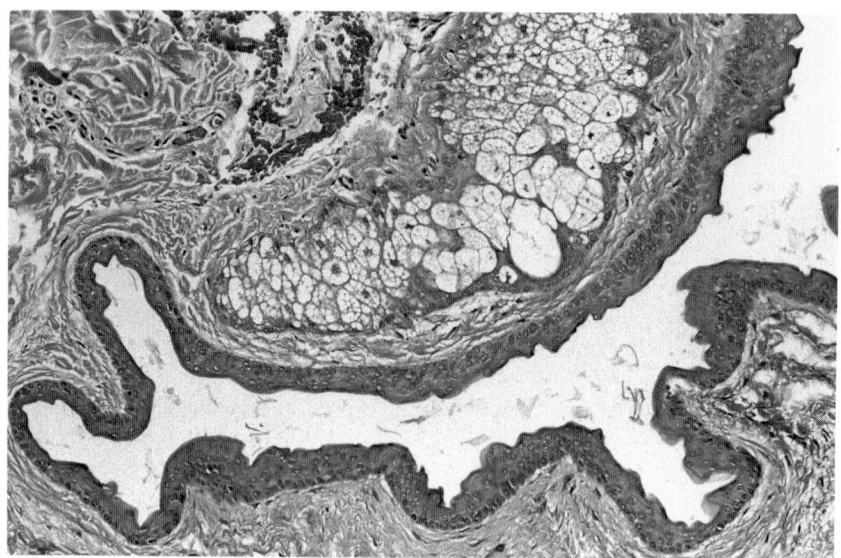

Figure 7.31 Steatocystoma multiplex with a thin, regular squamous epithelial lining which is much folded. Sebaceous glands are present in the wall.

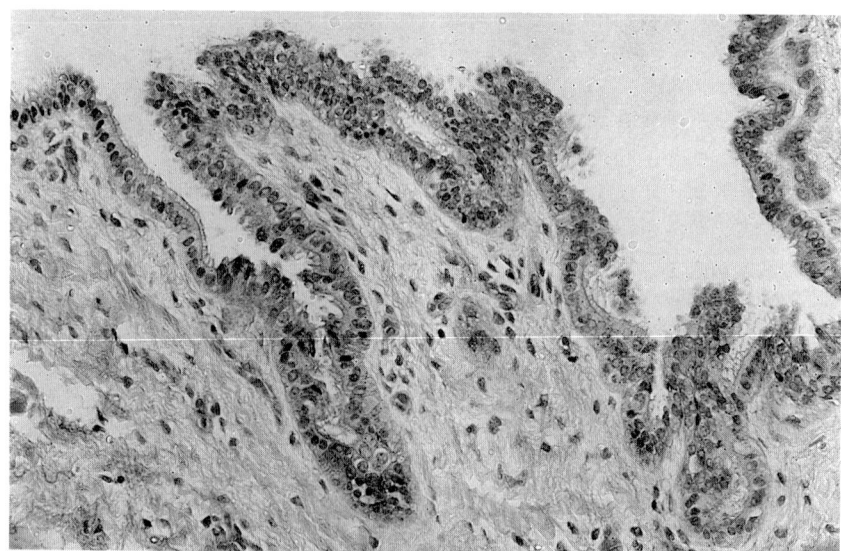

Figure 7.32 Ciliated cyst, with columnar ciliated epithelial lining.

cells. Eruptions of epidermal or pilar cysts occurring in adults raise the possibility of Gardner's syndrome, and the possibility of an underlying adenocarcinoma in the duodenum, or colo-rectum or of desmoid tumours in the peritoneum (Leppard and Sanderson, 1976; Leppard et al., 1977).

Less common cysts include the external angular dermoid, with hair follicle elements in its wall and its characteristic site at the external angle of the eye. The cysts of steatocystoma multiplex are similar but the epithelium usually has a folded profile. Very occasionally, one may come across the curious phenomenon of a ciliated cyst at the unlikely site of the ankle.

References

Ahmed, G. M. and Nath, D. K. (1988) Ceruminous gland tumour (a case report). *J. Laryngol. Otol.*, **102**, 346–9.

Alessi, E., Wong, S. N., Advani, H. H. and Ackerman, A. B. (1988) Nevus sebaceous is associated with unusual neoplasms. *An atlas. Am. J. Dermatopathol.*, **10**, 116–27.

Argenyi, Z. B., Balough, K. and Goeken, J.A. (1988) Immunohistochemical characterisation of chondroid syringomas. *Am. J. Clin. Pathol.*, **90**, 662–9.

Argenyi, Z. B., Goeken, J. A. and Balogh, K. (1989) Hyaline cells in chondroid syringomas. A light-microscopic, immunohistochemical, and ultrastructural study. *Am. J. Dermatopathol.*, **11**, 403–12.

Batsakis, J. G. and Brannon, R. B. (1981) Dermal analogue tumours of major salivary glands. *J. Laryngol. Otol.*, **95**, 155–64.

Beck, S. and Cotton, D. W. K. (1988) Recurrent solitary giant trichoepithelioma located in the perianal area; a case report. *Br. J. Dermatol.*, **118**, 563–6.

Brownstein, M. H., Mehregan, A. H., Bikowski, J. R., Lupulescu, A. and Patterson, J. C. (1979) The dermatopathology of Cowden's syndrome. *Br. J. Dermatol.*, **100**, 667–73.

Chow, W. C., Cockerell, C. J. and Geronemus, R. G. (1989) Microcystic adnexal carcinoma of the scalp. *J. Dermatol. Surg. Oncol.*, **15**, 768–71.

Cooper, P. H., Frierson, H. F. and Morrison, A. G. (1985a) Malignant transformation of eccrine spiradoma. *Arch. Dermatol.*, **121**, 1445–8.

Cooper, P. H., Mills, S. E., Leonard, D. D., Santa Cruz, D. J., Headington, J. T., Barr, R. J. and Katz, D. A. (1985b) Sclerosing sweat duct (syringomatous) carcinoma. *Am. J. Surg. Pathol.*, **9**, 422–33.

Cooper, P. H. (1986) Sclerosing carcinomas of sweat ducts (microcystic adnexal carcinomas). *Arch. Dermatol.*, **122**, 261–4.

Cotton, D. W. K., Kirkham, N. and Young, B. J. (1984) Immunoperoxidase anti-keratin staining of epidermal and pilar cysts. *Br. J. Dermatol.*, **111**, 63–8.

Cotton, D. W. K. and Braye, S. G. (1984) Dermal cylindromas originate from the eccrine sweat gland. *Br. J. Dermatol.*, **111**, 53–61.

Cotton, D. W. K. (1986) Immunohistochemical staining of normal sweat glands. *Br. J. Dermatol.*, **114**, 441–9.

Cotton, D. W. K., Slater, D. N., Rooney, N., Goepel, J. R. and Mills, P. M. (1986) Giant vascular eccrine spiradenomas, a report of two cases with histology, immunohistology and electron microscopy. *Histopathol.*, **10**, 1093–9.

Cotton, D. W. K. (1987) *An immunohistochemical study of benign eccrine sweat gland tumours.* MD Thesis. University of Sheffield.

Cotton, D. (1991) Troublesome tumours: 1. Adnexal tumours of the skin. *J. Clin. Pathol.*, **44**, 543–8.

Danks, J. A., Ebeling, P. R., Hatman, J., Chou, S. T., Moseley, J. M., Dunlop, J., Kemp, B. E. and Martin, T. J. (1989) Parathyroid hormone-related protein: immunohistochemical localisation in cancers and in normal skin. *J. Bone Min. Res.*, **4**, 273–8.

Darley, C. R., Pegum, J. S. and Pollock, D. J. (1983) Epidermotropic eccrine carcinoma. *J. R. Soc. Med.*, **76**, 616–18.

Dominguez Ingleias, F., Fresno Forcelledo, F., Soler Sanchez, T., Fernandez Garcia, L. and Herrero Zapatero, A. (1990) Chondroid syringoma: a histological and immunohistochemical study of 15 cases. *Histopathology*, **17**, 311–17.

Fahmy, A., Burgdorf, W. H. C., Schosser, R. H. and Pitha, J. (1982) Muir-Torre syndrome. *Cancer*, **49**, 1898–1903.

Gilks, C. B., Clement, P. B. and Wood, W. S. (1989) Trichoblastic fibroma. A clinicopathologic study of three cases. *Am. J. Dermatopathol.*, **11**, 397–402.

Goldstein, D. J., Barr, R. J. and Santa Cruz, D. J. (1982) Microcystic adnexal carcinoma, a distinct clinicopathologic entity. *Cancer*, **50**, 566–72.

Gould, E., Kurzon, R., Kowalczyk, A. P. and Saldana, M. (1984) Pilomatrix carcinoma with pulmonary metastasis. Report of a case. Cancer, **54**, 370–2.

Gromiko, N. (1927) Zur Kenntnis der Bosartigen unwandlung des Verkalkten Hautepitheliomas. *Arch. Pathol. Anat.*, **265**, 103–16.

Hassab-El-Naby, H. M., Tam, S., White W. L. and Ackerman, A. B. (1989) Mixed tumors of the skin. A histological and immunohistochemical study. *Am. J. Dermatopathol.*, **11**, 413–28.

Hayman, J. A., Danks, J. A., Ebling, P. R., Moseley, J. M., Kemp, B. E. and Martin, T. J. (1989) Expression of parathyroid hormone related protein in normal skin and in tumours of skin and skin appendages. *J. Pathol.*, **158**, 293–6.

Headington, J. T. (1976) Tumors of the hair follicle. A review. *Am. J. Pathol.*, **85**, 480–514.

Headington, J. T. (1980) Tricholemmoma. To be or not to be? *Am. J. Dermatopathol.*, **2**, 225–6.

Herbst, E. W. and Utz, W. (1984) Multifocal dermal-type basal cell adenomas of parotid glands with co-existing dermal cylindromas. *Virchows. Arch. (Pathol. Anat.)*, **403**, 95–102.

Hu, C.-H., Marques, A. S. and Winklemann, R. K. (1978) Dermal duct tumour. *Arch. Dermatol.*, **114**, 1659–64.

Hyman, A. B. and Brownstein, M. H. (1969) Eccrine poroma, an analysis of forty-five new cases. *Dermatologica*, **138**, 29–38.

Ito, M., Tazawa, T., Shimizu, N., Saito, A., Sato, Y. and Nonaka, I. (1988) Intraepidermal pilar epithelioma: a new dermatopathologic interpretation of a skin tumor. *J. Am. Acad. Dermatol.*, **18**, 123–32.

Jawarski, R. (1988) Malignant trichilemmal cyst. *Am. J. Dermatopathol.*, **10**, 276–7.

Jitsukawa, K., Sueki, H., Sato, S. and Anzai, T. (1987) Eccrine spiradenoma. An electron microscopic study. *Am. J. Dermatopathol.*, **9**, 99–108.

Jordan, D. R., Nerad, J. A. and Patrinely, J. R. (1989) Chondroid syringoma of the eyelid. *Can. J. Ophthalmol.*, **24**, 24–7.

Kanitakis, J., Zambruno, G., Euvrard, S., Hermier, C. and Thivolet, J. (1987) Eccrine syringofibroadenoma. Immunohistological study of a new case. *Am. J. Dermatopathol.*, **9**, 37–40.

Kariniemi, A.-L., Forsman, L. M., Wahlstrom, T. and Andersson, L. C. (1984) Expression of differentiating antigens in benign sweat gland tumours. *Br. J. Dermatol.*, **111**, 175–82.

Kato, H., Mizuno, N., Nakagawa, K., Furukawa, M. and Hamada, T. (1989) Microcystic adnexal carcinoma: a light microscopic, immunohistochemical and ultrastructural study. *J. Cutan. Pathol.*, **17**, 87–95.

Kohda, M., Manabe, T. and Ueki, H. (1990) Squamous islands in eccrine neoplasms. *Am. J. Dermatopathol.*, **12**, 344–9.

Kukreja, S. C., Shevrin, D. H., Wimbiscus, S. A., Ebeling, P. R., Danks, J. A., Rodda, C. P., Wood, W. I. and Martin, T. J. (1988) Antibodies to parathyroid hormone-related protein lower serum calcium in athymic mouse models of malignancy-associated hypercalcemia due to human tumors. *J. Clin. Invest.*, **82**, 1798–802.

Leppard, B. J. and Sanderson, K. V. (1976) The natural history of trichilemmal cysts. *Dermatologica*, **94**, 379–90.

Leppard, B. J., Sanderson, K. V. and Wells, R. S. (1977) Hereditary trichilemmal cysts. *Clin. Exp. Dermatol.*, **2**, 23–32.

Lopansri, S. and Mihm, M. C. (1980) Pilomatrix carcinoma or calcifying epithelio-carcinoma of Malherbe: a case report and review of the literature. *Cancer*, **45**, 2368–773.

Lupton, A. P. and McMarlin, S. L. (1986) Microcystic adnexal carcinoma. Report of a case with 30 year follow up. *Arch. Dermatol.*, **122**, 286–9.

Lynch, H. T., Lynch, P. M., Pester, J. and Fusaro, R. M. (1981) The cancer family syndrome, rare cutaneous phenotypic linkage of Torre's syndrome. *Arch. Int. Med.*, **141**, 607–11.

MacDonald, D. M., Wilson Jones, E. and Marks, R. (1977) Sclerosing epithelial hamartoma. *Clin. Exp. Dermatol.*, **2**, 153–60.

Malherbe, A. and Chenantais, J. (1985) Note sur l'epitheliome calcifie des glands sebacees. *Prog. Med.*, **8**, 826–8.

Massa, M. C. and Medenica, M. (1985) Cutaneous adnexal tumours and cysts: a review. Part 1 tumours with hair follicular and sebaceous glandular differentiation and cysts related to different parts of the hair follicle. *Pathology Annual*, **20 II**, 189–233.

McKee, P. H., Fletcher, C. D. M., Stavrinos, P. and Pambakian, H. (1990) Carcinosarcoma arising in eccrine spiradenoma. *Am. J. Dermatopathol.*, **12**, 335–43.

Mehregan, A. H. (1985a) Hair follicle tumors of the skin. *J. Cutan. Pathol.*, **12**, 189–95.

Mehregan, A. H. (1985b) Sebaceous tumours of the skin. *J. Cutan. Pathol.*, **12**, 196–9.

Moehlenbeck, F. W. (1973) Pilomatrixoma (calcifying epithelioma). *Arch. Dermatol.*, **108**, 532–4.

Moll, I., Heid, H. and Moll, R. (1988) Cytokeratin analysis of pilomatrixoma: changes in cytokeratin-type expression during differentiation. *J. Invest. Dermatol.*, **91**, 251–7.

Morioka, S. (1985) The natural history of *nevus sebaceous*. *J. Cutan. Pathol.*, **12**, 200–13.

Nakhleh, R. E., Swanson, P. E. and Wick, M. R. (1990) Cutaneous adnexal carcinomas with divergent differentiation. *Am. J. Dermatopathol.*, **12**, 325–34.

Nickoloff, B. J., Fleischmann, H. E., Carmel, J., Wood, C. C. and Roth, R. J. (1986) Microcystic adnexal carcinoma. Immunohistologic observations suggesting dual (pilar and eccrine). differentiation. *Arch. Dermatol.*, **122**, 290–4.

Noda, Y., Takai, Y., Iwai, Y., Meenaghan, M. A. and Mori, M. (1986) Immunohistochemical study of carbonic anhydrase in mixed tumours from major salivary glands and skin. *Virchows Archiv. A.*, **408**, 449–59.

Noda, Y., Horike, H., Tanimura, T., Tsujimura, T. and Mori, M. (1988) Immunohistochemical localization by monoclonal antibodies of S-100 alpha and beta proteins in mixed tumours and adenomas of the skin. *Virchows Archiv. B Cell Pathol.*, **54**, 371–80.

Penneys, N. S., Ackerman, A. B., Indigin, S. N. and Mandy, S. H. (1970) Eccrine poroma: two unusual variants. *Br. J. Dermatol.*, **82**, 613–15.

Penneys, N.S, Nadji, M. and Morales, M. (1982) Carcinoembryonic antigen in benign sweat gland tumours. *Arch. Dermatol.*, **118**, 225–7.

Penneys, N. S., Nadji, M., Ziegels-Weissman, J., Ketabchi, M. and Morales, A. R. (1982) Carcinoembryonic antigen in sweat gland carcinomas. *Cancer*, **50**, 1608–11.

Pinkus, H., Rogin, J. R. and Goldman, P. (1956) Eccrine poroma. *Arch. Dermatol.*, **74**, 511–21.

Pinkus, H. and Sutton, R. L. Jr. (1965) Trichofolliculoma. *Arch. Dermatol.*, **91**, 46–9.

Prandetsky, A. P. and Iuzuinkevich, A. K. (1969) Malherbe's epithelioma with sign of malignization. *Arkh. Patol.*, **31**, 64–6.

Puttick, L., Ince, P. and Comaish, J. S. (1986) Three cases of eccrine porocarcinoma. *Br. J. Dermatol.*, **115**, 111–16.

Pylyser, K., De Wolf-Peeters, C. and Marien, K. (1983) The histology of eccrine poromas: a study of 14 cases. *Dermatologica*, **167**, 243–9.

Rahbari, H. (1984) Syringoacanthoma: acanthotic lesion of the acrosyringium. *Arch. Dermatol.*, **120**, 751–6.

Rao, N. A., Hidayat, A. A., McLean, I. W. and Zimmerman, L. E. (1982) Sebaceous carcinomas of the ocular adnexa, a clinicopathologic study of 104 cases, with five-year follow-up data. *Hum. Pathol.*, **13**, 113–22.

Reed, R. J. and Lamar, L. M. (1966) Invasive hair matrix tumors of the scalp: invasive pilomatrixoma. *Arch. Dermatol.*, **94**, 310–16.

Requena, L., Requena, I., Romero, E., Sanchez, M. and Sanchez, Yus. E. (1990) Trichogenic trichoblastoma. An unusual neoplasm of hair germ. *Am. J. Dermatopathol.*, **12**, 175–81.

Revis, P., Chyu, J. and Medenica, M. (1988) Multiple eccrine spiradenoma: case report and review. *J. Cutan. Pathol.*, **15**, 226–9.

Rothman, D., Kendall, A. B. and Baldi, A. (1976) Giant pilomatrixoma (Malherbe's calcifying epithelioma). *Arch. Surg.*, **111**, 86–7.

Ryan, J. F., Darley, C. R. and Pollock, D. J. (1986) Malignant eccrine poroma: a report of three cases. *J. Clin. Pathol.*, **39**, 1099–104.

Sacks, E., Jakobiec, F. A., McMillan, R., Fraunfelder, F. and Iwamoto, T. (1987) Multiple bilateral apocrine cytadenomas of the lower eyelids. Light and electron microscopic studies. *Ophthalmology*, **94**, 65–71.

Sasaki, C. T., Yue, A. and Enriques, R. (1976) Giant calcifing epithelioma. *Arch. Otolaryngol.*, **102**, 753–5.

Sato, K. and Sato, F. (1987) Sweat secretion by human axillary apoeccrine sweat gland in vitro. *Am. J. Physiol.*, **252**, R181–7.

Sato, K., Leidal, R. and Sato, F. (1987) Morphology and development of an apoeccrine sweat gland in human axillae. *Am. J. Physiol.*, **252**, R166–80.

Shvili, D. and Rotham, A. (1986) Fulminant metastasising chondroid syringoma of the skin. *Am. J. Dermatopathol.*, **8**, 321–5.

Simpson, W., Garner, A. and Collin, J. R. (1989) Benign hair-follicle derived tumours in the differential diagnosis of basal cell carcinoma of the eyelids: a clinicopathological comparison. *Br. J. Ophthalmol.*, **73**, 347–53.

Slater, D. N. (1987) Trichoblastic fibroma: hair germ (trichogenic) tumours revisited. *Histopathol.*, **11**, 327–31.

Smith, J. L. S. and Coburn, J. B. (1956) Hidroacanthoma simplex. An assessment of a selected group of intraepidermal basal cell epitheliomata and their malignant homologues. *Br. J. Derm. Syph.*, **68**, 400–18.

Thomson, S. J. and Tanner, N. S. (1989) Carcinoma of the apocrine glands at the base of eyelashes, a case report and discussion of histological diagnostic criteria. *Br. J. Plast. Surg.*, **42**, 598–602.

Thyresson, H. N. and Doyle, J. A. (1981) Cowden's disease (multiple hamartoma syndrome). *Mayo Clin. Proc.*, **56**, 179–84.

Van der Walt, J. D. and Rohlova, B. (1984) Carcinomatous transformation in a pilomatrixoma. *Am. J. Dermatopathol.*, **6**, 63–9.

Varadi, D. P. and Saqueton, A. C. (1970) Perifollicular elsatolysis. *Br. J. Dermatol.*, **83**, 143–50.

Walsh, M. S. (1990) A case of eccrine porocarcinoma. *J. R. Soc. Med. Lond.*, **83**, 529–30.

Warner, T. F. C. S., Goell, W. S. and Cripps, D. J. J. (1982) Hidroacanthoma simplex: an ultrastructural study. *J. Cut. Pathol.*, **9**, 189–95.

Weedon, D. and Lewis, J. (1977) Acrosyringeal naevus. *J. Cutan. Pathol.*, **4**, 166–8.

Weedon, D., Bell, J. and Mayze, J. (1980) Matrical carcinoma of the skin. *J. Cut. Pathol.*, **7**, 39–42.

Wick, M. R., ed. (1985) *Pathology of unusual malignant cutaneous tumors*. Marcel Dekker, New York.

Wick, M. R., Swanson, P. E., Kaye, V. N. and Pittelkow, M. R. (1987) Sweat gland carcinoma *ex* eccrine spiradenoma. *Am. J. Dermatopathol.*, **9**, 90–8.

Winer, L. H. (1954) Dilated pore, trichoepithelioma. *J. Invest. Dermatol.*, **23**, 181–8.

Zackheim, H. S. and Pinkus, H. (1960) Perifollicular fibromas. *Arch. Dermatol.*, **82**, 913–17.

8 Dermal tumours

8.1 Mesenchymal tumours

The skin may be involved by many tumours which grow in the under-lying soft tissues. This chapter covers those tumours of mesenchyme which arise in the skin, together with some related tumours which present in similar ways. Any proposed diagnosis of a primary, soft-tissue sarcoma in the skin should be reconsidered and supported by reading specific accounts of soft tissue tumours. If the skin is involved, it will most usually be a secondary effect or, alternatively, the diagnosis may be wrong and alternative possibilities should be considered (Enzinger and Weiss, 1988).

8.1.1 Dermatofibroma

The terms dermatofibroma, histiocytoma cutis, cellular benign fibrous histiocytoma, and sclerosing haemangioma, have been used to varying extents as synonyms for this group of benign dermal nodules which have a number of features in common as well as showing individual variation. They present as small, firm dermal nodules, less than 1.5 cm in diameter, often with increased brown pigmentation of the overlying skin. Indeed, the lesions often present as pigmented lesions of worry-ing appearance and they require diagnostic excision biopsy.

The pigmentation seen in the biopsy is due to increased amounts of melanin within epidermal melanocytes. Pigmentary incontinence in the underlying dermis is uncommon. The epidermis also shows a varying degree of reactive hyperplasia, sometimes reaching the extent of 'pseu-doepitheliomatous' hyperplasia. This may be due to stimulation by growth factors released by the dermal lesion.

The lesion itself is a nodular collection of spindle cells, collagen and small blood vessels, sometimes with occasional foamy histiocytes, or xanthoma cells, and sometimes with histiocytic giant cells. Small amounts of haemosiderin may be present in the interstitium. Occa-

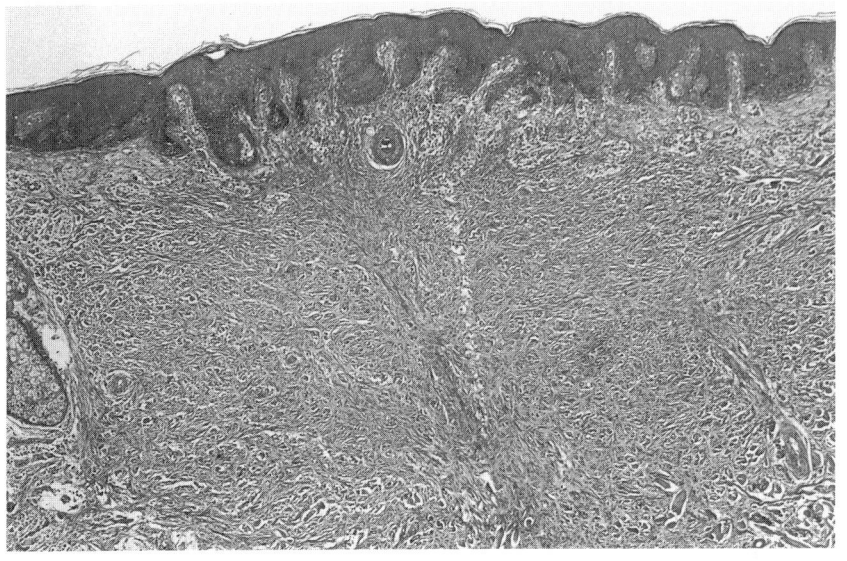

(a)

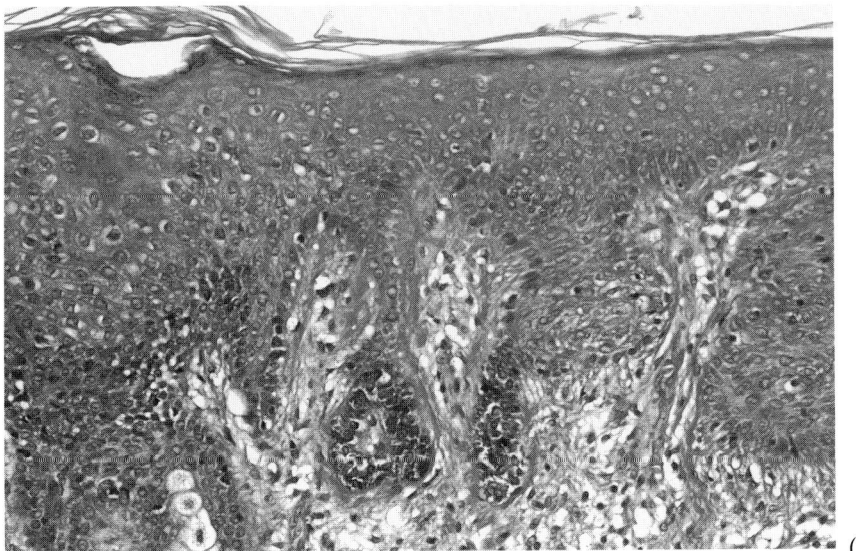

(b)

Figure 8.1 Dermatofibroma. (a) A moderately cellular, moderately circumscribed dermal nodule; (b) epidermal acanthosis and hyperpigmentation of basal melanocytes in the overlying epidermis.

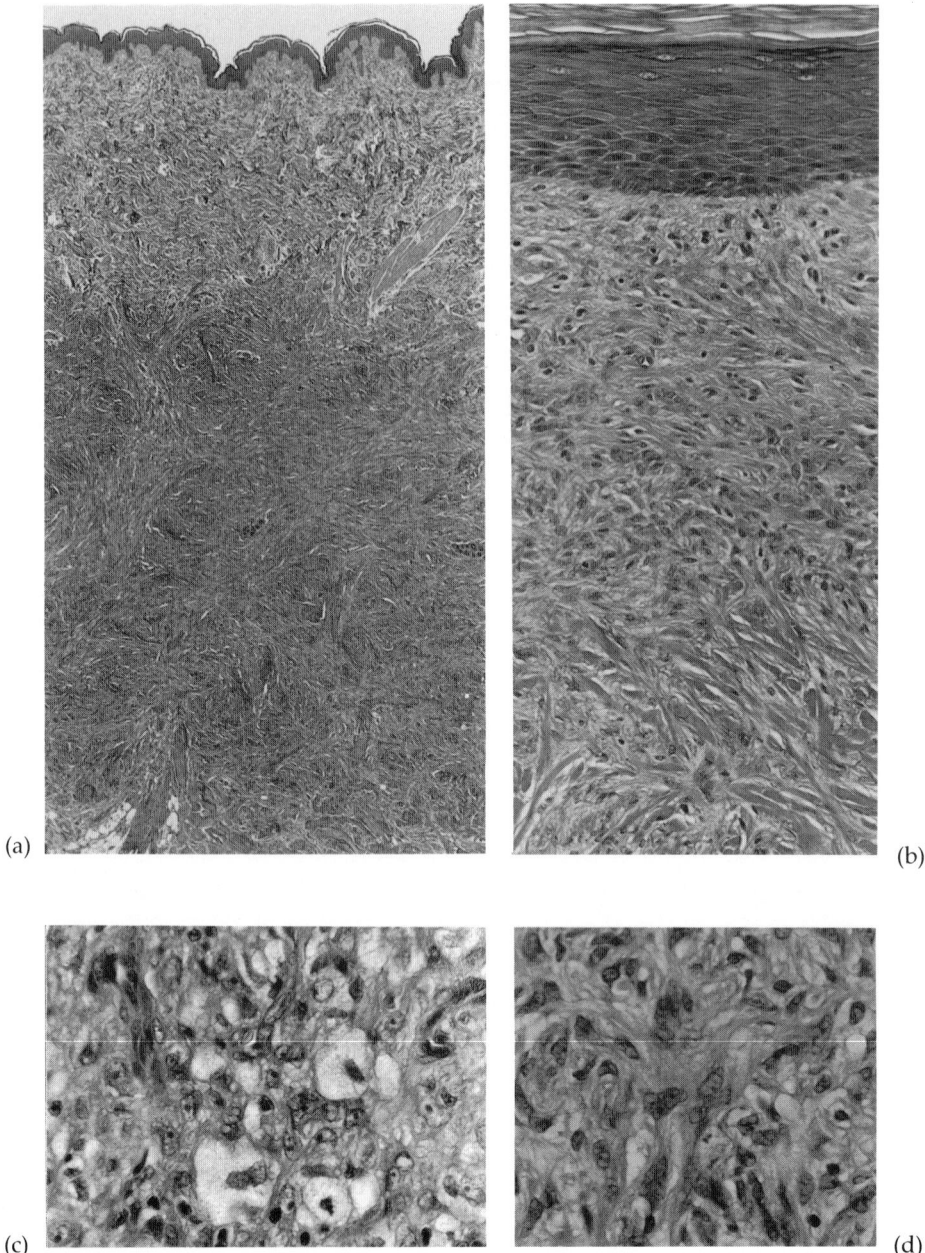

(a)

(b)

(c)

(d)

Figure 8.2 Dermatofibroma. (a) Moderately cellular dermal nodule; (b) ill-defined boundary between the lesion and adjacent normal dermis; (c) foam cells seen in some examples; (d) irregular arrangement of cells and stroma.

sional mitoses may also be seen and the cells may show a moderate degree of pleomorphism, but necrosis is an unlikely finding. The relative proportions of stroma and cells vary between lesions. The margins are indistinct, fading off into the surrounding dermis over a short distance. Extension into subcutaneous fat is distinctly uncommon.

Differential diagnosis is between other benign nodular lesions, of which neurofibroma is perhaps the commonest, and between other more malignant entities on the spectrum of dermal fibrohistiocytic tumours. Neurofibromas may show epidermal pigmentation, but the dermal lesion is more sharply circumscribed than dermatofibroma. When features such as mitoses, increased cellularity and subcutaneous invasion are seen, then one should consider dermatofibrosarcoma protuberans. Dermatofibromas may recur after incomplete excision, but to a much lesser extent than dermatofibrosarcoma protuberans.

The underlying cause of dermatofibromas remains unknown; they do not appear to be due to arthropod bites (Evans et al., 1989). The cells show immunoreactivity for factor XIIIa; a marker of dermal dendrocytes (Cerio et al., 1989). An epithelioid cell variant has recently been described (Wilson Jones et al., 1989).

8.1.2 Angiomatoid fibrous histiocytoma

A variant of benign cutaneous fibrous histiocytoma, although usually larger, the lesions are dark red, blue or black in colour and occur as painful, rapidly growing nodules on the extremities. Clinically, they may mimic melanoma, neurofibroma, haemangioma or a cyst. They contain large, blood-filled spaces, which may compose half of the lesion. The spaces have no endothelial lining but are lined and surrounded by histiocytes, with haemosiderin, fibroblasts and foam cells. The solid parts show typical appearances of cutaneous fibrous histiocytomas (Santa Cruz et al., 1981).

Table 8.1 Immunophenotypes of dermal spindle cell tumours

Tumour type	Vimentin	EMA	S100	Cytokeratin	Desmin
Dermatofibrosarcoma protuberans					
Atypical fibrous histiocytoma	+				
Malignant fibrous histiocytoma					
Squamous cell carcinoma		+		+	
Melanoma	+		+		
Leiomyosarcoma			+		+

8.1.3   Epithelioid cell histiocytoma

A further variant of dermatofibroma which occurs on the legs of adults as a solitary elevated nodule with a vascular appearance. The lesions have a collarette and contain large angulated cells which are factor XIIIa positive. The raised nodular profile, vascular component and epithelioid cells raise the possibility of Spitz naevus in differential diagnosis (Wilson Jones *et al.*, 1989).

8.1.4   Atypical fibroxanthoma

These are a group of spindle cell tumours which occur in damaged skin; the damage being most commonly caused by the sun, but also by radiotherapy or burns. They are seen as a solitary, rapidly growing nodule on the head or neck, usually in an older person, and they may ulcerate.

The dermis is filled with pleomorphic spindle cells, epithelioid cells and tumour giant cells, which extend up to the epidermis and may merge with the basal layer but without invading upwards (Helwig, 1963; Fretzin and Helwig, 1973; Dahl, 1976, Starink *et al.*, 1977; Leong and Milios, 1987).

The tumour has no positive diagnostic features. The diagnosis is made by excluding the major differential diagnoses, of which spindle cell melanoma, spindle cell squamous carcinoma, and malignant fibrous histiocytoma are, perhaps, the most important. Immunohistochemical phenotyping will show negative results with melanocyte markers such as S100, and may show positive immunoreactivity for vimentin, although not in all cases (Miettinen *et al.*, 1985; Silvis *et al.*, 1988). Large numbers of Langerhans cells may also be present within the tumour; they can be shown with S100 staining (Ricci *et al.*, 1988).

A diagnosis of atypical fibroxanthoma (AFX) is usually taken clinically to indicate an indolent tumour which can be managed conservatively. Certainly it should be better news than a melanoma of similar size, although malignant examples have been described (Helwig and May, 1986).

8.1.5   Dermatofibrosarcoma protuberans

Dermatofibrosarcoma protuberans (DFSP) lies in the spectrum of fibroblastic tumours between dermatofibroma and fibrosarcoma, and is an example of a soft-tissue tumour which is only found in the skin (Darier and Ferrand, 1924; Hoffmann, 1925). The lesions begin their development with a plaque stage before progressing after a period of years to a

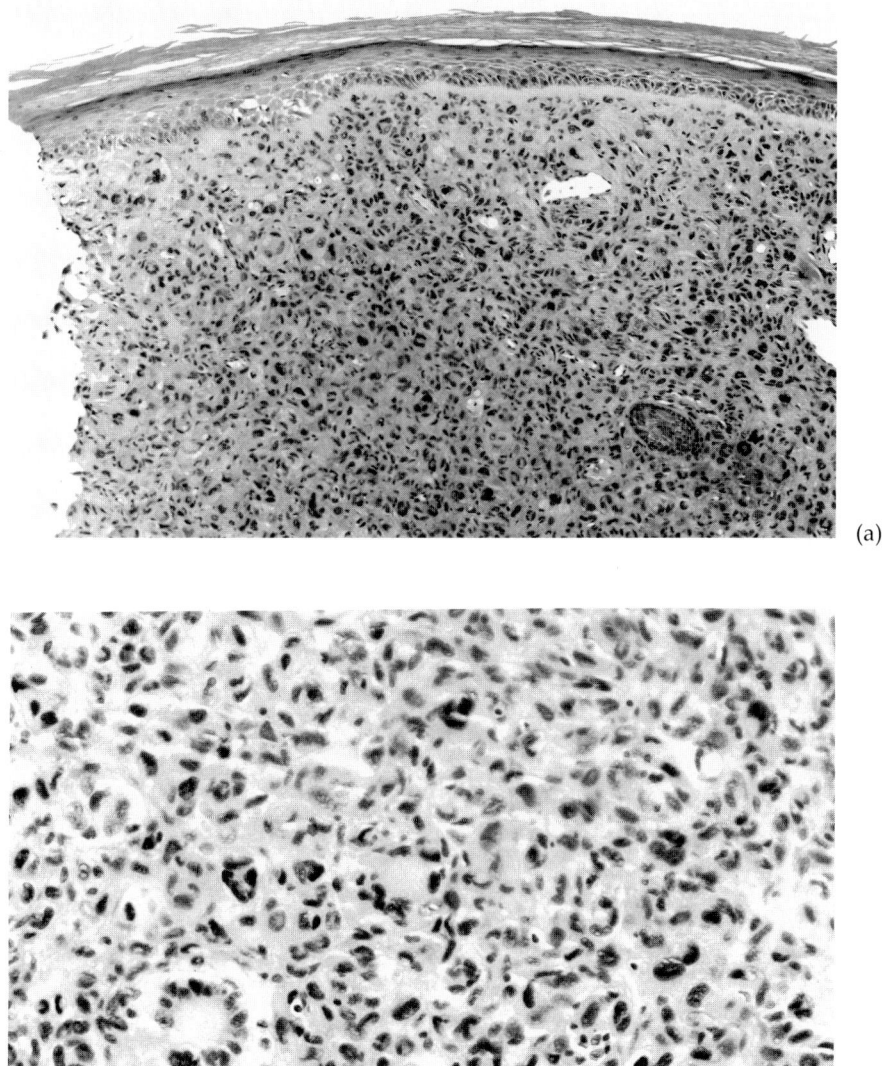

Figure 8.3 Atypical fibroxanthoma. (a) The dermis is filled by cells with moderately pleomorphic nuclei and eosinophilic cytoplasm; (b) Touton-type giant cells are a prominent feature.

nodular or multinodular stage. They are usually solitary, occur on the trunk or arms of men, and are prone to local recurrence after incomplete excision. Distant metastasis is most unusual.

The tumour cells have a uniform, monomorphic, thin spindle shape, usually arranged in a storiform pattern and infiltrating the dermis and subcutaneous fat. Appendages become enveloped without being destroyed. Strands of cells spread out sideways from the deeper parts of the tumour, making it difficult to be sure that the surgical margins are free of tumour. Mitoses may be present, but are infrequent and are not a guide to behaviour (Alguacil-Garcia et al., 1978; Fletcher et al., 1985).

Immunohistochemical studies show that the tumour cells react only with antibodies to vimentin, in keeping with a fibroblastic rather than a neural or histiocytic histogenesis (Lautier et al., 1990).

In about 5% of cases the tumour is colonized by melanocytes: the so-called 'storiform neurofibroma' or 'Bednar' tumour (Bednar, 1957). In other respects these pigmented variants are similar to usual dermatofibrosarcomas (Fletcher et al., 1988), despite claims of neural differentiation (Nakamura et al., 1987).

The more aggressive examples of DFSP have features overlapping with fibrosarcoma. If less than half of the tumour shows fibrosarcomatous change, no special action need be taken. The tumour could be called 'fibrosarcoma-like DFSP'. When more than half shows such change the tumour is best classified as a fibrosarcoma. No change is needed in the surgical approach because complete excision is the treatment of choice. Careful follow-up is worthwhile, however, so as to have a better chance of identifying any metastases at an early stage (Wrotnowski et al., 1988).

8.1.6   Granular cell tumour

Granular cell tumours of the skin are usually single lesions, although occasional examples of multiple lesions have been reported. They are benign lesions best treated by surgical excision if rapidly growing orsymptomatic. The granular cells show positive staining for S100 protein in nucleus and cytoplasm, and weak neurone specific enolase staining of cytoplasm (Mori et al., 1988). This can be a helpful way of delineating the tumour margins when examining an excision specimen for clearance.

The histogenesis is still debated, but it seems most likely that they are derived either directly from Schwann cells or from undifferentiated cells which develop a neural immunophenotype (Kyler et al., 1988). This is further supported by negative staining for epithelial and muscle markers (Buley et al., 1988).

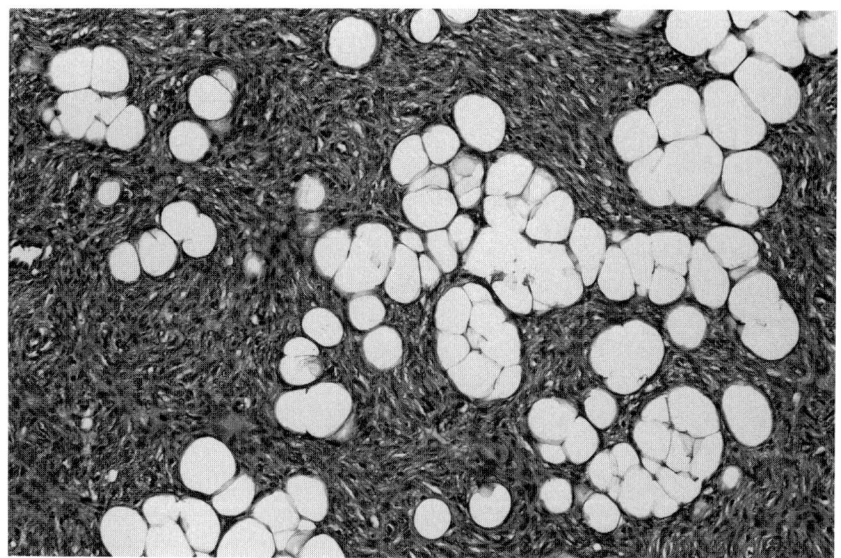

Figure 8.4 Dermatofibrosarcoma protuberans. Tumour cells extend into and infiltrate subcutaneous fat.

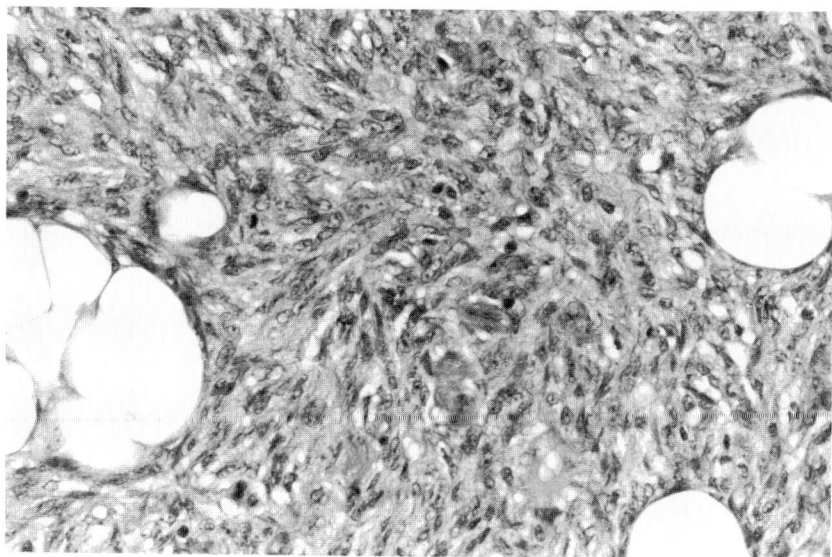

Figure 8.5 Dermatofibrosarcoma protuberans. Tumour cell nuclei are spindle shaped and occasional mitoses are present.

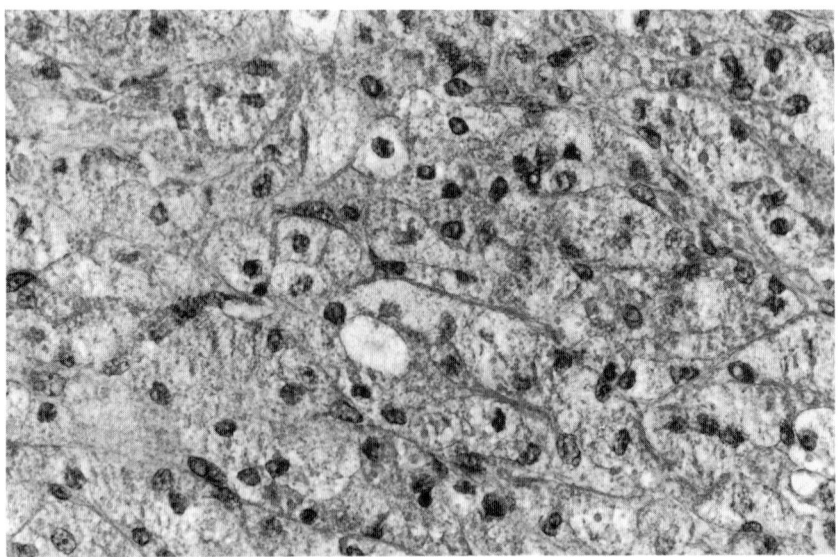

Figure 8.6 Granular cell tumour. Sheets of cells with regular nuclei and granular eosinophilic cytoplasm.

8.1.7 Fibrous papule of nose

These little lesions occur as small, sessile, flesh-coloured papules on the nose (Graham *et al.*, 1965). They contain stellate cells in the dermis, together with variable numbers of small blood vessels. One view is that these lesions represent involuting naevi, but the stellate cells show factor XIIIa immunoreactivity, which has been found in a variety of cell types, including dendritic reticulum cells and fibroblast-like mesenchymal cells, but not in naevus cells (Nemeth *et al.*, 1988). This finding supports the view that they are more likely to be of inflammatory rather than neoplastic origin, sharing as they do the perivascular fibrosis seen in angiofibromas and perifollicular fibrosis of perifollicular fibromas (Rosen and Suster, 1988; Zackheim and Pinkus, 1960).

8.1.8 Digital fibroma

Digital fibromas usually occur on the fingers of infants and often recur after local removal. They consist of poorly circumscribed dermal fibroblastic tumours, in which the spindle cells may contain inclusions. Although usually found in infancy, they can occur in adults and at sites other than the fingers (Santa Cruz and Reiner, 1978).

8.1.9   Xanthoma

Collections of foamy, lipid-filled macrophages can occur in a number of contexts, either with or without an associated systemic hyperlipidaemia. When associated with hyperlipidaemia biopsy is rarely performed. Xanthelasma of the eyelid may be excized for cosmetic reasons and shows an appearance of small focal collections of foam cells in the dermis.

8.1.10   Juvenile xanthogranuloma

This condition is one in which single or small numbers of raised red or yellow nodules develop in infants, but also in some older children and adults. They measure 0.5 to 1.0 cm across. They are usually quite typical clinically and so are often left in place, as in time they usually involute.

   If one is removed, the biopsy will show a granulomatous appearance with foamy macrophages and giant cells of both foreign-body and Touton type (Alterman *et al.*, 1988). Older lesions in the stage of involution will be less cellular and contain a fibroblastic and fibrotic component.

8.1.11   Myxoma

There is an increasingly heterogeneous variety of myxoid lesions of the skin, various examples of which either contain other elements or have other associations. Myxoid tumours include myxoid variants of lipoma, liposarcoma, neurofibroma, dermatofibrosarcoma protuberans and chordoma (Allen, 1980). More recently, it has been proposed that the lesions previously called trichodiscoma, fibrofolliculoma, perifollicular fibroma, trichofolliculoma, trichogenic adnexal tumour and cutaneous focal mucinosis all represent a single entity: the superficial angiomyxoma (Allen *et al.*, 1988). Whilst it is always a relief to be able to dispose of a few rarely seen differential diagnoses, this proposal has not been universally accepted.

   The lesion described as superficial angiomyxoma has variably demarcated margins and contains mucin which is PAS negative and Alcian blue positive at pH 1 to 4, with the staining being abolished by hyaluronidase digestion. Within the myxoid stroma, is a myriad of small blood vessels and also spindle and stellate stromal cells. Mitoses are only found occasionally. Some cases contain epithelial components, sometimes with cyst formation.

   Myxomas may also be found in association with the Carney complex

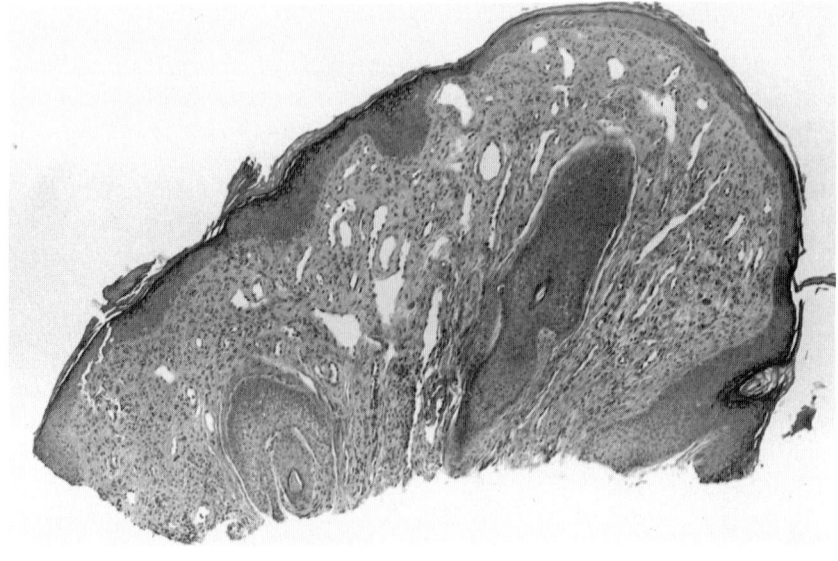

(a)

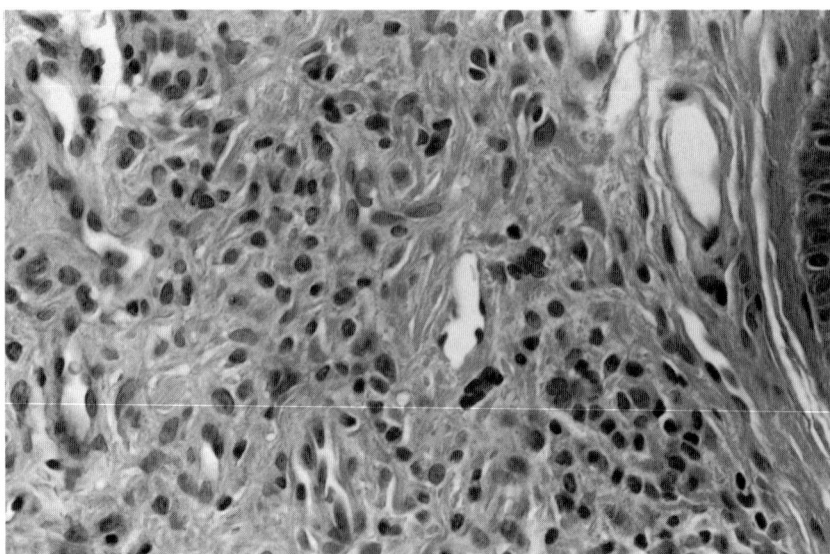

(b)

Figure 8.7 Fibrous papule of nose. (a) A shave biopsy showing (b) a moderately vascular lesion with sparse stromal cells and collagenous stroma.

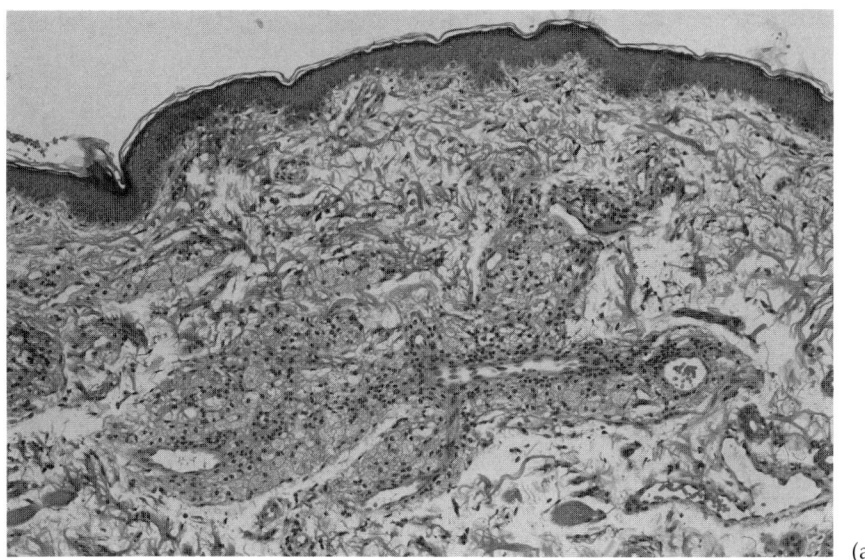

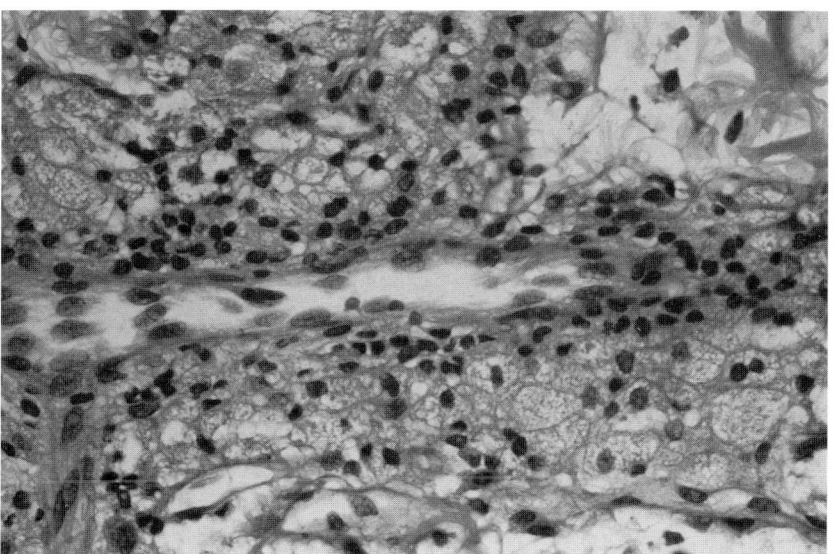

Figure 8.8 Xanthelasma. (a) The biopsy shows subtle changes, with (b) foam cells present around dermal vessels.

of spotty skin pigmentation, endocrine overactivity, especially nodular adrenal cortical hyperplasia and, more importantly, with atrial myxoma (Atherton *et al.*, 1980; Carney *et al.*, 1985; Carney, 1985). Death can result from the embolic complications of the atrial myxoma, which can also metastasize to the skin and mimic a primary tumour (Feldman and Keeling, 1989).

8.2   Vascular tumours

8.2.1   *Haemangioma*

Haemangiomas do not usually present much difficulty in biopsy diagnosis, although it can be difficult to distinguish them clinically from other pigmented lesions. Depending on the size of the vessels, they may be classified as capillary or cavernous, although intermediate types also occur. Variants include the verrucous haemangioma, with warty epidermal hyperplasia, and the angiokeratoma, which has cavernous vessels which lie in and fill the papillary dermis, abutting on the epidermal basement membrane. These lesions often show intravascular thrombosis. They may be associated with Fabry's disease.

8.2.2   *Vegetant intravascular haemangioendothelioma*

First described by Masson (1923), this appearance of papillary endothelial hyperplasia is generally considered to represent organizing intravascular thrombus. The lumen of the affected vessel is more or less filled by groups of proliferating capillaries, usually attached to the wall at one side.

A related lesion is the benign, acquired tufted angioma, which is seen in the first year of life, on the back of the neck and the back, and which shows an increased number of ectatic blood vessels within which endothelial cells proliferate and may form new lumina (Wilson Jones, 1976).

8.2.3   *Cirsoid aneurysm*

These curious lesions occur as small, pink or red papular lesions, usually less than 0.5 cm across, on the face, around the mouth and nose. They consist of a circumscribed collection of abnormally formed blood vessels showing variation in wall thickness from thick to thin. They are probably malformations rather than tumours.

The clinical impression is usually one of a small, pinkish naevus: consequently these lesions may turn up in shave biopsies. So if a

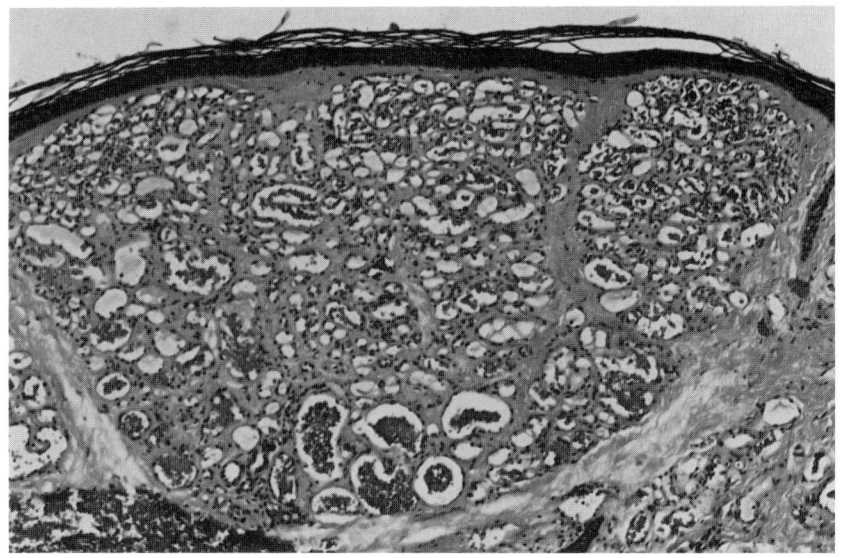

Figure 8.9 Capillary haemangioma. A circumscribed lobulated lesion with small, thin-walled vessels.

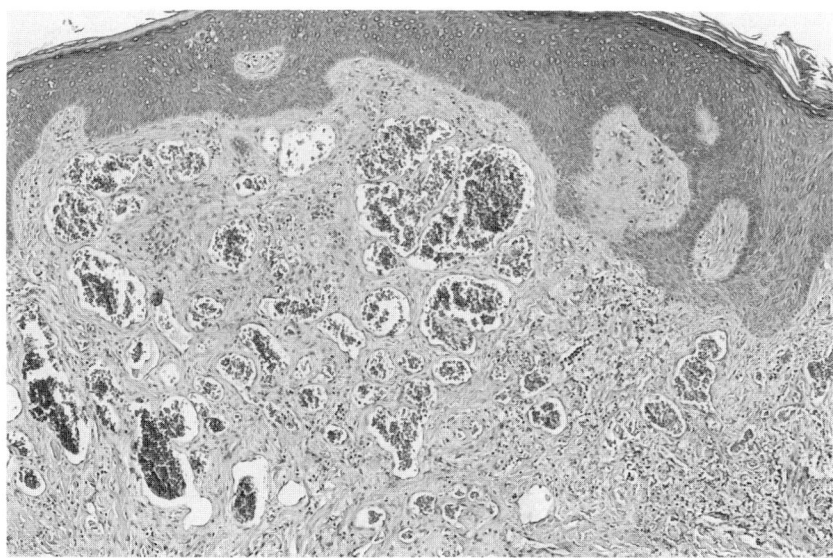

Figure 8.10 Haemangioma with capillary and cavernous, thin-walled vessels.

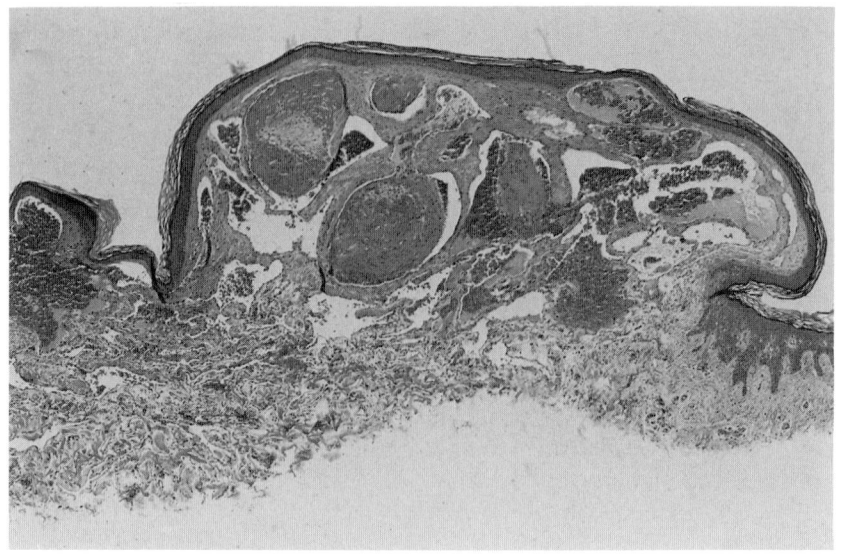

(a)

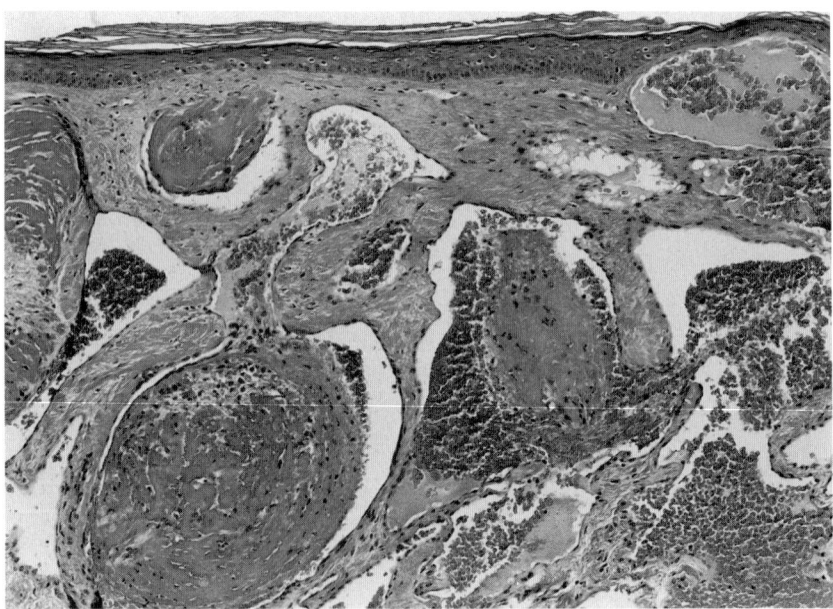

(b)

Figure 8.11 Cavernous haemangioma (a and b). Cavernous vascular spaces, many showing secondary thrombosis.

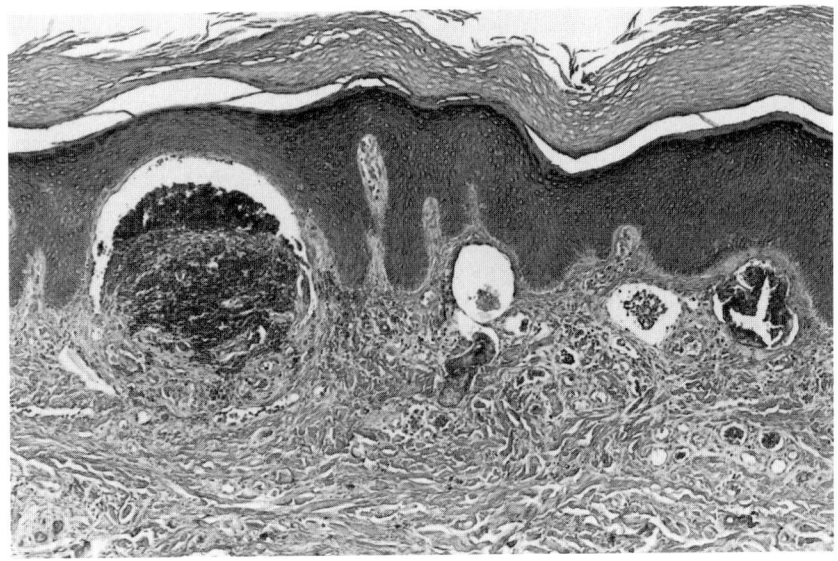

Figure 8.12 Angiokeratoma. Epidermal hyperkeratosis with cavernous vessels immediately beneath.

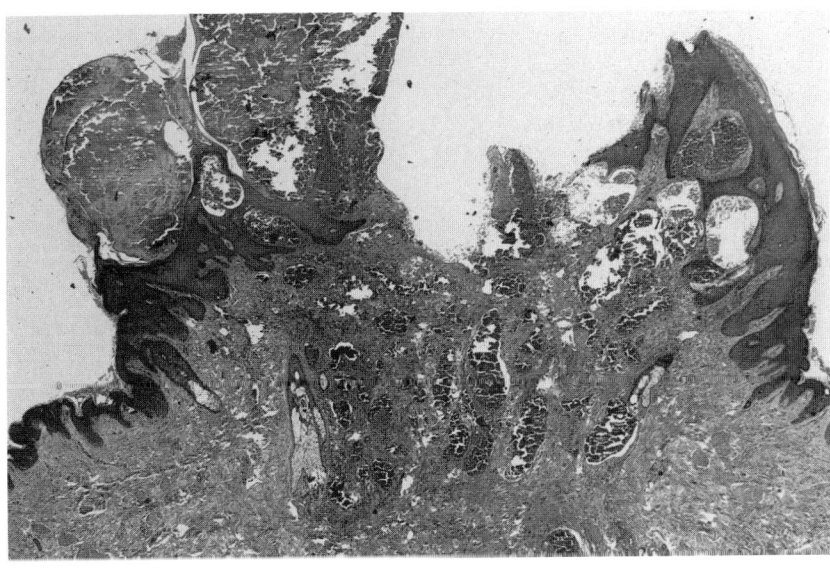

(a)

Figure 8.13 Verrucous haemangioma (a and b). In this example the top of the wart has become ulcerated. (Cont.)

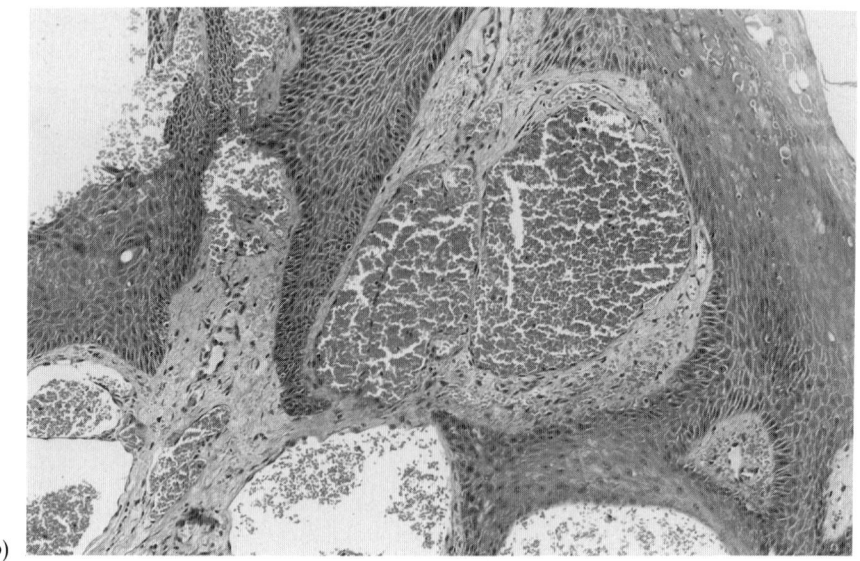

(b)

Figure 8.13 (Cont.)

biopsy of a putative naevus does not contain any naevus cells, even after looking at further levels, a fresh look at the deeper dermal vessels may reveal a cirsoid aneurysm.

8.2.4 *Pyogenic granuloma*

This is perhaps one of the commonest lesions, and is characterized by a lobular arrangement of leashes of small, thin-walled vessels, with little associated stroma. Occasional multiple lesions may be seen (De Kaminsky *et al.*, 1978). Differential diagnosis is usually from simple granulation tissue, although in HIV positive individuals the possibility of bacillary angiomatosis should be considered.

8.2.5 *Epithelioid haemangioendothelioma*

This occurs almost always in adults and is remarkable for rounded epithelioid endothelial cells with vacuolated eosinophilic cytoplasm. The vacuoles may represent attempts at lumen formation (Weiss and Enzinger, 1982).

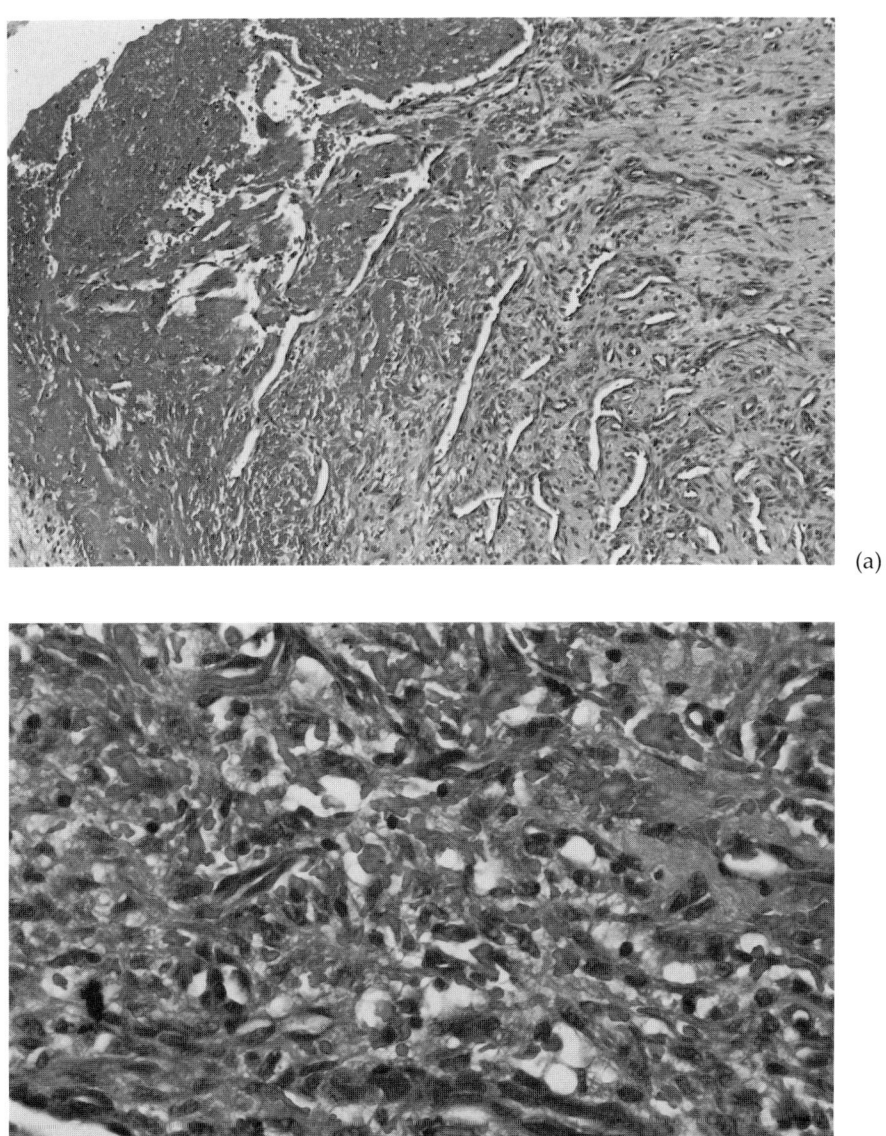

(a)

(b)

Figure 8.14 Masson's vegetant intravascular haemangioenothelioma (a and b). Organizing thrombus filling most of the lumen of a vessel.

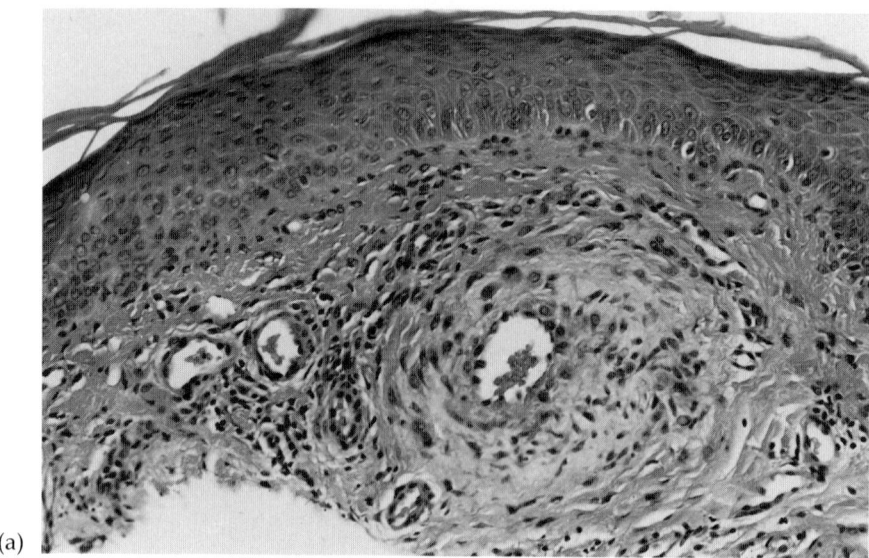

(a)

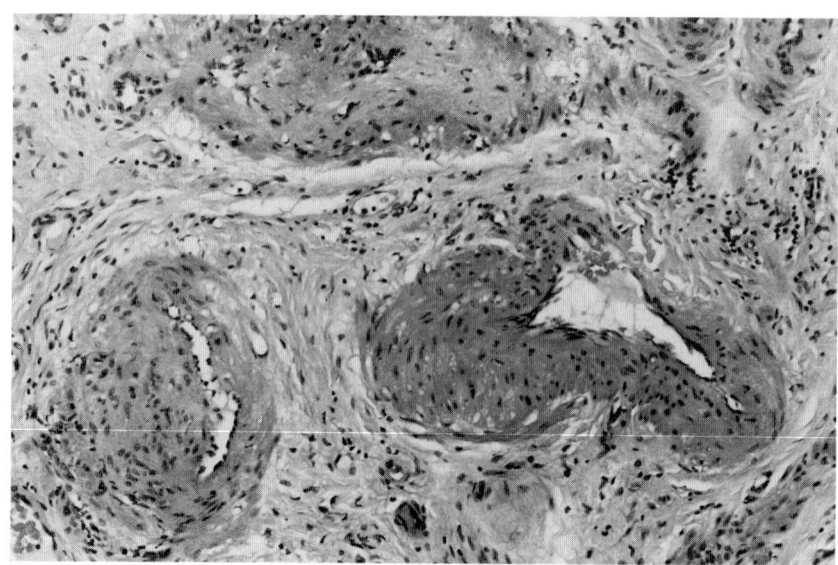

(b)

Figure 8.15 Cirsoid aneurysm (a and b). A localized collection of abnormal vessels showing variation in the thickness of vessel walls

8.2.6   Angiosarcoma

Cutaneous angiosarcoma is a highly aggressive malignancy with a median survival of 20 months and an overall 5-year survival of only 12%(Holden *et al.*, 1987). It occurs in association with post-mastectomy lymphoedema, in previously irradiated skin and in the sun-exposed skin of the face and scalp of the elderly. The tumour often has an insidious onset, looking at first like a bruise, then showing extensive local spread before developing distant metastases. The tumours vary in appearance from a well-differentiated type with developed vascular spaces and tumour cells dissecting between dermal collagen bundles, to less well-differentiated examples with undifferentiated spindle cells, prominent nuclear pleomorphism and frequent mitoses. The degree of differentiation does not appear to relate to the prognosis (Holden *et al.*, 1987).

The most widely used markers of vascular differentiation are factor-VIII related antigen and *Ulex europaeus* lectin (Ordonez and Batsakis, 1984). Electron microscopy shows features of endothelial differentiation and vascular lumena (Wilson Jones, 1976; Rosai *et al.*, 1976; Cooper, 1987).

8.2.7   Dabska tumour

Otherwise called malignant endovascular papillary angioendothelioma, this rare tumour consists of a proliferation in the dermis of well-formed, anastamosing vascular channels lined by atypical endothelial cells, which have a characteristic appearance of epithelioid cytoplasm with nuclei arrayed at the luminal pole of the cells. It may be present at birth. Both local spread into fat and muscle, and spread into regional lymph nodes, has been described. The tumour is generally considered to be of low-grade malignancy (Dabska, 1969; Morgan *et al.*, 1989).

8.2.8   Lymphangioma circumscriptum superficialis

Cutaneous lymphangiomas are usually either localized ectasias, or sometimes represent malformations. Malignant tumours occur almost exclusively as complications of long-standing lymphoedema following radical mastectomy operations, which are now, thankfully, of historical interest only (Stewart and Treves, 1948; Drachman *et al.*, 1988).

8.2.9   Glomus tumour

Glomus tumours occur as small dermal nodules, which, especially if sub-ungal, may be painful. They are derived from specialized epithe-

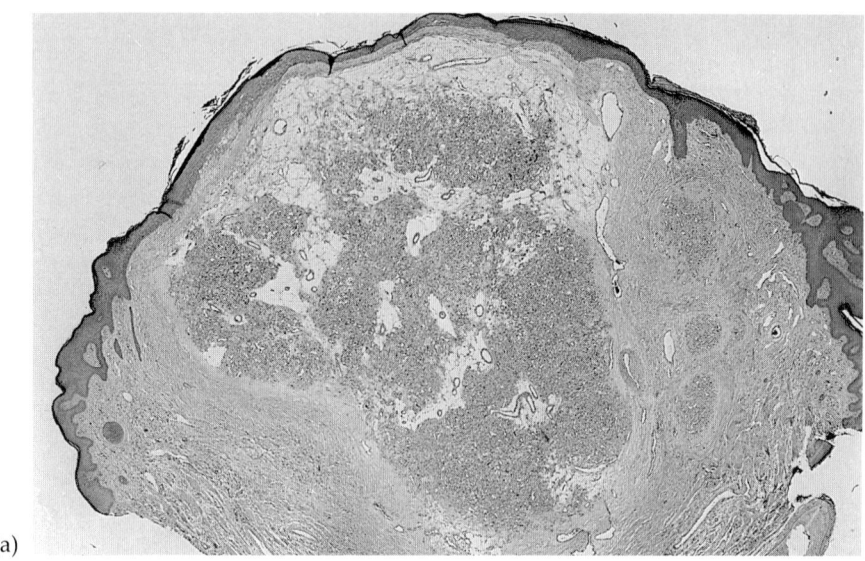

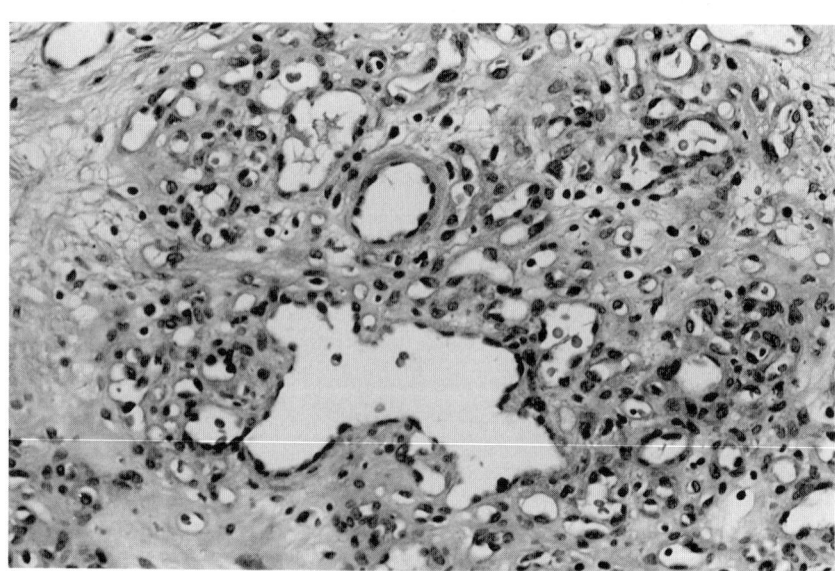

Figure 8.16 Pyogenic granuloma (a and b). An exophytic lesion containing lobulated leashes of small, thin-walled vessels.

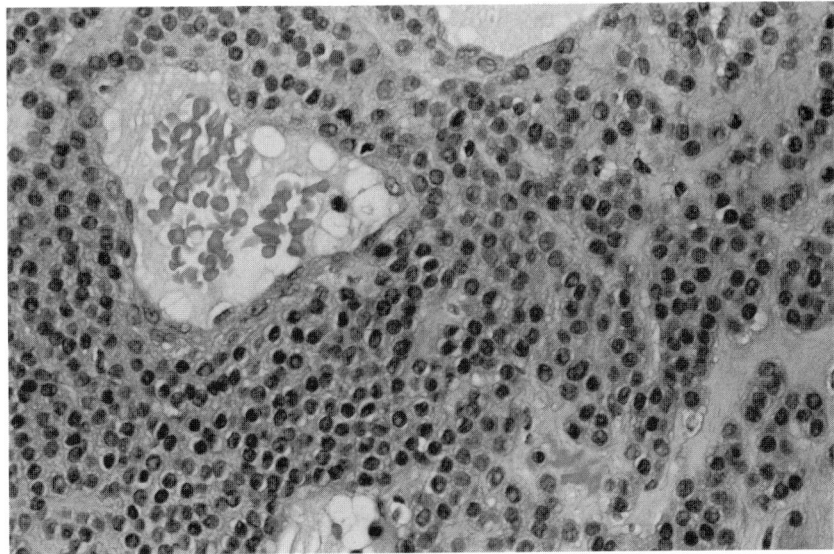

Figure 8.17   Glomus tumour. Regular glomus cells are arrayed around dilated blood vessels.

lioid cells in the wall of myoarterial glomus tissue, and in biopsies appear as perivascular collections of cells, in an orderly arrangement, without mitoses or other features of malignancy (Pepper *et al.*, 1977).

Multiple lesions may be present (Alos Ribera *et al.*, 1989). Immunohistochemical staining shows that the tumour cells are immunoreactive for muscle-specific actin and vimentin, with other keratin and intermediate filament markers negative. There are many small nerve fibres in the connective tissue septae between the packets of glomus cells. This observation may have a bearing on the frequently painful nature of these lesions (Dervan *et al.*, 1989).

A related lesion is the cutaneous myofibroma, which has a biphasic pattern with central vascular or glomus-like features surrounded by actin-positive cells. It occurs in young adults and is cured by simple excision (Smith *et al.*, 1989).

8.3   Neural tumours

8.3.1   *Neurofibroma*

Neurofibromas are typically small dermal tumours which are well circumscribed, with delicate spindle cells and also with mast cells interspersed in the stroma. Differential diagnosis is from the sparsely cellular neuronaevus and sometimes from dermatofibroma. The biopsy may be from a patient with neurofibromatosis, in which case lesions of tuberous sclerosis may also be present (Nickel and Reed, 1962).

8.3.2   Neurilemmoma

Nerve sheath tumours are uncommon in the skin, but one that is worth remembering is the nerve sheath myxoma, which occurs as a nodule about 1 cm in diameter, on the face and arms and is commoner in women. The lesions lie in the reticular dermis and consist of fascicles of spindle cells which are S100 positive. They lie in an Alcian blue-positive myxoid matrix. The lesions are benign and cured by simple excision (Pulitzer and Reed, 1985; Fletcher et al., 1986).

8.3.3   Cellular neurothekeoma

This entity occurs as unremarkable papules and nodules on the head and neck of young adults. The biopsy shows fascicles of pale polygonal and spindle cells extending deep into the dermis. Mild cytological atypia and occasional mitoses may be present, but the lesion behaves in a benign fashion. All immunohistochemical markers, including S100, are negative. The lesion is probably derived from perineurium and has to be distinguished from Spitz naevi and melanoma (Barnhill and Mihm, 1990).

8.3.4   Solitary circumscribed neuroma

This lesion typically occurs on the face or around the mouth in middle-aged adults, and is less than 5 mm in diameter. The central nodule of interlacing fascicles of Schwann cells and axons is surrounded by an incomplete capsule of epithelial membrane antigen (EMA) positive perineural cells. There is no known association with von Recklinghausen's disease or type IIb multiple endocrine neoplasia syndrome (Reed et al., 1972; Fletcher, 1989). A traumatic origin has been suggested (Dover et al., 1989).

8.3.5   Meningioma

Nodules of heterotopic meningeal tissue occur rarely on the scalp or back. They usually present in childhood (in otherwise normal children), although they can be associated with spinal closure defects. The architecture of individual lesions varies, but they all have in common the cytological appearance of a meningioma, with meningothelial cells,

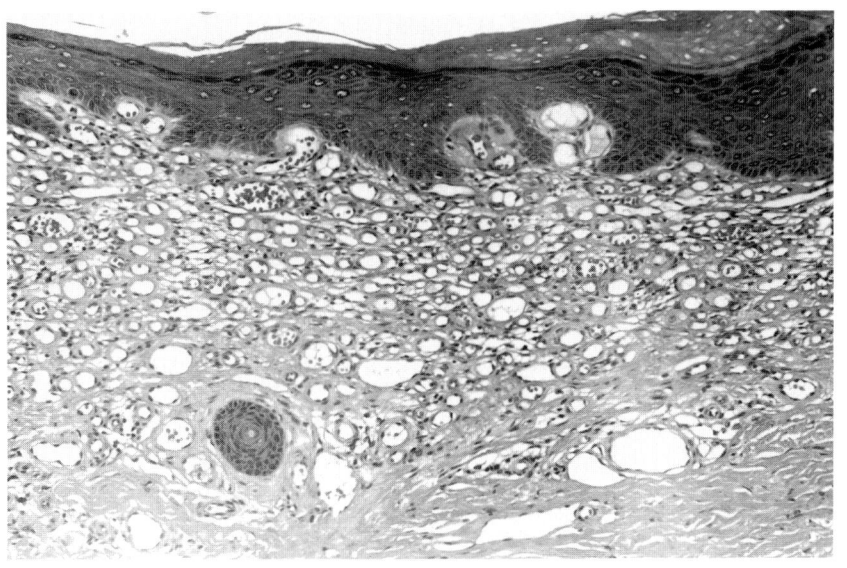

(a)

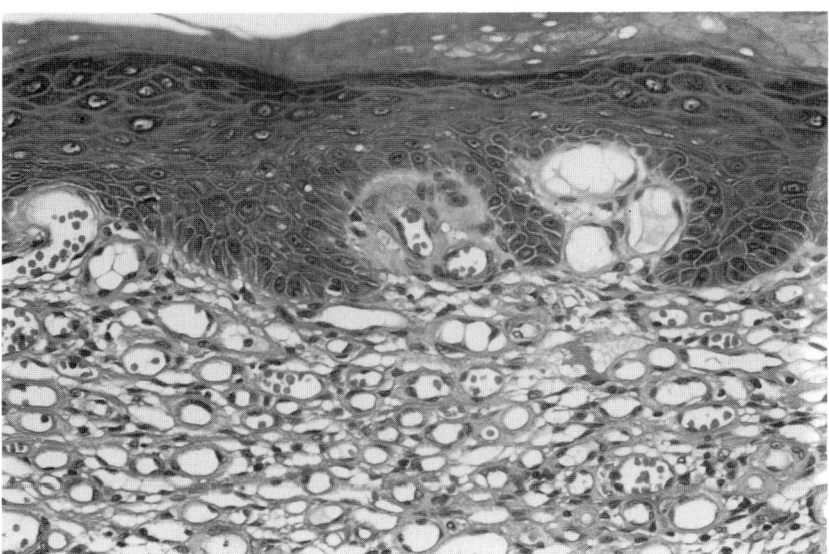

(b)

Figure 8.18 Solitary circumscribed lymphangioma. (a) The dermis is filled by closely packed vessels. (b) The vessels have thin walls with inconspicuous lining cells (Courtesy of Dr K. Blessing).

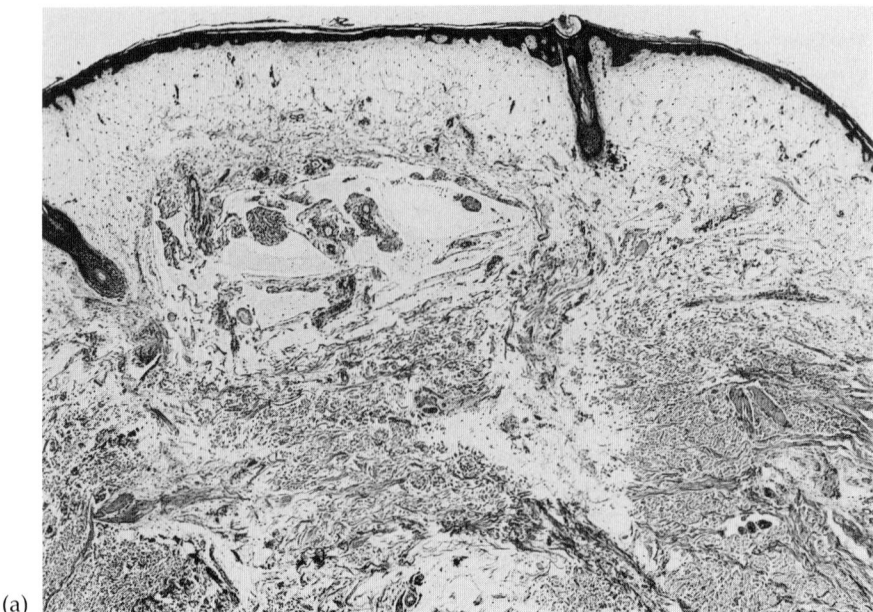

(a)

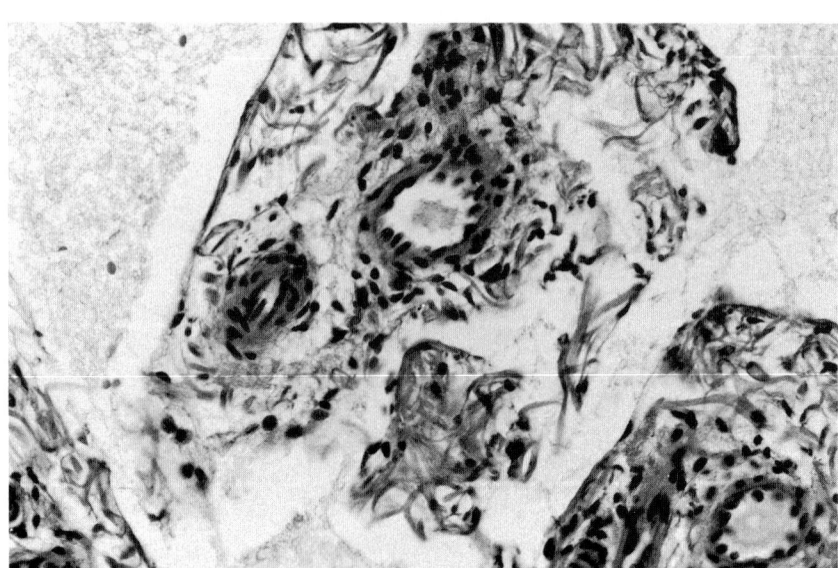

(b)

Figure 8.19 Lymphangioma circumscriptum. (a) The epidermis is raised, with underlying dermal oedema, and (b) a central lesion with leashes of thin-walled lymphatic vessels.

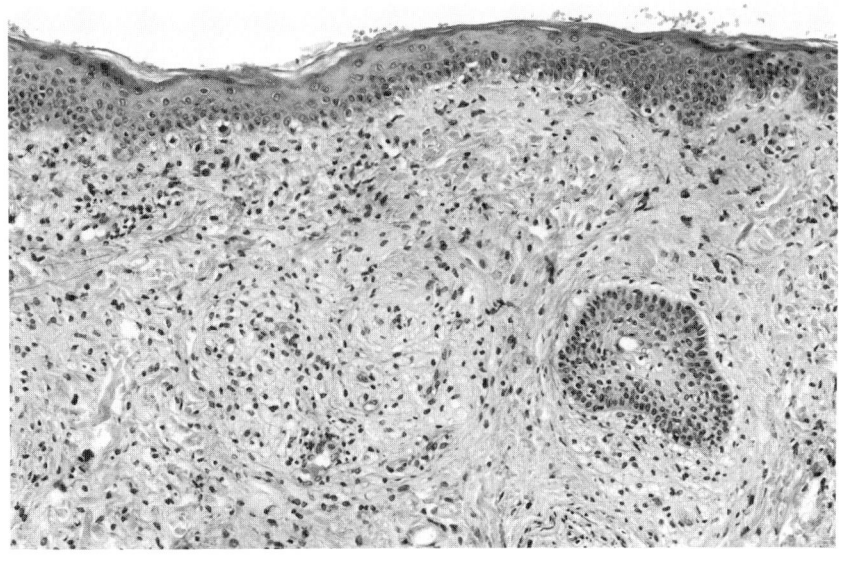

(a)

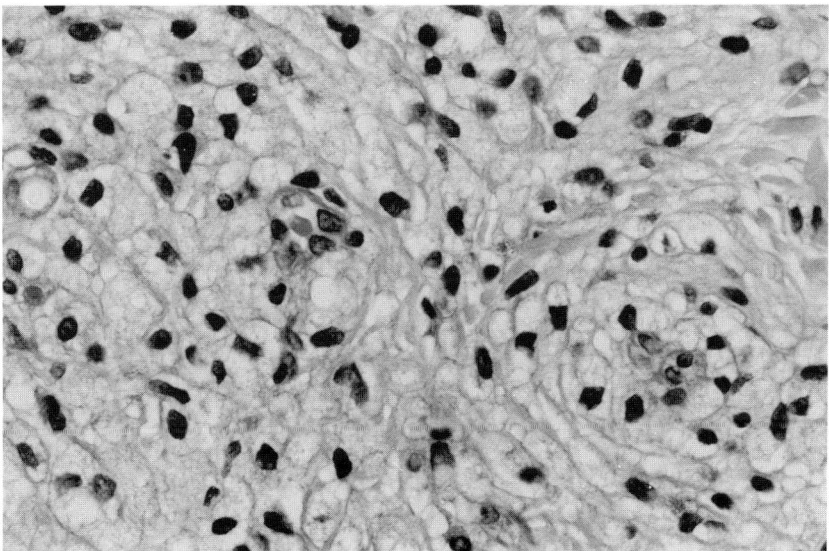

Figure 8.20 Neurofibroma. (a) The dermis contains a well circumscribed lesion, with (b) a delicated arrangement of cells with pale cytoplasm filling the dermis.

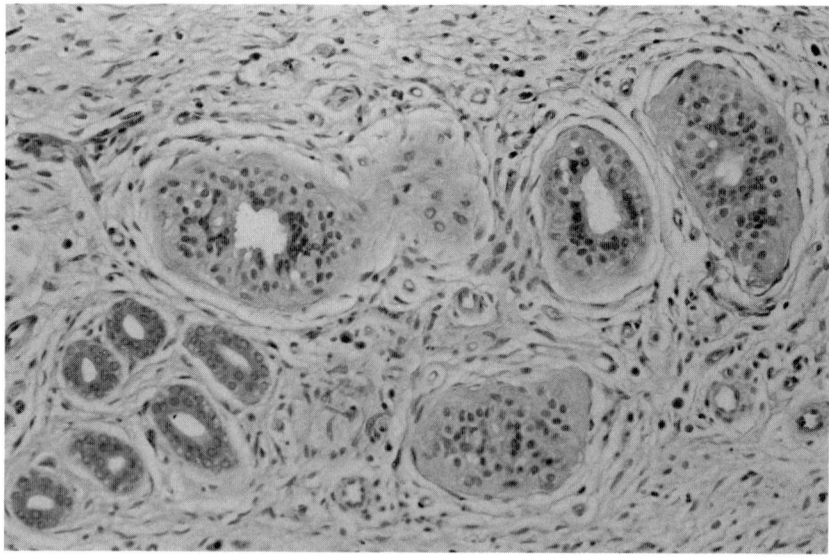

Figure 8.21   Neurofibroma. Appendages are surrounded by the tumour cells.

psammoma bodies and small collagenous bodies. Immunohistochemical staining shows vimentin in the meningothelial cells, sometimes associated with epithelial membrane antigen immunoreactivity in the same cells. The lesions appear to be entirely benign (Lopez *et al.*, 1974; Theaker *et al.*, 1990).

8.4   Neuroendocrine carcinoma

The description by Toker (1972) of trabecular carcinoma led to a flurry of publications as the entity of primary cutaneous neuroendocrine carcinoma was recognized and characterized. These are tumours of the middle-aged and elderly, which usually have quite a short history of a rapidly enlarging, rounded exophytic nodule. The limbs are the commonest site, followed by the face. The tumour lies in the dermis and usually has a few prominent, thin-walled vessels coursing over its surface.

The histological appearance is characteristic, and as is often the case, is best seen in well prepared and fixed material (Kirkham and Cole, 1983). Three sub-types have been described: trabecular, solid and diffuse (Pilotti *et al.*, 1988). The tumour cells are medium sized and have pale nuclei with inconspicuous nucleoli and cytoplasm, resembling lymphoblasts. These cells are arranged in cords and nests in a tumour which contains many small, thin-walled blood vessels and in varying proportions according to the predominant sub-type. Plasma cells are often present in the perivascular spaces.

The tumours show a high mitotic rate and also a high apoptotic rate. A minority of tumours may show other forms of differentiation, such as the formation of ductular structures resembling acrosyringium, or areas of squamous differentiation (Gould *et al.*, 1988; Szadowska *et al.*, 1989). Differential diagnosis is from metastatic small cell carcinoma from primary sites such as the bronchus, cutaneous deposits of lymphoblastic lymphoma and other adnexal carcinomas.

Ultrastructural studies show small numbers of cytoplasmic dense core neurosecretory granules (Kirkham and Cole, 1983; Warner *et al.*, 1983). Because the number of granules is low, the tumours are almost always negative when stained with Grimelius' method for argyrophilic granules.

It is important to distinguish this tumour from malignant lymphoma (Wick *et al.*, 1986). Immunohistochemical studies show cytoplasmic staining for neurone-specific enolase (Kirkham and Isaacson, 1983) and calcitonin. The most useful differential test, however, is to stain for low-molecular weight cytokeratin, with an antibody such as CAM 5.2, which shows characteristic focal cytoplasmic dot positivity. This appearance corresponds to the whorls of intermediate filaments, which can be seen in the cytoplasm of tumour cells by electron microscopy (Balaton *et al.*, 1989). The tumours may also stain for chromogranin (Weiler *et al.*, 1988).

8.5   Smooth muscle tumours

8.5.1   *Leiomyoma*

The commonest form of cutaneous, smooth muscle tumour is that derived from the arrector pili muscles. Rather than forming discrete, circumscribed tumours the lesions consist of multiple fascicles of well-differentiated muscle growing between the collagen bundles of the reticular dermis.

8.5.2   *Angioleiomyoma*

These are one of the painfull nodular lesions of the extremity. They occur in the middle-aged and 67% are painful. They are usually less than 1 cm in diameter and consist of well-circumscribed nodules containing tortuous vascular channels with thick muscular walls. They are

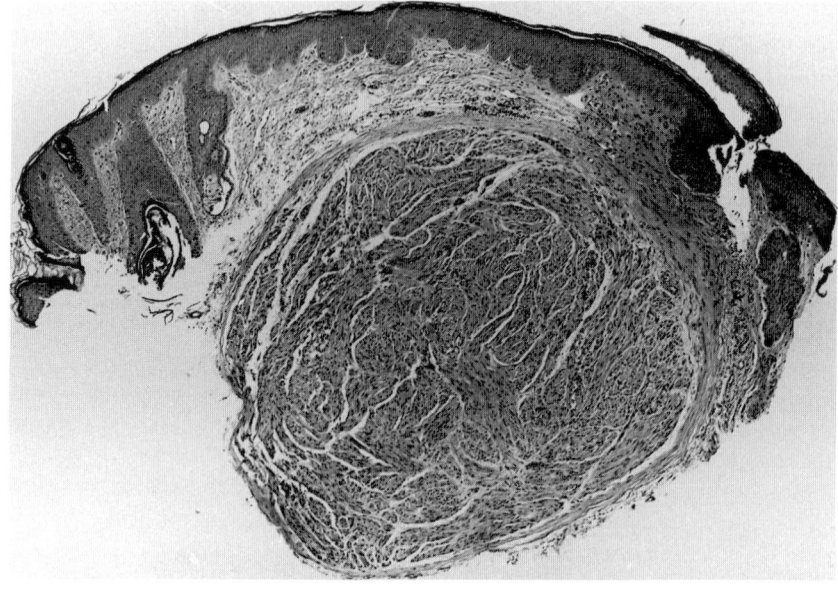

(a)

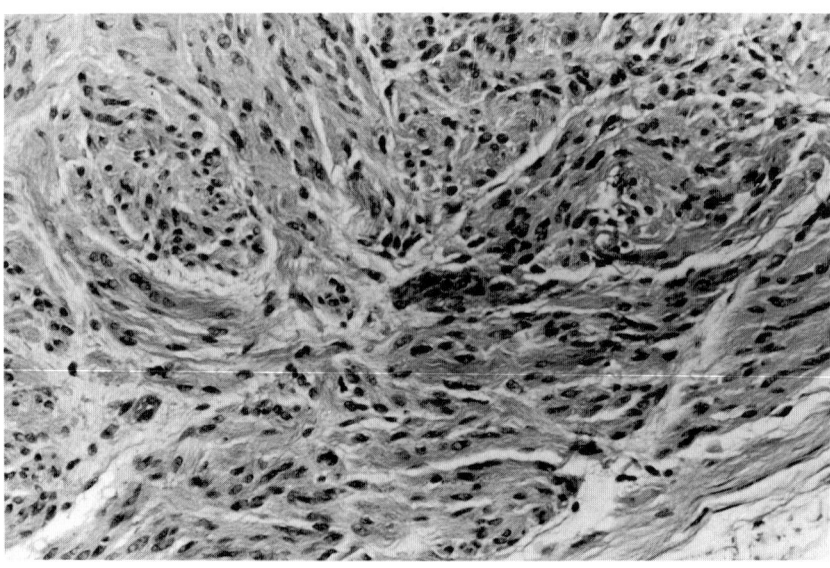

(b)

Figure 8.22 Solitary circumscribed neuroma. (a) The dermis contains a small, well-circumscribed nodule with (b) well-differentiated spindle cells.

cured by simple excision (MacDonald and Sanderson, 1974; Freedman and Meland, 1989).

8.5.3   Leiomyosarcoma

Malignant leiomyosarcomas do occur but are most unusual. Spread from an underlying, soft-tissue sarcoma is more likely to be seen but even that is rare (Dahl and Angervall, 1974; Headington et al., 1977; Jegasothy et al., 1981; Fields and Helwig, 1981; Iacobucci et al., 1987). It should be considered in the differential diagnosis of poorly differentiated skin tumours, when immunoreactivity for desmin and vimentin should be demonstrable. A case with abundant granular eosinophilic cytoplasm has been reported as a complication of radiotherapy (Suster et al., 1988).

8.6 Naevus lipomatosus superficialis

There are two clinical types of naevus lipomatosus superficialis. The classic type has multiple lesions in one area, and occurs most often in the lumbar region, buttocks and thighs and has been described on the scalp (Chanoki et al., 1989). The other type presents as a solitary papule or nodule and has no favoured location. An excision biopsy will show ectopic adipose tissue in the dermis, possibly extending up to the papillary dermis (Abel and Dougherty, 1962; Wilson Jones et al., 1975).

8.7   Cutaneous metastases

When examining a biopsy in which there is a tumour which is difficult to classify, one should always consider the possibility of metastasis. Cutaneous metastases are relatively uncommon, but are associated with a relatively limited number of primary sites (McKee, 1985). Carcinoma of the bronchus must always be high on the list, especially in the differential diagnosis of neurendocrine carcinoma.

In men, two possibilities are particularly important. In younger men, the syndrome of 'metastatic adenocarcinoma of unknown primary (ACUP)' is due to metastasis from a primary, malignant, germ-cell tumour of the testis. The primary tumour is usually a teratoma, but an interesting phenomenon is that the primary may be very small, or may even consist of a small scar with little or no apparent tumour component. The metastasis may mark for human chorionic gonadotrophin (HCG) in addition to epithelial markers.

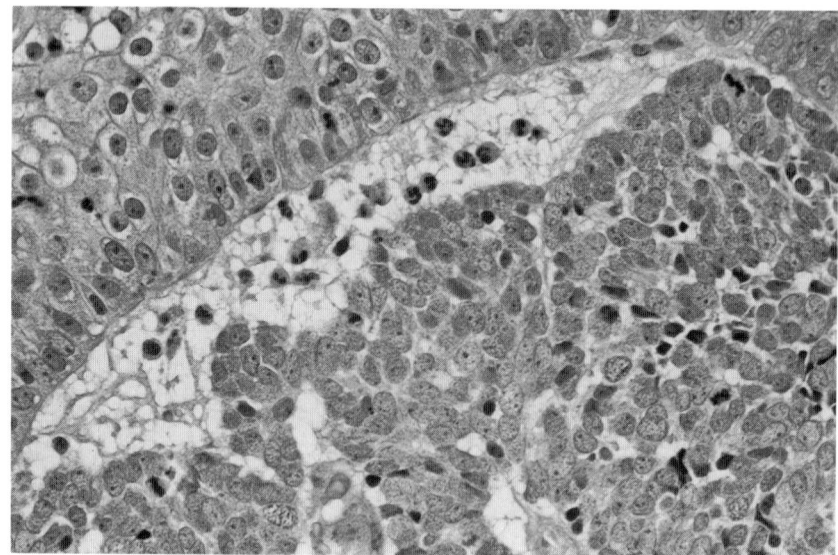

(a)

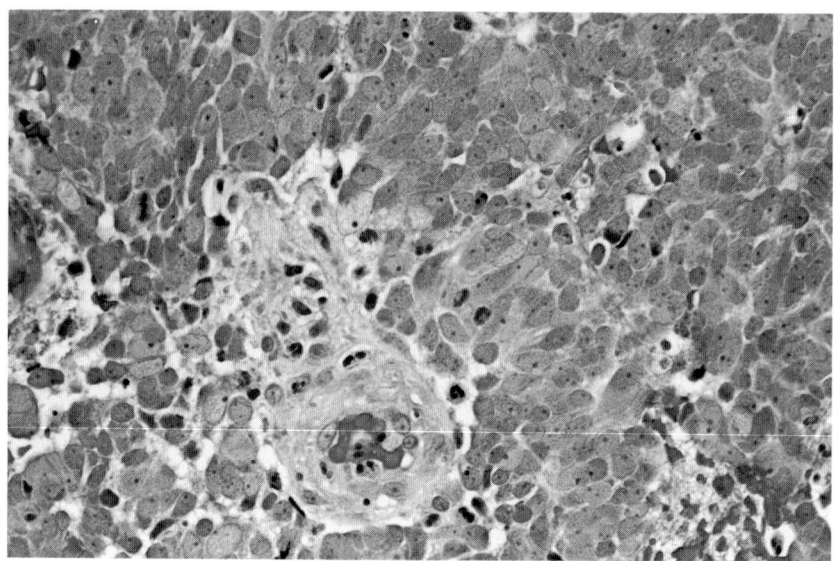

(b)

Figure 8.23 Neuroendocrine carcinoma. (a) Tumour cell nuclei are larger than those of keratinocytes and have smaller nucleoli; (b) small numbers of lymphocytes and plasma cells are present in perivascular spaces.

In older men, the prostate is a prominent source of cutaneous metastases, which are usually found in the skin of the lower abdomen or genitalia, and will mark with antibodies to prostate-specific antigen or prostatic acid phosphatase (Katake *et al.*, 1982; Scupham *et al.*, 1988).

A related phenomenon is that of penile squamous carcinoma metastatic to the skin of the leg and growing in continuity with the epidermis, giving the apparent appearance of a primary tumour (Youngberg *et al.*, 1989).

In women, local recurrence and both regional and distant metastases from primary breast carcinoma are, perhaps, the most commonly seen tumours. Lobular carcinoma can mimic a naevus in the skin. Metastases from ovarian or uterine tumours may present around the umbilicus or in the vulva, at the side of the vagina. Melanoma can be confused with breast carcinoma; a reminder always to think of melanoma. The differential diagnosis can be made using epithelial markers, such as CAM 5.2 and HMFG2, and melanoma markers, such as HMB-45, S100 and NKI/C3 (Barker and Girling, 1989).

Metastatic papillary carcinoma of the thyroid can be specifically diagnosed with antibodies to thyroglobulin (Doutre *et al.*, 1988). Malignant mesothelioma may extend through the chest wall and present as a cutaneous tumour (Berkowitz *et al.*, 1989). Renal cell carcinoma and gastric adenocarcinoma may also spread to the skin (Menter *et al.*, 1989; Fujiwara *et al.*, 1989).

Other reports of even rarer possibilities, such as left atrial cardiac myxoma (in which embolic manifestations may occur in up to 40% of cases and can mimic a peripheral vasculitis or connective tissue disease as a result of arterial tumour embolism), emphasize that when a dermal tumour is difficult to classify, the possibility of metastasis should always be considered (Feldman and Keeling, 1989; Reed *et al.*, 1989).

Non-metastatic manifestations of malignancy may also turn up occasionally. Examples include necrolytic migratory erythema in association with glucagonoma (Verbov, 1981; Kheir *et al.*, 1986; Price *et al.*, 1989), erythema gyratum repens, cutaneous icthyosis or bullous disease in association with bronchial or mediastinal tumours, and fat necrosis in association with pancreatic carcinoma.

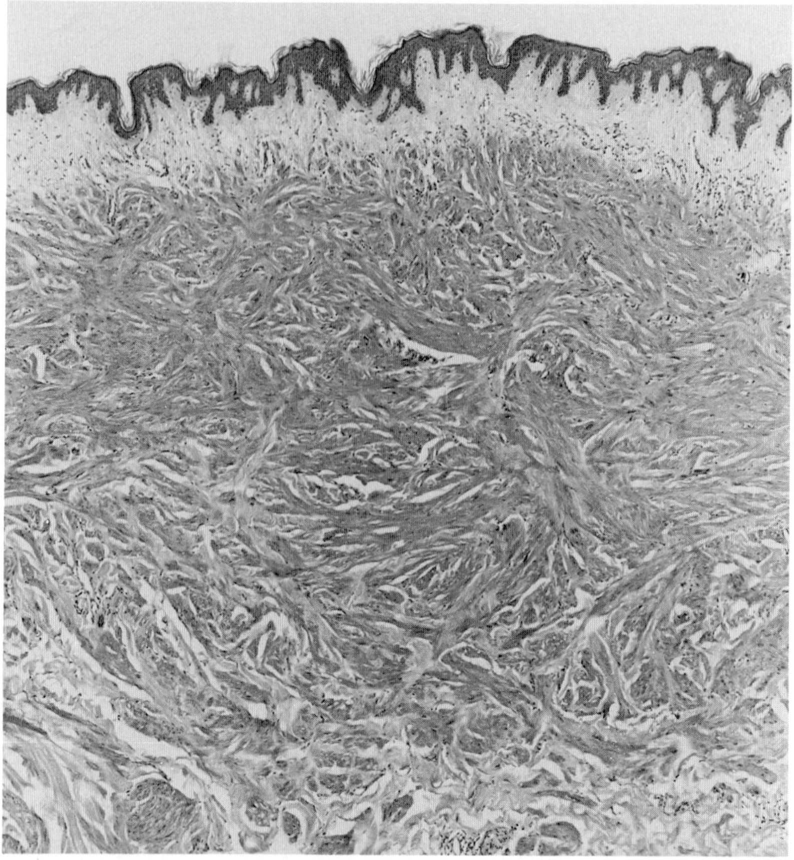

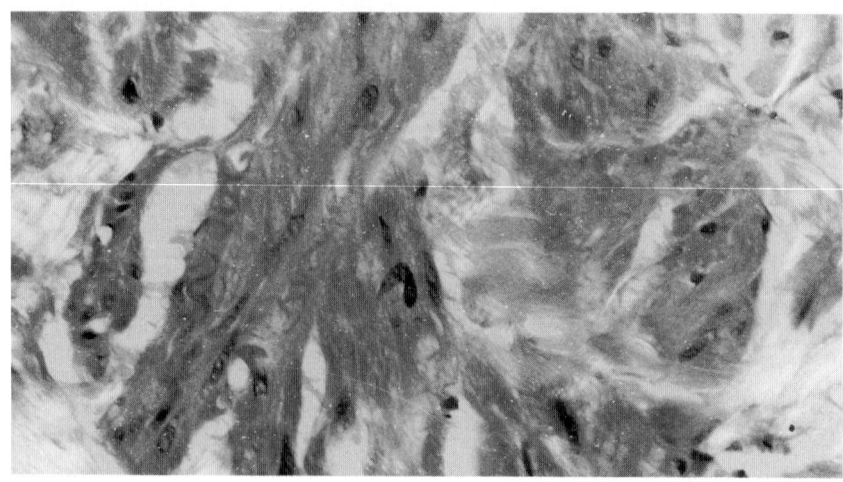

(a)

(b)

Figure 8.24   Leiomyoma. (a) The biopsy contains a poorly circumscribed lesion with (b) eosinophilic fascicles of well-differentiated smooth muscle.

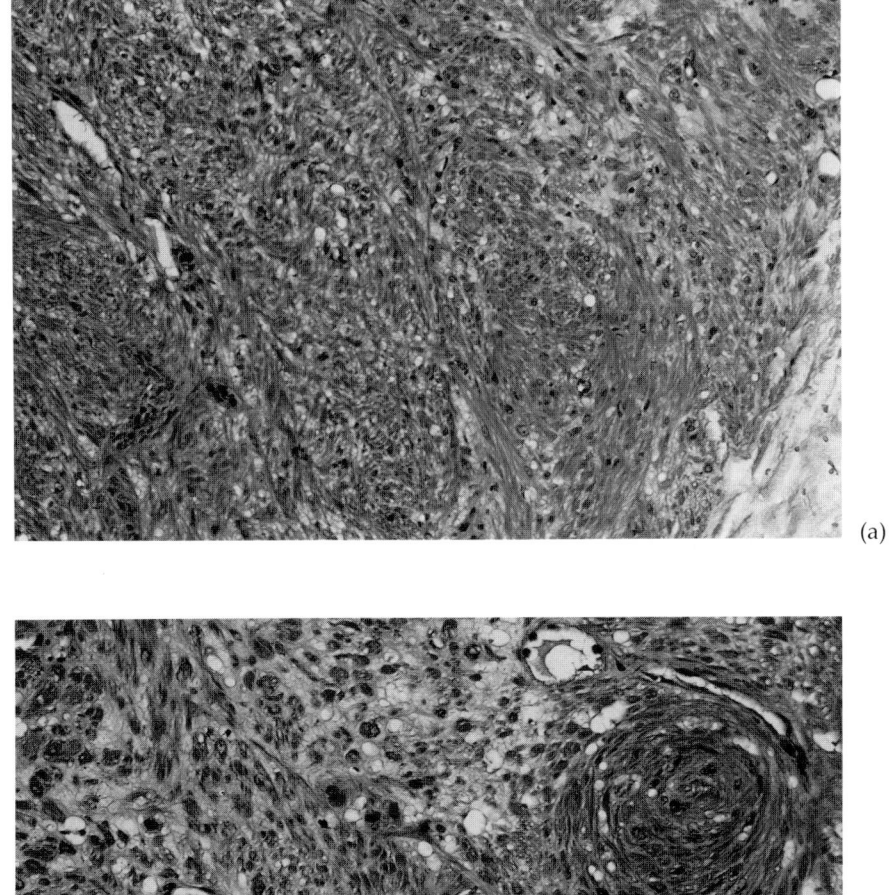

Figure 8.25 Angioleiomyoma. (a) A well-circumscribed nodule with (b) a mixture of thick-walled vessels and stromal spindle cells.

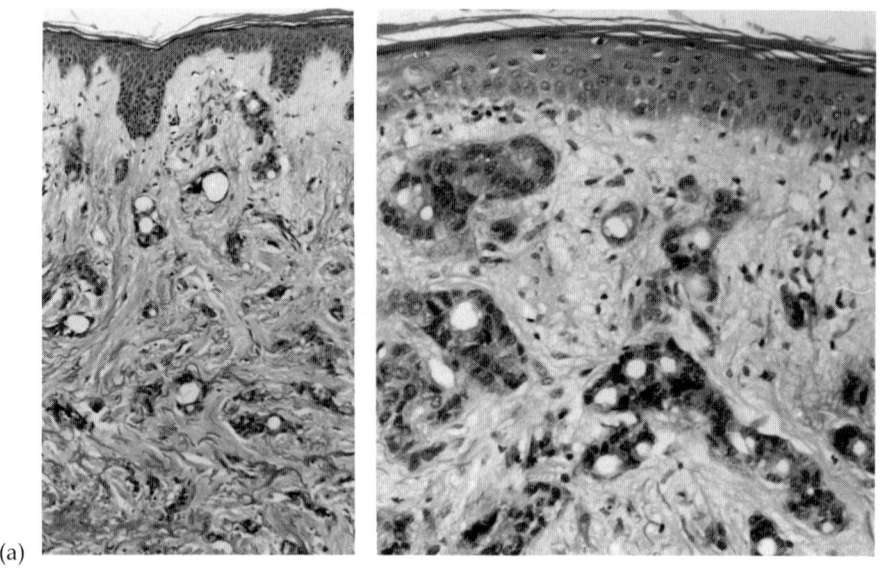

(a) (b)

Figure 8.26 Alopecia mucinosa (a and b). Invasive ductal carcinoma of the breast metastatic to the scalp, with resulting alopecia.

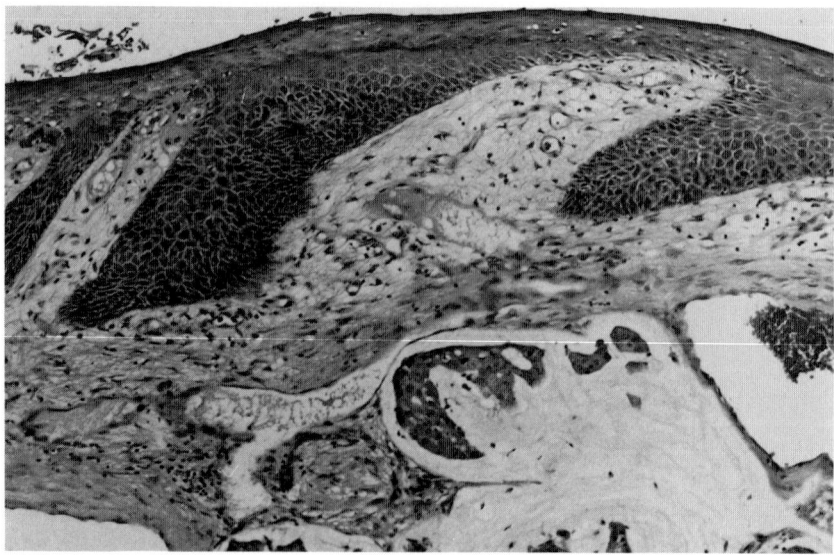

Figure 8.27 Mucinous carcinoma of the breast showing direct extension into the dermis.

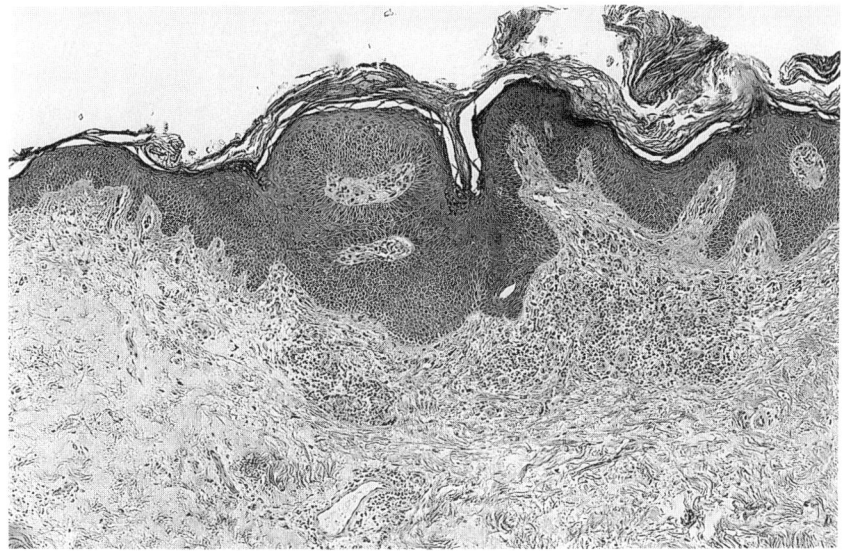

Figure 8.28 Sign of Leser Trelat. Small eruptive seborrhoeic keratosis-like lesions are a marker of underlying malignancy.

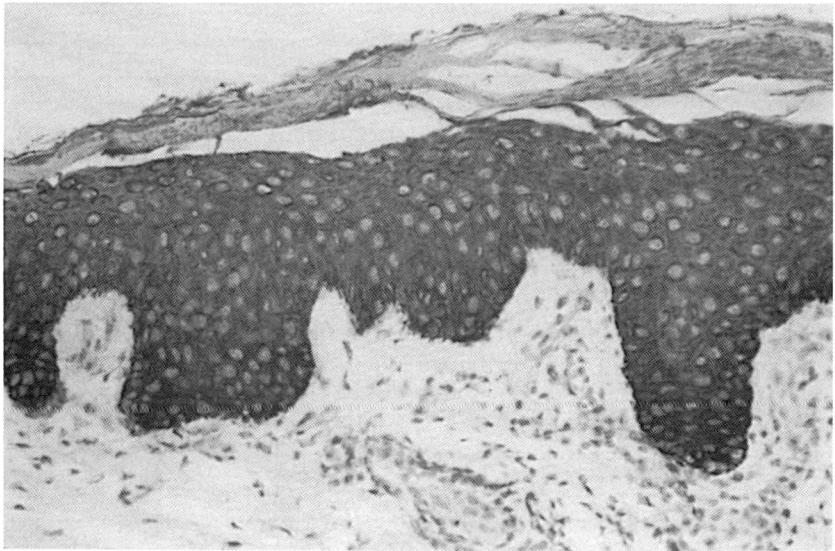

Figure 8.29 Erythema gyratum repens. Acanthosis and parakeratosis in the scaly zone of this cancer associated rash, with characteristic 'tree ring' clinical appearance.

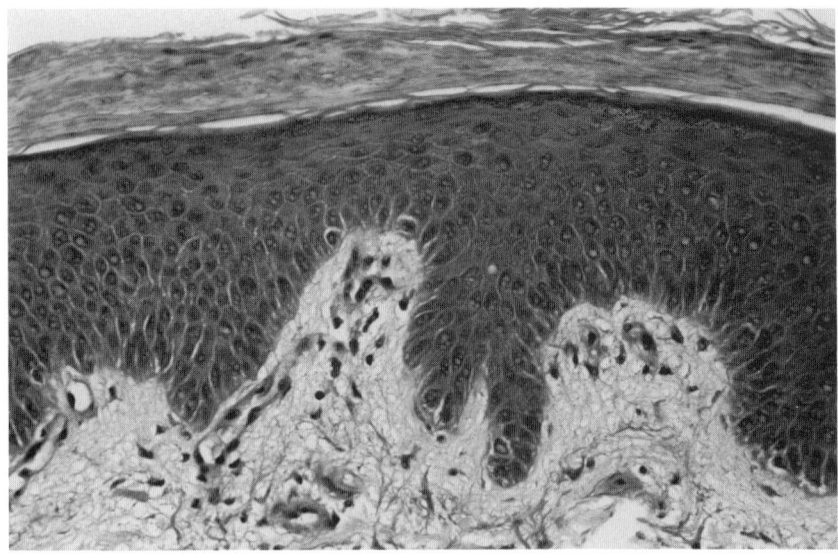

Figure 8.30   Necrolytic migratory erythema. Parakeratotic scale separates from the epidermis in this patient with a glucagonoma.

References

Abel, R. and Dougherty, J. W. (1962) Nevus lipomatosus cutaneus superficialis (Hoffman-Zurhalle). *Arch. Dermatol.*, **85**, 524–6.

Alguacil-Garcia, A., Unni, K. K. and Goellner, J. R. (1978) Histogenesis of dermatofibrosarcoma protuberans: an ultrastructural study. *Am. J. Clin. Pathol.*, **69**, 427–34.

Allen, P. W. (1980) Myxoid tumours of soft tissues. *Pathol. Annu.*, **15**, 133–92.

Allen, P. W., Dymock, R. B. and MacCormac, L. B. (1988) Superficial angiomyxomas with and without epithelial components. Report of 30 tumours in 28 patients. *Am. J. Surg. Pathol.*, **12**, 519–30.

Alos Ribera, J. L., Umbert, I. and Umbert, P. (1989) [Multiple glomangiomas]. *Med. Cutan. Ibero. Lat. Am.*, **17**, 183–5.

Alterman, K., Remmele, W. and Smith, M. (1988) Karl Touton and his "Xanthelasmic giant cell". A selective review of multinucleated giant cells. *Am. J. Dermatopathol.*, **10**, 257–69.

Atherton, D. J., Pitcher, D. W., Wells, R. S. and MacDonald, D. M. (1980) A syndrome of various cutaneous pigmented lesions, myxoid neurofibromata and atrial myxoma: the NAME syndrome. *Br. J. Dermatol.*, **103**, 421–9.

Balaton, A. J., Capron, F., Baviera, E. E., Meyrignac, P., Vaury, P. and Vuong, P. N. (1989) Neuroendocrine carcinoma (Merkel cell tumour?) presenting as a subcutaneous tumor. An ultrastructural and immunohistochemical study of three cases. *Path. Res. Pract.*, **184**, 211–16.

Barker, J. N. W. N. and Girling, A. C. (1989) A case of metastatic malignant melanoma masquerading as disseminated mammary carcinoma. *Histopathol.*, **14**, 219–21.

Barnhill, R. L. and Mihm, M. C. (1990) Cellular neurothekeoma. A distinctive variant of neurothekeoma mimicking nevomelanocytic tumors. *Am. J. Surg. Pathol.*, **14**, 113–20.

Bednar, B. (1957) Storiform neurofibroma, pigmented and non-pigmented. *Cancer*, **10**, 368–76.

Berkowitz, R. K., Longley, J., Buchness, M. R., Silvers, D. N., Ozzello, L. and Grossman, M. E. (1989) Malignant mesothelioma: diagnosis by skin biopsy. *J. Am. Acad. Dermatol.*, **21**, 1068–73.

Buley, I. D., Gatter, K. C., Kelly, P. M. A., Heryet, A. and Millard, P. R. (1988) Granular cell tumours revisited. An immunohistochemical and ultrastructuralstudy. *Histopathol.*, **12**, 263–74.

Carney, J. A. (1985) Differences between non-familial and familial cardiac myxoma. *Am. Surg. Pathol.*, **9**, 53–5.

Carney, J. A., Gordon, H., Carpenter, P. C., Shenoy, B. V. and Go, V. L. W. (1985) The complex of myxomas, spotty pigmentation, and endocrine over-activity. *Medicine*, **64**, 270–83.

Cerio, R., Spaull, J. and Wilson Jones, E. (1989) Histiocytoma cutis: a tumour of dermal dendrocytes (a dermal dendrocytoma). *Br. J. Dermatol.*, **120**, 197–206.

Chanoki, M., Sugamoto, I., Suzuki, S. and Hamada, T. (1989) Nevus lipomatosus cutaneus superficialis of the scalp. *Cutis*, **43**, 143–4.

Cooper, P. H. (1987) Angiosarcoma of the skin. *Semin. Diagn. Pathol.*, **4**, 2–17.

Dabska, M. (1969) Malignant endovascular papillary angioendothelioma of skin on childhood. Clinicopathological study of 6 cases. *Cancer*, **24**, 503–9.

Dahl, I. and Angervall, L. (1974) Cutaneous and subcutaneous leiomyosarcoma, a clinicopathologic study of 47 patients. *Pathol. Eur.*, **9**, 307–15.

Dahl, L. (1976) Atypical fibroxanthoma of the skin: a clinicopathological study of 57 cases. *Acta. Pathol. Microbiol. Scand.*, **84**, 183–97.

Darier, J. and Ferrand, M. (1924) Dermatofibrosarcoma progressifs et recidivants ou fibrosarcomas de la peau. *Ann. Dermatol. Syphil.*, **5**, 545–62.

De Kaminsky, A. R., Otero, A. C., Kaminsky, C. A., Shaw, M., Formentini, E. and Abulafia, J. (1978) Multiple disseminated pyogenic granuloma. *Br. J. Dermatol.*, **98**, 461–4.

Dervan, P. A., Tobbia, I. N., Casey, M., O'Loughlin, J. and O'Brien, M. (1989) Glomus tumours: an immunohistochemical profile of 11 cases. *Histopathol.*, **14**, 483–91.

Doutre, M. S., Beylot, C., Baquey, A., Bonnemaison, D., Bezian, J. H., Bioulac, P. and Carteyron, M. (1988) Cutaneous metastasis from papillary carcinoma of the thyroid. A case confirmed by monoclonal antithyroglobulin antibody. *Dermatologica*, **177**, 241–3.

Dover, J. S., From, L. and Lewis, A. (1989) Palisaded encapsulated neuromas. A clinicopathologic study. *Arch. Dermatol.*, **125**, 386–9.

Drachman, D., Rosen, L., Sharaf, D. and Weissman, A. (1988) Postmastectomy low-grade angiosarcoma. An unusual case, clinically resembling a lymphangioma circumscription. *Am. J. Dermatopathol.*, **10**, 247–51.

Enzinger, F. M. and Weiss, S. W. (1988) *Soft tissue tumours*; 2nd edn, Mosby, St Louis.

Evans, J., Clarke, T., Mattacks, C. A. and Pond, C. M. (1989) Dermatofibromas and arthropod bites: is there any evidence to link the two. *Lancet*, **ii**, 36–7.

Feldman, A. R. and Keeling, J. H. 3d. (1989) Cutaneous manifestation of atrial myxoma. *J. Am. Acad. Dermatol.*, **21**, 1080–4.

Fields, J. P. and Helwig, E. B. (1981) Leiomyosarcoma of the skin and subcutaneous tissue. *Cancer*, **47**, 156–69.

Fletcher, C. D. M., Evans, B. J., MacArtney, J. C., Smith, N., Jones, E. W. and McKee, P. H. (1985) Dermatofibrosarcoma protuberans: a clinicopathological and immunohistochemical study with review of the literature. *Histopathology*, **9**, 921–38.

Fletcher, C. D. M., Chan, J. K.-C. and McKee, P. H. (1986) Dermal nerve sheath myxoma: a study of three cases. *Histopathology*, **10**, 135–45.

Fletcher, C. D. M., Theaker, J. M., Flanagan, A. and Krausz, T. (1988) Pigmented dermatofibrosarcoma protuberans (Bednar tumour): melanocytic colonization or neuroectodermal differentiation? A clinicopathological and immunohistochemical study. *Histopathol.*, **13**, 631–43.

Fletcher, C. D. M. (1989) Solitary circumscribed neuroma of the skin (so-called palisaded, encapsulated neuroma). *Am. J. Surg. Pathol.*, **13**, 574–80.

Freedman, A. M. and Meland, N. B. (1989) Angioleiomyomas of the extremities: report of a case and review of the Mayo Clinic experience. *Plast. Reconstr. Surg.*, **83**, 328–31.

Fretzin, D. F. and Helwig, E. B. (1973) Atypical fibroxanthoma of the skin. *Cancer*, **31**, 1541–52.

Fujiwara, S., Ichikawa, H., Matsunaga, E., Shinkai, H., Takayasu, S., Wada, K. and Sekine, H. (1989) Delayed cutaneous metastasis of gastric carcinoma. *J. Dermatol.*, **16**, 242–6.

Gould, E., Albores-Saavedra, J., Dubner, B., Smith, W. and Payne, C. M. (1988) Eccrine and squamous differentiation in Merkel cell carcinoma. An immunohistochemical study. *Am. J. Surg. Pathol.*, **12**, 768–72.

Graham, J. H., Sanderl, J. B., Johnson, W. C. and Helwig, E. B. (1965) Fibrous papule of nose. *J. Invest. Dermatol.*, **45**, 194–203.

Headington, J. T., Beals, T. F. and Niederhuber, J. E. (1977) Primary leimyosarcoma of skin: a report and critical appraisal. *J. Cutan. Pathol.*, **4**, 308–17.

Helwig, E. B. (1963) Atypical fibroxanthoma. *Tex. J. Med.*, **59**, 664–7.

Helwig, E. B. and May, D. (1986) Atypical fibroxanthoma with metastasis. *Cancer*, **57**, 368–76.

Hoffmann, E. (1925) Uber das knollentreibende Fibrosarkom der Haut (Dermatofibrosarkoma protuberans). *Dermatol. Z.*, **43**, 1–28.

Holden, C. A., Spittle, M. F. and Wilson Jones, E. (1987) Angiosarcoma of the face and scalp, prognosis and treatment. *Cancer*, **59**, 1046–57.

Iacobucci, J. J., Stevenson, T. R., Swanson, N. A. and Headington, J. T. (1987) Cutaneous leiomyosarcoma. *Ann. Plast. Surg.*, **19**, 552–4.

Jegasothy, B. V., Gilgor, R. S. and Hull, M. (1981) Leiomyosarcoma of the skin and subcutaneous tissue. *Arch. Dermatol.*, **117**, 478–81.

Katake, R., Waisman, J. and Lupu, A. (1982) Cutaneous and subcutaneous metastasis from carcinoma of the prostate. *Urology*, **19**, 373–6.

Kheir, S. M., Omura, E. F., Grizzle, W. E., Herrera, G. A. and Lee, I. (1986) Histologic variation in the skin lesions of the glucagonoma syndrome. *Am. J. Surg. Pathol.*, **10**, 445–53.

Kirkham, N. and Cole, M. D., (1983) Merkel cell carcinoma: a malignant neuroendocrine tumour of the eyelid. *Br. J. Ophthalmol.*, **67**, 600–3.

Kirkham, N. and Isaacson, P. (1983) Merkel cell carcinoma: a report of three case with neurone-specific enolase activity. *Histopathol.*, **7**, 251–9.

Kyler, J. R., Krause, S. E., Mallory, S. B. and Johnston, Y. E. (1988) Multiple cutaneous granular cell tumors in childhood. *South. Med. J.*, **81**, 1583–6.

Lautier, R., Wolff, H. H. and Jones, R. E. (1990) An immunohistochemical study of dermatofibrosarcoma protuberans supports its fibroblastic character and contradicts neuroectodermal or histiocytic components. *Am. J. Dermatopathol.*, **12**, 25–30.

Leong, A. S. Y. and Milios, J. (1987) Atypical fibroxanthoma of the skin: a clinicopathological and immunochemical study and discussion of its histogenesis. *Histopathology*, **11**, 463–75.

Lopez, D. A., Silvers, D. N. and Helwig, E. B. (1974) Cutaneous meningiomas – a clinicopathologic study. *Cancer*, **34**, 728–44.

MacDonald, D. M., Sanderson, K. V. (1974) Angioleiomyoma of the Skin. *Br. J. Dermatol.*, **91**, 161–8.

Masson, P. (1923) Hemangioendotheliome vegetant intravasculaire. *Bull. Soc. Anat.* (Paris), **93**, 517–32.

McKee, P. H. (1985) Cutaneous metastases. *J. Cutan. Pathol.*, **12**, 239–50.

Menter, A., Boyd, A. S. and McCaffree, D. M. (1989) Recurrent renal cell carcinoma presenting as skin nodules: two case reports and review of the literature. *Cutis.*, **44**, 305–8.

Miettinen, M., Lehto, V.-P., and Virtanen, I. (1985) Antibodies to intermediate filament proteins: the differential diagnosis of cutaneous tumours. *Arch. Dermatol.*, **121**, 736–41.

Morgan, J., Robinson, M. J., Rosen, L. B., Unger, H. and Niven, J. (1989) Malignant endovascular papillary angioendothelioma (Dabska tumor). *Am. J. Dermatopathol.*, **11**, 64–8.

Mori, O., Hachisuka, H., Sakamoto, F., Nomura, H. and Sasai, Y. Immunohistochemical observations of S-100 protein and neuron specific enolase in the tumour cells of granular cell tumour. *Acta Histochem.* (Jena), **83**, 33–8.

Nakamura, T., Ogata, H. and Katsuyama, T. (1987) Pigmented dermatofibrosarcoma protuberans. Report of two cases as a variant of dermatofibrosarcoma protuberans with partial neural differentiation. *Am. J. Dermatopathol.*, **9**, 18–25.

Nemeth, A. J., Penneys, N. S. and Bernstein, H. B. (1988) Fibrous papule: a tumor of fibrohistiocytic cells that contain factor XIIIa. *J. Am. Acad. Dermatol.*, **19**, 1102–6.

Nickel, W. R. and Reed, W. B. (1962) Tuberous sclerosis. Special reference to the microscopic alterations in the cutaneous hamartomas. *Arch. Dermatol.*, **85**, 209–26.

Ordonez, N. G. and Batsakis, J. G. (1984) Comparison of Ulex europaeus I lectin and factor VIII-related antigen in vascular lesions. *Arch. Pathol. Lab. Med.*, **108**, 129–32.

Pepper, M. C., Laubenheimer, R. and Cripps, D. J. (1977) Multiple glomus tumours. *J. Cutan. Pathol.*, **4**, 244–57.

Price, M. L., Darley, C. R. and Kirkham, N. (1989) The glucagonoma syndrome. *J. R. Soc. Med.*, **82**, 553–4.

Pilotti, S., Rilke, F., Bartoli, C. and Grisotti, A. (1988) Clinicopathologic correlations of cutaneous neuroendocrine Merkel cell carcinoma. *J. Clin. Oncol.*, **6**, 1863–73.

Pulitzer, D. R. and Reed, R. J. (1985) Nerve sheath myxoma (perineural myxoma). *Am. J. Dermatopathol.*, **7**, 409–21.

Reed, R. J., Fine, R. M. and Meltzer, H. D. (1972) Palisaded, encapsulated neuromas of the skin. *Arch. Dermatol.*, **106**, 865–70.

Reed, R. J., Utz, M. P. and Terezakis, N. (1989) Embolic and metastatic cardiac myxoma. *Am. J. Dermatopathol.*, **11**, 157–65.

Ricci, A. Jr., Cartun, R. W. and Zakowski, M. F. (1988) Atypical fibroxanthoma. A study of 14 cases emphasizing the presence of Langerhans' histiocytes with implications for differential diagnosis by antibody panels. *Am. J. Surg. Pathol.*, **12**, 591–8.

Rosai, J., Summer, H. W., Major, M. C., Kostianovsky, M. and Peres-Uresa, C. (1976) Angiosarcoma of the skin. A clinicopathologic and fine structural study. *Hum. Pathol.*, **7**, 83–109.

Rosen, L. B. and Suster, S. (1988) Fibrous papules. A light microscopic and immunohistochemical study. *Am. J. Dermatopathol.*, **10**, 109–15.

Santa Cruz, D. J. and Reiner, C. B. (1978) Recurrent digital fibroma of child-hood. *J. Cutan. Pathol.*, **5**, 339–46.

Santa Cruz, D. J. and Kyriakus, M. (1981) Aneurysmal ("angiomatoid") fibrous histiocytoma of the skin. *Cancer*, **47**, 2053–61.

Scupham, R., Beckman, E. and Fretzin, D. (1988) Carcinoma of the prostate metastatic to the skin. *Am. J. Dermatopathol.*, **10**, 178–80.

Silvis, N. G., Swanson, P. E., Manivel, J. C., Kaye, V. N. and Wick, M. R. (1988) Spindle-cell and pleomorphic neoplasms of the skin. *Am. J. Dermato-pathol.*, **10**, 9–19.

Smith, K. J., Skelton, H. G., Barrett, T. L., Lupton, G. P. and Graham, J. H. (1989) Cutaneous myofibroma. *Mod. Pathol.*, **2**, 603–9.

Starink, T., Hausman, R., Van Delden, L. and Neering, H. (1977) Atypical fibroxanthoma of the skin. Presentation of 5 cases and a review of the literature. *Br. J. Dermatol.*, **97**, 167–77.

Stewart, F. and Treves, N. (1948) Lymphangiosarcoma in postmastectomy lymphedema. *Cancer*, **1**, 64–81.

Suster, S., Rosen, L. B. and Sanchez, J. C. (1988) Granular cell leiomyosarcoma of the skin. *Am. J. Dermatopathol.*, **10**, 234–9.

Szadowska, A., Wozniak, L., Lasota, J., Giryn, I., Mirecka, B. and Wolska, H. (1989) Neuroendocrine (Merkel cell). carcinoma of the skin: a clinico-mor-phological study of 13 cases. *Histopathol.*, **15**, 483–93.

Theaker, J. M., Fletcher, C. D. M. and Tudway, A. J. (1990) Cutaneous hetero-topic meningeal nodules. *Histopathology*, **16**, 475–9.

Toker, C. (1972) Trabecular carcinoma. *Arch. Dermatol.*, **105**, 107–10.

Verbov, J. (1981) Necrolytic migratory erythema associated with an islet cell tumour of the pancreas. *Dermatologica*, **163**, 189–94.

Wrotnowski, U., Cooper, P. H. and Shmookler, B. M. (1988) Fibrosarcomatous change indermatofibrosarcoma protuberans. *Am. J. Surg. Pathol.*, **12**, 287–93.

Warner, T. F. C. S., Uno, M., Hafez, G. R., Burgess, J., Bolles, C., Lloyd, R. V. and Oka, M. (1983) Merkel cells and Merkel cell tumours: ultrastructure, immunohistochemistry and review of the literature. *Cancer*, **52**, 238–45.

Weiler, R., Fischer-Colbrie, R., Schmid, K. W., Feichtinger, H., Bussolati, G., Grimelius, L., Krisch, K., Kerl, H., O'Connor, D. and Winkler, H. (1988) Immunological studies on the occurrence and properties of chromogranin A and B and secretogranin II in endocrine tumors. *Am. J. Surg. Pathol.*, **12**, 877–84.

Weiss, S. M. and Enzinger, F. M. (1982) Epithelioid hemangioendothelioma: a vascular tumor often mistaken for carcinoma. *Cancer*, **50**, 970–81.

Wick, M. R., Kaye, V. N., Sibley, R. K., Tyler, R. and Frizzera, G. (1986) Primary neuroendocrine carcinoma and small cell malignant lymphoma of the skin. A descriminant immunohistochemical comparison. *J. Cutan. Pathol.*, **13**, 347–58.

Wilson Jones, E., Marks, R. and Pongsehirun, D. (1975) Naevus superficialis lipomatosus. *Br. J. Dermatol.*, **93**, 121–33.

Wilson Jones, E. (1976) Malignant vascular tumours. *Clin. Exp. Dermatol.*, **1**, 287–312.

Wilson Jones, E., Cerio, R. and Smith, N. P. (1989) Epithelioid cell histiocytoma: a new entity. *Br. J. Dermatol.*, **120**, 185–95.

Wrotnowski, U., Cooper, P. H. and Shmookler, B. M. (1988) Fibrosarcomatous change in dermatofibrosarcoma protuberans. *Am. J. Surg. Pathol.*, **12**, 287–93.

Youngberg, G. A., Berro, J., Young, M. and Leicht, S. S. (1989) Metastatic epidermotropic squamous carcinoma histologically simulating primary carcinoma. *Am. J. Dermatopathol.*, **11**, 457–65.

Zackheim, H. S. and Pinkus, H. (1960) Perifollicular fibromas. *Arch. Dermatol.*, **82**, 913–17.

9 Eczematous, psoriasiform and lichenoid reactions

This chapter deals with a relatively small number of inflammatory conditions: those which mainly involve the epidermis. Other rashes, which have a prominent dermal component, are dealt with in Chapter 10.

9.1 Eczema

Eczema is a clinical description of an inflammatory condition whose biopsy appearances vary depending upon the stage in the development of the disease at which the biopsy takes place (Mihm, *et al.*, 1976; Tong, 1976; Willis, *et al.*, 1986). Briefly, the process starts with the accumulation of lymphocytes around upper dermal vessels, leading to spread of lymphocytes into the interstitial papillary dermis, with a varying degree of associated oedema. The process continues with lymphocytes entering the epidermis (exocytosis), with the accompanying development of interstitial oedema (spongiosis). This is associated with changes in the maturation of the epidermis, manifested by persistant nucleation of cells in the cornified layer (parakeratosis). The development of parakeratosis corresponds to the clinical appearance of scaling, which tends to be seen in the later stages of the evolution of most inflammatory lesions.

The early lesion will show a characteristic combination of superficial perivascular and interstitial dermatitis with epidermal exocytosis, spongiosis and parakeratosis. As the disease progresses, the dermal changes may become less marked, whilst the epidermis becomes more markedly hyperplastic. This is the process of lichenification. The prickle cell layer is increased in thickness (acanthosis), as is the cornified layer (hyperkeratosis). With time, the inflammatory component of the lesion may become less obvious, leaving only epidermal acanthosis and hyperkeratosis. Examination of serial sections may show a very occasional focus of spongiosis or exocytosis. This is lichenified eczema.

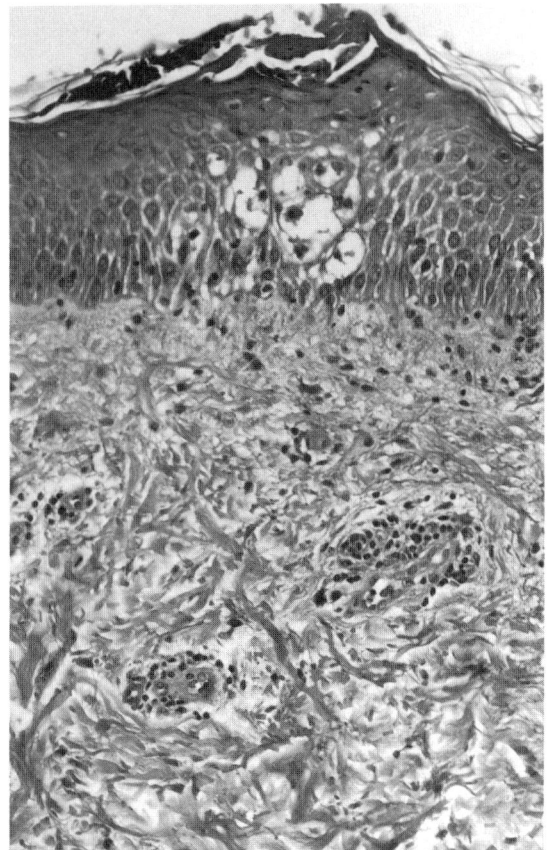

Figure 9.1   Eczema. Superficial perivascular and interstitial lymphocytic infiltration with the formation of a spongiotic vesicle.

The lichenification is exacerbated by scratching or rubbing. Similar lesion can be produced in this way without intervening inflammation, producing lesions of lichen simplex.

The use of 1 micron plastic-embedded sections allows the process to be seen in greater detail and individual cell types to be identified with a greater degree of certainty. Acute vesicular lesions show epidermal spongiosis and dermal lymphocytic infiltration, some of which are activated and most of which are CD4 positive T-cells.

Mast cells are present in normal numbers and show varying degrees of hypogranulation. Eosinophils, neutrophils, and basophils are rarely seen. Endothelial cell hypertrophy, without necrosis, is seen in venules.

Lichenified lesions show acanthosis with a dermal inflammatory in-

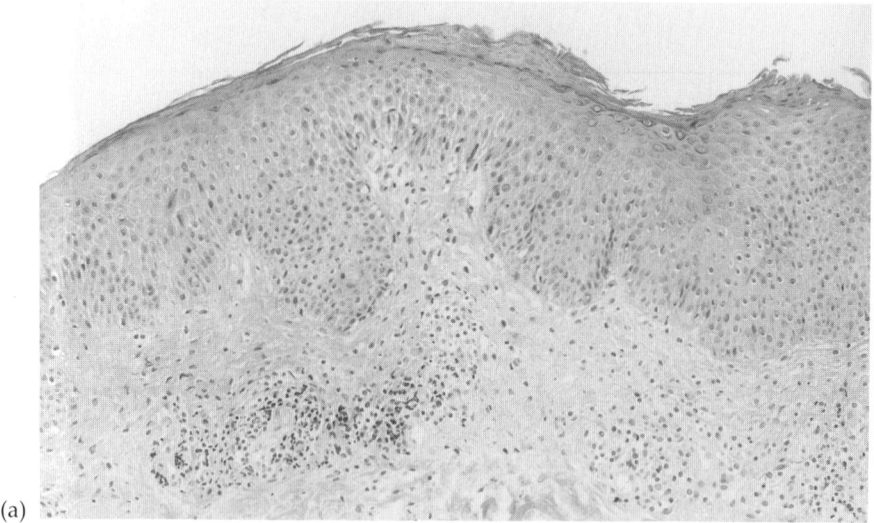

(a)

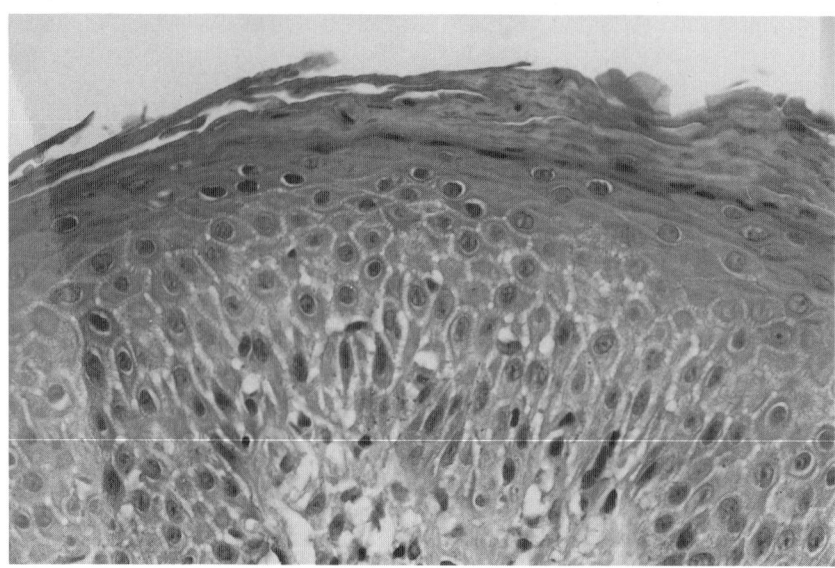

(b)

Figure 9.2 Eczema. (a) The dermis shows a superficial perivascular and interstitial lymphocytic infiltrate, whilst the epidermis (b) shows spongiosis, exocytosis and parakeratosis.

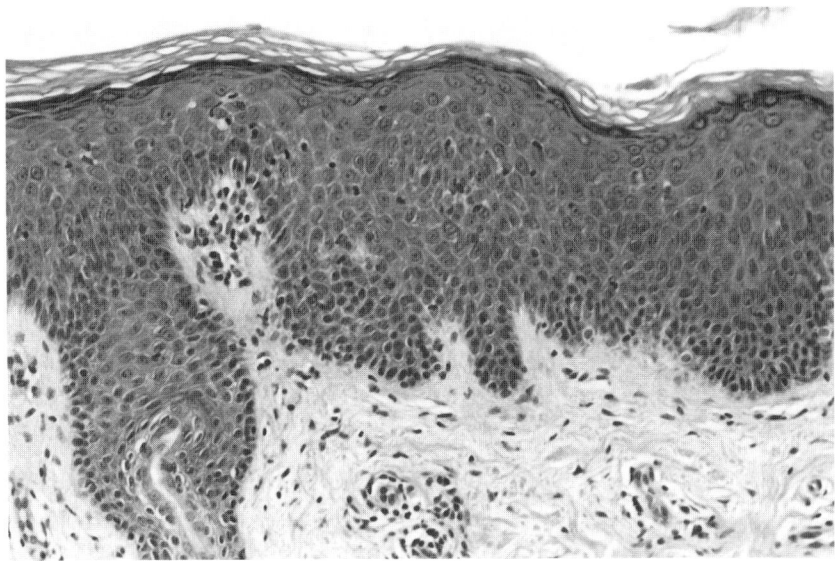

Figure 9.3   Eczema. A chronic lesion showing acanthosis and only sparse exocytosis and spongiosis.

filtrate in which the mast cells are increased in number and fully granulated, together with increased numbers of lymphocytes and monocyte-macrophages. The venules show marked endothelial cell hypertrophy and basement membrane thickening.At this, stage dermal nerves show demyelination and fibrosis, and epidermal Langerhans cells are increased in number. Eosinophils are not a feature of licheni-fied lesions, but the major basic protein of their granules has been demonstrated in the dermis by direct immunofluorescence (Bos, *et al.*, 1986; Soter, 1989).

9.2   Psoriasis

Although there are detailed descriptions of the histopathology of psoriasis, this condition is rarely biopsied. In the majority of cases, the clinical diagnosis is obvious. Biopsies are usually only done in problem cases where the clinical picture is atypical in some way (Chowaniec, *et al.*, 1981). The consequence is that the biopsy probably will not show typical or diagnostic features, thus compounding the problem.

Psoriasis is process of epidermal hyperplasia, in which the granular cell layer may be lost and the stratum corneum shows parakeratosis (Barr, 1985; Wright, 1985). The precise appearances will depend upon

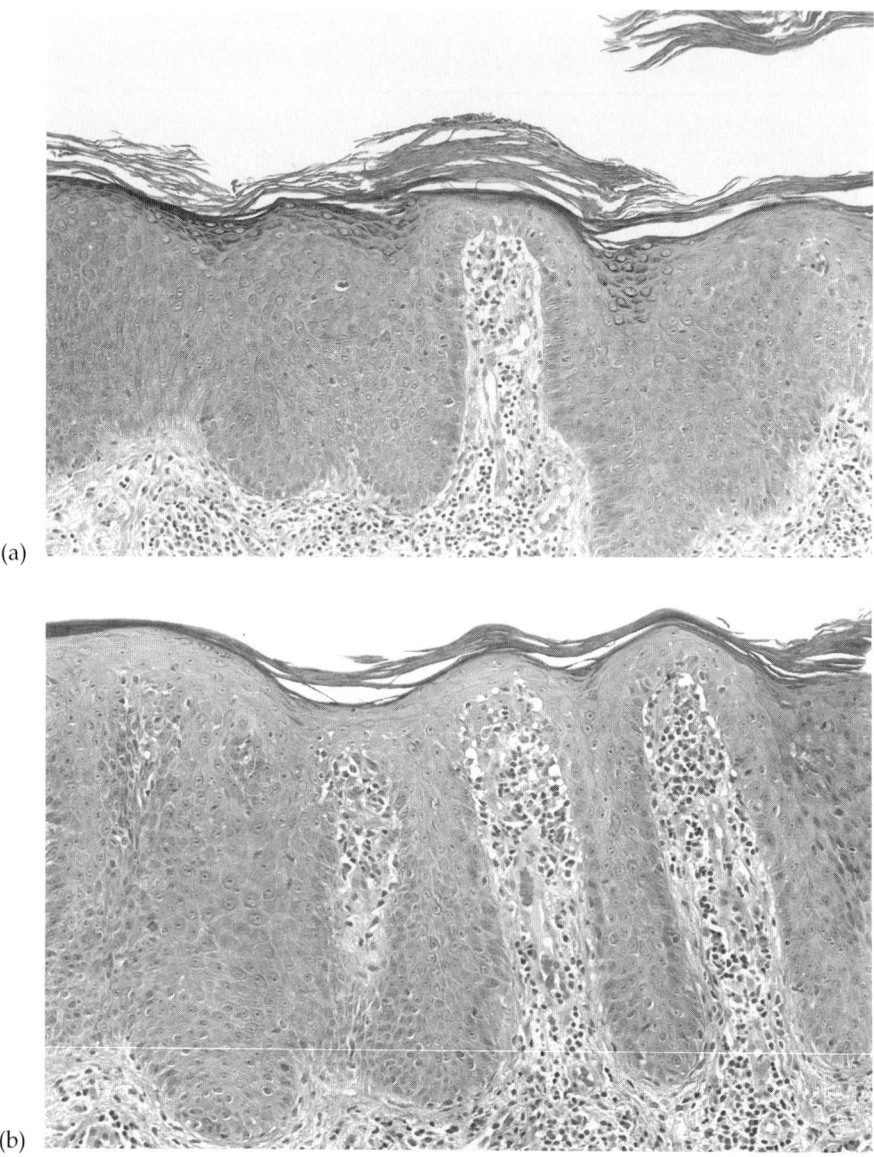

(a)

(b)

Figure 9.4 Psoriasis showing (a) parakeratotic scale and epidermal thinning over the dermal papillae, and (b) regular prolongation of rete ridges.

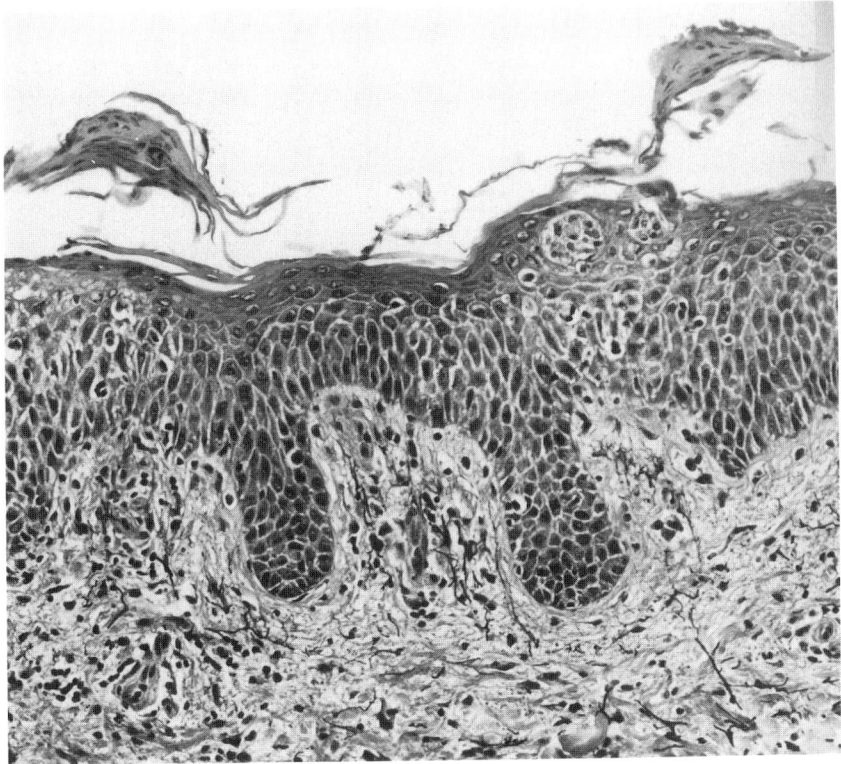

Figure 9.5   An acute lesion of psoriasis showing prominent exocytosis over dermal papillae, with capping by parakeratotic scale.

the age of the lesion and the site of the biopsy (Pinkus and Mehregan, 1966). The profile of the epidermis in a typical lesion will show regular elongation of the dermal papillae, with a relatively thin epidermis at the top of the papillae. There may be intercelluiar oedema and infiltration with lymphocytes and neutrophils here in association with the phenomenon of the 'squirting papilla' (Pinkus and Mehregan, 1966). This part of the reaction may be quite prominent, producing spongiform pustules of Kogoj. These can extend into the overlying parakeratotic keratin to produce Munro microabscesses, containing pyknotic neutrophils.

The last two features together with the parakeratotic scale are the most reliable features for diagnosis. In many biopsies, it may only be possible to say that the changes are 'psoriasiform', and a confident distinction from other possible diagnoses, of which eczema is high on the list, may be impossible.

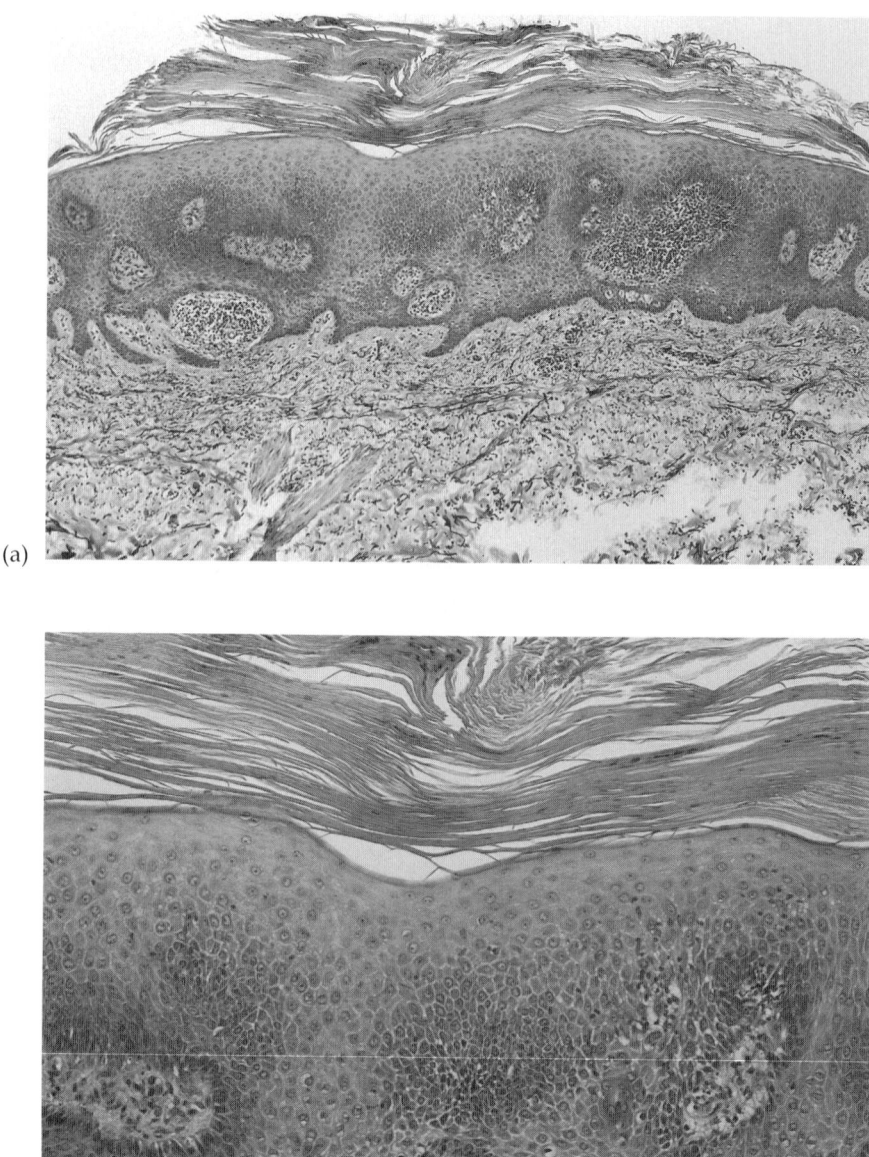

Figure 9.6 Guttate psoriasis. (a) A circumscribed lesion, showing (b) parakeratosis and loss of the granular layer.

The pathogenesis of psoriasis continues to keep researchers busy. It seems clear that the keratinocytes are essentially normal and are subject to abnormal stimuli (Watt *et al.*, 1988). The disease has been seen to resolve after bone marrow transplantation and cyclosporin therapy, so it seems likely that cell mediated factors play a part (Jowitt and Liu Yin, 1990).

9.3   Seborrhoeic dermatitis

'Seb. derm' shows features seen in both eczema and psoriasis: the lower epidermis will show exocytosis and spongiosis in the manner of eczema, whilst the upper dermis will show psoriasiform acanthosis surmounted by parakeratotic scale in which there may be small numbers of pyknotic neutrophils (Pinkus and Mehregan, 1966). The presence of neutropils in the keratin layer should always alert one to the possibility of superficial fungal infection, even if another diagnosis seems likely. The PAS stain is often advocated as the best way of identifying fungi, but we find that Grocott's methanamine silver technique is better. The dermis will show a moderate, superficial perivascular and interstitial lymphocytic infiltrate.

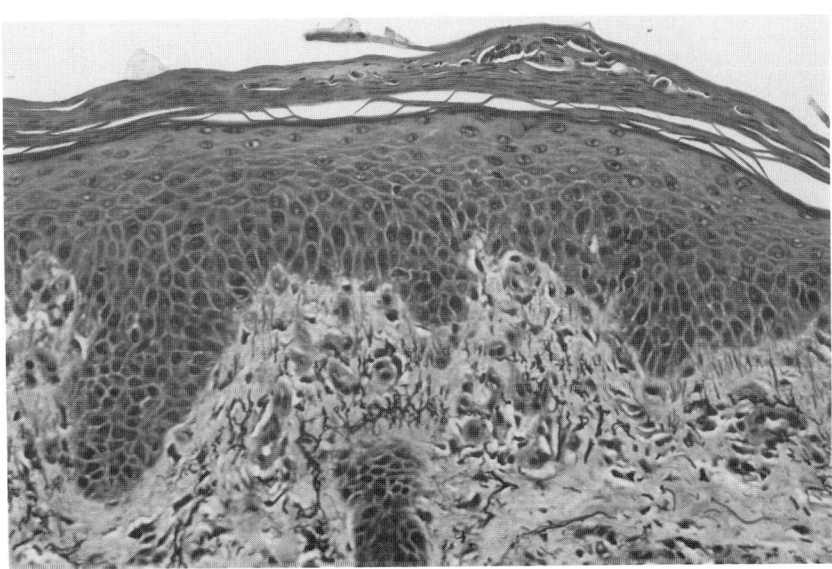

Figure 9.7   Seborrhoeic dermatitis with acanthotic epidermis and pyknotic neutrophils in the scale.

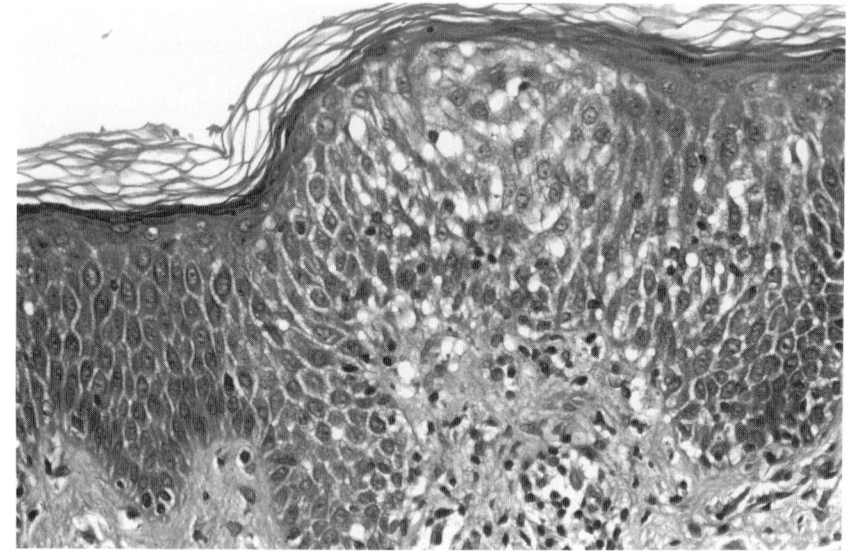

(a)

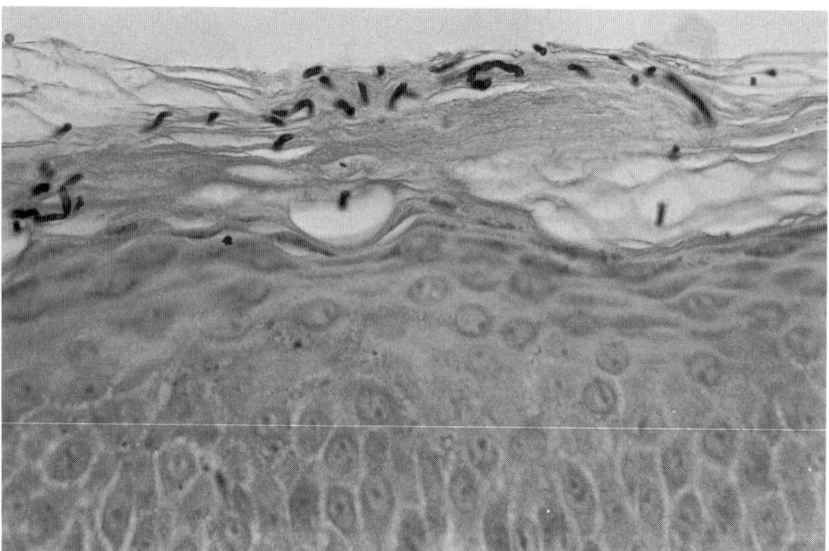

(b)

Figure 9.8 Superficial fungal infection. (a) The H and E stain shows a spongiotic, acanthotic epidermis, whilst (b) Grocott's stain reveals the hyphae of tinea versicolor.

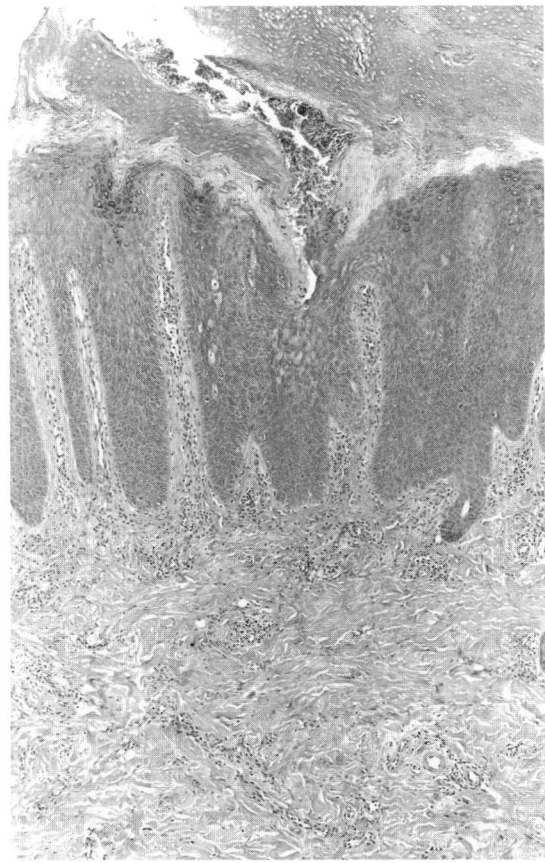

Figure 9.9 Lichen simplex. The lesion shows marked acanthosis, hypergranulosis and hyperkeratosis, without cellular atypia and with only sparse dermal lymphocytic infiltration.

9.4 Lichen simplex

Chronic rubbing of the skin results in reactive hyperplasia, with acanthosis, elongated rete ridges, hyperkeratosis and variable parakeratosis, which can progress to the point that a lesion develops which merits biopsy. Differential diagnosis is from other hyperplastic and dysplastic warty lesions of the skin, but in the absence of atypia the presence of entirely hyperplastic changes should make the diagnosis reasonably plain.

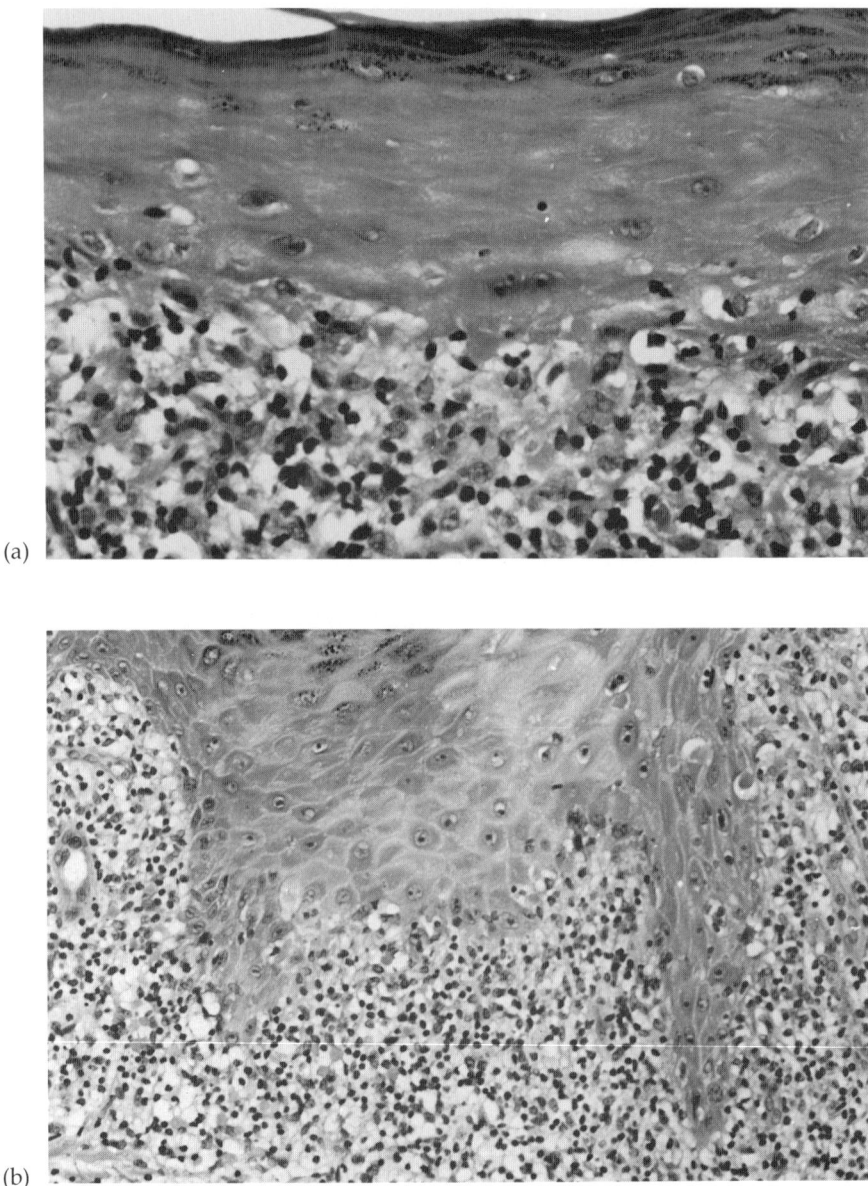

(a)

(b)

Figure 9.10 Lichen planus. (a) Interface dermatitis, with (b) the formation of eosinophilic Civatte bodies.

9.5   Lichen planus

The third main kind of inflammatory condition which mainly involves the epidermis is lichen planus and the related lichenoid reactions (Pinkus, 1973; Shiohara, 1988; Weedon, 1985). These all have in common the appearance of interface dermatitis: that is, there is a lymphocytic infiltration of the papillary dermis which extends in a band through the extent of the lesion. The lesions themselves may be very sharply circumscribed. The infiltrate extends into the lower epidermis, where individual cells may be damaged, producing the so-called 'Civatte' bodies, which are characterisitc of this reaction. In time, these may also be seen in the upper dermis.

The changes in an individual biopsy will depend upon the stage at which a biopsy was performed (Ragaz and Ackerman, 1978). Early lesions will be very infiltrated. With time, localized hyperkeratosis develops, in association with epidermal hyperplasia. This is also manifested by the appearance of the so-called 'saw tooth' profile to the basal cell layer. As the reaction wanes, little infiltration will be seen but pigmentary incontinence will be seen in the underlying papillary dermis.

As well as idiopathic lichen planus, similar changes may be seen in a lichenoid drug eruption, which can be essentially similar although

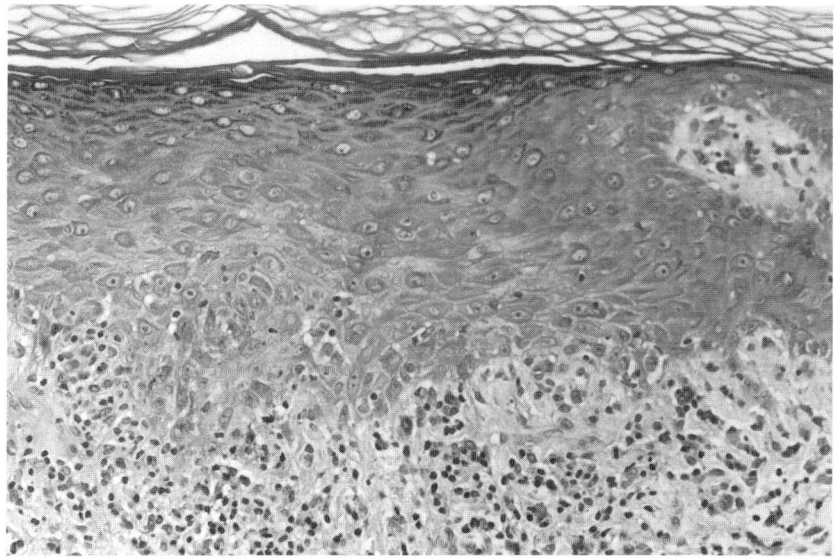

Figure 9.11   Lichen planus. A hypertrophic lesion with acanthosis as well as interface activity.

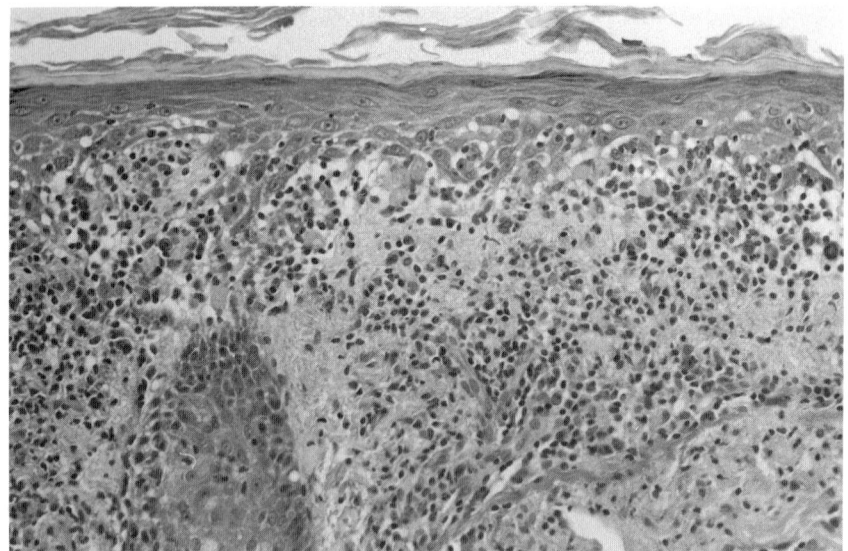

Figure 9.12 Lichen planus. An atrophic example with many Civatte bodies.

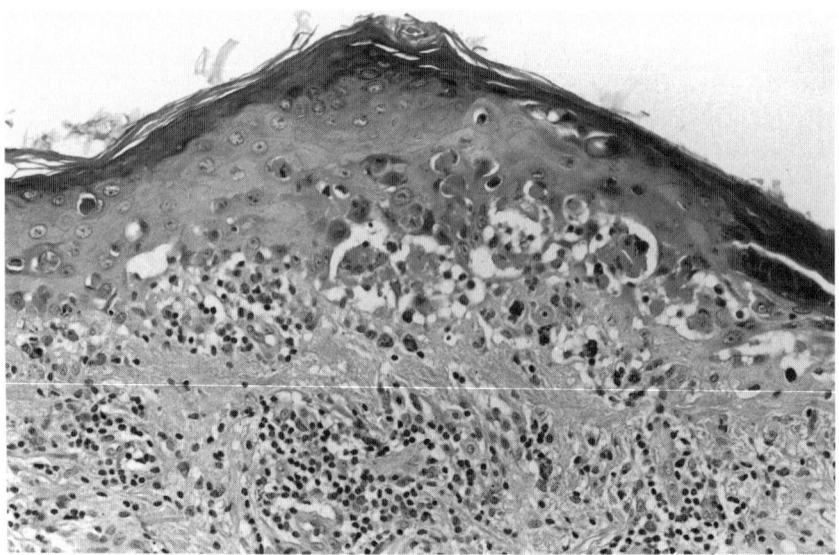

Figure 9.13 Lichenoid drug eruption. This is essentially similar to lichen planus but more florid than usual and with plentiful Civatte bodies.

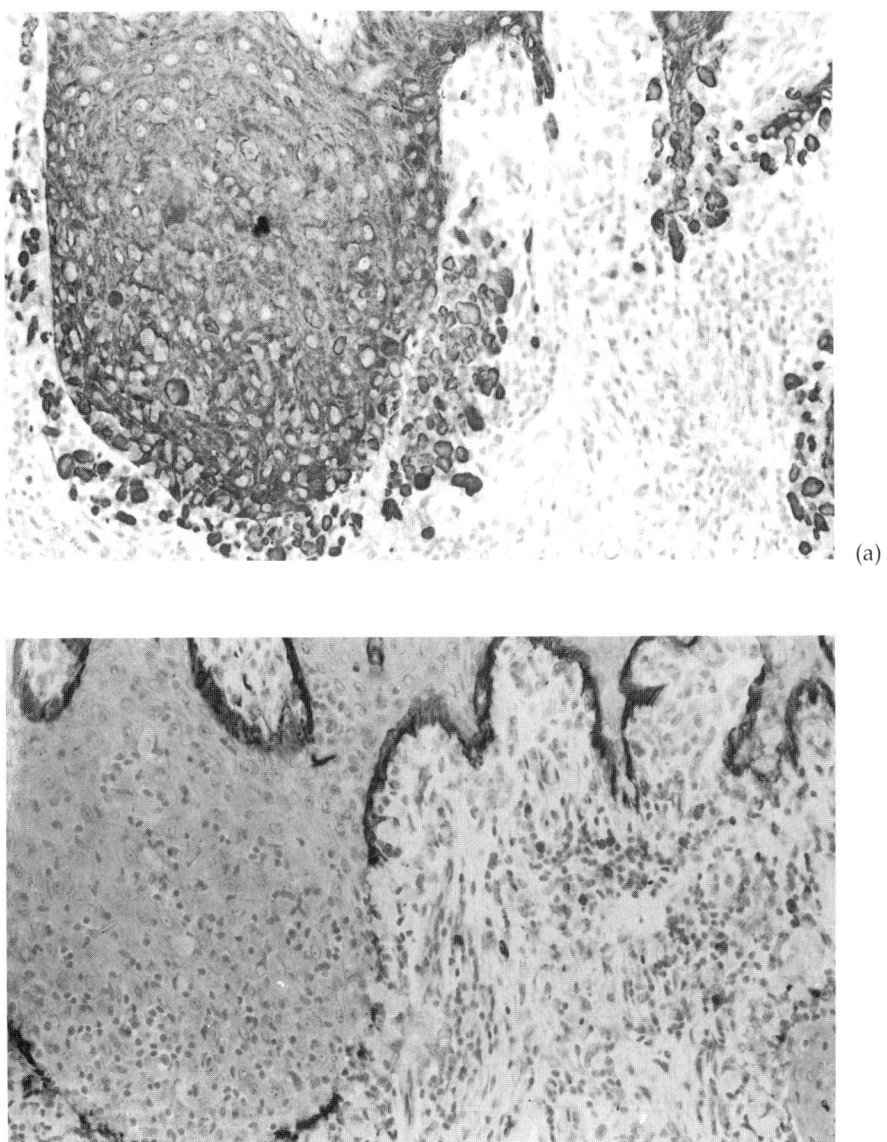

(a)

(b)

Figure 9.14 Lichen planus. Frozen sections showing (a) Civatte bodies extending into the upper dermis (high molecular weight cytokeratin, LP34, immunoperoxidase), and (b) disrupted epidermal basement membrane at the site of active interface dermatitis (Type VII collagen, LH 7.2 and immunoperoxidase).

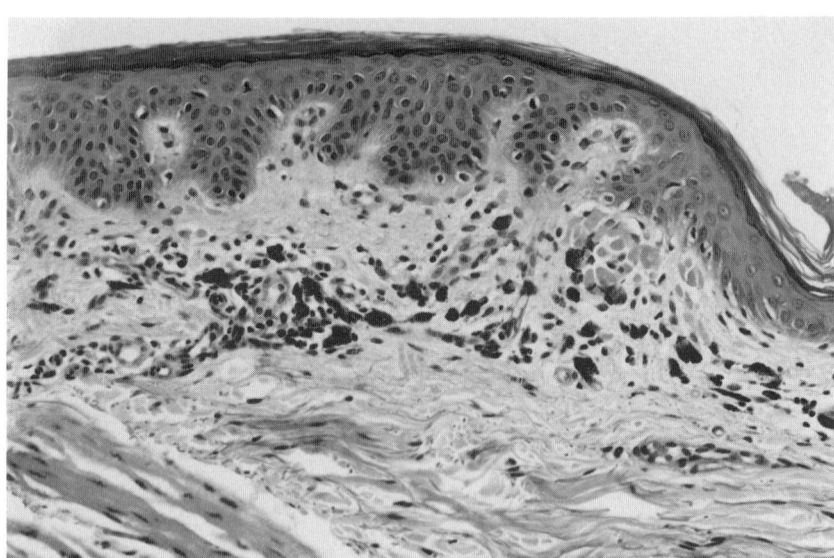

Figure 9.15   Lichen planus. A burnt out lesion showing pigmentary incontinence and residual Civatte bodies in the dermis.

maybe even more vigorous in the reaction and the number of Civatte bodies produced.

9.6   Lichen plano-pilaris

Occasionally the changes of lichen planus will be seen around the lower part of a hair follicle whose infundibulum is plugged with keratin: the changes of lichen plano-pilaris. With time the inflammation subsides leading to atrophy and scarring of the epidermis, at which stage it can be indistinguishable from scarring alopecia of other cause.

References

Barr, R. J. (1985) Psoriasiform and related papulasquamous disorders. *J. Cutan. Pathol.*, **12**, 412–25.

Bos, J. D., van Garderen, I. D., Krieg, S. R. and Poulter, L. W. (1986) Different in situ distribution patterns of dendritic cells having Langerhans (T6+) and interdigitating (RFD 2+) cell. Immunophenotype in psoriasis, atopic dermatitis, and other inflammatory dermatoses. *J. Invest. Dermatol.*, **87**, 358–61.

Chowaniec, O., Jablonska, S., Beutner, E. H., Proniewska, M., Jarzabek, Chorzelska, M. and Rzesa, G. (1981) Earliest clinical and histological changes in psoriasis. *Dermatologica*, **163**, 42–51.

Jowitt, S. N. and Liu Yin, J. A. (1990) Psoriasis and bone marrow transplantation. *Br. Med. J.*, **300**, 1398–9.

Mihm, M. C. Jr, Soter, N. A., Dvorak, H. F. and Austen, K. F. (1976) The structure of normal skin and the morphology of atopic eczema. *J. Invest. Dermatol.*, **67**, 305–12.

Pinkus, H. and Mehregan, A. H. (1966) The primary histologic lesions of seborrhoeic dermatitis and psoriasis. *J. Invest. Dermatol.*, **46**, 109–16.

Pinkus, H. (1973) Lichenoid tissue reactions. *Arch. Dermatol.*, **107**, 840–6.

Ragaz, A. and Ackerman, A. B. (1978) Evolution, maturation and regression of lesions of lichen planus. New observations and corrections of chemical and histologic findings. *Am. J. Dermatopathol.*, **3**, 5–25.

Shiohara, T. (1988) The lichenoid tissue reaction. An immunological perspective. *Am. J. Dermatopathol.*, **10**, 252–6.

Soter, N. A. (1989) Morphology of atopic eczema. *Allergy*, **44** (suppl. 9), 16–9.

Tong, A. K. (1986) The pathology of atopic dermatitis. *Clin. Rev. Allergy*, **4**, 27–42.

Weedon, D. (1985) The lichenoid tissue reaction. *J. Cutan. Pathol.*, **12**, 279–81.

Willis, C. M., Young, E., Brandon, D. R. and Wilkinson, J. D. (1986) Immunopathological and ultrastructural findings in human allergic and irritant contact dermatitis. *Br. J. Dermatol.*, **115**, 305–16.

Wright, N. A. (1985) Changes in epidermal cell proliferation in proliferative skin disease. In *Dermatopathology*, (ed. C. L. Berry), Springer-Verlag, Berlin, pp. 142–66.

10 Benign lymphoid infiltrates

The benign lymphoid infiltrates of the skin cover many processes, conditions and appearances. This chapter is by necessity selective. Whole books have been written on this topic alone, so a balance has been attempted between those conditions which are reasonably common, such as lupus erythematosus, and others, such as Lyme disease and Sweet's syndrome, where there have been advances either in the recognition of the condition, as in the first, or where confusion is rife in the face of an uncommon condition and where an analysis of the available information may help resolve one or two misconceptions.

The interpretation of inflammatory cell infiltrations of the skin is perhaps the part of dermatopathology which is least well done by pathologists, but this need not be the case. Credibility is soon lost if the dermatologist receives too many biopsy reports describing non-specific dermatitis. This can be a legitimate statement but only in a minority of cases. In the majority it is possible to go further. This process is eased when there is a good level of communication between pathologist and dermatologist so that one is aware of the clinical details of the patient, the appearance of the rash, its symptoms and history. It is not possible to unravel these biopsies if they are submitted innocent of clinical information, in the splendid isolation of the pathologist's office.

Ackerman has offered a system for analysing dermal infiltrates which is a useful way of approaching the problem (Ackerman, 1978). He divided the dermis into the superficial and deep perivascular compartments and added the interstitial one. These infiltrates can be described as superficial perivascular, superficial and deep perivascular, superficial perivascular and interstitial, and so forth. One must also decide whether the blood vessels are actively or passively involved in the process. That is whether vasculitis is present or not. This is a thorny problem which is discussed in detail in Chapter 15. Also one must look for involvement of the epidermis, hair follicles and sweat glands in the inflammatory process.

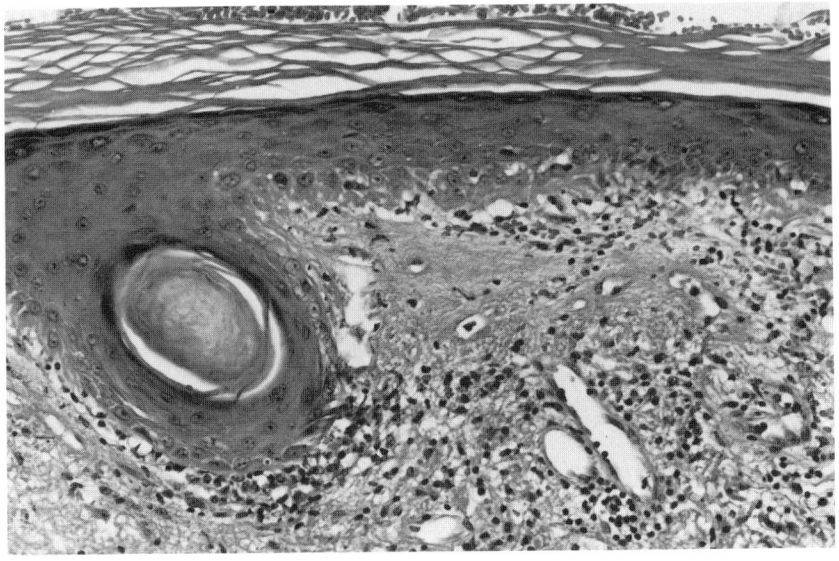

(a)

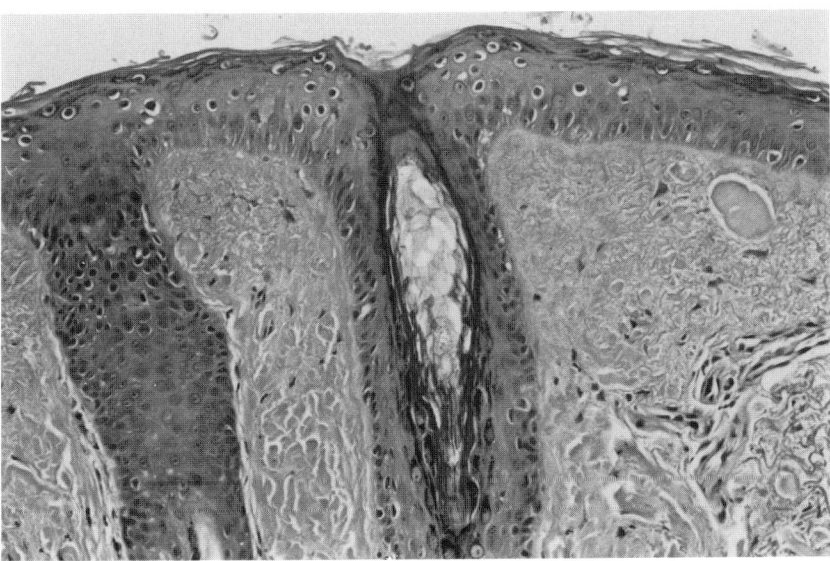

(b)

Figure 10.1 Lupus erythematosus. (a) Acute lesion with prominent basal hydropic changes and lymphocytic reaction, and (b) a more chronic lesion showing widening of the basement membrane which appears as a pale band at the dermal-epidermal junction.

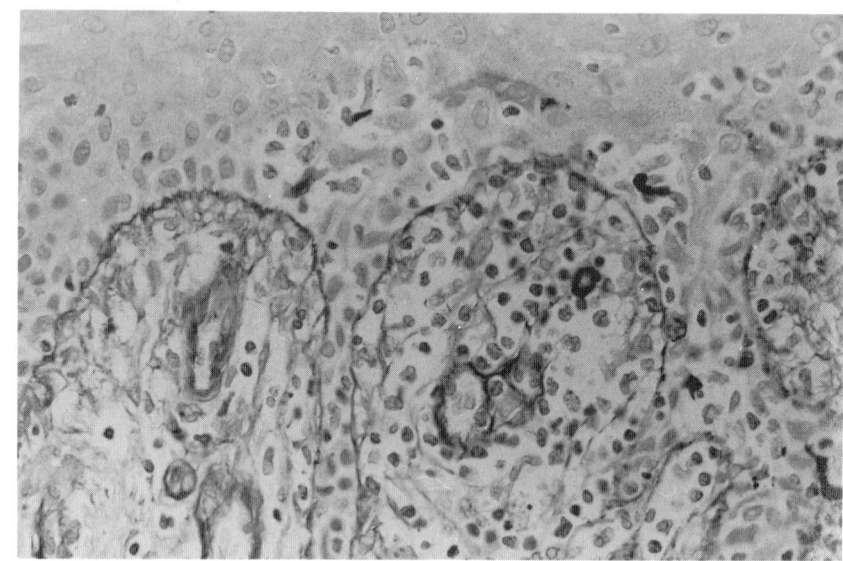

(a)

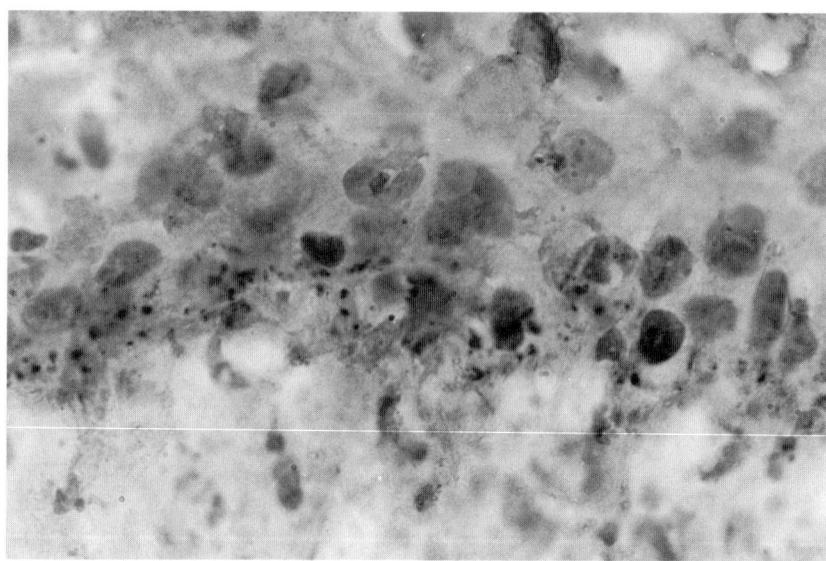

(b)

Figure 10.2 Lupus erythematosus (a and b). Granular deposition of IgG at the dermo-epidermal junction (immunoperoxidase).

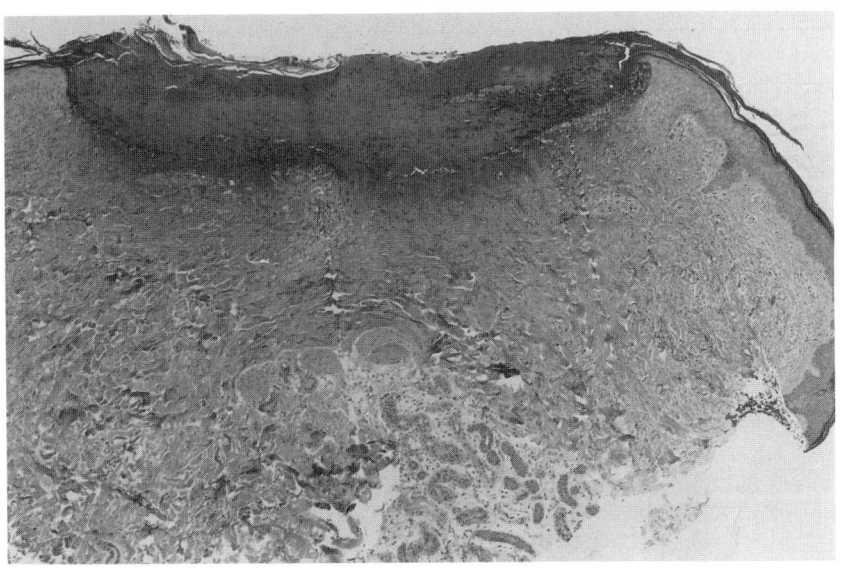

(a)

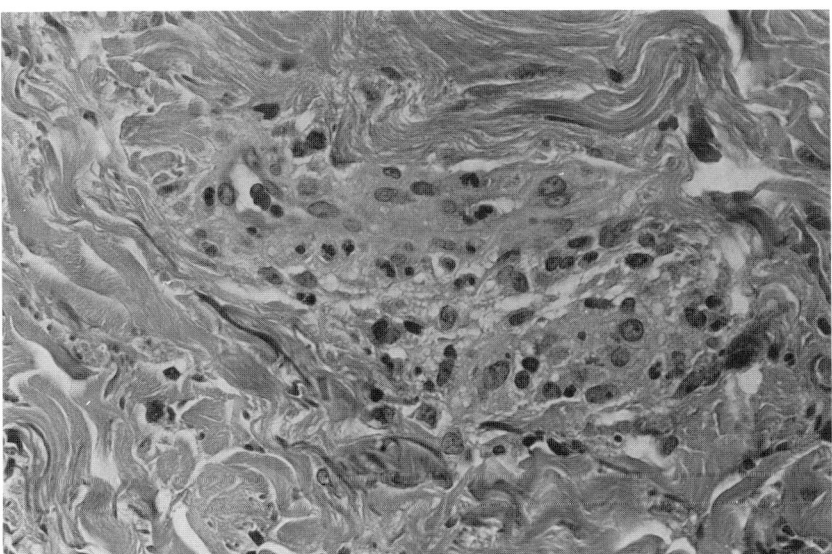

(b)

Figure 10.3 Systemic lupus erythematosus. (a) A dermal infarct, with (b) lymphocyte and macrophage infiltration around dermal vessels at the base of the lesion.

Much store is placed in the character of the infiltrating cells but, by and large, T-lymphocytes will almost always predominate; B-lymphocytes are unusual inhabitants of the skin even when there is clear evidence of immune complex formation in conditions such as pemphigoid or dermatitis herpetiformis. The exceptions include Sweet's syndrome where neutrophils predominate, syphilis where plasma cells predominate, and the various granulomas where macrophages will be seen either infiltrating, palisading or forming giant cells.

10.1   Lupus erythematosus

Lupus erythematosus is a disease which presents in several clinical and serological forms, representing a wide spectrum with a common underlying pathogenesis. The different forms cannot be reliably distinguished histologically (Clark *et al.*, 1973). The lesions are localized inflammatory papulosquamous plaques, which begin with a perivascular mononuclear cell infiltrate and subsequently, involve the epidermis and appendages. The appearances in a particular biopsy will depend upon the age of the lesion (Hood and Farmer, 1985).

In the active phase, the biopsy will show well-developed follicular plugging and epidermal hyperkeratosis with areas of parakeratosis. The main abnormalities are at the dermo-epidermal junction, where there is apparent thickening of the basement membrane and hydropic change of the basal keratinocytes, together with lymphocytic infiltration of the dermis beneath.

Immunohistochemical studies show immune complexes present at the dermo-epidermal junction, usually containing at least IgG and C3. The biopsy appearances are the same as those seen in patients with systemic lupus erythematosus (SLE), as is the finding of immune complexes at the dermo-epidermal junction. An IgM band may also be found in up to 55% of cases, but is not specific, being found in many other inflammatory dermatoses including lichen planus and eczema (Wojnarowska *et al.*, 1986). SLE and discoid lupus erythematosus (DLE) cannot be separated on biopsy appearances alone. Serological abnormalities are often lacking in DLE however: only about 20% of patients have detectable, anti-nuclear antibodies.

Cytomegalovirus infection can mimic the appearances of collagen vascular disease and cytomegalovirus (CMV) vasculitis has been described in association with SLE (Bulpitt and Brahn *et al.*, 1989).

10.2   Polymorphic light eruption

Polymorphic light eruption is characterized clinically by a persistent, acquired reaction to sunlight, which is delayed in onset and varied in its appearance (Haxthausen, 1919). It usually starts in the second or third decade and may affect up to 10–21% of those living in temperate climes. Biopsies are best done after the patient has been sat out in the sun for a while to bring out the rash and thus ensure that the pathologist has something to look at in the biopsy.

A lymphocytic infiltrate is seen densely aggregated around dermal vessels, resembling the changes seen in cases of allergic contact dermatitis. The lymphocytes start to accumulate within 5 hours of sun exposure and are preceded by an influx of dermal lymphocytes. In the first 72 hours after sun exposure, CD4 positive helper lymphocytes predominate; after which CD8 positive suppressor lymphocytes appear and then predominate, probably contributing to the resolution of the rash (Norris *et al.*, 1989). Immune complexes are not a feature of this process.

10.3   Jessner's lymphocytic infiltrate

In Jessner's original case report, he described a condition which he thought to be a variation or early stage of DLE or polymorphic light eruption (PLE). There has been sufficient confusion over the years to make it worthwhile quoting from his original paper. He stated that

> the lesions are flat, discoid, more or less elevated pinkish to reddish brown, starting as small papules, expanding peripherally, sometimes clearing in the centre, sometimes showing a circinate arrangement. The surface is smooth, occasionally uneven. There is no follicular hyperkeratosis. The consistency is firm, there may only be one, a few, or numerous lesions. They persist for weeks or months or longer, disappear without sequelae, and may recur in the same or other areas and cause practically no subjective symptoms. The face is obviously the area of predilection, but other parts of the body may or may not be affected.
>
> Histologically, the findings are rather consistent. The epidermis may be stretched, but is otherwise uninvolved. There may be edema in the sub-papillary regions on fresh lesions; older ones show none. Distributed through the cutis are rather sharply circumscribed lymphocytic infiltrations, sometimes extending to the subcutaneous fat, frequently, but not always, around vessels or appendages. The infiltrates consist of lymphocytes, mostly small ones and a few histiocytes and plasma cells. The infiltrates are often enmeshed in a fine reticulum. There are no eosinophiles, no germinal centres or germinal centre-like formations

(Jessner, 1953)

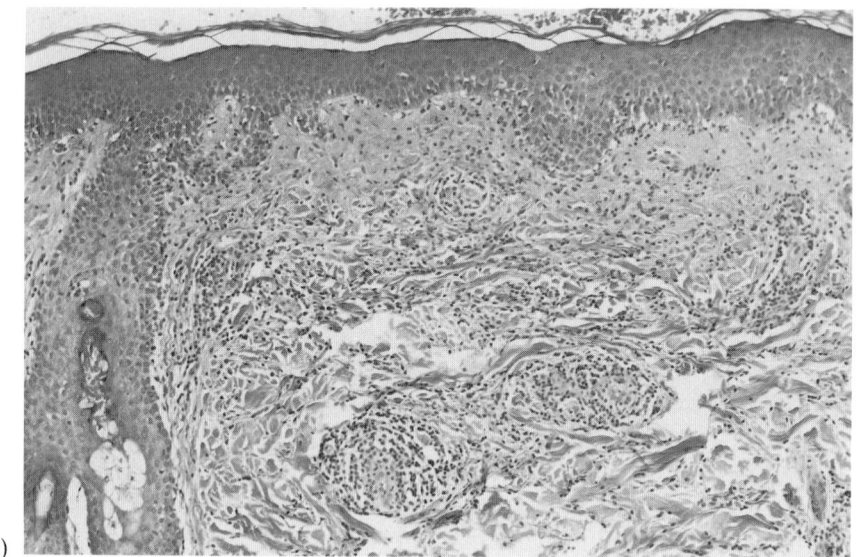

(a)

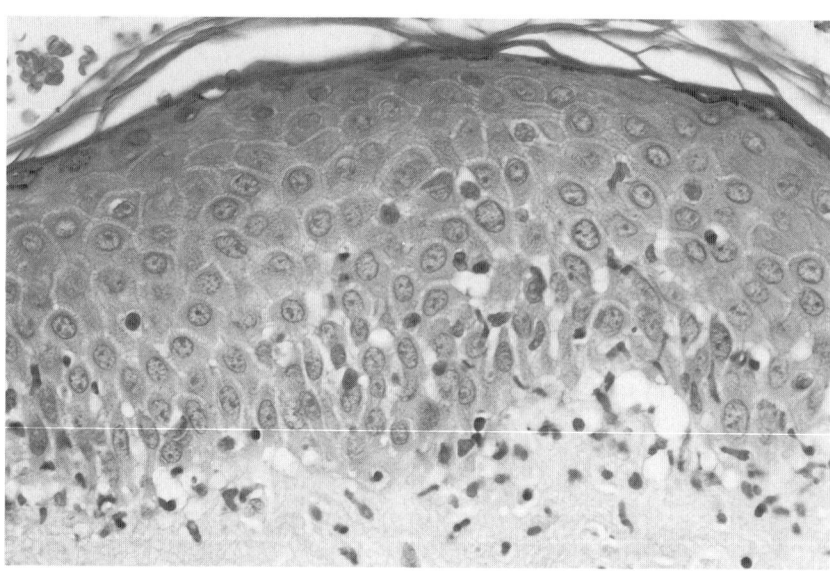

(b)

Figure 10.4 Polymorphic light eruption. (a) Predominantly dermal perivascular lymphocytic infiltration, but (b) also showing basal epidermal changes in this acute lesion.

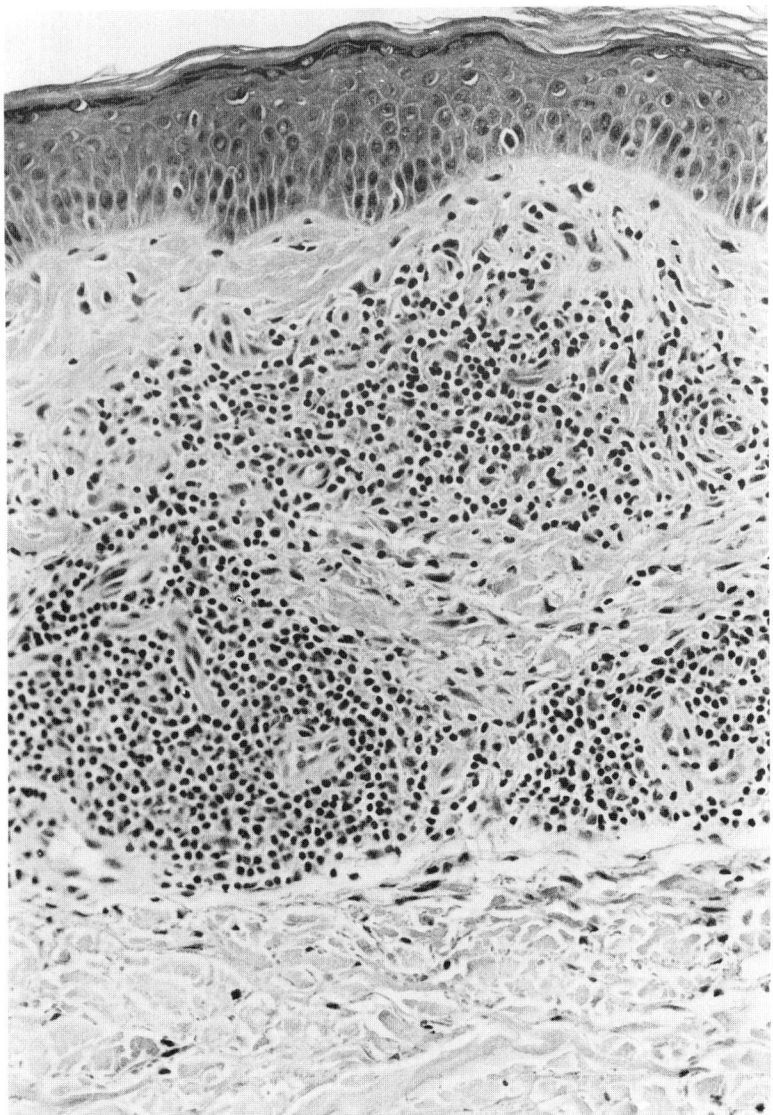

Figure 10.5   Jessner's lymphocytic infiltrate with prominent perivascular lymphocytic infiltration extending deeply into the dermis, but without extension to the epidermis.

The debate about whether or not Jessner's lymphocytic infiltrate exists continues to rumble on, but it does appear to be a reasonably well characterized condition and is worth separating from LE because of its better outlook. Both conditions have T-cells in their infiltrates,

(Konttinen *et al.*, 1981, 1987), with only a few cells positive for immuno-globulin (Willemze *et al.*, 1984). More recently, it has been shown that the T-cells do not proliferate within the dermal infiltrates but merely accumulate from the circulation. There is no immunoglobulin or complement at the dermo-epidermal junction (Konttinen *et al.*, 1987). It does not progress to lymphoma or polymorphic light eruption, although it can co-exist with the latter (Toonstra *et al.*, 1989).

10.4   Erythema multiforme

This is a self-limiting or episodic reaction which may involve the skin and sometimes also the mucous membranes. The individual lesions show a concentric appearance of peripheral erythema, with more marked changes in the centre, giving a target or iris lesion in well-developed lesions. Individual lesions last for up to 7 days and an episode may last as long as 6 weeks. The biopsy will show necrosis of keratinocytes and sub-epidermal separation in the centre of the lesion, with dermal oedema, vascular dilatation and perivascular lymphocytic infiltration towards the edge. Sometimes, the changes at the centre may lead to the actual development of a bulla, which may need to be distinguished from other causes of subepidermal blisters.

Lesions may develop as a complication of herpes simplex infection, when less severe changes, mainly spongiosis, exocytosis and basal cell liquefaction degeneration are seen. In the past sulphonamides have provoked more severe lesions, with mucosal involvement (Howland *et al.*, 1984).

10.5   Lymphocytoma cutis

Localized collections of lymphoid tissue may simulate lymphoma in the dermis, but with good sections, supplemented by immunohisto-chemical studies, it should be possible to identify those lesions which are reactive. When follicles with germinal centres are a feature, the follicles should be well developed and show evidence of polyclonal proliferation of B-cells (Smolle *et al.*, 1990). There should not be any evidence of invasion of or damage to appendages or blood vessel walls (Hulinska *et al.*, 1989). The underlying cause may be difficult to identify, but possibilities, such as infection, should be considered. Lympho-cytoma has been reported as a manifestation of Lyme disease (Abele *et al.*, 1989).

Southern blot analysis of DNA from lesions to detect the presence of a monoclonal rearrangement of immunoglobulin genes allows a distinction to be made between those lesions which are clonal and carry a

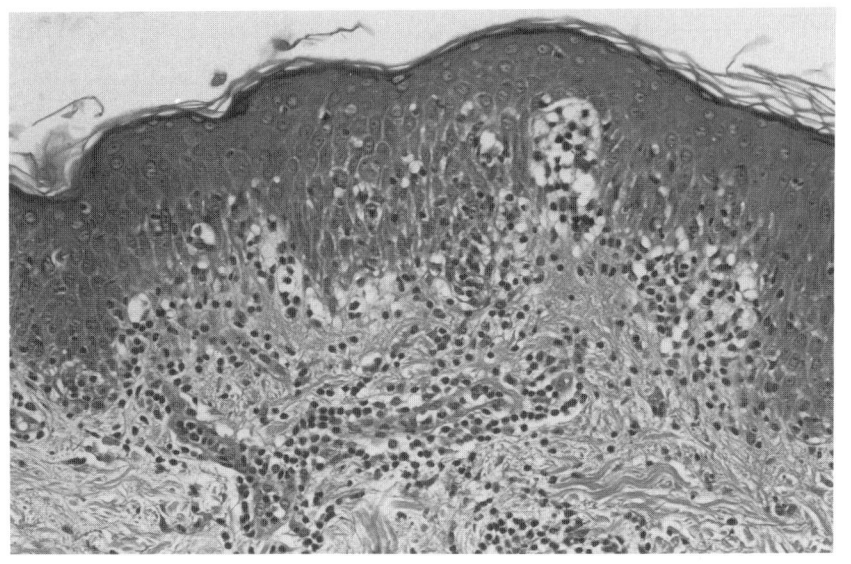

(a)

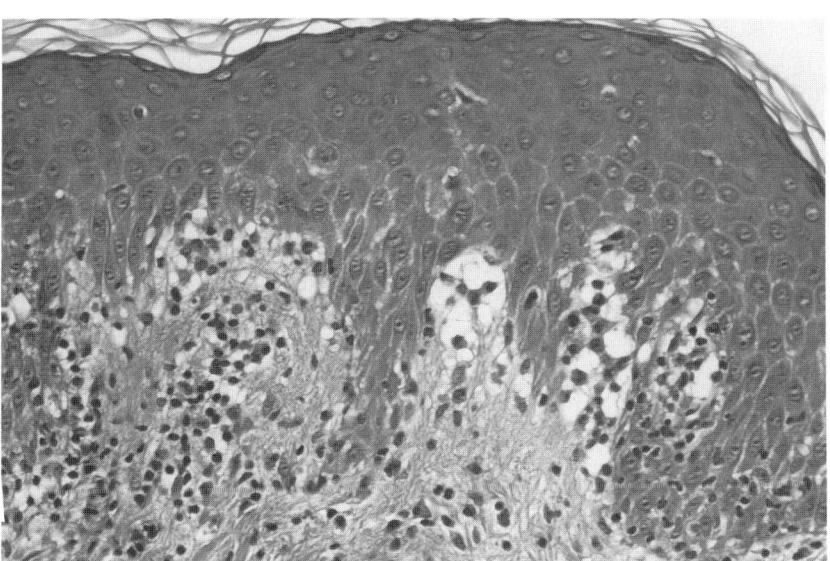

(b)

Figure 10.6 Erythema multiforme. (a) Extensive lymphocytic infiltration and oedema, with (b) epidermal extension and keratinocyte necrosis.

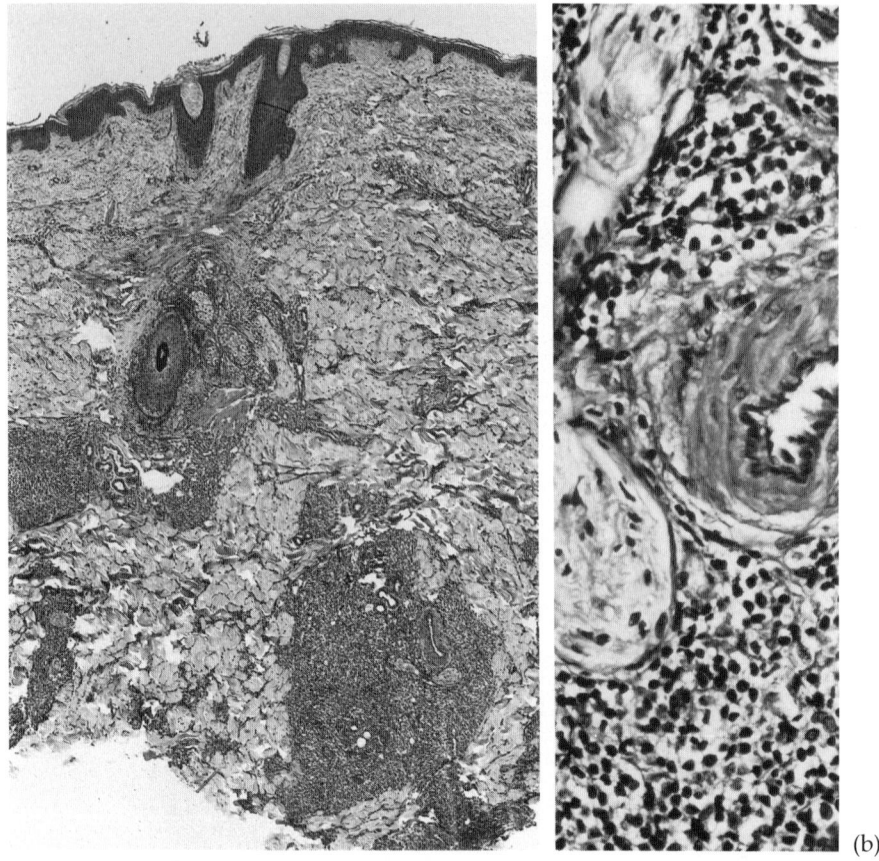

(a)
(b)

Figure 10.7 Lymphocytoma cutis. (a) Large lymphoid aggregates in the dermis, composed of small lymphocytes, and (b) without vasculitis or neural infiltration.

risk of progression to lymphoma, and a second group which are entirely reactive (Cleary and Sklar, 1989; Wood *et al.*, 1989).

10.6 Pityriasis lichenoides acuta

The acute form of pityriasis lichenoides or, to give it its full title, pityriasis lichenoides acuta et varioliformis acuta (PLEVA), shows an acute picture of interface dermatitis, with dermal perivascular infiltration extending into the epidermis, with associated intercellular oedema, keratinocyte necrosis and extravasation of erythrocytes, which can also extend into the epidermis (Willemze and Scheffer, 1985). Vasculitis is not a feature of this condition.

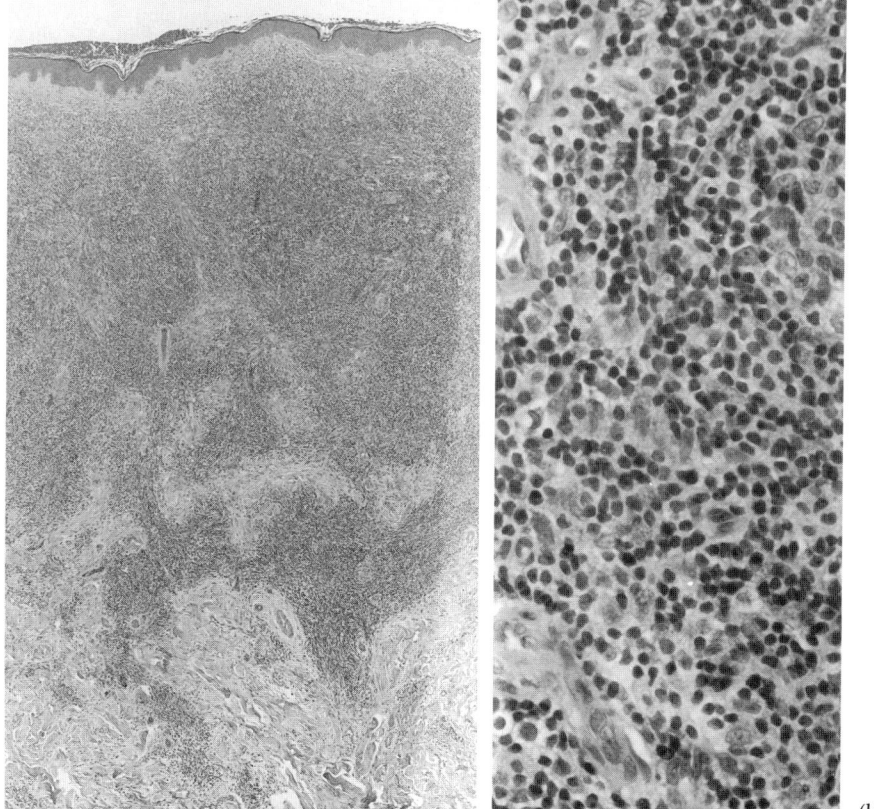

(a)   (b)

Figure 10.8   Persistent insect bite. (a) Dense lymphocytic dermal infiltration, with more lymphocytes in the upper than the lower dermis; (b) the infiltrate contains uniform, small lymphocytes.

10.7   Pityriasis lichenoides chronica

The chronic form of pityriasis lichenoides shows similar but less marked, features to the acute form. The infiltrate can be quite subtle, distributed around upper dermal vessels, with associated extravasation of erythrocytes.

In the past there has been a degree of semantic overlap between pityriasis lichenoides chronica and small plaque parapsoriasis. The nomenclature of parapsoriasis has in itself been confusing, but there is probably only a need for two types: small plaque parapsoriasis, or digitate dermatosis, which is a benign, self-limiting condition, and large plaque parapsoriasis, which is a premycotic stage of cutaneous T-

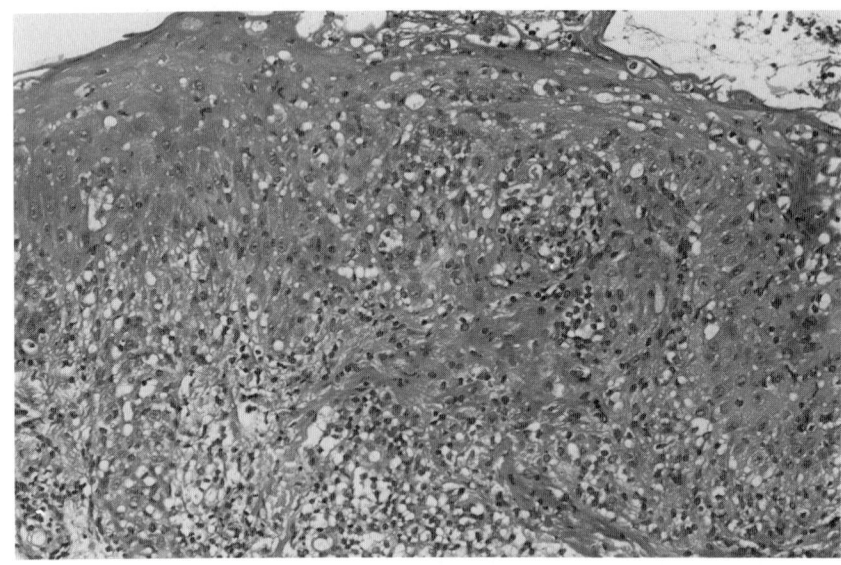

Figure 10.9 Pityriasis lichenoides acuta. An extensive acute interface dermatitis with extension into the upper epidermis.

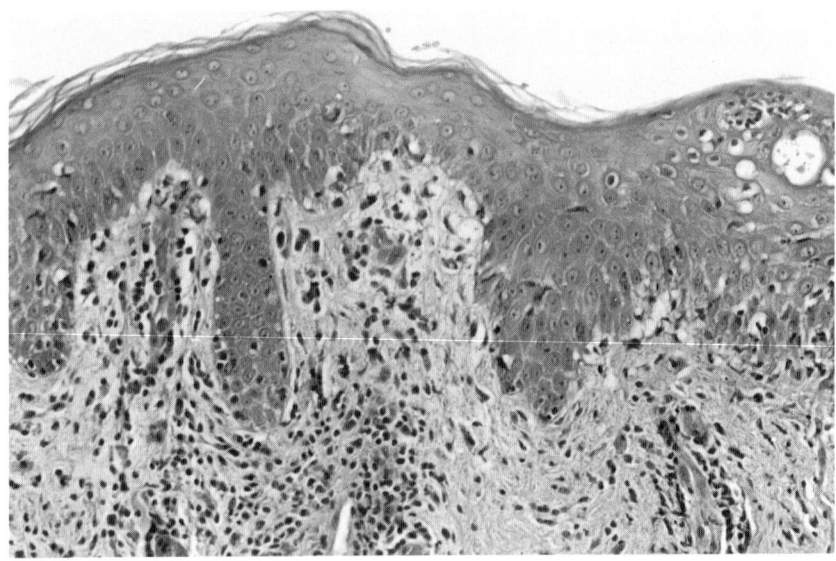

Figure 10.10 Pityriasis lichenoides acuta. Less acute than in Fig. 10.9, but showing dermal and epidermal involvement and intraepidermal vesiculation.

cell lymphoma in many cases. Guttate, lichenoid and reteform parapsoriasis are terms which can be abandoned (Benmaman and Sanchez, 1988).

10.8   Pityriasis rubra pilaris

This condition has clinical similarities with psoriasis, but the biopsy appearances differ. The epidermis shows acanthosis with short rete ridges and a thick layer of cells above the dermal papillae. The granular layer is preserved and may be thickened, with associated hyperkeratosis, sometimes with parakeratosis. The hyperkeratosis extends to fill follicular infundibulae (Soeprono, 1986).

10.9   Gyrate erythema

There is a related group of erythemas which are mainly diagnosed by their clinical rather than biopsy appearances (White, 1985). Erythema gyratum repens is a marker of underlying internal malignancy, with a most striking appearance of a widespread change resembling wood grain, which is most marked in the intertriginous areas (Appell et al., (1988). Although found in association with pulmonary tuberculosis (Barber et al., 1978), and without any evidence of malignancy (Langlois et al., 1985), it is most usually seen as a manifestation of malignancy of which bronchogenic carcinoma is perhaps the commonest (Levine et al., 1985; Ingber and Sandbank, 1986; Skolnick and Mainman, 1975; Olsen et al., 1984). It may result from some form of immunological activation, but remains largely unexplained (Holt and Davies, 1977).

The biopsy shows mild patchy spongiosis with parakeratosis, corresponding to the wood grain appearance of the rash, and with mild to moderate dermal perivascular lymphocytic infiltration.

Erythema annulare centrifugum is a generic term which encompases most of the other gyrate erythemas (Shelley and Hurley, 1960). Biopsies may show predominantly superficial or superficial and deep dermal infiltration. Erythema chronicum migrans is an example of the deep type.

10.10   Lyme disease – erythema chronicum migrans

Lyme disease is associated with infection by the spirochaete *Borrelia burgdorferi*, which is transmitted by the bite of *Ixodes* ticks (Parke, 1987). Although first recognized in New England, cases have now been seen in many countries, including southern England (Williams et al., 1986; Bateman et al., 1987). It is a multisystem disease, with cutaneous

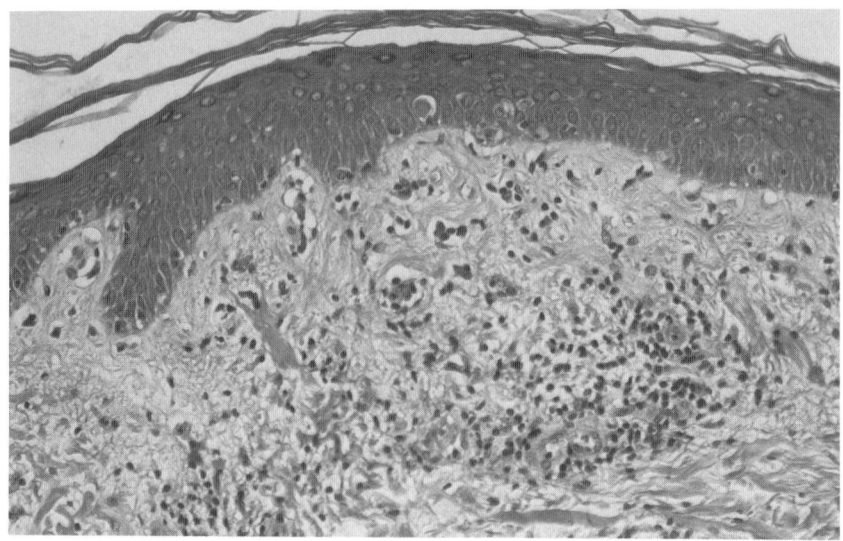

Figure 10.11 Pityriasis lichenoides chronica. The chronic stage with
lymphocytic infiltration around upper dermal vessels and occasional
extravasated erythrocytes.

manifestations which are a consequence of a cell mediated immune
reaction to the spirochaetes. Within a few weeks of the bite, a rapidly
expanding lesions of erythema chronicum migrans can develop
(Muhlemann, 1984; Berger, 1989).

The biopsy will show a superficial and deep perivascular and interstitial infiltrate consisting mostly of lymphocytes. Towards the advancing edge of the lesion, plasma cells may be seen, whereas at the
centre, eosinophils are present. Spirochaetes are visible in a minority of
lesions when sections are stained by the Warthin-Starry method (Berger,
1984), although this is a difficult technique to use. Monoclonal antibodies to the organism are now available. The organisms are 5–30
microns long, 0.12–0.25 microns thick, and have 8 or 11 flagella arising
from both ends of the body (Hulinska *et al.*, 1989). Later in the development of the disease, septal panniculitis has been described (Kramer
et al., 1986).

Serological confirmation of the diagnosis is unreliable, possibly
because of the predominantly cell mediated nature of the reaction
(Editorial, 1989), and also because the presence of antibodies does not
necessarily indicate disease (Guy *et al.*, 1989). As well as the erythema
migrans, other skin lesions including granuloma annulare, erythema
nodosum, papular urticaria, Henoch-Schonlein-like purpura, and morphea have been found, although whether these are due to Lyme

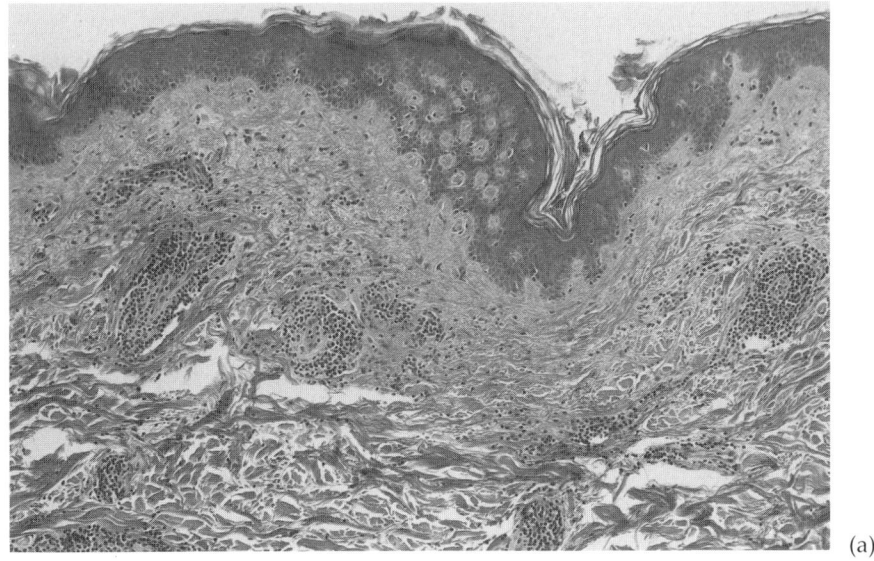

(a)

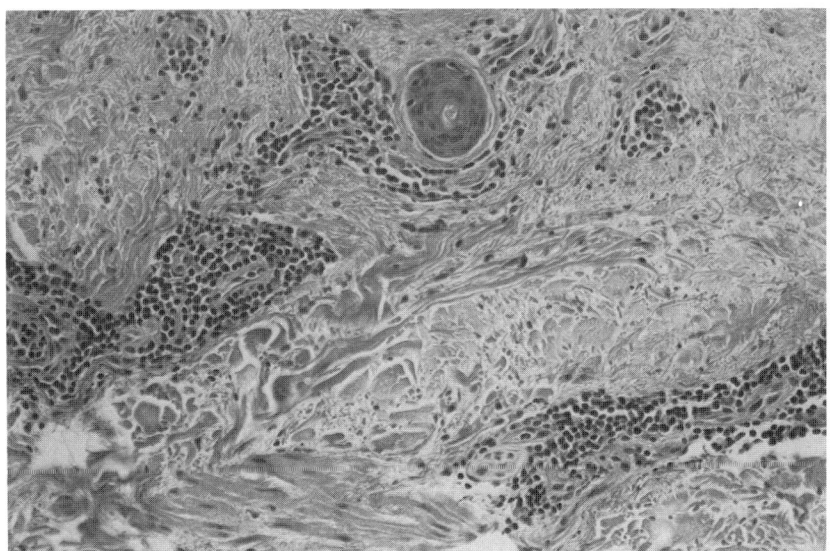

(b)

Figure 10.12   Erythema annulare centrifugum. An erythema with lymphocytic reaction confined around dermal vessels.

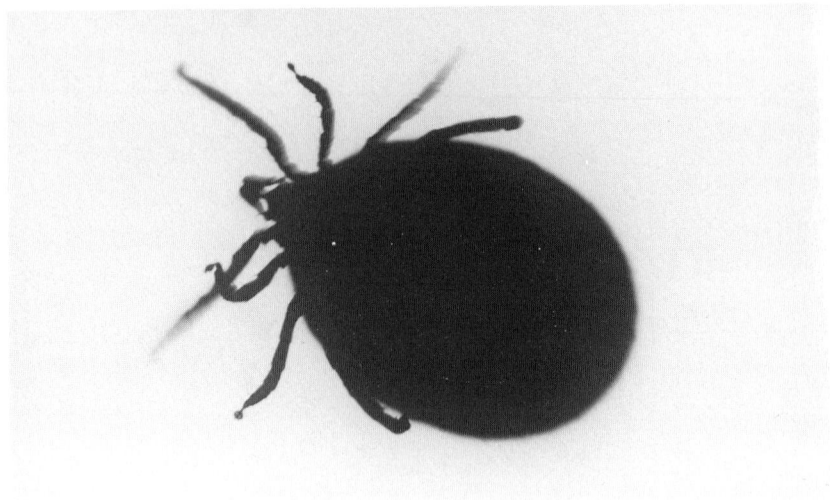

Figure 10.13   Adult female *Ixodes ricinus*, the tick responsible for the transmission of the spirochaete Borrelia burgdorferi. The tick is engorged by a blood meal and carries the spirochaete in her mid-gut.

disease or are coincidental findings is yet to be determined (Berger, 1989). Systemic infection can produce arthritis (Macallan *et al.*, 1987), or meningitis (Bourke *et al.*, 1988).

It is important to make the diagnosis because it can be treated with antibiotics. Early treatment can prevent or diminish the cell mediated reaction (Parke, 1987), and late disease can progress to an appearance of acrodermatitis chronica atrophicans (Kaufman *et al.*, 1989).

10.11   Sweet's syndrome

In 1964 Sweet described 8 cases assembled over 15 years of a condition characterized by fever, a neutrophil polymorphonuclear leukocytosis in the peripheral blood, raised, painful plaques on the limbs, face and neck and a biopsy appearance of a dense dermal infiltrate of neutrophils without vasculitis (Sweet, 1964; Gunawardena *et al.*, 1975; Storer *et al.*, 1983). Dermal vessels may show endothelial cell swelling. The dermis shows a variable degree of oedema possibly leading to the formation of subepidermal bullae, the epidermis may show focal secondary spongiosis and parakeratosis. Although there is no actual leukocytoclastic vasculitis, the presence of so many neutrophils may be associated with small amounts of apoptotic nuclear dust. Immune

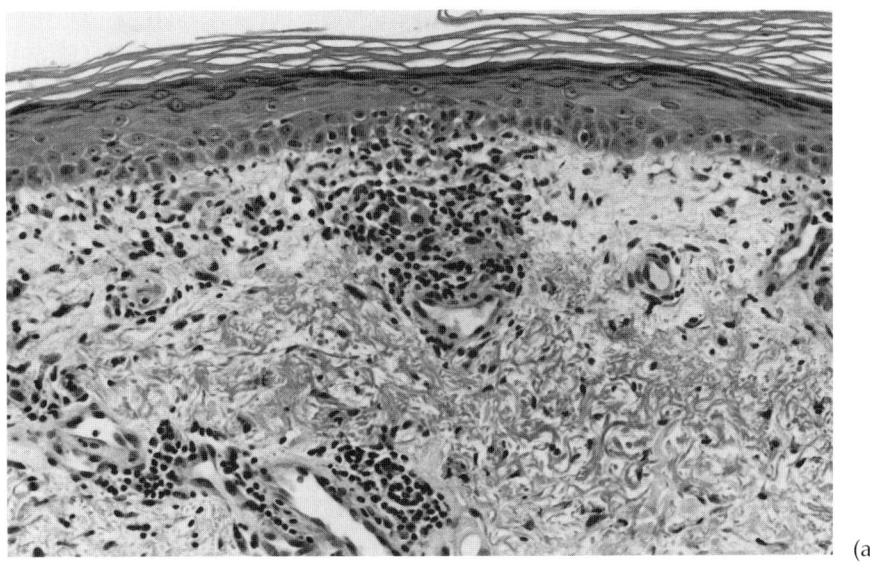

(a)

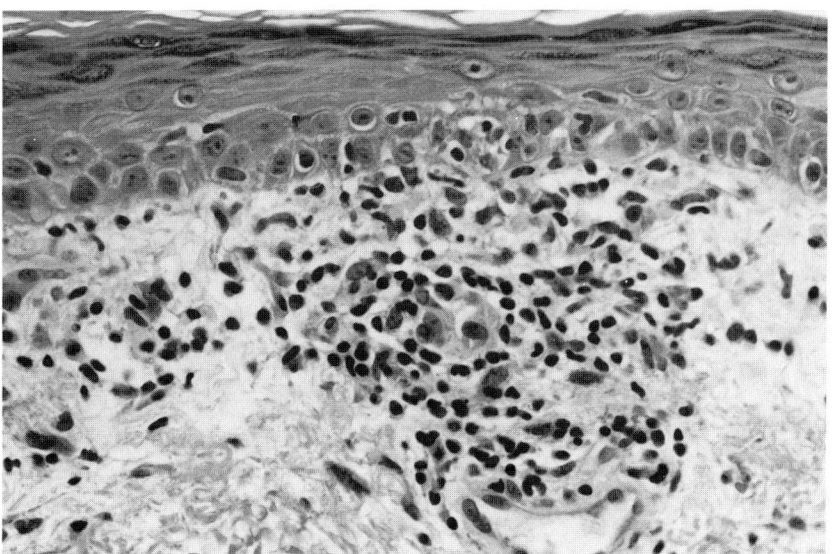

(b)

Figure 10.14 Meningitis. (a) The acute erythema of meningococcal septicaemia, with (b) lymphocytic reaction around upper dermal vessels and focal extension into the epidermis.

complexes are not demonstrable. Treatment is with systemic cortico-steroids. Sweet's syndrome has been reported in association with a number of conditions including subacute thyroid disease, subacute lupus erythematosus, Sjogren's syndrome, Crohn's disease (Kemmett *et al.*, 1988; Becuwe *et al.*, 1989), ulcerative colitis (Sweet, 1964; Benton *et al.*, 1985), myeloproliferative disease, where the degree of activity of the eruption is not an index of the activity of the myelodysplastic syndrome, and malignancy in general (Cooper *et al.*, 1983; Caughman *et al.*, 1989; Cohen and Kuzrock, 1987; Hasegawa *et al.*, 1989; Furukawa *et al.*, 1989).

The association with myeloproliferative disease is mainly with granu-locytic leukaemia, being commoner than lymphocytic or monocytic leukaemia, where the association is usually with poor prognosis. There appears to be a wide spectrum of acute neutrophilic dermatoses, with typical Sweet's syndrome at one end and pyoderma gangrenosum at the other. In the middle there is an overlap of blistering and ulcerative skin lesions which are difficult to classify into one or the other ends (Dereure *et al.*, 1988).

Su and Lui (1986) have suggested diagnostic criteria: both major criteria (abrupt onset of tender or painful erythematous or violaceous plaques or nodules; predominantly neutrophilic infiltration of the der-mis without leukocytoclastic vasculitis) and at least two minor criteria (illness preceded by fever or infection; accompanying fever, arthralgia, conjunctivitis, or underlying malignancy; leukocytosis; good response to systemic steroids and lack of response to antibiotics) are required to make the diagnosis.

The subject has been well reviewed by Jordaan (1989) who emphas-izes that the well-described neutrophilic phase is preceded by a pre-dominantly lymphocytic phase and is succeeded by a histiocytic phase. Differential diagnosis therefore varies according to the stage of develop-ment of the lesion at the time of biopsy, and depends upon close clinico-pathological liason, to consider problems such as the overlap between Sweet's disease and erythema elevatum diutinum.

10.12   Papular urticaria and mastocytosis

Chronic urticarial skin conditions are often a problem to pathologist and dermatologist alike (Kaplan *et al.*, 1987). The biopsy may, at first sight, show little change. A second look will show variable but increased numbers of mast cells – normal skin contains few mast cells. They are better seen in Giemsa stained sections (Lennert and Parwaresch, 1979). They will be found both around the dermal vessels and in the dermal stroma. Vasculitis is not a feature of chronic urticaria and immune complexes are not found (Winklemann, 1985; Boon *et al.*, 1986).

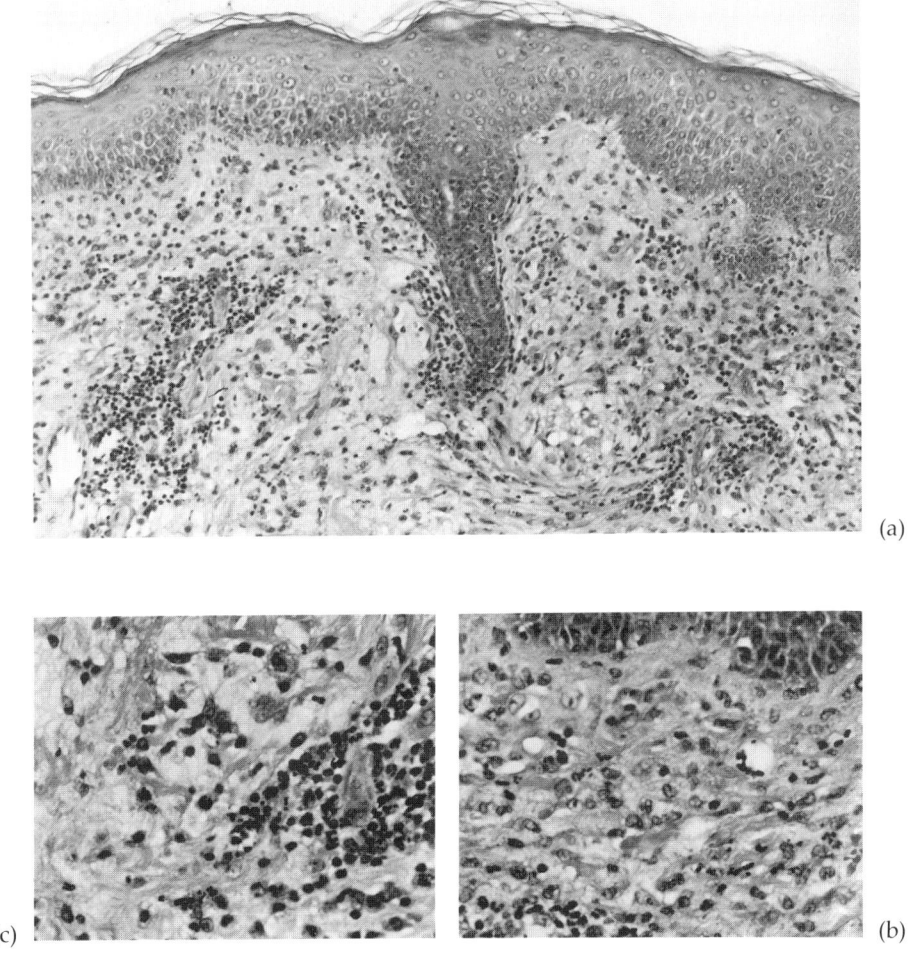

Figure 10.15 Sweet's disease. (a) Extensive dermal perivascular and interstitial infiltration with (b and c) neutrophils predominating.

Biopsies usually come from patients with irritating papular eruptions where the differential diagnosis lies between dermatitis herpetiformis, papular urticaria and prurigo simplex. The first of these can be excluded by the lack of IgA in papillary microabscesses. The differentiation of the latter two can be more of a problem, with localized epidermal acanthosis and fewer mast cells being features more in favour of prurigo.

Systemic mastocytosis can involve the skin, where the appearance is that of urticaria pigmentosum: macular lesions with many mast cells around dermal vessels (Monheit *et al.*, 1979).

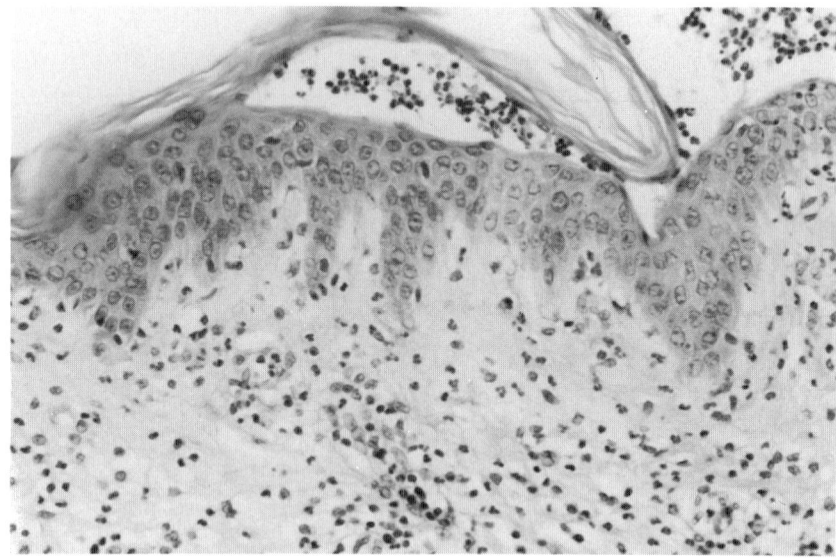

Figure 10.16   Impetigo. Neutrophil infiltration of dermis and epidermis, with the formation of a superficial blister.

10.13   Incontinentia pigmenti

Incontinentia pigmenti is inherited as an X-linked dominant condition, and is lethal in males (Spallone, 1987). In the acute stage, the epidermis contains vesicles, with large numbers of eosinophils in and around them. The epidermis also shows dyskeratotic cells and whorls of keratinocytes. The condition progresses to a stage of patchy pigmentation and depigmentation, associated with pigmentary incontinence (Ashley and Burgdorf, 1987). Dermal nerves appear to be abnormal and may play a part in the transfer of melanin to the dermis (Worret *et al.*, 1988).

10.14   Graft versus host disease

The development of bone marrow transplantation as a form of therapy has produced a new disease in which the graft CD8 positive lymphocytes attack the host skin (Lampert *et al.*, 1982; Lever *et al.*, 1986). The changes seen vary with the intensity of the reaction, from a simple lichenoid reaction with focal or diffuse vacuolar changes of basal cells, through a spongiotic and dyskeratotic reaction to the development of subepidermal clefts and even complete loss of the epidermis (Sloane *et al.*, 1984; Hymes *et al.*, 1985). The process also involves endothelial cell injury in the underlying dermis, as well as the more obvious epidermal cell changes (Dumler *et al.*, 1989).

The differential diagnosis includes rashes associated with infections

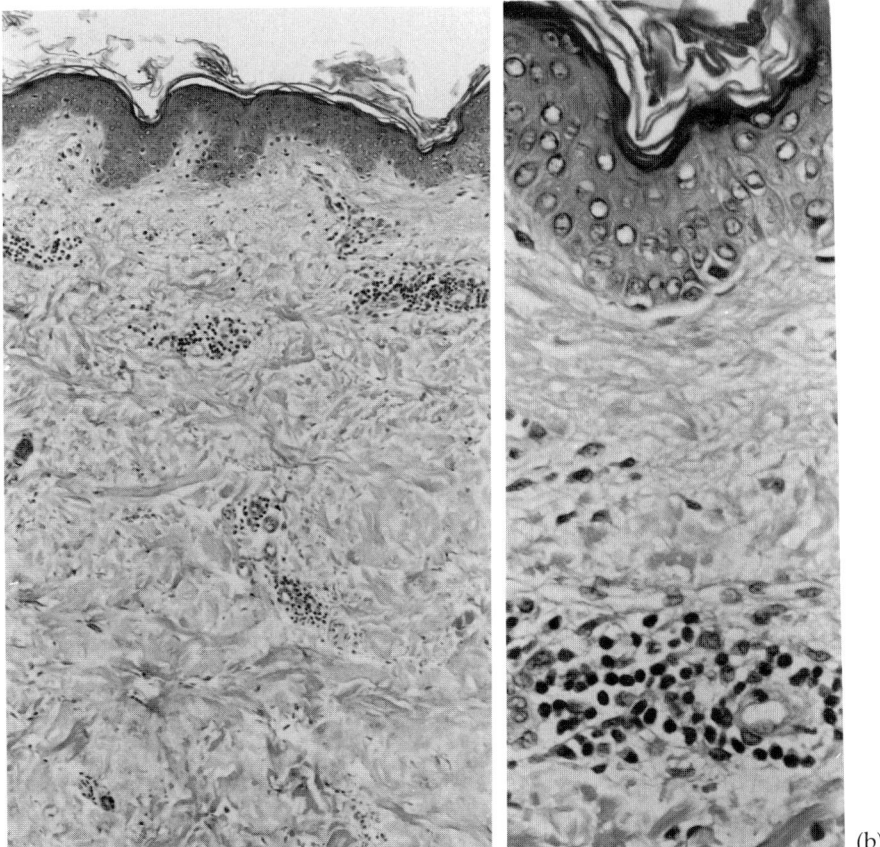

(a)   (b)

Figure 10.17   Papular urticaria. (a) Dermal oedema, with (b) sparse lymphocyte and mast cell infiltration around superficial and deep dermal vessels.

and drug reactions. A macular and papular rash associated with a superficial perivascular lymphocytic dermal infiltrate has also been described in patients on chemotherapy, the rash developing as the patients recover from the immunosupressive effects of the therapy and immunocompetent T-cells return to the skin (Horn *et al.*, 1989).

10.15   Alopecia – technical note

The differential diagnosis of alopecia revolves around the problem of differentiating remediable from irremediable processes. Despite the many claims to the contrary, male pattern baldness is a marker of the unstoppable march of time, without any inflammatory component in

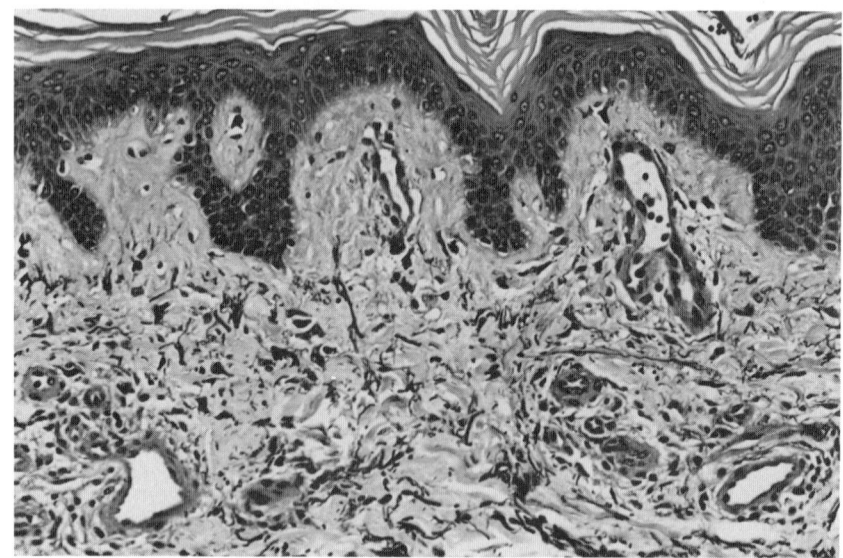

(a)

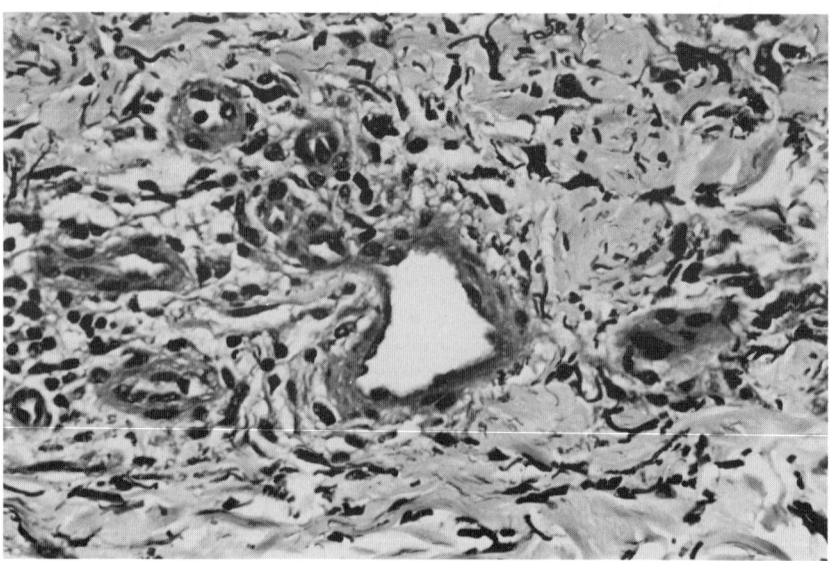

(b)

Figure 10.18 Urticaria pigmentosum. (a) Many mast cells are present around vessels, and (b) in the dermal interstitium (AOG).

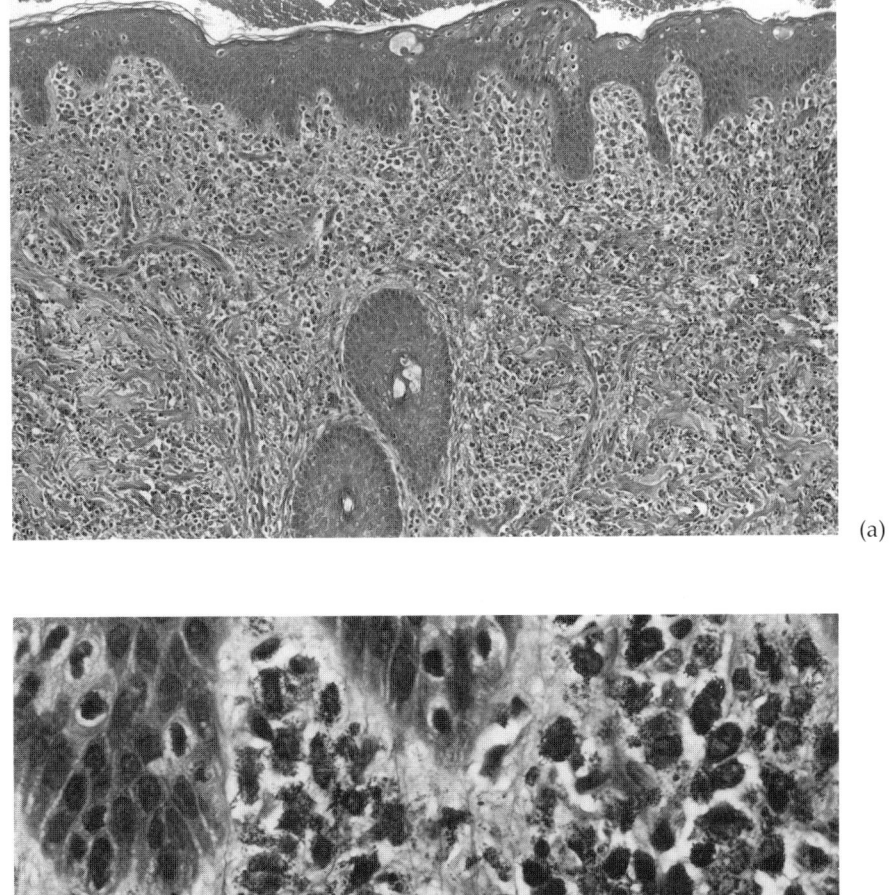

Figure 10.19 Cutaneous mastocytoma. (a) A tumourous infiltration of the dermis by (b) mast cells (AOG).

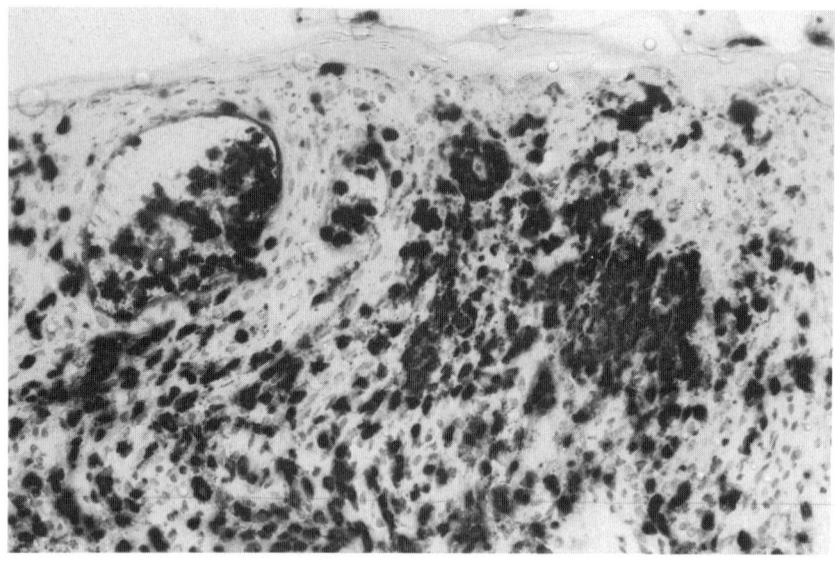

Figure 10.20   Incontinentia pigmenti. In this frozen section, the large numbers of eosinophils present in epidermal vesicles and between keratinocytes are stained as a result of the action of their endogenous peroxidase (immunoperoxidase).

biopsies. Other conditions may have an underlying inflammatory process which can be potentially reversible.

When approaching the diagnosis of an alopecia it is important to remind oneself of the special anatomy of the hair follicle and its growth cycle. In short, there are three stages in the cycle: the active growth phase is anagen, the early stage of evolution is catagen and the resting phase is telogen.

The biopsy will usually be taken with a punch and should be orientated so as to be able to cut transverse sections at different levels through the block, so that, first, all of the follicles in the biopsy can be seen, and, second, that changes in different levels of the follicles can be identified. This technique was proposed by Headington and is described in detail in his article (Headington, 1984). A computer-aided approach to morphometric quantification of the changes in alopecia has also been described (Gibbons *et al.*, 1986). This same approach has also been applied to the study of acne keloidalis (Herzberg *et al.*, 1990).

10.16   Alopecia areata

The biopsy will show miniature anagen follicles, which do not extend deeply into the dermis, with an inflammatory infiltrate of variable degree around the follicles, more prominent in newer lesions (Messenger *et al.*, 1986). This is associated with the abnormal expression of class I and II major histocompatibility antigens on follicular epithelial cells (Brockner *et al.*, 1987), which appears to be induced by the lymphocytic infiltrate (Khoury *et al.*, 1988).

10.17   Trichotillomania

This form of artefact, produced by pulling hair out, produces predictable changes: there are empty follicles interspersed between others which may contain broken hairs, or may be normal. There may be traction damages to the follicular epithelium, but dermal inflammation should be absent.

10.18   Scarring alopecia

Also known as 'pseudopelade of Broque' is an inflammatory process which leads to follicle destruction. In the active phase, lymphocytes are found around the upper two-thirds of the follicles and extend into the epithelium and associated sebaceous glands. Later on, the inflamma-

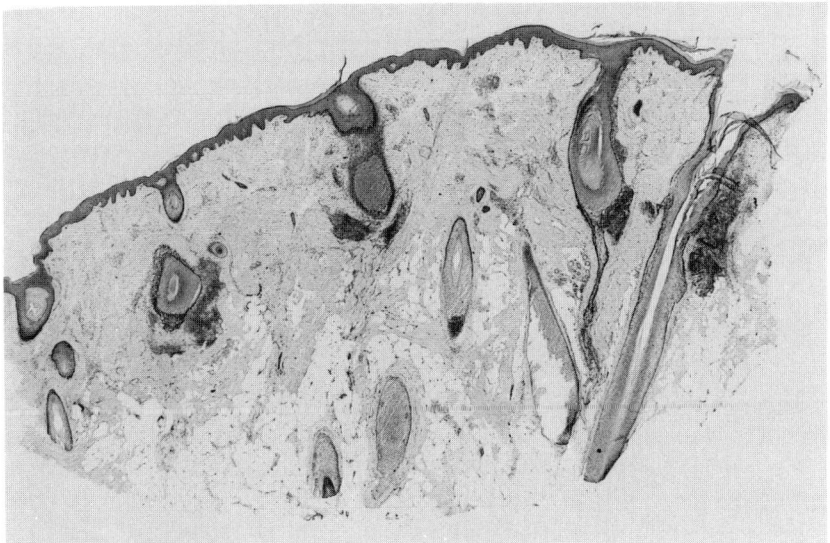

Figure 10.21   Scarring alopecia. In this frozen section stained for basement membrane with the antibody LH 7.2, the inflammatory infiltration around the dilated, and keratin-filled, upper portions of the hair follicles can be seen (immunoperoxidase).

tion subsides and the destroyed follicles are marked by fibrous scars, which extend down into the dermis and contain elastic fibres, which can be best seen in AOG stained sections.

The differential diagnosis is from conditions such as lichen plano-pilaris, which involves the whole follicle, lupus erythematous, which should show basal hydropic change and immune complexes at the dermo–epidermal junction, and localized scleroderma, which shows more generalized dermal fibrosis.

10.19   Follicular mucinosis

The accumulation of Alcian blue-positive mucin in the outer root sheath of the follicle and in the associated sebaceous gland, may be a merely reactive process or may be associated with lymphoma. Differential diagnosis is not straightforward, but reactive follicular mucinosis is more likely when mucin is easily seen and eosinophils are present in the associated infiltrate. When the infiltrate is dense, shows marked epidermotrophism and contains hyperconvoluted or hyperchromatic cells, then the mucinosis is probably a manifestation of lymphoma (Logan and Headington, 1988).

10.20   Erosive pustular dermatosis of the scalp

This condition is a chronic pustular inflammatory process of the scalp, which is found in elderly women and consists of extensive crusted lesions with scarring alopecia. The biopsies show varying degrees of chronic inflammatory cell infiltration, often with plasma cells in the reticular dermis and with varying degrees of follicular atrophy. Stains for bacteria and fungi are negative. The lesions may be responsive to steroid therapy (Pye *et al.*, 1979). A similar condition has been described in socially deprived young patients in the Sudan (Jacyk, 1988).

10.21   Subcorneal pustular dermatosis

Subcorneal pustular dermatosis (Sneddon-Wilkinson disease) is a van-ishingly rare condition characterized by intraepidermal pustules, which lie in the prickle cell layer and usually do not elevate the overlying keratin to any great extent. The disease may be associated with other conditions, such as rheumatoid arthritis, and is usually responsive to dapsone therapy (Murphy and Griffiths, 1989; Roger *et al.*, 1990).

References

Abele, D. C., Anders, K. H. and Chandler, F. W. (1989) Benign lymphocytic infiltration (Jessner-Kanof): another manifestation of borreliosis? *J. Am. Acad. Dermatol.*, **21**, 795–7.

Ackerman, A. B. (1978) Histologic diagnosis of inflammatory skin diseases. Lea and Febiger.

Appell, M. L., Ward, W. Q. and Tyring, S. K. (1988) Erythema gyratum repens. A cutaneous marker of malignancy. *Cancer*, **62**, 548–50.

Ashley, J. R. and Burgdorf, W. H. (1987) Incontinentia pigmenti: pigmentary changes independent of incontinence. *J. Cutan. Pathol.*, **14**, 248–50.

Barber, P. V., Doyle, L., Vickers, D. M. and Hubbard, H. (1978) Erythema gyratum repens with pulmonary tuberculosis. *Br. J. Dermatol.*, **98**, 465–8.

Bateman, D. E., White, J. E., Elrington, G. and Lawton, N. F. (1987) Three further cases of Lyme disease. *Br. Med. J.*, **294**, 548–9.

Becuwe, C., Delaporte, E., Colombel, J. F., Piette, F., Cortot, A. and Bergoend, H. (1989) Sweet's syndrome associated with Crohn's disease. *Acta. Derm. Venereol. (Stockh.)*, **69**, 444–5.

Benmaman, O. and Sanchez, J. C. (1988) Comparative clinicopathologic study on pityriasis lichenoides chronica and small plaque parapsoriasis. *Am. J. Dermatopathol.*, **10**, 189–96.

Berger, B. W. (1984) Erythema chronicum migrans of Lyme disease. *Arch. Dermatol.*, **120**, 1017–21.

Berger, B. W. (1989) Dermatologic manifestations of Lyme disease. *Rev. Infect. Dis.*, **11** (suppl. 6), S1475–81.

Benton, E. C., Rutherford, D. and Hunter, J. A. A. (1985) Sweet's syndrome and pyoderma gangrenosum associated with ulcerative colitis. *Acta. Derm. Venereol. (Stockh.)*, **65**, 77–80.

Boon, W. J., Nieboer, C. and Huijgens, P. C. (1986) Pathogenetic studies in chronic urticaria. Failure to demonstrate vasculitis, complement activation and fibrinolysis. *Dermatologica*, **173**, 264–70.

Bourke, S. J., Baird, D. R., Bone, F. J., Baird, D. R. and Stevenson, R. D. (1988) Lyme disease with acute purulent meningitis. *Br. Med. J.*, **297**, 460–1.

Brockner, E.-B., Echternacht-Happle, K., Hamm, H. and Happle, R. (1987) Abnormal expression of class I and class II major histocompatibility antigens in alopecia areata: modulation by topical immunotherapy. *J. Am. Acad. Dermatol.*, **88**, 564–8.

Bulpitt, K. J. and Brahn, E. (1989) Systemic lupus erythematosus and concurrent cytomegalovirus vasculitis: diagnosis by antemortem skin biopsy. *J. Rheumatol.*, **16**, 677–80.

Caughman, W., Stern, R. and Haynes, H. (1989) Neutrophilic dermatosis of myeloproliferative disorders. *Am. J. Dermatopathol.*, **11**, 99–111.

Clark, W. H., Reed, R. J. and Mihm, M. C. (1973) Lupus erythematosus. Histopathology of cutaneous lesions. *Hum. Pathol.*, **4**, 157–63.

Cleary, M. L. and Sklar, J. (1989) Clonal rearrangements of immunoglobulin genes and progression to B cell lymphoma in cutaneous lymphoid hyperplasia. *Am. J. Pathol.*, **135**, 13–19.

Cohen, P. R. and Kuzrock, R. (1987) Sweet's syndrome and malignancy. *Am. J. Med.*, **82**, 1220–6.

Cooper, P. H., Innes, D. J. and Greer, K. E. (1983) Acute febrile neutrophilic dermatosis (Sweet's syndrome) and myeloproliferative disorders. *Cancer*, **51**, 1518–26.

Dereure, O., Guillot, B., Bareon, G., Zabarino, P. and Guilhou, J. J. (1988) [Acute febrile neutrophilic dermatosis and malignant hematologic diseases: report of a new bullous case and review of the literature]. *Ann. Dermatol. Venereol.*, **115**, 689–701.

Dumler, J. S., Beschorner, W. E., Farmer, E. R., Di Gennaro, K. A., Saral, R. and Santos, G. W. (1989) Endothelial-cell injury in cutaneous acute graft-versus-host disease. *Am. J. Med.*, **135**, 1097–103.

Editorial (1989) Diagnosis of Lyme disease. *Lancet*, **ii**, 198–9.

Furukawa, Y., Inoue, T., Yamane, T., Hiyoshi, M., Sasaki, A., Kishida, T., Kojima, K., Im, T. and Tatsumi, N. (1989) [Sweet's syndrome associated with myelodysplastic syndrome]. *Rinsho Ketsueki*, **30**, 764–7.

Gibbons, R. D., Fiedler-Weiss, V. C., West, D. P. and Lapin, G. (1986) Quantification of scalp hair – a computer-aided methodology. *J. Am. Acad. Dermatol.*, **86**, 78–82.

Gunawardena, D. A., Gunawardena, K. A., Ratnayaka, R. M. R. S. and Vasanthanathan, N. S. (1975) The clinical spectrum of Sweet's syndrome (acute febrileneutrophilic dermatosis) – a report of eighteen cases. *Br. J. Dermatol.*, **92**, 363–73.

Guy, E. C., Bateman, D. E., Martyn, C. N., Heckels, J. E. and Lawton, N. F. (1989) Lyme disease: prevalence and clinical importance of *Borrelia burgdorferi* specific IgG in forestry workers. *Lancet*, **i**, 484–6.

Hasegawa, Y., Tomiyama, J., Ninomiya, H. and Abe, T. [Appearance of Sweet's syndrome in a patient with myelodysplastic syndrome (MDS) without relation to the hematological findings of MDS]. *Rinsho Ketsueki*, **30**, 863–7.

Haxthausen, H. (1919) *Hudsygdomme Freankaldt af Lyset.* Copenhagen: Pios Boghandel, 109–61.

Headington, J. T. (1984) Transverse microscopic anatomy of the scalp. A basis for a morphometric approach to disorders of the hair follicle. *Arch. Dermatol.*, **120**, 449–56.

Herzberg, A. J., Dinehart, S. M., Kerns, B. J. and Pollack, S. V. (1990) Acne keloidalis. Transverse microscopy, immunohistochemistry and electron microscopy. *Am. J. Dermatopathol.*, **12**, 109–21.

Holt, P. J. A. and Davies, M. G. (1977) Erythema gyratum repens – an immunologically mediated dermatosis? *Br. J. Dermatol.*, **96**, 343–7.

Horn, T. D., Redd, J. V., Karp, J. E., Beschorner, W. E., Burke, P. J. and Hood, A. F. (1989) Cutaneous eruptions of lymphocyte recovery. *Arch. Dermatol.*, **125**, 1512–17.

Hood, A. F. and Farmer, E. R. (1985) Histopathology of cutaneous lupus erythematosus. *Clin. Dermatol.*, **3**, 36–48.

Howland, W. W., Golitz, L. E., Weston, W. L. and Huff, J. C. (1984) Erythema multiforme: clinical, histopathologic, and immunologic study. *J. Am. Acad. Dermatol.*, **10**, 438–46.

Hulinska, D., Jirous, J., Valesova, M. and Herzogova, J. (1989) Ultrastructure of Borrelia burgdorferi in tissues of patients with Lyme disease. *J. Basic Microbiol*, **29**, 73–83.

Hymes, S. R., Farmer, E. R., Lewis, P. G., Tutschka, P. J. and Santos, G. W. (1985) Cutaneous graft-versus-host reaction: prognostic features seen by light microscopy. *J. Am. Acad. Dermatol.*, **12**, 468–74.

Ingber, A. and Sandbank, M. (1986) Erythema figuratum versus erythema gyratum repens. *J. Am. Acad. Dermatol.*, **15**, 111–12.

Jacyk, W. K. (1988) Pustular ulcerative dermatosis of the scalp. *Br. J. Dermatol.*, **118**, 441–4.

Jessner, M. and Kanof, N. B. (1953) Lymphocytic infiltration of the skin. *Arch. Dermatol.*, **68**, 447–9.

Jordaan, H. F. (1989) Acute febrile neutrophilic dermatosis. A histological study of 37 patients and a review of the literature. *Am. J. Dermatopathol.*, **11**, 99–111.

Kaplan, A. P., Buckley, R. H. and Mathews, K. P. (1987) Allergic skin disorders. *JAM*, **258**, 2900–9.

Kaufman, L. D., Gruber, B. L., Phillips, M. E. and Benach, J. L. (1989) Late cutaneous Lyme disease: acrodermatitis chronica atrophicans. *Am. J. Med.*, **86**, 828–30.

Kemmett, D., Gawkrodger, D. J., Wilson, G. and Hunter, J. A. A. (1988) Sweet's syndrome in Crohn's disease. *Br. Med. J.*, **297**, 1513–14.

Khoury, E. L., Price, V. H. and Greenspan, J. S. (1988) HLA-DR expression by hair follicle keratinocytes in alopecia areata: evidence that it is secondary to the lymphoid infiltration. *J. Am. Acad. Dermatol.*, **90**, 193–200.

Konttinen, Y. T., Reitamo, S., Ranki, A. and Segerberg-Konttinen, M. (1981) T-lymphocytes and mononuclear phagocytes in the skin infiltrate of systemic and discoid lupus erythematosus and Jessner's lyphocytic infiltrate. *Br. J. Dermatol.*, **104**, 141–5.

Konttinen, Y. T., Bergroth, V., Johansson, E., Nordstrom, D. and Mahnstrom, M. (1987) A long-term clinicopathologic survey of patients with Jessner's lymphocytic infiltration of the skin. *J. Invest. Dermatol.*, **89**, 205–8.

Kramer, N., Rickert, R. R., Brodkin, R. H. and Rosenstein, E. D. Septal panniculitis as a manifestation of Lyme disease. *Am. J. Med.*, **81**, 149–52.

Langlois, J. C., Shaw, J. M. and Odland, G. F. (1985) Erythema gyratum repens unassociated with internal malignancy. *J. Am. Acad. Dermatol.*, **12**, 911–13.

Lampert, I. A., Janossy, G., Suitters, A. J., Bofill, M., Palmer, S., Gordon-Smith, E., Prentice, H. G. and Thomas, J. A. (1982) Immunological analysis of the skin in graft versus host disease. *Clin. Exp. Immunol.*, **50**, 123–31.

Lennert, K. and Parwaresch, R. (1979) Mast cells and mast cell neoplasia. *Histopathology*, **3**, 349–65.

Levine, L. E., Morgan, N. E., Fretzin, D. and Rubenstein, D. (1985) Erythema gyratum repens. *Arch. Dermatol.*, **121**, 170–1.

Lever, R., Turbitt, M., Mackie, R., Hann, I., Gibson, B., Burnett, A. and Willoughby, M. (1986) A prospective study of the histological changes in the skin in patients receiving bone marrow transplants. *Br. J. Dermatol.*, **114**, 161–70.

Logan, R. A. and Headington, J. T. (1988) Follicular mucinosis (alopecia mucinosa): a histologic study of 80 cases (abstr). *J. Cutan. Pathol.*, **15**, 324.

Macallan, D. C., Hughes, C. A. and Bradlow, A. (1987) Lyme arthritis in southern England. *Br. Med. J.*, **294**, 1062–3.

Messenger, A. G., Slater, D. N. and Bleehen, S. S. (1986) Alopecia areata: alterations in the hair growth cycle and correlation with follicular pathology. *Br. J. Dermatol.*, **114**, 337–47.

Monheit, G. D., Murad, T. and Conrad, M. (1979) Systemic mastocytosis and the mastocytosis syndrome. *J. Cut. Pathol.*, **6**, 42–52.

Muhlemann, M. F. (1984) Thirteen cases of erythema chronicum migrans in Britain. *Br. J. Dermatol.*, **111**, 335–9.

Murphy, G. M. and Griffiths, W. A. (1989) Subcorneal pustular dermatosis. *Clin. Exp. Dermatol.*, **14**, 165–7.

Norris, P. G., Morris, J., McGibbon, D. M., Chu, A. C. and Hawk, J. L. M.

(1989) Polymorphic light eruption: an immunopathological study of evolving lesions. *Br. J. Dermatol.*, **120**, 173–83.

Olsen, T. G., Milroy, S. K. and Jones-Olsen, S. (1984) Erythema gyratum repens with associated squamous cell carcinoma of the lung. *Cutis*, **34**, 351–5.

Parke, A. (1987) From New to old England: the progress of Lyme disease. *Br. Med. J.*, **294**, 525–6.

Pye, R. J. (1979) Erosive pustular dermatosis of the scalp. *Br. J. Dermatol.*, **100**, 559–66.

Roger, H., Thevenet, J. P., Souteyrand, P. and Sauvezie, B. (1990) Subcorneal pustular dermatosis associated with rheumatoid arthritis and raised IgA: simultaneous remission of skin and joint involvements with dapsone treatment. *Ann. Rheum. Dis.*, **49**, 190–1.

Shelley, W. B. and Hurley, H. J. (1960) An unusual autoimmune syndrome. Erythema annulare centrifugum, generalized pigmentation and breast hypertrophy. *Arch. Dermatol.*, **81**, 889–97.

Skolnick, M. and Mainman, E. R. (1975) Erythema gyratum repens with metastatic adenocarcinoma. *Arch. Dermatol.*, **111**, 227–9.

Sloane, J. P., Thomas, J. A., Imrie, S. F., Easton, D. F. and Powles, R. L. (1984) Morphological and immunohistochemical changes in the skin in allogeneic bone marrow recipients. *J. Clin. Pathol.*, **37**, 919–30.

Smolle, J., Torne, R., Soyer, H. P. and Kerl, H. (1990) Immunohistochemical classification of cutaneous pseudolymphomas: delineation of distinct patterns. *J. Cutan. Pathol.*, **17**, 149–59.

Soeprono, F. F. (1986) Histologic criteria for the diagnosis of pityriasis rubra pilaris. *J. Am. Acad. Dermatol.*, **8**, 277–83.

Spallone, A. (1987) Incontinentia pigmenti: pigmentary changesindependent of incontinence. *J. Cutan. Pathol.*, **14**, 248–50.

Storer, J. S., Nesbitt, L. T., Galen, W. K. and DeLeo, V. A. (1983) Sweet's syndrome. *Int. J. Dermatol.*, **22**, 8–12.

Su, W. P. D. and Lui, H. H. H. (1986) Diagnostic criteria for Sweet's syndrome. *Cutis*, **37**, 167–74.

Sweet, R. D. (1964) An acute neutrophilic dermatosis. *Br. J. Dermatol.*, **76**, 349–56.

Toonstra, J., Wildschut, A., Boer, J., Smeenk, G., Willemze, R., van der Putte, S. C. J., Boonstra, H. and van Vloten, W. A. (1989) Jessner's lymphocytic infiltration of the skin. A clinical study of 100 patients. *Arch. Dermatol.*, **125**, 1525–30.

White, J. W. (1985) Gyrate erythema. *Dermatologic Clinics*, **3**, 129–39.

Willemze, R., Vermeer, B. J. and Meijer, C. J. L. M. (1984) Immunohistochemical studies of the skin (Jessner) and discoid lupus erythematosus. *J. Am. Acad. Dermatol.*, **11**, 832–40.

Willemze, R. and Scheffer, E. (1985) Clinical and histologic differentiation between lymphomatoid papulosis and pityriasis lichenoides. *J. Am. Acad. Dermatol.*, **13**, 418–28.

Williams, D., Rolles, C. J. and White, J. E. (1986) Lyme disease in a Hampshire child – medical curiosity or beginning of an epidemic? *Br. Med. J.*, **292**, 1560–1.

Winklemann, R. K. (1985) Cholinergic urticaria shows neutrophilic inflammation. *Acta. Derm. Venereol.* (Stockh.), **65**, 432–4.

Wojnarowska, F., Bhogal, B. and Black, M. M. (1986) The significance of an IgM band at the dermo-epidermal junction. *J. Cutan. Pathol.*, **13**, 359–62.

Wood, G. S., Ngan, B. Y., Tung, R., Hoffman, T. E., Abel, E. A., Hoppe, R. T., Warnke, R. A., Cleary, M. L. and Sklar, J. (1989) Clonal rearrangements of immunoglobulin genes and progression to B cell lymphoma in cutaneous lymphoid hyperplasia. *Am. J. Pathol.*, **135**, 13–19.

11 Cutaneous lymphoma and other malignant lymphoid infiltrates

For many years there was only one kind of skin lymphoma, generically known as mycosis fungoides, with a variant in which blood involvement could be shown: the Sezary syndrome. In the late 1970s we started to be able to label T-cells and their subsets in skin biopsies, and it was shown that this was a disease in which OKT4 positive cells predominated (Kung *et al.*, 1981). At this time, the generic title was changed to 'cutaneous T-cell lymphoma', which was defined as a neoplastic disorder of functional helper/inducer T-cells that show a marked affinity for the epidermis (Edelson, 1980). Cytogenetic studies helped to establish the concept that the tumours arose from a single clone of malignant T-cell, even when present at multiple sites (Edelson *et al.*, 1979). The disease has come to be regarded as one more kind of non-Hodgkin lymphoma, which must be staged and treated in a similar way to lymphomas presenting at other sites in the body (Hamminga *et al.*, 1982; Lamberg *et al.*, 1984).

In the past decade we have developed a wider view of the phenotypic features which unify and at the same time subdivide the various kinds of skin lymphoma (Picker *et al.*, 1987; Slater, 1987). We now know that there are also primary B-cell lymphomas in the skin and that there are some rather indolent conditions which resemble lymphoma when seen in biopsies.

The arrival of the techniques of molecular biology has given some prospect of resolving thorny problems by offering a way of identifying T-cell clonality, by showing rearrangements of the beta chain of the T-cell receptor gene, on the basis that monoclonal proliferations are most likely to be malignant (Berger *et al.*, 1988; Bignon *et al.*, 1989). Thus cases of lymphomatoid papulosis were shown to be monoclonal (Weiss *et al.*, 1986), although so were cases of pityriasis lichenoides et varioliformis acuta (Weiss *et al.*, 1987). It is likely that cutaneous T-cell lymphomas arise from a specialized subpopulation of CD4 positive T-cells. There is an excess of tumours which react with monoclonal antibodies to the Vbeta8 family of beta chain variable region genes of the T-cell antigen receptor. This population may be selected by antigen or viruses (Jack *et al.*, 1990). The possibility of an underlying viral factor in pathogenesis has also been postulated as a common factor in the development of lymphomatoid papulosis, mycosis fungoides and some types of Hodgkin's disease (Kadin, 1985).

These various techniques have also seen the demise of the pseudolymphoma, a condition which, to paraphrase the old adage, is a pseudocondition which causes pseudodeaths in pseudopatients. We now have the tools to decide in the majority of cases whether we are dealing with a lymphoma or a reactive process. Indeed, T-cell receptor beta chain gene rearrangement studies have been used to discriminate between nine patients who had reactive lymphoid proliferations and a germ line configuration of the gene, and one patient who showed a clonal rearrangement 1 year before a cutaneous T-cell lymphoma became clinically evident (Griesser *et al.*, 1990). Let us hope to see as little as possible of the pseudolymphoma in the future.

What follows is a brief account of the spread of conditions which can occur. As with lymphoma at any site, the important thing as far as treatment and prognosis is concerned is to make a clear biopsy diagnosis in the knowledge of the clinical picture, and to review or revise the diagnosis in light of further clinical or staging information, the lymphoma being treated on the basis of tumour type, grade and clinical stage. As the clinicopathological features of cutaneous lymphomas are diverse, they should be classified and studied in a similar way to their nodal counterparts (van Vloten and Willemze, 1985; Mukai *et al.*, 1988).

11.1   Cutaneous T-cell lymphoma (CTCL)

Of the many botanical names used in the traditional nomenclature of dermatology, mycosis fungoides is perhaps the most colourful. The search for Alibert's fungating mushrooms is not, however, of much use in the interpretation of biopsies from patients with a possible diagnosis of lymphoma. The precursor lesions of mycosis fungoides and their evolution into overt disease are a constant source of interest and debate. It is at the earliest stage of the development of the disease that treatment is likely to be most effective, but diagnosis is most difficult (Sterry, 1985).

Immunophenotyping clearly has its limitations in the diagnosis of cutaneous lymphoma, as it is not possible to easily establish the presence or absence of a monoclonal population in tissue sections (Slater, 1990). A reasonable panel would include antibodies to CD1, CD3, CD4,

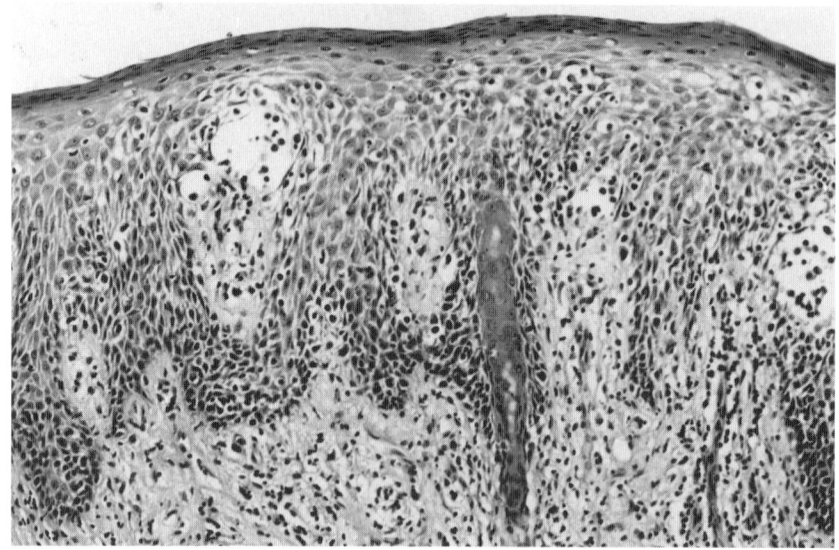

Figure 11.1   Cutaneous T-cell lymphoma showing epidermotrophism of tumour lymphocytes.

CD8 and Ki-67, with the possible addition of CD15 and CD30 when considering the possibility of lymphomatoid papulosis. Large cell lymphomas of CD30 positive T-cell type have a better prognosis than Cd30 negative cases (Beljaards *et al.*, 1989).

The erythematous stage is characterized by a diffuse interstitial infiltration of the papillary dermis by lymphocytes, which are predominantly CD4 positive. They extend into the epidermis where they form small aggregates in association with CD1 positive Langerhans cells. The presence of Langerhans cells in the epidermis in densities of less than $90/mm^2$ is an adverse prognostic feature (Meissner *et al.*, 1990).

At the earliest stage, the epidermal basal cells will show vacuolar degeneration. As the number of T-cells in the epidermis increases, the epidermis will show a variable degree of hyperplasia, which led to the now little-used description of parapsoriasis. If you are lucky you may see some well-defined Pautrier's microabsesses in the epidermis, where a cluster of T-cells and Langerhans cells lie in a loose vesicular space (Everett, 1985). The CD8 positive cells which are present tend to cluster around the dermal blood vessels. In many biopsies, however, it is impossible to be certain whether one is looking at a biopsy of eczema or of early lymphoma (Sanchez and Ackerman, 1979). In these circum-

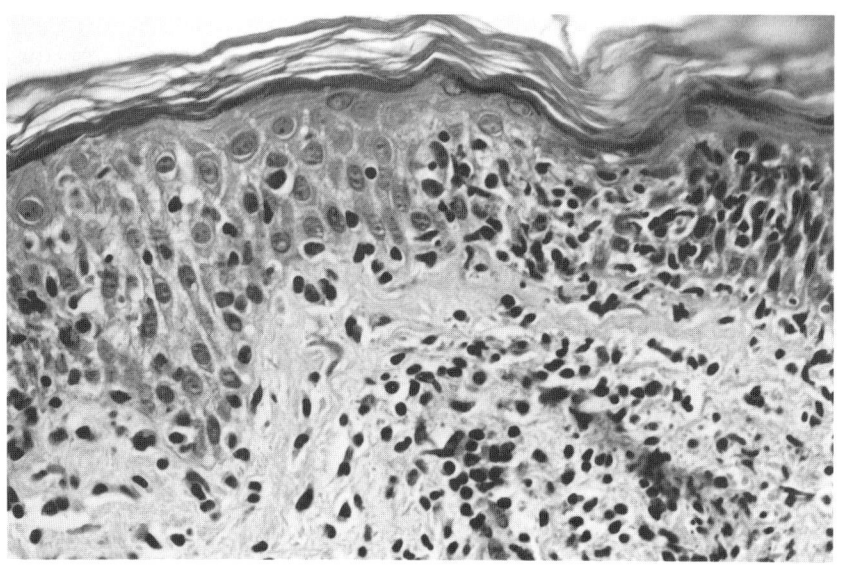

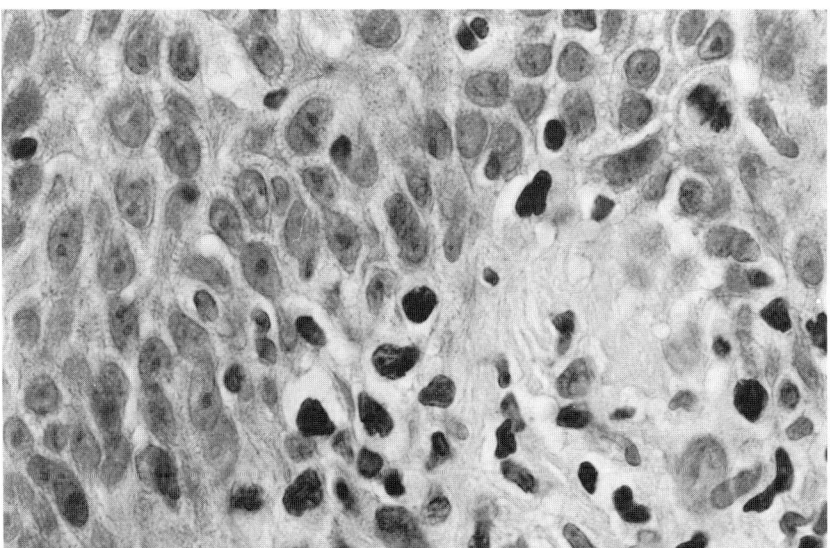

Figure 11.2 Cutaneous T-cell lymphoma (a and b). Epidermal invasion by atypical lymphocytes.

stances, the biopsy acts as a baseline for comparison with later ones.

Plaque parapsoriasis is the next stage in the spectrum. This area has been confused in the past by descriptors such as guttate, lichenoid or retiform parapsoriasis: terms which could be usefully eliminated (Samman, 1972). The biopsy from this sort of lesion must be distinguished from psoriasis rather than eczema. Features in favour of lymphoma are the presence of epidermotropism by single cells or groups of cells, the presence of hyperconvoluted, hyperchromatic cerebriform cells and the presence of irregular epidermal hyperplasia rather than the regular hyperplasia seen in psoriasis.

The problem of differential diagnosis remains. For instance, in one series 30% of patients with large plaque parapsoriasis eventually developed frank cutaneous lymphoma. On average, it took four biopsies and 22 months to arrive at the diagnosis, showing that large plaque parapsoriasis is an important precursor of mycosis fungoides and could, indeed, be better called premycosis fungoides (Lazar *et al.*, 1989). On the other hand, the other 70% had benign reactive epidermal hyperplasias which did not progress to lymphoma.

At a later stage, when tumour nodules start to develop, this epidermotropism is a less prominent feature and may even be absent. Immunohistochemical staining of frozen sections from these biopsies is of some help in diagnosis. As well as the CD4 predominance, there is also a variable expression of the Ki-67 nuclear proliferation antigen on the tumour lymphocytes, in keeping with the low grade nature of the process. This Ki-67 immunoreactivity seems to be mainly restricted to the intraepidermal component of the T-cell infiltrate, the dermal cells not apparently being in the cell cycle (Nickoloff and Griffiths, 1990).

Much has been written about the large atypical cells with hyperconvoluted, cerebriform nuclei which are said to characterize mycosis fungoides and distinguish it from its benign differential diagnoses. However, it has been the author's experience that these are rarely seen in routine sections of biopsies, except in the more advanced cases.

It may be possible to differentiate benign from malignant with the help of electron microscopy and measurement of the nuclear contour index. This approach may also be of help in identifying hyperconvoluted lymphocyte nuclei in lymph node biopsies, when trying to see whether the changes present are merely reactive dermatopathic lymphadenopathy or represent involvement of regional nodes by the lymphoma.

Typical cases of small cell CTCL can transform to a large cell variant which corresponds to a change from a low- to high-grade disease, more aggressive behaviour and poorer survival. When the clinical stage also advances, with the development of extracutaneous involvement, the prognosis will be poorer than with cutaneous transformation alone.

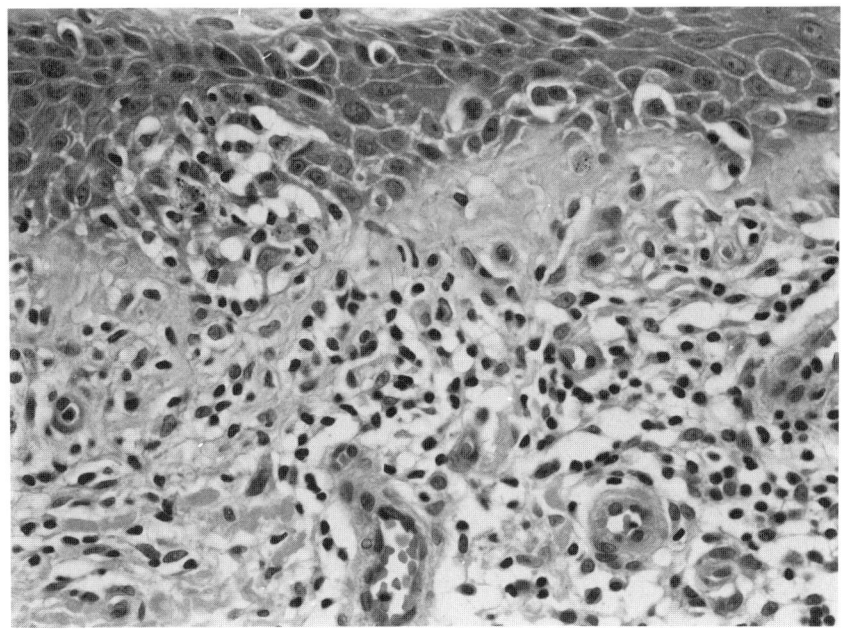

Figure 11.3 Cutaneous T-cell lymphoma with Pautrier's microabcesses within the epidermis.

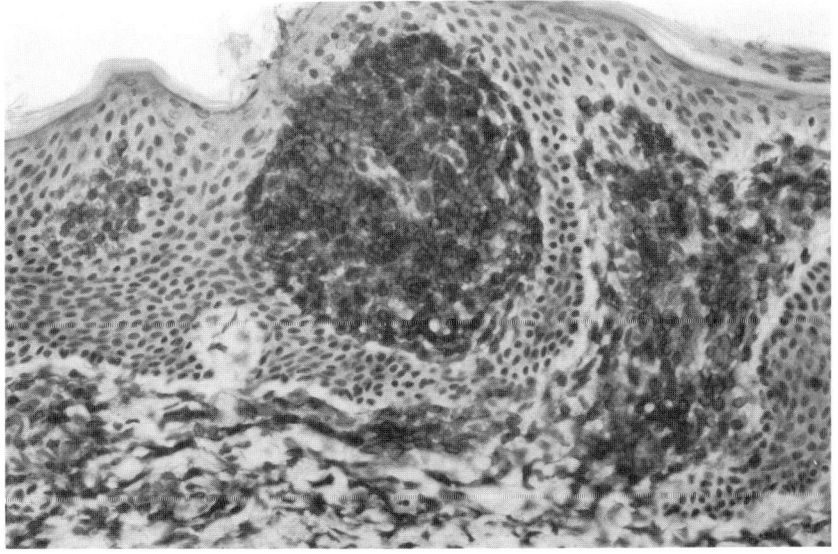

Figure 11.4 Cutaneous T-cell lymphoma. A frozen section showing pan-T-cell CD3 immunoreactivity (immunoperoxidase).

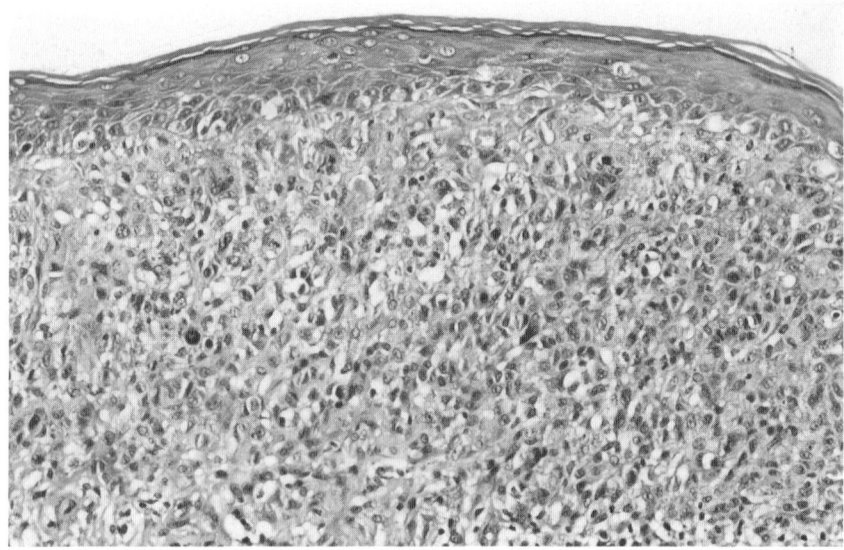

Figure 11.5   Cutaneous T-cell lymphoma. Tumour stage with reduced epidermotrophism.

The T-cell phenotype should be maintained, but some antigens may be lost and new ones expressed (Salhany *et al.*, 1988; Horiuchi *et al.*, 1988).

11.2   Angiocentric lymphoma

A further variant of cutaneous T-cell lymphoma is one in which the infiltrate is not epidermotropic but, instead, is centered around vessels in mid and deep dermis and subcutis. There has been a certain degree of reticence in abandoning the term 'lymphomatoid granulomatosis' in the face of overwhelming evidence that this condition is a lymphoma and not a form of vasculitis, that is, lymphomatoid granulomatosis and angiocentric lymphoma are one and the same (Nichols *et al.*, 1982; Wood *et al.*, 1984; Chan and Ng, 1989). For instance, an overlap between angiocentric lymphoma and so-called lymphomatoid granulomatosis of the skin has been described (Kessler *et al.*, 1981), as well as an apparent transformation from a necrotizing granulomatous vasculitis to overt lymphoma (Foley, 1987). Pulmonary involvment may occur (Bluefarb and Steinberg, 1952). Lung biopsies taken from patients with this condition were interpreted in the past as showing a necrotizing angiitis (Liebow *et al.*, 1972). The angiocentric lymphoma of the lung is an indistinguishable disease as far as the vascular lesions are concerned (Addis *et al.*, 1988).

The patients are middle-aged and have nodular lesions, some of which may be painful, and usually involve more than one part of the body and often include extracutaneous sites. The skin is involved in 20–60% of cases and skin lesions may be the first to develop. The nodules may develop and spread into annular lesions, with the central area of skin returning to a normal appearance without scarring (Bender et al., 1978), whilst nodules on the legs may ulcerate (Minars *et al.*, 1975). The lesions may resemble sarcoidosis clinically, but the presence of a polymorphic, angiocentric and angiodestructive infiltrate with atypical lymphocytes should differentiate this condition from this and other differential diagnoses, such as lupus erythematosus or figurate erythema.

Tumour cells have a T-cell phenotype and are of variable size, but 'cerebriform cells' are uncommon. The cells infiltrate the walls of vessels within the lesions, sometimes with associated coagulative necrosis – angioinvasive and angiodestructive.

The disease may well be refractory to therapy, and has much in common with nasal and nasopharyngeal T-cell lymphomas: the so-called 'lethal midline granuloma' (Chan *et al.*, 1988). As such, early diagnosis and treatment offers the best hope for the patient (Fauci *et al.*, 1982; Brolell *et al.*, 1986).

11.3 Lymphomatoid papulosis

In 1968, Macauley described a condition which is characterized by transient, self-healing papulonodular eruptions. The process is of clinical importance because of the possibility that it may develop from an apparently benign, reactive granulomatous dermatitis and progress to overt malignancy (Bender, 1978; Espinoza *et al.*, 1985). Clinically, the lesions are more common in men and develop as papules 1–2 cm in diameter, usually on the extremities. They may occur in crops over a prolonged course of many years before transforming to lymphoma (Braun-Falco *et al.*, 1983).

The biopsy shows a superficial and deep dermal infiltrate in which there are variable numbers of large atypical cells. The appearances vary from case to case. Willemze *et al.* (1982, 1983a) defined two types (A and B), which do not represent different entities but rather different ends of the same spectrum. The type A lesion has a mixed dermal infiltrate with variable numbers of large atypical cells. The degree of infiltration corresponds to the age of the lesion with sparse perivascular infiltration in early lesions and a dense, wedge-shaped infiltrate in fully developed lesions. The atypical cells have polymorphic nuclei with prominent nucleoli and abundant cytoplasm. Cells resembling

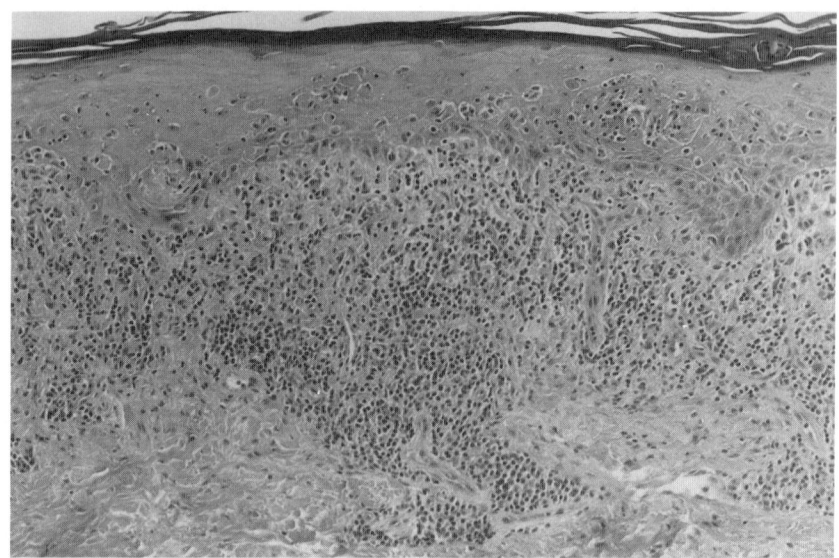

(a)

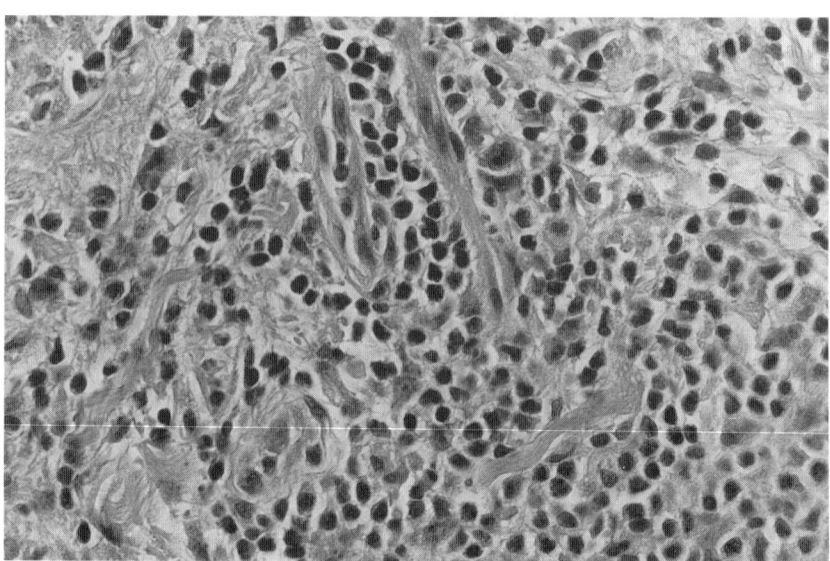

(b)

Figure 11.6 Lymphomatoid papulosis. (a) Infiltration of dermis and epidermis with associated keratinocyte necrosis, and (b) large, atypical cells in dermal infiltrate.

Reed-Sternberg cells are not uncommon, and the whole picture may resemble Hodgkin's disease. Papules and nodules of Type A lymphomatoid papulosis usually involute spontaneously in 3–8 weeks. The type B form of the disease shows a predominance of small, medium-sized and large mononuclear cells with cerebriform nuclei infiltrating around dermal vessels and in the basal and parabasal epidermis. In contrast to the type A form of the disease, these lesions to not appear to show a relationship between the histological pattern and the age of the lesion. Transitional appearances between type A and type B may be seen. Predominant involvement of hair follicles has also been reported (Requena et al., 1990).

Immunohistochemistry shows that the large atypical cells have the phenotype of activated T-cells in that they are Ki-1 (CD30) positive and they also mark for CD3, CD4, HLA-DR and IL-2 receptor (CD25) (Ralfkaeir et al., 1985; Kaudewitz et al., 1986). T-cell receptor gene rearrangement studies have also show evidence of clonality in these lesions (Kadin et al., 1987).

The main problem is one of differential diagnosis. The type A lesion has features resembling Hodgkin's disease and probably accounts for occasional descriptions of primary cutaneous Hodgkin's disease in the past (Brehmer-Andersson, 1976). There are occasional reports of Hodgkin's disease developing in patients with lymphomatoid papulosis (Dowd et al., 1981; Scheen et al., 1981; Willemze et al., 1983a). There may also be confusion with mycosis fungoides. Indeed, lymphomatoid papulosis can develop in patients with established mycosis fungoides, and up to 10% of patients with lymphomatoid papulosis may subsequently develop a non-Hodgkin's lymphoma (Weinman and Ackerman, 1981). Diagnosis must depend on a combination of a clinical picture of self-healing papulonecrotic eruptions usually on the trunk, but also possibly on the limbs, head and neck, together with a biopsy containing atypical Ki-1 or Ber-H2 positive cells. In the differential diagnosis from pityriasis lichenoides et varioliformis acuta, cases of lymphomatoid papulosis show CD30 positive cells, whilst pityriasis biopsies show diffuse epidermal cytoplasmic staining for HLA-DR and a predominance of CD8 positive cells in the infiltrate at the dermo-epidermal junction (Varga et al., 1990). At present, treatment is unsatisfactory and a long follow-up is needed to detect the possible onset of lymphoma – in a minority of patients after an interval of up to 25 years.

A related case described as 'follicular lymphoid hyperplasia of skin with high content of activated T-helper cells', showed a heterogeneous dermal infiltrate with large atypical cells in and around the dermal follicles which were CD30, CD25, CD2, CD3 and CD4 positive. Some cells were also CD15 positive. The lesion regressed spontaneously

(Bournerias *et al.*, 1989). A similar case of a localized, cutaneous, large cell lymphoma with a Ki-1-positive 'aberrant' T-helper/inducer pheno-type and a demonstrated clonal rearrangement of the T-cell receptor gene also behaved in an indolent fashion despite the high grade appearance seen in the biopsy (Lindholm *et al.*, 1989). Cases such as these probably account for occasional reports of primary cutaneous Hodgkin's disease in the older literature; such cases were also associated with a good prognosis (Banerjee *et al.*, 1991).

11.4   Regressing atypical histiocytosis

This condition is one of those which is more worrying to the patho-logist than the patient (Headington, 1987a). The patients have nodular lesions which ulcerate, regress spontaneously, recur without systemic involvement and generally behave in an indolent fashion. Biopsies show atypical histiocytes, mononuclear or multinuclear, with malignant cytological appearances, many mitoses, and with associated epidermal hyperplasia (Flynn *et al.*, 1982). T-cell receptor gene rearrangement studies suggest that this is, in fact, a form of T-cell lymphoma (Head-ington *et al.*, 1987b). A more acute and widespread case has been reported (Horiguchi *et al.*, 1989). A T-cell, signet-ring cell proliferation, with a histiocytic morphology, but with a benign, self-healing course, is also recorded (van der Putte *et al.*, 1987).

11.5   Woringer-Kolopp disease

This is a rare condition originally described in a case report of a 13-year-old boy, with solitary verrucous lesions on the distal parts of the limbs, which were interesting because although the patient's disease had a benign course, the appearance of the biopsy was more worrying (Woringer and Kolopp, 1939). The lesions show a predominantly epidermal infiltrate of T-lymphocytes, which have the ultrastructural characteristics of Sezary cells, suggesting that this is an epidermotrophic variant of mycosis fungoides (Braun-Falco *et al.*, 1973; Degreef *et al.*, 1976; Natarajan and Wilson, 1985). These cells lie close to Langerhans cells in the epidermis (Geerts *et al.*, 1982). There has been some debate about their phenotype. Most reported cases are CD4 positive but CD8 positive cases have been described, suggesting either two subtypes of disease or, possibly, some functional difference from mycosis fungoides (Deneau *et al.*, 1984; Mackie and Turbitt, 1984).

In differentiating it from mycosis fungoides, one should bear in mind that the lesions are mostly limited to the distal limbs, and are character-ized by hyperkeratosis with spotty parakeratosis, without hypergranulosis. The epidermis may show irregular acanthosis alternating with focal epidermal atrophy. The Pagetoid infiltrate of T cells is limited to the lower third of the epidermis, especially at the tips of rete ridges (Braun-Falco et al., 1973; Mandojana and Helwig, 1983).

The condition is best regarded as a rather benign variant of mycosis fungoides. The intraepidermal T-cells show evidence of proliferation and of loss of pan-T-cell antigens and of monoclonality (Mielke et al., 1989). The lesions are extremely radio-sensitive and have also been treated by surgical excision (Mandojana and Helwig, 1983), but follow-up is recommended because the process can progress to overt lymphoma (Lacour et al., 1986).

11.6   Histiocytosis X

The conditions eosinophilic granuloma, Hand-Schüller-Christian disease and Letterer-Siwe disease form a spectrum collectively known as histiocytosis X. They are characterized by a dermal infiltrate of cells which share features of epidermal Langerhans cells: they are positive for CD1 (T6), S100 protein and HLA-DR, and contain cytoplasmic Birbeck granules (Murphy et al., 1981; Birbeck et al., 1961). The tumour cells also may react with antibodies to interferon gamma: a reaction not seen with normal Langerhans cells (Neumann et al., 1988). The skin lesions usually take the form of papules in which there is quite extensive infiltration with tumour cells which have pale, medium-sized nuclei, often with longitudinal grooves. Eosinophils are interspersed within the infiltrate.

Related to this are the so-called 'non-X histiocytoses', which include rare lesions that appear to be derived from interdigitating reticulum cells rather than Langerhans cells (Miracco et al., 1988; Hui et al., 1987). These present as multiple papular tumours on the face, limbs and upper trunk. The tumour cells have irregularly folded nuclei, an immunophenotype which is identical to that of Langerhans or interdigitating reticulum cells, but Birbeck granules are absent. The lesions do not appear to have an aggressive clinical course.

11.7   Cutaneous B-cell lymphoma

Whilst the majority of primary cutaneous lymphomas are of T-cell type, immunohistochemical staining allows the small group of B-cell skin lymphomas to be identified (Faure et al., 1990). One group of B-cell tumours has been well characterized. Called primary cutaneous large cell lymphomas of follicular centre cell origin, the tumours usually have a long history of a slowly progressive localized nodule on the trunk, scalp or lower legs. They are raised up and the larger ones may be umbilicated. The process may extend into surrounding skin producing a plaque (Willemze, 1987a, b).

The biopsy shows a diffuse, large cell lymphoma filling the dermis, but without involving the epidermis. The tumour cells are of both cleaved and non-cleaved type and express monotypic surface immunoglobulin and HLA-DR and B-cell antigens. The tumours have a favourable prognosis; the majority are localized to the primary site and respond to local radiotherapy.

Occasional, high-grade primary B-cell lymphomas of the skin may also occur, and tend to behave aggressively, with the development of extracutaneous involvement (Prost *et al.*, 1987).

11.8 Secondary cutaneous involvement by follicular lymphoma

The skin can become secondarily involved by a systemic B-cell lymphoma. This can take a variety of forms, ranging from a band of dermal infiltration, mimicking T-cell lymphoma, through a nodular type with the formation of tumour nodules, to a deeper diffuse or infiltrating pattern.

The onset of cutaneous involvement may be either in keeping with a

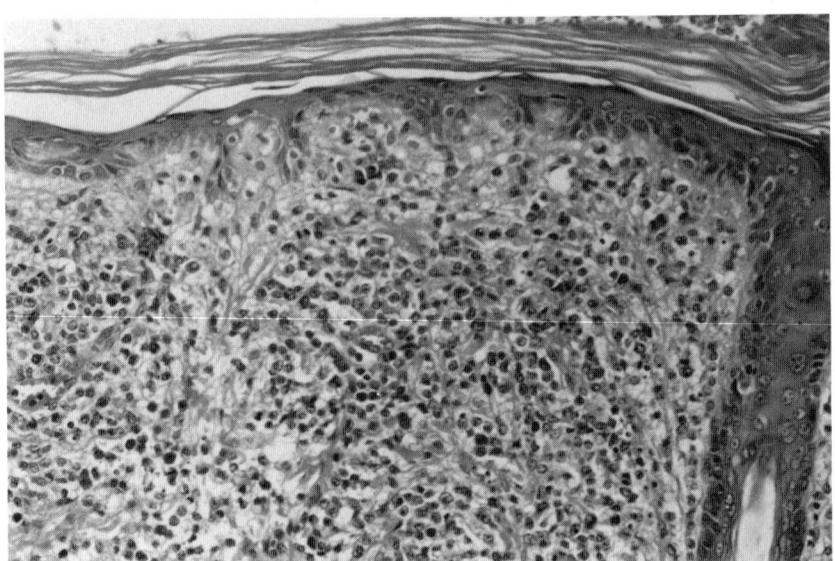

Figure 11.7 Cutaneous B-cell lymphoma (a, b and c). Dermis filled with tumour cells, without substantial epidermotrophism.

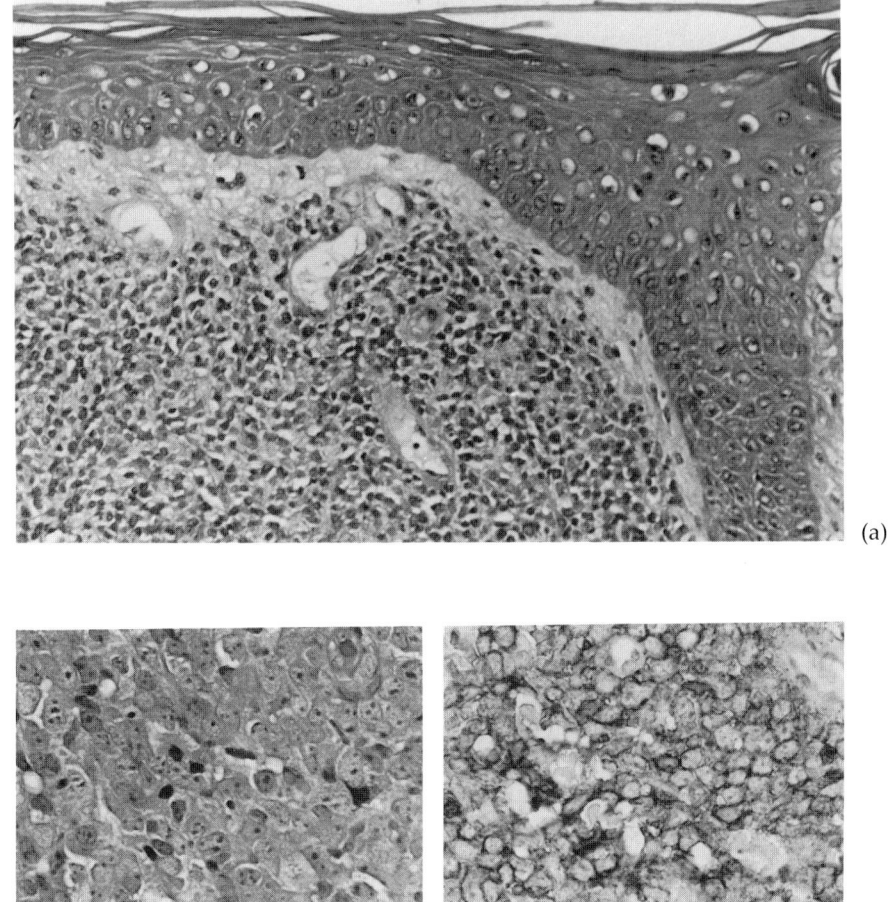

Figure 11.8   Cutaneous B-cell lymphoma (a) Tumour in dermis, (b) high-grade appearance of tumour cell nuclei, and (c) positive membrane staining with pan-B cell CD20 marker L26 (immunoperoxidase).

high-grade primary nodal lyphoma, or may indicate transformation of the disease from low to high grade. This is more likely to be the case if some time has passed from the original diagnosis and treatment of low-grade disease. Patients with transformed tumours have a poorer prognosis, with only a 60% 5-year survival compared to 100% for low-grade disease.

Tumour nodules can be distinguished from reactive follicles by the same features used in diagnosis of the primary disease. The follicle centre will not show subdivision into centroblastic and centrocytic compartments, tingible body macrophages will be absent and monotypic surface immunoglobulin should be demonstrable on the tumour cells (Dabski *et al.*, 1989).

11.9 Cutaneous involvement by leukaemia

Leukaemic skin involvement may take the form of red-brown papules and nodules, possibly with associated purpura, which on biopsy show infiltration of the reticular dermis by tumour cells resembling the phenotype of the primary tumour (Ricevuti *et al.*, 1985). Sometimes in granulocytic leukaemia, the biopsy may show the neutrophilic infiltration described as Sweet's disease. The most frequently involved sites are the trunk, arms and legs (Stawski, 1978). The possibility of tumorous infiltration should be considered in the differential diagnosis of children with a blueberry muffin appearance (Gottesfeld *et al.*, 1989).

References

Addis, B. J., Hyjek, E. and Isaacson, P. G. (1988) Primary pulmonary lymphoma. A re-appraisal of its histogenesis and its relationship to pseudolymphoma and interstitial pneumonia. *Histopathol.*, **13**, 1–17.

Banerjee, S. S., Heald, J. and Harris, M. (1991) Twelve cases of Ki-1 positive anaplastic large cell lymphoma of the skin. *J. Clin. Pathol.*, **44**, 119–25.

Beljaards, R. C., Meijer, C. J. L. M., Scheffer, E., Toonstra, J., van Vloten, W. A., van der Putte, C. J. Geerts, M.-L. and Willemze, R. (1989) Prognostic significance of CD30 (Ki-1/Ber-H2) expression in primary cutaneous large-cell lymphomas of T-cell origin. *Am. J. Pathol.*, **135**, 1169–78.

Bender, B. L., Kapadia, S. B., Synkowski, D. R. and Zitelli, J. A. (1978) Lymphomatoid granulomatosis preceded by chronic granulomatous dermatitis. *Arch. Dermatol.*, **114**, 1547–9.

Berger, C. L., Eisenberg, A., Soper, L., Chow, J., Simone, J., Gapas, Y., Cacciapaglia, B., Bennett, L., Edelson, R. L., Warburton, D. and Benn, P. (1988) Dual genotype in cutaneous T cell lymphoma: immunoglobulin gene rearrangement in clonal T cell malignancy. *J. Am. Acad. Dermatol.*, **90**, 73–7.

Bignon, Y. J., Roger, H., Souteyrand, P., Fonck, Y., D'incan, M., Bernard, D., Chassagne, J., Dastugue, B. and Plagne, R. (1989) Study of T-cell antigen receptor gene rearrangement: a useful tool for early diagnosis of mycosis fungoides. *Acta. Derm. Venereol. (Stockh.)*, **69**, 217–22.

Bluefarb, S. M. and Steinberg, H. I. (1952) Pulmonary manifestations of mycosis fungoides. *Ann. Intern. Med.*, **36**, 625–39.

Braun-Falco, O., Marghescu, S. and Wolff, U. H. (1973) Pagetoid reticulose Morbus Woringer-Kolopp. *Hautarzt*, **24**, 11–21.

Braun-Falco, O., Nikolowski, J., Burg, G. and Schmoeckel, C. Lymphomatoide papulose. Ubersicht und eigene Beobachtungen an vier Patienten. *Hautarzt*, **34**, 59–65.

Brehmer-Andersson, E. (1976) Mycosis fungoides and its relation to the Sezary syndrome, lymphomatoid papulosis and primary cutaneous Hodgkin's disease: a clinical, histopathologic and cytologic study of fourteen cases and a critical review of the literature. *Acta. Derm. Venereol. (Stockh.)*, **56** (suppl. 75), 1–142.

Brodell, R. T., Miller, C. W. and Eisen, A. Z. Cutaneous lesions of lymphomatoid granulomatosis. *Arch. Dermatol.*, **122**, 303–6.

Chan, J. K., Ng, C. S., Ngan, K. C., Hui, P. K., Lo, S. T. and Lau, W. H. (1988) Angiocentric T-cell lymphoma of the skin. An aggressive lymphoma distinct from mycosis fungoides. *Am. J. Surg. Pathol.*, **12**, 861–76.

Chan, J. K. and Ng, C. S. (1989) Trends in lymphoma diagnosis. *Lancet*, **i**, 837.

Dabski, K., Banks, P. M. and Winkelmann, R. K. (1989) Clinicopathologic spectrum of cutaneous manifestations in systemic follicular lymphoma. A study of 11 patients. *Cancer*, **64**, 1480–5.

Degreef, H., Holvoet, C., Van Vloten, W. A., Desmet, V. and De Wolf-Peeters, K. (1976) Woringer-Kolopp disease. An epidermotrophic variant of mycosis fungoides. *Cancer*, **38**, 2154–65.

Deneau, D. G., Wood, G. S., Beckstead, J., Hoppe, R. T. and Price, N. (1984) Woringer-Kolopp disease (Pagetoid reticulosis). *Arch. Dermatol.*, **120**, 1045–51.

Dowd, P. M., Munro, D. D. and Stansfeld, A. G. (1981) Lymphomatoid papulosis and primary cutaneous Hodgkin's disease. *J. R. Soc. Med.*, **74**, 68–71.

Edelson, R. L., Berger, C. L., Raafat, J. and Warburton, D. (1979) Karyotype studies of cutaneous T cell lymphoma: evidence for clonal origin. *J. Invest. Dermatol*, **73**, 548–50.

Edelson, R. L. (1981) Cutaneous T-cell lymphoma. J. Dermatol. *Surg. Oncol.*, **6**, 358–68.

Espinoza, C. G., Erkman-Balis, B. and Fenske, N. A. (1985) Lymphomatoid papulosis: a premalignant T cell disorder. *J. Am. Acad. Dermatol.*, **13**, 736–43.

Everett, M. A. (1985) Early diagnosis of *Mycosis fungoides*: vacuolar interface dermatitis. *J. Cut. Pathol.*, **12**, 271–8.

Fauci, A. S., Haynes, B. F., Costa, J., Katz, P. and Wolff, S. M. (1982) Lymphomatoid granulomatosis. Prospective clinical and theraputic experience over 10 years. *N. Engl. J. Med.*, **306**, 68–74.

Faure, P., Chittal, S., Gorguet, B., Caveriviere, P., Brousset, P., Viraben, R., Mazerolles, C. and Delsol, G. (1990) Immunohistochemical profile of cutaneous B-cell lymphoma on cryostat and paraffin sections. *Am. J. Dermatopathol.*, **12**, 122–33.

Foley, J. F. (1987) Cutaneous necrotizing granulomatous vasculitis with evolution to T cell lymphoma. *Am. J. Med.*, **82**, 839–44.

Flynn, K. J., Dehner, L. P., Gajl-Peczalska, K. J., Dahl, M. V., Ramsay, N. and Wang, N. (1982) Regressing atypical histiocytosis: a cutaneous proliferation of atypical neoplastic histiocytes with unexpectedly indolent biologic behavior. *Cancer*, **49**, 959–70.

Geerts, M. L., Kaiserling, E. and Kirt, A. (1982) Microenvironment of Woringer-Kolopp disease. *Dermatologica*, **164**, 15–29.

Gottesfeld, E., Silverman, R. A., Coccia, P. F., Jacobs, G. and Zaim, M. T. (1989) Transient blueberry muffin appearance of a newborn with congenital monoblastic leukemia. *J. Am. Acad. Dermatol.*, **21**, 347–51.

Griesser, H., Feller, A. C. and Sterry, W. (1990) T-cell receptor and immunoglobulin gene rearrangements in cutaneous T-cell-rich pseudolymphomas. *J.*

Invest. Dermatol., **95**, 292–5.

Hamminga, L., Hermans, J., Noordijk, E. M., Meijer, C. J. L. M., Schefter, E. and van Vloten, W. A. (1982) Cutaneous T-cell lymphoma: clinicopathological relationships, therapy and survival in ninety-two patients. *Br. J. Dermatol*, **107**, 145–56.

Headington, J. T., Roth, M. S. and Schnitzer, B. (1987a) Regressing atypical histiocytosis: a review and critical appraisal. *Semin. Diagn. Pathol.*, **4**, 28–37.

Headington, J. T., Roth, M. S., Ginsburg, D., Lichter, A. S., Hyder, D. and Schnitzer, B. (1987b) T-cell receptor gene rearrangement in regressing atypical histiocytosis. *Arch. Dermatol.*, **123**, 1183–7.

Horiuchi, Y., Tone, T., Umezawa, A. and Takezaki, S. (1988) Large cell mycosis fungoides of tumor stage. Unusual T8, T4, T6 phenotype expression. *Am. J. Dermatopathol.*, **10**, 54–8.

Horiuchi, Y., Tanaka, T., Toda, K., Oguchi, M., Komura, J., Ozaki, M., Nakashima, Y., Miyachi, Y. and Imamura, S. (1989) Regressing ulcerative histiocytosis. *Am. J. Dermatopathol.*, **11**, 166–71.

Hui, P. K., Feller, A. C., Kaiserling, E., Hesse, G., Rodermund, O.-E., Haneke, E., Weber, L. and Lennert, K. (1987) Skin tumor of T accessory cells (interdigitating reticulum cells) with high content of T lymphocytes. *Am. J. Dermatopathol.*, **9**, 129–37.

Jack, A. S., Boylston, A. W., Carrel, S. and Grigor, I. (1990) Cutaneous T-cell lymphoma cells employ a restricted range of T-cell antigen receptor variable region genes. *Am. J. Pathol.*, **136**, 17–21.

Kadin, M. E. (1985) Common activated helper-T-cell origin for lymphomatoid papulosis, mycosis fungoides, and some types of Hodgkin's disease. *Lancet*, **ii**, 864–5.

Kadin, M. E., Vonderheid, E. C., Sako, D., Clayton, L. K. and Olbricht, S. (1987) Clonal composition of T cells in lymphomatoid papulosis. *Am. J. Pathol.*, **126**, 13–17.

Kaudewitz, P., Stein, H., Burg, G., Mason, D. Y. and Braun-Falco, O. (1986) Atypical cells in lymphomatoid papulosis express the Hodgkin cell-associated antigen Ki-1. *J. Invest. Dermatol.*, **86**, 350–4.

Kessler, S., Lund, H. Z. and Leonard, D. D. (1981) Cutaneous lesions of lymphomatoid granulomatosis. Comparison with lymphomatoid papulosis. *Am. J. Dermatopathol.*, **3**, 115–27.

Kung, P. C., Berger, C. L., Goldstein, G., Lo Gerfo, P. and Edelson, R. L. (1981) Cutaneous T cell lymphoma: characterisation by monoclonal antibodies. *Blood*, **57**, 261–6.

Lacour, J. P., Juhlin, L., El Baze, P., Barety, M. and Ortonne, J. P. (1986) Disseminated pagetoid reticulosis associated with mycosis fungoides: immunomorphologic study. *J. Am. Acad. Dermatol.*, **14**, 898–901.

Lamberg, S. I., Green, S. B., Byar, D. P., Block, J. B., Clendenning, W. E., Douglas, M. C., Epstein, E. H., Fuks, Z. Y., Golitz, L. E., Lorincz, A. L., McBurney, E. I., Michel, B., Roenigk, H. H., Van Scott, E. J. and Vonderheid, E. C. (1984) Clinical staging of cutaneous T-cell lymphoma. *Ann. Intern. Med.*, **100**, 187–92.

Lazar, A. P., Caro, W. A., Roenigk, H. H. Jr and Pinski, K. S. (1989) Parapsoriasis and mycosis fungoides: the Northwestern University experience, 1970 to 1985. *J. Am. Acad. Dermatol.*, **21**, 919–23.

Liebow, A. A., Carrington, C. R. B. and Friedman, P. J. (1972) Lymphomatoid granulomatosis. *Hum. Pathol.*, **3**, 457–558.

Lindholm, J. S., Barron, D. R., Williams, M. E. and Swerdlow, S. H. (1989) Ki-1-positive cutaneous large cell lymphoma of T cell type: report of an indolent subtype. *J. Am. Acad. Dermatol.*, **20**, 342–8.

Mackie, R. M. and Turbitt, M. L. (1984) A case of pagetoid reticulosis bearing the T cytotoxic suppressor surface marker on the lymphoid infiltrate:further evidence that pagetoid reticulosis is not a variant of mycosisfungoides. *Br. J. Dermatol.*, **110**, 89–94.

Macaulay, W. L. (1968) Lymphomatoid papulosis. A continuing self-healing eruption, clinically benign – histologically malignant. *Arch. Dermatol.*, **97**, 23–30.

Mandojana, R. M. and Helwig, E. B. (1983) Localised epidermotrophic reticulosis (Woringer-Kolopp disease). *J. Am. Acad. Dermatol.*, **8**, 813–29.

Meissner, K., Michaelis, K., Rehpenning, W. and Loning, T. (1990) Epidermal Langerhans' cell densities influence survival in mycosis fungoides and Sezary syndrome. *Cancer*, **65**, 2069–73.

Mielke, V., Wolff, H. H., Winzer, M. and Sterry, W. (1989) Localized and disseminated Pagetoid reticulosis. Diagnostic immunophenotypic findings. *Arch. Dermatol.*, **125**, 402–6.

Minars, N., Kays, S. and Escobar, M. R. (1975) Lymphomatoid granulomatosis of skin: a new clinicopathologic entity. *Arch. Dermatol.*, **111**, 493–502.

Miracco, C., Raffaelli, M., de Santi, M. M., Fimiani, M. and Tosi, P. (1988) Solitary cutaneous reticulum cell tumor. Enzyme-immunohistochemical and electron-microscopic analogies with IDRC sarcoma. *Am. J. Dermatopathol.*, **10**, 47–53.

Mukai, K., Sato, Y., Watanabe, S., Ishihara, K., Shimoyama, M. and Shimosato, Y. (1988) Non-Hodgkin lymphoma of the skin excluding mycosis fungoides and cutaneous involvement of adult T-cell leukaemia/lymphoma. *J. Cutan. Pathol.*, **15**, 193–200.

Murphy, F. G., Bhan, A. K., Sato, S., Harrist, T. J. and Mihm, M. C. Jr (1981) Characterization of Langerhans cells by the use of monoclonal antibodies. *Lab. Invest.*, **45**, 465–8.

Natarajan, S. and Wilson, P. D. (1985) Pagetoid reticulosis (Woringer-Kolopp disease): histiocyte marker (lysozyme) study and ultrastructural observations. *Dermatologica*, **171**, 332–7.

Neumann, C., Schaumburg-Lever, G., Dopfer, R. and Kolde, G. (1988) Interferon gamma is a marker for histiocytosis X cells in the skin. *J. Invest. Dermatol.*, **91**, 280–2.

Nichols, P. W., Koss, M., Levine, A. M. and Lukes, R. J. (1982) Lymphomatoid granulomatosis: a T-cell disorder? *Am. J. Med.*, **72**, 467–71.

Nickoloff, B. J. and Griffiths, C. E. M. (1990) Intraepidermal but not dermal T lymphocytes are positive for a cell-cycle-associated antigen (Ki-67) in mycosis fungoides. *Am. J. Pathol.*, **136**, 261–6.

Picker, L. J., Weiss, L. M., Medeiros, L. J., Wood, G. S. and Warnke, R. A. (1987) Immunophenotypic criteria for the diagnosis of non-Hodgkin's lymphoma. *Am. J. Pathol.*, **128**, 181–201.

Prost, C., Reyes, F., Wechsler, J., Gaston, A., Richard, I. and Poirier, J. (1987) High-grade malignant cutaneous plasmacytoma metastatic to the central nervous system. *Am. J. Dermatopathol.*, **9**, 30 6.

Ralfkaier, E., Stein, H., Lange Wantzin, G., Thomson, K., Ralfkaier, N. and Mason, D. Y. (1985) Lymphomatoid papulosis: characterisation of skin infiltrates by monoclonal antibodies. *Am. J. Clin. Pathol.*, **84**, 587–93.

Requena, L., Sanchez, M., Coca, S. and Sanchez Yus, E. (1990) Follicular lymphomatoid papulosis. *Am. J. Dermatopathol.*, **12**, 67– 75.

Ricevuti, G., Mazzone, A., Rossini, S., Rizzo, S. C., Ricevuti, G., Bosatra, M., Jucci, A., Dell'Acqua, R. and Sacchi, S. (1985) Skin involvement in hemopathies: specific cutaneous manifestations of acute nonlymphoid leukemias and non-Hodgkin lymphomas. *Dermatologica*, **171**, 250–4.

Salhany, K. E., Cousar, J. B., Greer, J. P., Casey, T. T., Fields, J. P. and Collins, R. D. (1988) Transformation of cutaneous T cell lymphoma to large cell lymphoma. A clinicopathologic and immunologic study. *Am. J. Pathol.*, **132**, 265–77.

Samman, P. D. (1972) The natural history of parapsoriasis en plaque (chronic superficial dermatitis) and pre-reticulotic poikiloderma. *Br. J. Dermatol.*, **87**, 405–11.

Sanchez, J. L. and Ackerman, A. B. (1979) The patch stage of mycosis fungoides. *Am. J. Dermatopathol.*, **1**, 5–26.

Scheen, S. R., Doyle, J. A. and Winkelmann, R. K. (1981) Lymphoma-associated papulosis: lymphomatoid papulosis associated with lymphoma. *J. Am. Acad. Dermatol.*, **4**, 451–7.

Seleznick, M. J., Aguilar, J. L., Rayhack, J., Fenske, N. and Espinoza, L. R. (1989) Polyarthritis associated with cutaneous T cell lymphoma. *J. Rheumatol.*, **16**, 1379–82.

Slater, D. N. (1987) Recent developments in cutaneous lymphoproliferative disorders. *J. Pathol.*, **153**, 5–19.

Slater, D. (1990) Clonal dermatoses: a conceptual and diagnostic dilemma. *J. Pathol.*, **162**, 1–3.

Stawski, M. Skin manifestations of leukaemias and lymphomas. *Cutis*, **21**, 814–18.

Sterry, W. (1985) Mycosis fungoides. In *Dermatopathology* (ed. C. L. Berry) Springer Verlag, p.p. 167–223.

van der Putte, S. C. J., Toonstra, J., Bruns, H. M., van Wichen, D. F., van Unnik, J. A. M. and van Vloten, W. A. (1987) T-cell signet-ring cell proliferation in the skin simulating true histiocytic lymphoma. *Am. J. Dermatopathol.*, **9**, 120–8.

van Vloten, W. A. and Willemze, R. (1985) New techniques in the evaluation of cutaneous T-cell lymphoma. *Dermatol. Clin.*, **3**, 665–72.

Varga, F. J., Vonderheid, E. C., Olbricht, S. M. and Kadin, M. E. (1990) Immunohistochemical distinction of lymphomatoid papulosis and pityriasis lichenoides et varioliformis acuta. *Am. J. Pathol.*, **136**, 979–87.

Weinman, V. F. and Ackerman, A. B. (1981) Lymphomatoid papulosis. A critical review and new findings. *J. Am. Acad. Dermatol.*, **3**, 129–63.

Weiss, L. M., Wood, G. S., Trela, M., Warnke, R. A. and Sklar, J. (1986) Clonal T-cell populations in lymphomatoid papulosis. *New Engl. J. Med.*, **315**, 475–9.

Weiss, L. M., Wood, G. S., Ellisen, L. F., Reynolds, T. C. and Sklar, J. (1987) Clonal T-cell populations in pityriasis lichenoides et varioliformis acuta (Mucha-Habermann disease). *Am. J. Pathol.*, **126**, 417–21.

Willemze, R., Meijer, C. J. L. M., van Vloten, W. A. and Scheffer, E. (1981) The clinical and histological spectrum of lymphomatoid papulosis. *Br. J. Dermatol.*, **107**, 131–44.

Willemze, R., Scheffer, E., Ruiter, D. J., van Vloten, W. A. and Meijer, C. J. L. M. (1983a) Immunological, cytochemical and ultrastructural studies in lymphomatoid papulosis. *Br. J. Dermatol*, **108**, 381–94.

Willemze, R., de Graaf-Reitsma, C. B., van Vloten, W. A. and Meijer, C. J. L. M. (1983b) The cell populations of cutaneous B-cell lymphomas. *Br. J. Dermatol.*, **108**, 395–409.

Willemze, R., Meijer, C. J. L. M., Sentis, H. J., Scheffer, E., van Vloten, W. A., Toonstra, J. and van der Putte, S. C. J. (1987a) Primary cutaneous large cell lymphomas of follicular center cell origin. *J. Am. Acad. Dermatol.*, **16**, 518–26.

Willemze, R., Meijer, C. J. L. M., Scheffer, E., Kluin, P. M., van Vloten, W. A., Toonstra, J. and van der Putte, S. C. J. (1987b) Diffuse large cell lymphomas of follicular center cell origin presenting in the skin. *Am. J. Pathol.*, **126**, 325–33.

Wood, M. L., Harrington, C. I., Slater, D. N., Rooney, N. and Clark, A. (1984) Cutaneous lymphomatoid granulomatosis: a rare cause of recurrent skin ulceration. *Br. J. Dermatol.*, **110**, 619–25.

Woringer, F. and Kolopp, P. (1939) Lésion érythématosquameuse polycyclique de l'avant-bras évoluant depuis six ans chez un garconnet de trieze ans: histologiquement infiltrat intraepidermique d'appearance tumerale. *Ann. Derm. Vénér.*, **10**, 945–58.

12 Vesiculo-bullous diseases

In this chapter the principle varieties of blistering skin diseases will be described. Whilst due weight must be given to the clinical aspects of each patient, this is one area where particular attention must be given to biopsy and laboratory technique (Millikan, 1987).

The biopsy must be taken carefully and should, whenever possible, be taken to include a whole, fresh blister. The older the blister the less clear will be the changes, and if the blister has burst the appearances will be confused by the associated secondary reaction.

In the past, immunofluorescent techniques have been used to localize immune complexes within, or in association with, the epidermis and its basement membrane. Recent advances in immunohistochemical methods have now rendered this approach largely redundant. The whole fresh biopsy, with its blister intact, can be frozen on the cryostat chuck. By trimming into the block it is then possible to get sections showing the intact blister, which can be stained with H and E to show the morphology and stained immunohistochemically to search for localization of immune complexes. If the biopsy is trimmed in the unfrozen state then, of course, the blister will burst and much of the morphology will be lost.

We have been using the indirect immunoperoxidase method on frozen sections for immunohistochemical staining. Not only is this of comparable sensitivity to immunofluorescence, but also it allows a permanent preparation to be made which can be viewed on an ordinary light microscope. This has the double advantage of not only avoiding the unpopular trip to the stuffy claustrophobia of the darkroom, but also of producing a result which can be demonstrated easily at a later date. The method on frozen sections does not include a step to block endogenous peroxidase, so the eosinophils stain very strongly and are easily seen as a consequence. This can be quite helpful in differential diagnosis. For example, eosinophils are a feature of pemphigoid but not eczema. Other newer immunohistochemical methods, such as the avidin-biotin and streptavidin-biotin methods, are applicable to paraffin sections, where satisfactory results can be obtained in the majority of cases.

12.1 Pemphigus

In pemphigus, the blisters form within the epidermis in association with deposition of IgG and/or C3 along epidermal cell membranes. Circulating antibodies are often detectable, especially in the more advanced cases of pemphigus vulgaris; their titre correlate with the extent and severity of the disease.

There are several subcategories of the disease. Pemphigus vulgaris has blisters forming at a suprabasal level. Pemphigus vegetans Neumann and pemphigus vegetans Hallopeau are clinical variants of pemphigus vulgaris; the three conditions forming points on a spectrum of disease (Lever, 1965).

Pemphigus foliaceous has blisters at a more superficial level, usually in the granular layer, and has variants including pemphigus erythematosus, and Brazilian pemphigus foliaceous, which is endemic in central and southern areas of South America and occurs in epidemics. It may have an infective cause, possibly viral, which is transmitted intradermally by flies (Castro et al., 1982, 1983; Robledo et al., 1988; Editorial, 1988).

Neonatal pemphigus occurs in the first few months of life and is probably caused by maternal IgG passed through the placenta (Storer et al., 1982), and, indeed there are reports of pemphigus in the children of women suffering from pemphigus in pregnancy.

Amongst drugs, penicillamine is the best characterized inducer of pemphigus; usually pemphigus foliaceus but also pemphigus vulgaris (Troy et al., 1981). Pemphigus has also been linked with treatment with single agents such as penicillin, ampicillin (Feller and Marks, 1980; Ruocco et al., 1979), captopril (Parfrey et al., 1980), nifampitin (Gange et al., 1976; Lee et al., 1984), and pyrazolon derivatives (Chorzelski et al., 1966), and with combination therapy with propranolol and meprobamate (Goddard et al., 1980), and indomethacin and aspirin (DeMento and Grover, 1973).

In the early lesion there should be an accumulation of eosinophils in the dermis, with extension into the epidermis. Associated with this, there will be a variable degree of intercellular oedema. This appearance has been called eosinophilic spongiosis (Lever, 1965, 1983; DeMento and Grover, 1973). At the next stage, the spongiosis becomes more marked and intercellular prickles disappear, resulting in a loss of cell-to-cell adhesion and the consequent development of a cleft, and then a

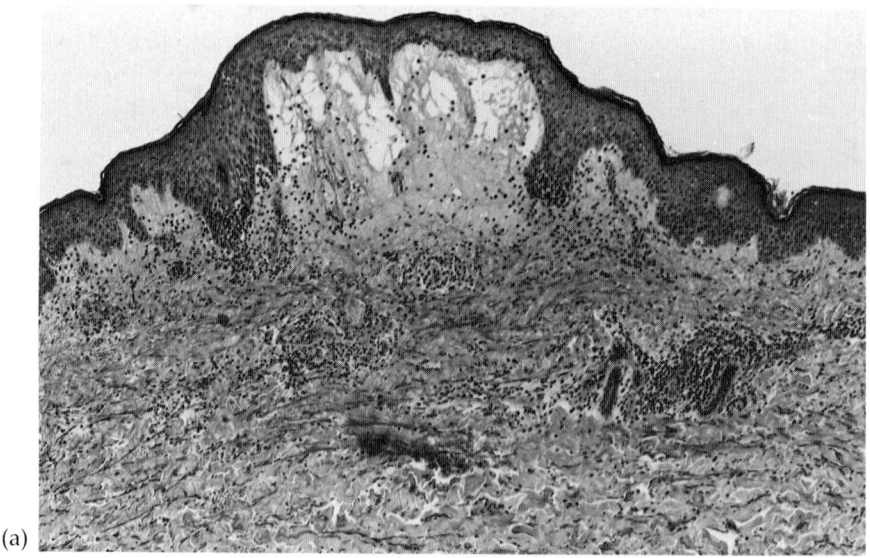

(a)

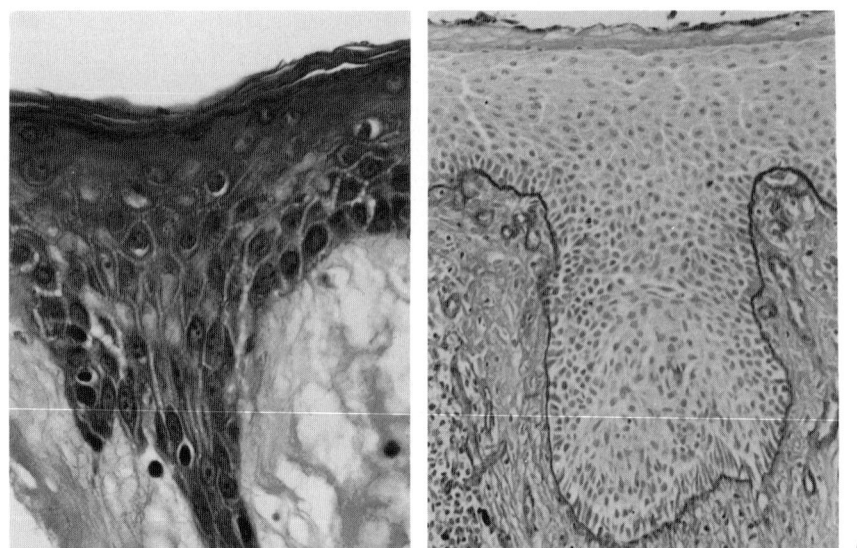

(b)   (c)

Figure 12.1 Bullous pemphigoid. (a) Subepidermal blister, with moderate cellular infiltration of dermis, (b) roof of blister, and (c) linear deposition of IgG (immunoperoxidase).

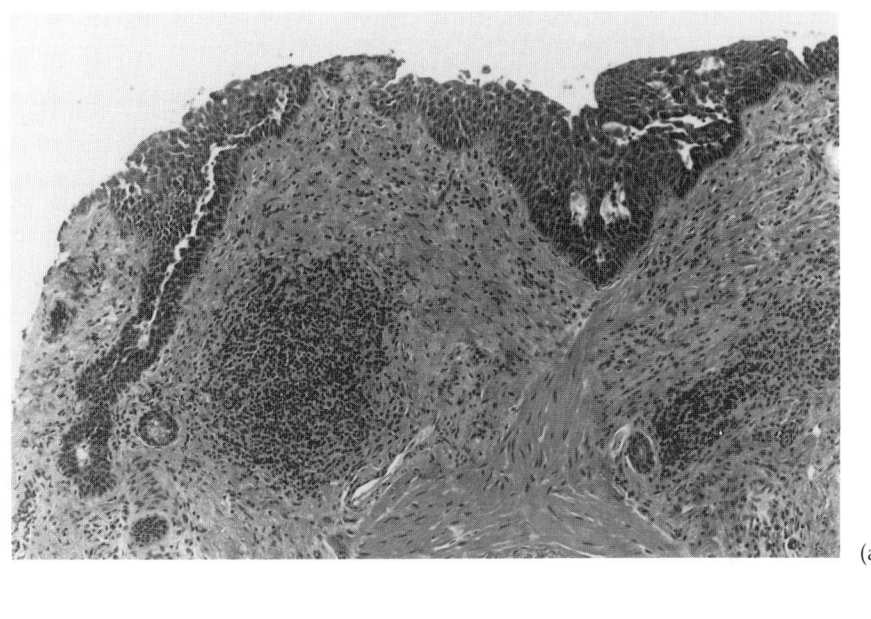

(a)

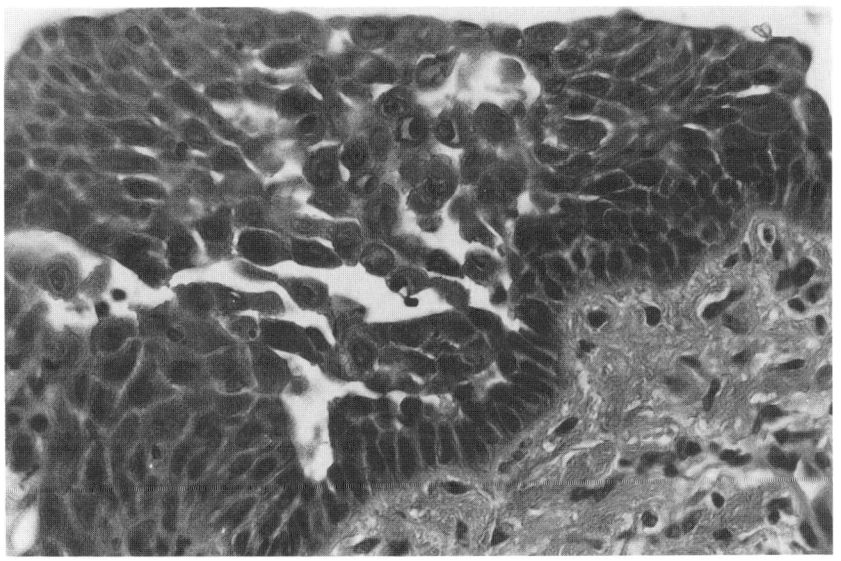

(b)

Figure 12.2 Pemphigus vulgaris, with intraepidermal acantholysis (a, b and c).

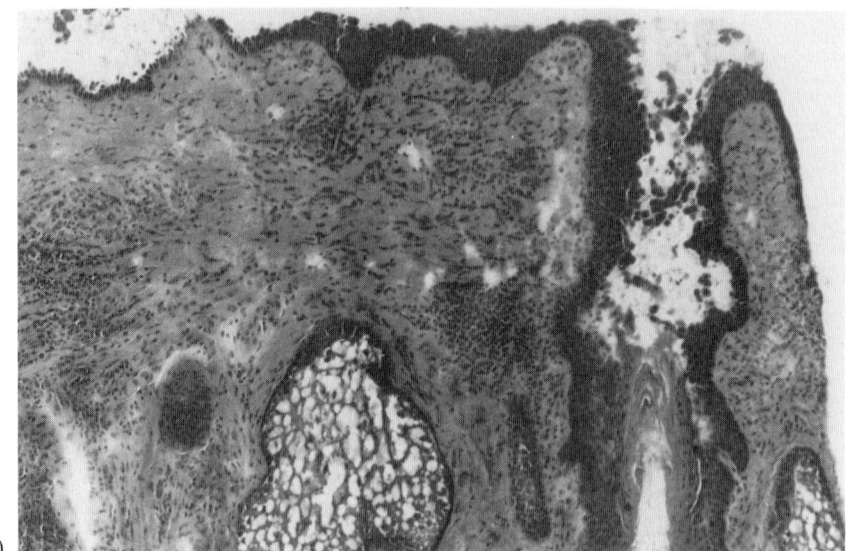

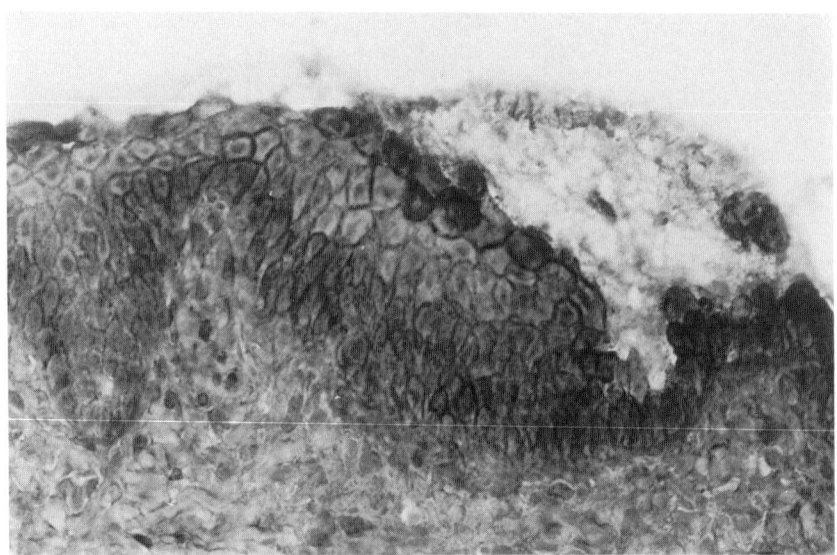

Figure 12.3 Pemphigus vulgaris. Frozen sections showing (a) extension of acantholysis into hair follicle infundibulum, and (b) intercellular staining for IgG (immunoperoxidase)

blister in the layer above the basal cells. This process is driven by antibodies binding to epidermal antigens, which fix complement and thereby signal the synthesis and release of plasminogen activator. The subsequent conversion of plasminogen to plasmin leads to acantholysis and blister formation.

In pemphigus foliaceus and its variants, a similar process is seen, but taking place at a higher level, usually subcorneal or within the granular cell layer. The superficial nature can make diagnosis difficult, first, because the tops of the blisters are easily lost and, second, because there is often an accumulation of neutrophil polymorphs in the cleft which then looks just like impetigo (Lever, 1983).

The immunohistochemical findings are necessary to confirm the diagnosis. Intercellular IgG deposits are present in over 90% of patients with pemphigus vulgaris (Ackerman, 1978; Beutner et al., 1965). Pemphigus foliaceus may show positive staining restricted to the upper epidermis, but this is not necessarily the case (Jordan et al., 1971; Bystryn et al., 1974). In Brazilian pemphigus, complement (C3) and immunoglobulins are present in the epidermal intercellular spaces and, in addition, granular deposits of C3 may also be present in the basement membrane zone (de Messias et al., 1988).

The presence of intercellular deposits of IgG can only be taken to suggest a diagnosis of pemphigus NOS: differential diagnosis between the various forms of pemphigus must be made on morphological and clinical grounds. For instance, if dyskeratotic cells are present, then the diagnosis is unlikely to be pemphigus vulgaris and familial benign chronic pemphigus should be considered (Steffen, 1987).

The development of immunoblot analysis offers the prospect of an alternative way of differentiating sub types of pemphigus by identifying the antigen against which circulating antibodies are directed (Hashimoto et al., 1990).

12.2   Bullous pemphigoid

Bullous pemphigoid is both commoner and less lethal than pemphigus vulgaris. The blisters that form are subepidermal and are associated with the deposition of immune complexes at the dermo-epidermal junction. The disease is part of a spectrum which includes cicatricial pemphigoid, localized scarring pemphigoid (Brunsting-Perry) and pemphigoid gestationis. The majority of patients are over 60 years old when the disease starts (Lever, 1965). Cases have been recorded in infants and children, with essentially similar clinical and biopsy appearances to those seen in adults (Senear and Usher, 1926; Castro and Proenca, 1982), following penicillamine therapy (Rasmussen et al.,

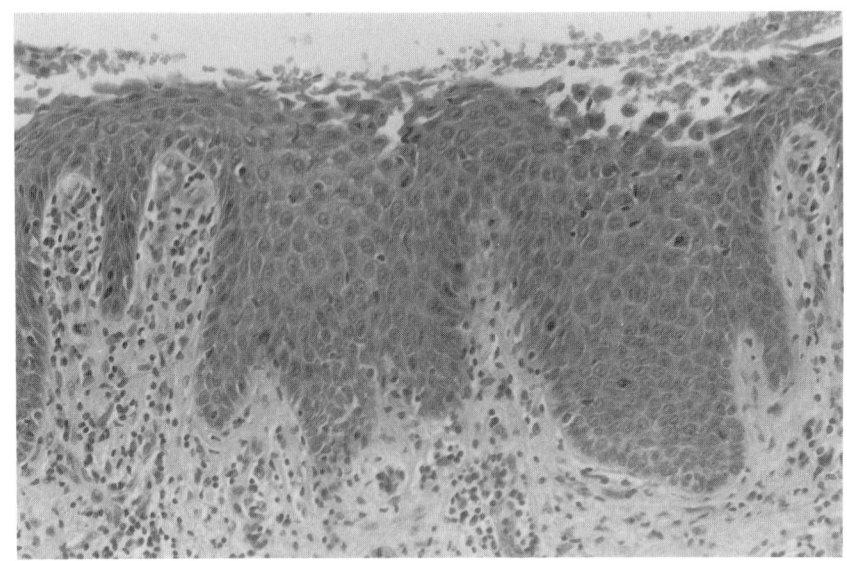

(a)

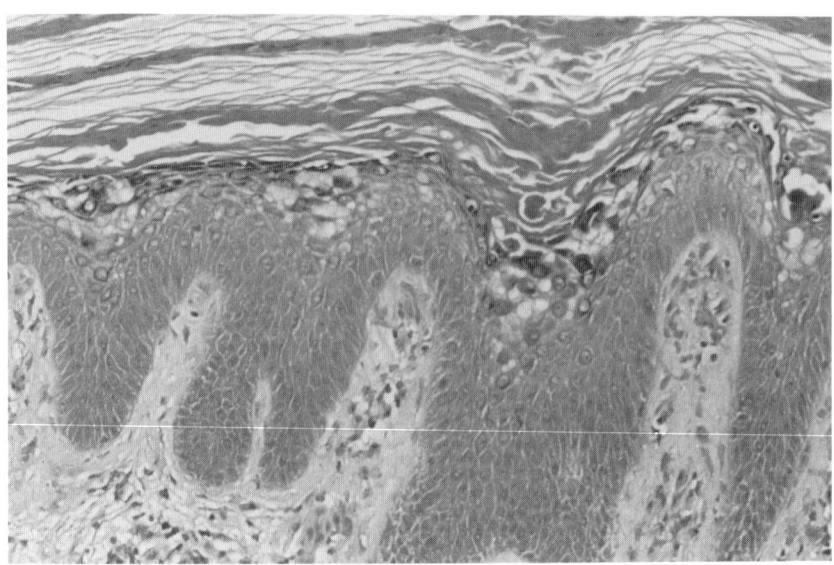

(b)

Figure 12.4 Pemphigus foliaceus. (a) Superficial acantholysis with loss of blister roof, and (b) incipient blister formation immediately above the granular layer.

1989), and even in a patient given injections of human placental extracts to provide 'biological stimulation' (Saurat *et al.*, 1988).

Pemphigoid may also present as a non-metastatic manifestation of malignancy. It has been reported in association with malignant lymphoma, and malignant tumours of skin, lung, breast, pancreas, kidney, gastrointestinal tract and genito-urinary system (Stone and Schroeter, 1975).

The blisters may be large and tense, arising either on normal or inflamed skin (Lever, 1965; Castro *et al.*, 1983). The eruption can be preceded by a prodromal phase lasting from weeks to years, during which time the skin appears inflamed but not blistered (Amato *et al.*, 1988). Mucous membrane involvement is relatively common (Silverman *et al.*, 1986).

The biopsy should show the blister forming at the level of the epidermal basement membrane. Linear deposition of IgG and C3 along the basement membrane at either side of the blister should be readily demonstrable. In the dermis and blister there will be numerous eosinophils as well as neutrophils.

Amongst the variants is one in which the blisters are small and vesicular, resembling dermatitis herpetiformis. This has been called 'polymorphic pemphigoid', and shows the same linear IgG and C3 pattern as bullous pemphigoid (Storer *et al.*, 1982).

Nodular pemphigoid is a condition in which there is a blistering and linear IgG and C3 deposition superimposed upon nodules and plaques which resemble nodular prurigo (Troy *et al.*, 1981; Feller and Mark, 1980; Ruocco *et al.*, 1979).

There are a number of conditions to be considered in the differential diagnosis. Most problems are easily resolved, however, if a fresh biopsy is stained for IgG, IgA, IgM and C3. Thus a negative result in a patient with an indeterminable rash may be suggestive of eczema rather than early bullous pemphigoid. Occasional solitary acantholytic lesions resembling Hailey-Hailey disease can coexist with pemphigoid, but probably do not mean that the patient has both diseases (Mehregan *et al.*, 1989).

The mechanism of blister formation remains to be completely elucidated, but eosinophils and occasional macrophages appear to be responsible for selective damage to components of the lamina lucida, caused by the release of their proteolytic enzymes (Dubertret *et al.*, 1980).

The bullous pemphigoid antigen is a normal component of basement membrane, which is ultrastructurally very intimately associated with the hemidesmosomes (Mutasim *et al.*, 1989). It is a 220 kd protein which is synthesized by keratinocytes in culture and is distinct from laminin. The cicatricial pemphigoid antigen remains unidentified, but appears to lie in a different part of the lamina lucida to the bullous pemphigoid antigen (Fine *et al.*, 1984). The antigens involved in the subepidermal bullous disorders must be identified before a final classification can be achieved. Western blotting offers a more sensitive method for the detection of circulating bullous pemphigoid antibodies than immunofluorescence, and may also allow this heterogenous group of subepidermal bullous dermatoses to be subclassified more accurately (Bernard *et al.*, 1989).

12.3   Cicatricial pemphigoid

Bullous pemphigoid has been separated on clinical grounds from a variant known as cicatricial pemphigoid: a condition particularly involving mucous membranes and resistant to treatment. However, there appears to be considerable overlap between the two conditions. Whilst bullous pemphigoid has been said to mainly affect skin, frequent and widespread mucosal and conjunctival involvement may be found when specifically sought, making the differentiation between the two conditions on clinical grounds difficult or impossible (Venning *et al.*, 1988). Cicatricial pemphigoid is found almost exclusively in middle-aged and elderly people, but a small number of cases have been described in childhood (Laskaris *et al.*, 1988). The cicatricial pemphigoid antigen appears to be similar to the bullous pemphigoid antigen, but it is expressed in a different way in the dermal–epidermal junction, which may account for the development of scarring, which distinguishes this condition from bullous pemphigoid (Bernard *et al.*, 1990).

The biopsy should show subepidermal blister formation with IgA, IgG and C3 localization in the basement membrane zone. Some cases show IgA alone, and these tend to have a higher frequency of mucous membrane and ocular involvement (Peters and Rogers, 1989).

12.4   Pemphigoid gestationis

This condition, previously known as herpes gestationis, is an interesting disease from the point of view of its pathogenesis. It is characterized by subepidermal bullae, which form in association with immunoglobulin and complement deposition at the dermal–epidermal junction (Kelly *et al.*, 1988). Although usually seen in pregnancy, it also occurs in association with trophoblastic tumours (Karvonen *et al.*, 1984).

The antibodies cross react with antigen in the chorionic epithelium and amnion of the placenta. The antigen is a 180 kDa glycoprotein which is present in the lamina lucida of the basement membrane of both the skin and the amnion. Although the biopsy appearance is essentially indistinguishable from bullous pemphigoid, the antigen is distinct from the 220 kDa antigen recognized in pemphigoid.

Pemphigoid gestationis appears to have a unique mechanism of pathogenesis. The 180 kDa glycoprotein is probably presented to the maternal immune system as paternal antigen in association with paternal major histocompatability complex (MHC) class II antigens, where it is the subject of an allogeneic reaction, with subsequent antibody mediated reaction. This seems to be a unique mechanism amongst organ-specific autoimmune diseases (Kelly *et al.*, 1989).

12.5   Linear IgA disease

Linear deposition of IgA in the basement membrane zone is almost always associated with subepidermal bullous disease, and is found in three clinical conditions: adult linear IgA bullous dermatosis, chronic bullous disease of childhood, and cicatricial pemphigoid (Chorzelski and Jablonska, 1979; Peters and Rogers, 1989). All three conditions are manifestations of the same disease. The antigen is identical and is different from the antigens seen in bullous pemphigoid and epidermolysis bullosa acquisita (Pothupitiya *et al.*, 1988).

Mucosal and ocular involvement is present in over 60% of patients. The IgA lacks a secretory component and J chain, and is not produced by mucosal-associated lymphoid tissue. There is no association with gluten-sensitive enteropathy, although some adults with the disease do also develop lymphoma. The IgA deposition can be demonstrated in biopsies from skin or oral mucosa, but is not found in the conjunctiva even in the presence of severe cicatrizing conjunctivitis or symblepharon. The blister forms through a split in the basement membrane, either at the level of the lamina densa or the lower part of the lamina lucida.

12.6   Epidermolysis bullosa acquisita

Epidermolysis bullosa acquisita (EBA) has attracted attention recently as a chronic subepidermal blistering disease which must be distinguished from pemphigoid and the bullous variant of lupus erythematosus. It is a rare condition which affects both skin and mucous membranes in both children and adults, and is associated with increased skin fragility, involvement of more easily traumatized areas of the body, and healing with the formation of scars and milia (Nieboer *et al.*, 1980; Yaoita *et al.*, 1981; Briggaman *et al.*, 1985). Morphological distinction from pemphigoid is probably not possible. The blisters are sub-

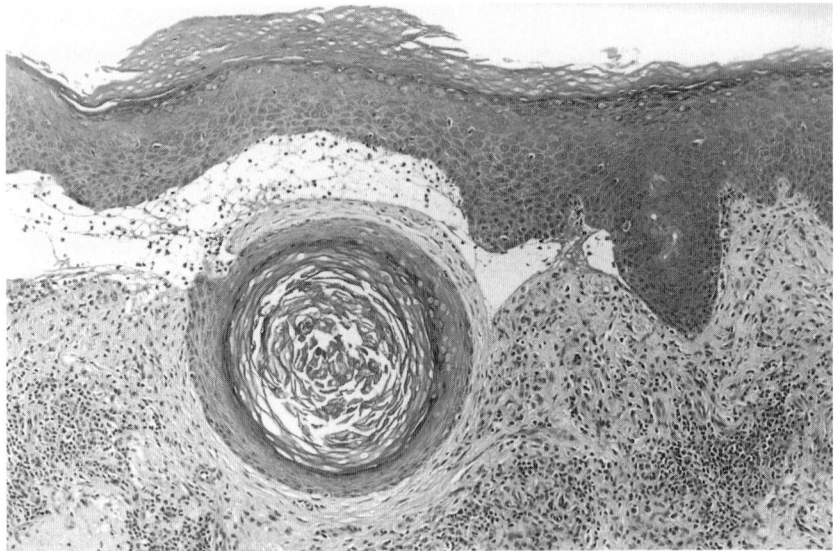

Figure 12.5　Epidermolysis bullosa aquisita. Subepidermal blister formation with associated secondary development of milia cyst.

epidermal and are accompanied by IgG deposition in the basement membrane zone, beneath the lamina densa. The antibodies are directed against the alpha chains and carboxy-terminals of type VII collagen, which is present in the lamina densa (Woodley *et al.*, 1988). There appears to be some degree of genetic predisposition in that the HLA class II haplotype DR2 is significantly increased in both black and white EBA patients (Gammon *et al.*, 1988). The disease usually responds poorly to therapy; patients with intractable pemphigoid may, on review, be found to have EBA.

12.7　Dystrophic epidermolysis bullosa

This group of rare and disabling inherited conditions includes many variants, and is divided into three major categories: epidermolysis bullosa simplex shows blister formation within the epidermis, junctional epidermolysis bullosa shows a split through the lamina lucida, with the lamina densa in the base of the blister; and dystrophic epidermolysis bullosa has the split beneath the lamina densa (Pearson,1962).

The latter group is divided into recessive and dominantly inherited variants. Recently, antenatal biopsy diagnosis has started to become possible. Using antibodies to type VII collagen (LH 7.2 and KF-1) on fetal skin biopsies, there is a marked reduction or complete absence of staining of the epidermal basement membrane in fetuses with the recessive variant, whilst those with the dominant variant show normal staining (Fine *et al.*, 1988; Leigh *et al.*, 1988). The underlying defect in recessive dystrophic epidermolysis bullosa appears to be an abnormality of type VII collagen synthesis with resulting defective formation of anchoring fibrils (Smith and Sybert, 1990), possibly due to defective packaging or transport of type VII collagen within the cytoplasm of basal keratinocytes (Fine *et al.*, 1990).

The antibodies GB3 and AA3 can be used in a similar way to diagnose junctional epidermolysis bullosa. Electron microscopy is, however, still the preferred way of identifying the changes in the basement membrane in this group of conditions (Eady *et al.*, 1987; Fine *et al.*, 1987).

12.8 Dermatitis herpetiformis

This pruritic rash is associated with gluten sensitive enteropathy and with the deposition of IgA in dermal papillae. In the early stages, the skin has an erythematous appearance, without blisters, but IgA may be present. The blisters develop at the tips of dermal papillae, in association with accumulations of neutrophils and as the lesions develop, with the inclusion of eosinophils.

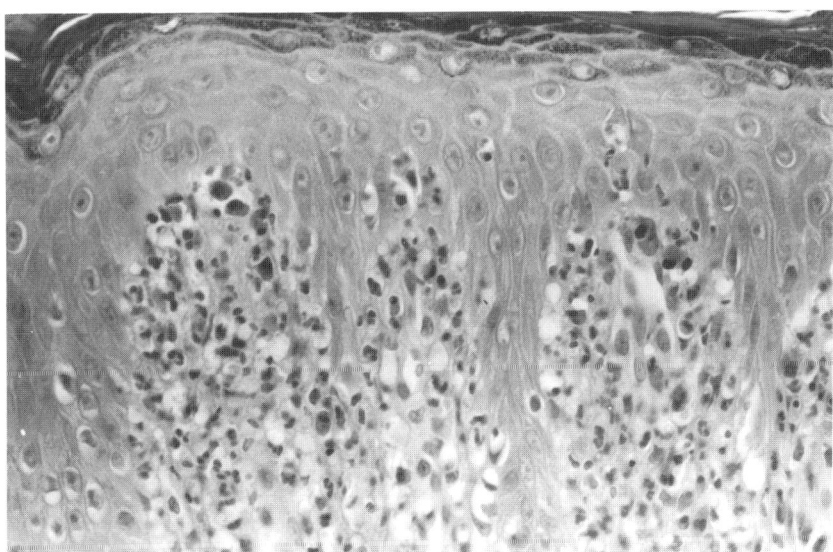

Figure 12.6 Dermatitis herpetiformis. Eosinophilic papillary microabscesses without acantholysis.

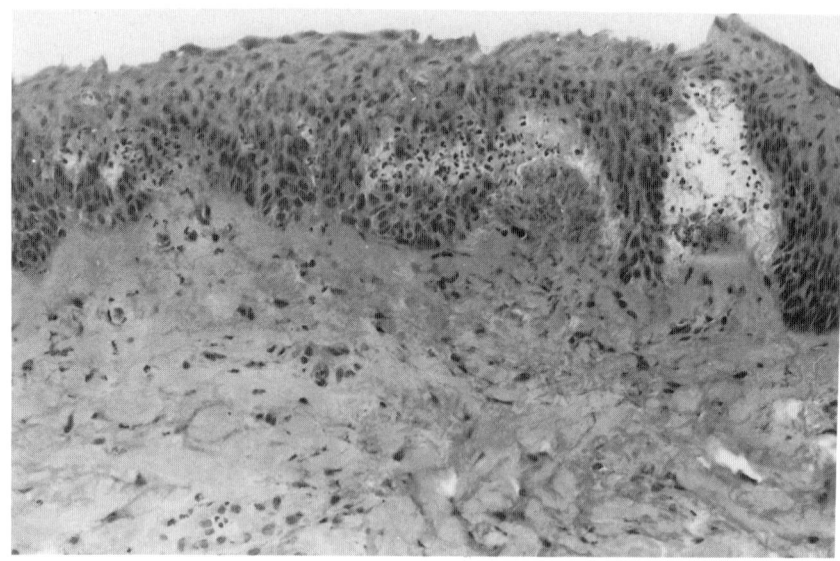

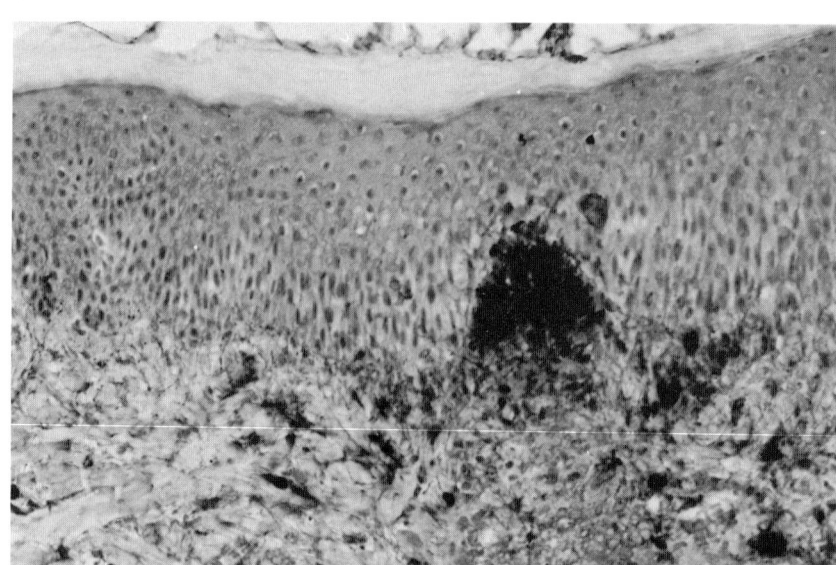

Figure 12.7 Dermatitis herpetiformis. Frozen sections showing (a) papillary subepidermal blisters, and (b) associated IgA localization (immunoperoxidase).

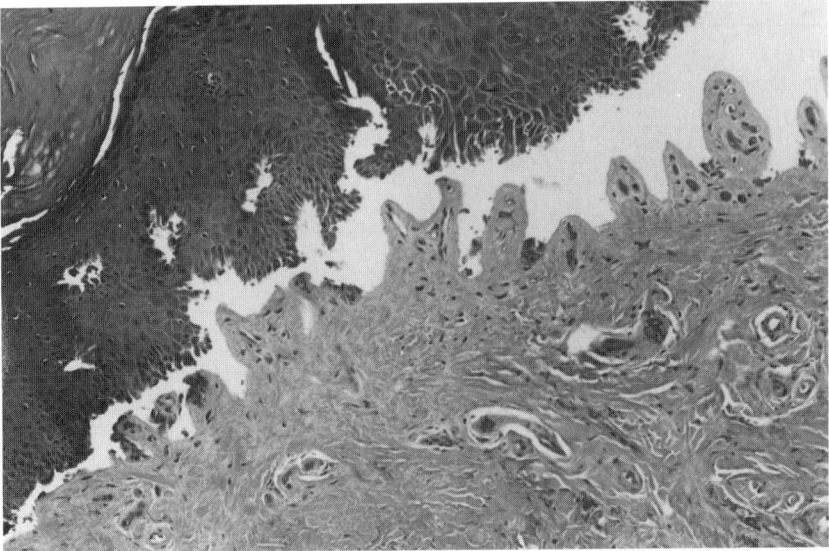

Figure 12.8 Porphyria cutanea tarda. Subepidermal blister formation without cellular reaction and with preservation of dermal papillae.

The immunoglobulin which is deposited is almost exclusively of IgA 1 subclass (Egelrud, 1986). It is dimeric, with the inclusion of J chain, and appears to be produced by mucosal associated lymphoid tissue as part of the associated enteropathy (Unsworth *et al.*, 1982). Renal deposits may lead to an associated glomerulonephritis (Heironimus and Perry, 1986). The antigen in the papillary dermis or basement membrane remains unidentified, although it may share an epitope with gliadin.

12.9 Porphyria cutanea tarda

There are several varieties of porphyria, but this is the one most likely to be seen in biopsy practice. Two features may be seen. First, there may be subepidermal blisters which show a characteristic appearance of the epidermis being 'ripped-off' the dermis, leaving the dermal papillae intact. There is sparse inflammatory cell reaction and immune complexes are absent. Second, hyaline-like material may be found around dermal blood vessels. The blisters occur in sun-exposed skin.

12.10 Pseudoporphyria

An identical appearance to the blistering of porphyria may also be seen as an adverse reaction to drugs, including etretinate (McDonagh and

Harrington, 1989) and chlorthalidone (Baker *et al.*, 1989). In these circumstances there is no associated evidence of abnormal porphyrin metabolism.

12.11   Bullous amyloidosis

Amyloidosis can involve a variety of organ systems, with skin involvement being relatively common. Very occasionally, skin involvement can present as a bullous disease. The blisters are subepidermal and resemble pemphigoid or epidermolysis bullosa aquisita, but without immune complex deposition in the basement membrane zone (Muller *et al.*, 1969; Johnson *et al.*, 1989).

References

Ackerman, A. B. (1978) *Histologic Diagnosis of Inflammatory Skin Diseases*, Lea and Febiger, Philadelphia, pp. 525–32.

Amato, D. A., Silverstein, J. and Zitelli, J. (1988) The prodrome of bullous pemphigoid. *Int. J. Dermatol.*, **27**, 560–3.

Baker, E. J., Reed, K. D. and Dixon, S. L. (1989) Chlorthalidone-induced pseudoporphyria: clinical and microscopic findings of a case. *J. Am. Acad. Dermatol.*, **21**, 1026–9.

Bernard, P., Didierjean, L., Denis, F., Saurat, J.-H. and Bonnetblanc, J.-M. (1989) Heterogeneous bullous pemphigoid antibodies: detection and characterization by immunoblotting when absent by indirect immunofluorescence. *J. Invest. Dermatol.*, **92**, 171–4.

Bernard, P., Prost, C., Lecerf, V., Intrator, L., Combemale, P., Bedane, C., Roujeau, J.-C., Revuz, J., Bonnetblanc, J.-M. and Dubertret, L. (1990) Studies of cicatricial pemphigoid autoantibodies using direct immunoelectron microscopy and immunoblot analysis. *J. Invest. Dermatol.*, **94**, 630–5.

Beutner, E. H., Lever, W. F., Witebsky, E., Jordon, R. and Chertock, B. (1965) Autoantibodies in pemphigus vulgaris. *JAMA*, **192**, 682–8.

Briggaman, R. A., Gammon, W. R. and Woodley, D. T. (1985) Epidermolysis bullosa acquisita of the immunopathogical type (dermolytic pemphigoid). *J. Invest. Dermatol.*, **85**, 79s–84s.

Burge, S. M., Fenton, D. A., Dawber, R. P. R. and Leigh, I. M. (1988) Darier's disease: an immunohistochemical study using monoclonal antibodies to human cytokeratins. *Br. J. Dermatol.*, **118**, 629–40.

Bystryn, J. C., Abel, E. and DeFeo, C. (1974) Pemphigus foliaceus. Subcorneal intercellular antibodies of unique specificity. *Arch. Dermatol.*, **110**, 857–61.

Castro, R. M. and Proenca, N. G. (1982) Ahnlichkeiten und Unterschiede zwischen brasilianischem "Fogo selvagem" und Pemphigus foliaceus Cazenave. *Hautarzt*, **33**, 574–7.

Castro, R. M., Roscoe, J. T. and Sampaio, S. A. P. (1983) Brazilian pemphigus foliaceus. *Clinics in Dermatol.*, **1**, 22–41.

Chorzelski, T. P., Jablonska, S., and Blaszczyk, D. M. (1966) Autoantibodies in pemphigus. *Acta. Derm. Venereol.*, **46**, 26.

Chorzelski, T. P. and Jablonska, S. (1979) IgA linear dermatosis of childhood (chronic bullous disease of childhood). *Br. J. Dermatol.*, **101**, 535–42.

de Messias, I. T., von Kluster, L. C., Santamaria, J. and Kajdacsy-Balla, A. (1988) Complement and antibody deposition in Brazilian pemphigus foliaceus and correlation of disease activity with circulating antibodies. *Arch. Dermatol.*, **124**, 1664–8.

DeMento, F. J. and Grover, R. W. (1973) Acantholytic herpetiform dermatitis. *Arch. Dermatol.*, **107**, 883–7.

Dubertret, L., Bertaux, B., Fosse, M. and Touraine, R. (1980) Cellular events leading to blister formation in bullous pemphigoid. *Br. J. Dermatol.*, **104**, 615–24.

Eady, R. A. J., Tidman, M. J., Heagerty, A. H. M. and Kennedy, A. R. (1987) Approaches to the study of epidermolysis bullosa. *Curr. Prob. Derm.*, **17**, 127–41.

Editorial (1988) South American pemphigus foliaceous. *Lancet*, **ii**, 1120.

Egelrud, T. (1986) Dermatitis herpetiformis: selective deposition of immunoglobulin A1 in granular deposits in clinically normal skin. *Acta. Derm. Venereol. (Stockh.)*, **66**, 11–15.

Feller, M. J. and Mark, A. S. (1980) Penicillamine- and ampicillin-induced pemphigus vulgaris. *Int. J. Dermatol.*, **7**, 392–3.

Fine, J.-D., Neises, G. R. and Katz, S. I. (1984) Immunofluorescence and immuno-electron microscopic studies in cicatricial pemphigoid. *J. Invest. Dermatol.*, **82**, 39–43.

Fine, J.-D. (1987) Altered basement membrane antigenicity in epidermolysis bullosa. *Curr. Prob. Derm.*, **17**, 111–26.

Fine, J.-D., Eady, R. A. J., Levy, M. L., Hejtmancik, F., Courtney, K. B., Carpenter, R. J., Holbrook, K. A. and Hawkins, H. K. (1988) Prenatal diagnosis of dominant and recessive dystrophic epidermolysis bullosa: application and limitations in the use of KF-1 and LH 7.2 monoclonal antibodies and immunofluorescence mapping techniques. *J. Invest. Dermatol.*, **91**, 465–71.

Fine, J.-D., Horiguchi, Y., Stein, D. H., Esterly, N. B. and Leigh, I. M. (1990) Intraepidermal type VII collagen. *J. Am. Acad. Dermatol.*, **22**, 188–95.

Gammon, W. R., Heise, E. R., Burke, W. A., Fine, J.-D., Woodley, D. T. and Briggaman, R. A. (1988) Increased frequency of HLA-DR2 in patients with autoantibodies to epidermolysis bullosa acquisita antigen: evidence that the expression of autoimmunity to type VII collagen is HLA class II allele related. *J. Invest. Dermatol.*, **91**, 228–32.

Gange, W., Rhodes, E. L., Edwards, C. O. and Powell, M. E. A. (1976) Pemphigus induced by rifampicin. *Br. J. Dermatol.*, **95**, 445–8.

Goddard, W., Lambert, D., Gavanou, J. and Chapius, J. L. (1980) Pemphigus inquit apres treatment par l'association propanolol-mepbromate. *Ann. Dermatol. Venerol.*, **107**, 1213–16.

Hashimoto, T., Ogawa, M. M., Konohana, A. and Nishikawa, T. (1990) Detection of pemphigus vulgaris and pemphigus foliaceus antigens by immunoblot analysis using different antigen sources. *J. Invest. Dermatol.*, **94**, 327–31.

Heironimus, J. D. and Perry, E. L. (1986) Dermatitis herpetiformis and glomerulonephritis. (1986) Case report and review of the literature. *Am. J. Med.*, **80**, 508–10.

Johnson, T. M., Rapini, R. P., Hebert, A. A., Lowe, L., Verani, R. and Evanoff, G. (1989) Bullous amyloidosis. *Cutis*, **43**, 346–52.

Jordon, R. E., Triftshauser, C. T. and Schroeter, A. L. (1971) Direct immuno-fluorescent studies of pemphigus and bullous pemphigoid. *Arch. Dermatol.*, **103**, 486–91.

Karvonen, J., Ilonen, J., Reunala, T. and Tiilikainen, A. (1984) Autoimmunity in herpes gestationis: inhibition of mixed lymphocyte culture by patient's sera. *Br. J. Dermatol.*, **111**, 183–9.

Kelly, S. E., Bhogal, B. S., Wojnarowska, F. and Black, M. M. (1988) Expression of a pempgigoid gestationis related antigen by human placenta. *Br. J. Dermatol.*, **118**, 605–11.

Kelly, S. E., Black, M. M. and Fleming, S. (1989) Pemphigoid gestationis: a unique mechanism of initiation of an autoimmune response by MHC Class II molecules? *J. Pathol.*, **158**, 81–2.

Laskaris, G., Triantafyllou, A. and Economopoulou, P. (1988) Gingival manifestations of childhood cicatricial pemphigoid. *Oral Surg. Oral Med. Oral Pathol.*, **66**, 349–52.

Lee, C. W., Lim, J. H. and Kang, H. J. (1984) Pemphigus foliaceus induced by rifampicin. *Br. J. Dermatol.*, **111**, 619–22.

Leigh, I. M., Eady, R. A. J., Heagerty, A. H. M., Purkis, P. E., Whitehead, P. A. and Burgeson, R. E. (1988) Type VII collagen is a normal component of epidermal basement membrane, which shows altered expression in recessive dystrophic epidermolysis bullosa. *J. Invest. Dermatol.*, **90**, 639–42.

Lever, W. F. (1965) *Pemphigus and Pemphigoid*, Charles C. Thomas, Springfield, Il.

Lever, W. F. (1983) *Histopathology of the Skin*, 6th edn, J. B. Lippincott, Philadelphia pp. 104–13.

McDonagh, A. J. and Harrington, C. I. (1989) Pseudoporphyria complicating etretinate therapy. *Clin. Exp. Dermatol.*, **14**, 437–8.

Mehregan, D. A., Umbert, I. J. and Peters, M. S. (1989) Histologic findings of Hailey-Hailey disease in a patient with bullous pemphigoid. *J. Am. Acad. Dermatol.*, **21**, 1107–12.

Millikan, L. E. (1987) Vesiculobullous skin disease with prominent immunologic feature. *JAMA*, **258**, 2910–15.

Muller, S. A., Sams, W. M. and Dobson, R. L. (1969) Amyloidosis masquerading as epidermolysis bullosa acquisita. *Arch. Dermatol.*, **99**, 739–47.

Mutasim, D. F., Morrison, L. H., Takahashi, Y., Labib, R. S., Skouge, J., Diaz, L. A. and Anhalt, G. J. (1989) Definition of bullous pemphigoid antibody binding to intracellular and extracellular antigen associated with hemidesmosomes. *J. Invest. Dermatol.*, **92**, 225–30.

Nieboer, C., Boorsma, D. M., Woerdeman, M. J. and Kalsbeek, G. L. (1980) Epidermolysis bullosa aquisita. *Br. J. Dermatol.*, **102**, 383–92.

Parfrey, P. S., Clement, M., Vandenburg, M. J. and Wright, P. (1980) Captopril-induced pemphigus. *Br. Med. J.*, **281**, 194.

Pearson, R. W. (1962) Studies on the pathogenesis of epidermolysis bullosa. *J. Invest. Dermatol.*, **39**, 551–75.

Peters, M. S. and Rogers, R. S. (1989) Clinical correlations of linear IgA deposition at the cutaneous basement membrane zone. *J. Am. Acad. Dermatol.*, **20**, 761–70.

Pothupitiya, G. M., Wojnarowska, F., Bhogal, B. S. and Black, M. M. (1988) Distribution of the antigen in adult linear IgA disease and chronic bullous dermatosis of childhood suggests that it is a single and unique antigen. *Br. J. Dermatol.*, **118**, 175–82.

Rasmussen, H. B., Jepsen, L. V. and Brandrup, F. (1989) Penicillamine-induced bullous pemphigoid with pemphigus-like antibodies. *J. Cutan. Pathol.*, **16**, 154–7.

Robledo, M. A., Prado de, C. S., Jaramillo, D. and Leon, W. (1988) South American pemphigus foliaceus: study of an epidemic in El Bagre and Nechi, Columbia 1982 to 1986. *Br. J. Dermatol.*, **118**, 737–44.

Ruocco, V., Rossi, A., Pisani, M., Astarita, C. and Alviggi, L. (1979) An abortive form of pemphigus vulgaris probably induce by penicillin. *Dermatologica*, **159**, 266–73.

Saurat, J.-H., Didierjean, L., Merot, Y. and Salomon, D. (1988) Blistering skin disease in a man after injections of human placental extracts. *Br. Med. J.*, **297**, 775.

Senear, F. E. and Usher, B. (1926) An unusual type of pemphigus combining features of lupus erythematosus. *Arch. Dermatol.*, **13**, 761–81.

Smith, L. T. and Sybert, V. P. (1990) Intra-epidermal retention of type VII collagen in a patient with recessive dystrophic epidermolysis bullosa. *J. Invest. Dermatol.*, **94**, 261–4.

Silverman, S., Gorsky, M., Lozada-Nur, F. and Liu, A. (1986) Oral mucous membrane pemphigoid. *Oral Surg. Oral Med. Oral Pathol.*, **61**, 233–7.

Stanley, J. R., Hawley-Nelson, P., Yaar, M., Martin, G. R. and Katz, S. I. (1982) Laminin and bullous pemphigoid antigen are distinct basement membrane proteins synthesised by epidermal cells. *J. Invest. Dermatol.*, **78**, 456–9.

Steffen, C. G. (1987) Familial benign chronic pemphigus. *J. Am. Acad. Dermatol.*, **9**, 58–73.

Stone, S. P. and Schroeter, A. L. (1975) Bullous pemphigoid and associated malignant neoplasms. *Arch. Dermatol.*, **111**, 991–4.

Storer, J. S., Galen, W. K., Nesbitt, L. T. and DeLeo, V. A. (1982) Neonatal pemphigus vulgaris. *J. Am. Acad. Dermatol.*, **6**, 929–32.

Troy, J. L., Silvers, D. N., Grossman, M. E. and Jaffe, I. A. (1981) Penicillamine-associated pemphigus: is it really pemphigus? *J. Am. Acad. Dermatol.*, **4**, 547–55.

Unsworth, D. J., Payne, A. W., Leonard, J. N., Fry, L. and Holborrow, E. J. (1982) IgA in dermatitis herpetiformis skin is dimeric. *Lancet*, **ii**, 478–80.

Venning, V. A., Frith, P. A., Bron, A. J., Millard, P. R. and Wojnarowska, F. (1988) Mucosal involvement in bullous and cicatricial pemphigoid. A clinical and immunopathological study. *Br. J. Dermatol.*, **118**, 7–15.

Woodley, D. T., Burgeson, R. E., O'Keefe, E. J., Inman, A. O., Queen, L. L. and Gammon, W. R. (1988) Identification of the skin basement membrane autoantigen in epidermolysis bullosa aquisita. *N. Engl. J. Med.*, **310**, 1007–13.

Yaoita, H., Briggaman, R. A., Lawley, T. J., Provost, T. T. and Katz, S. I. (1981) Epidermolysis bullosa aquisita: ultrastructural and immunological studies. *J. Invest. Dermatol.*, **76**, 288–92.

13 Infective and non-infective granulomas

Dr S. Lucas and Dr N. Kirkham

This chapter describes a number of granulomatous processes, in some of which an infective cause has been identified, such as leprosy and leishmaniasis, and others which remain idiopathic. The description 'granulomatous' has both clinical and pathological connotations, which do not always overlap. Clinically, a granuloma is a reddish, indurated area, usually present for some time. Histologically, this is taken to be a chronic inflammatory process in which the cellular infiltrate contains epithelioid macrophages and variable numbers and types of giant cells. The infiltrate becomes organized or aggregated into granulomas of varying size and shape, varying from the small, discrete epithelioid granulomas of sarcoidosis to the large palisading granulomas seen in necrobiosis lipoidica.

Giant cells form from the fusion of macrophages and take up several different appearances. Foreign-body giant cells are associated with a reaction to foreign material and may even contain particles of the material. Langhans giant cells are found in epithelioid cell granulomas in several conditions, including actinic granuloma and sarcoidosis. Touton giant cells are formed when the stimulus to cell fusion is accompanied by a factor which stimulates lipid uptake, but which is missing in the development of other kinds of giant cell (Alterman *et al.*, 1988).

Granulomas can, therefore, be classified according to their size, appearance, position in the dermis or subcutis, presence or absence of necrosis or necrobiosis in their centres, and the presence or absence of infective organisms or foreign bodies within them. There are, in addition, some conditions which are called by the name but do not show true granulomas histologically. These are varieties of vasculitis and are dealt with in Chapter 14.

13.1   Infective granulomas

13.1.1   *Leprosy*

Leprosy is caused by *Mycobacterium leprae*. The mode of transmission in man is not certain; currently an inhalational route is favoured, but direct infection through the epidermis is by no means excluded. Since the *M. leprae* bacillus is non-toxic, the clinical pathology of leprosy results from the host's cellular reaction to infection (e.g. granulomatous infiltration) and, in heavily infected people, from the space-occupying effect of billions of bacilli in macrophages and nerves in the superficial parts of the body. Only a small minority of those infected with *M. leprae* ever develop lesions of leprosy.

The diagnostic dermatopathology of leprosy may be divided into three aspects: early leprosy, determined leprosy, and leprosy reactions (Ridley 1974, 1985; Lucas and Ridley, 1989). The most critical aspect in evaluating possible leprosy skin pathology is a good technique for staining acid-fast bacilli (AFB): modified Ziehl-Neelsen methods are numerous, and a laboratory should determine which works most consistently. Control slides are essential, but it is advisable not to use a heavily bacillated sample, since even if only 1% of the AFB stain, it will still give the appearance of good positivity.

Indeterminate (early) leprosy

Clinically, the earliest detectable skin lesions are single or a few flat macules, hypopigmented and erythematous, often with reduced sensation. The histology is a mild lymphocytic and histiocytic infiltrate around superficial and deep vessels, nerves and the skin appendages; focal sites of intra-epidermal lymphocytes with spongiosis are common, but marked melanin incontinence is not a feature. The Schwann cells in dermal nerves may have a mild endoneural as well as perineural lymphocytic infiltrate and show hyperplasia (but this is highly subjective). If the clinical features suggest leprosy, this histology is supportive, but not diagnostic unless one or more AFB are found in critical sites. The sites to study are: (1) the Schwann cells of dermal nerves; (2) macrophages around vessels; (3) the upper dermal connective tissue between the epidermis and the superficial vascular plexus. At least five stained sections should be examined before quitting the search. If many AFB are seen, the patient will probably become lepromatous without treatment (q.v.); if few or one are seen, the prognosis is uncertain.

The differential diagnosis of early leprosy is obviously large. Major

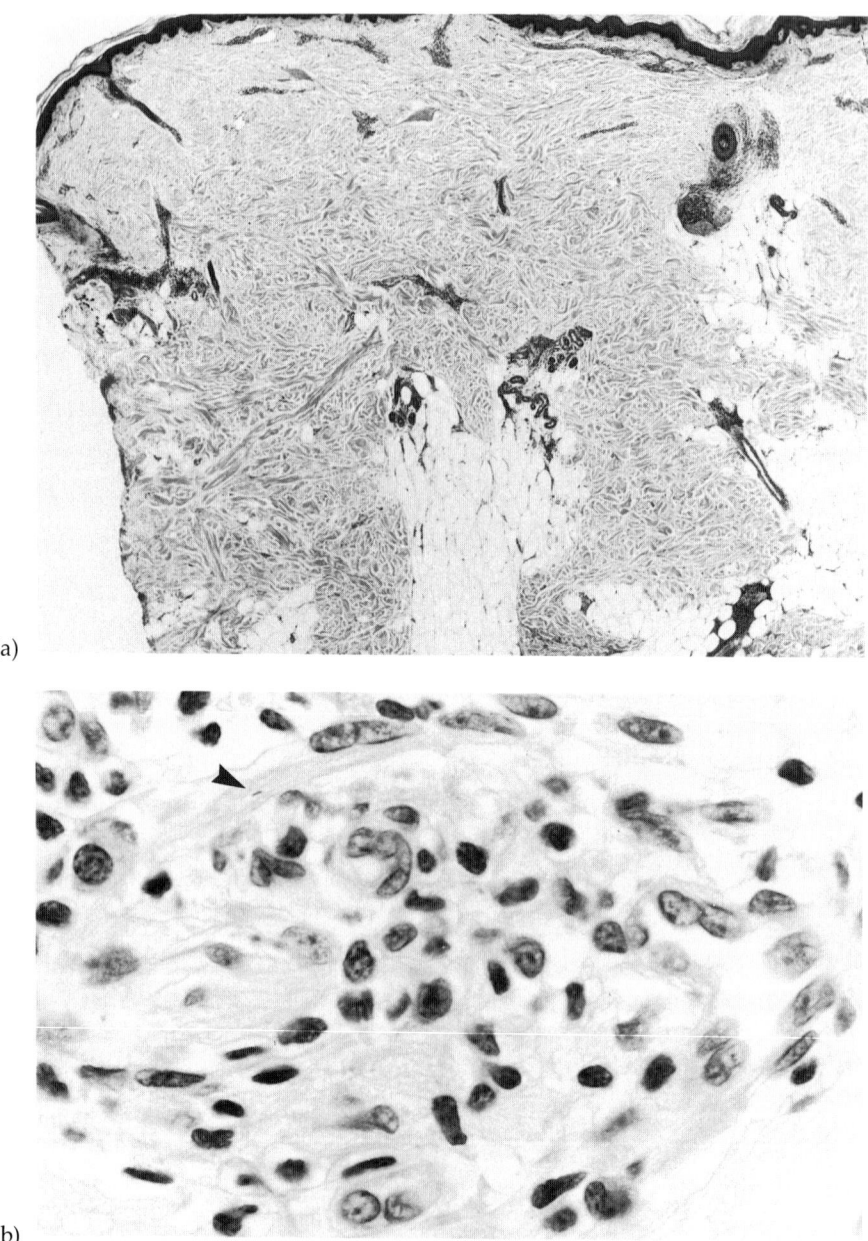

(a)

(b)

Figure 13.1 Indeterminate, early leprosy. (a) Mild lymphocytic infiltrate around skin appendages, vessels and nerves throughout the dermis, and (b) indeterminate, early leprosy. Neurovascular bundle with a single AFB (arrowed) in a Schwann cell (Wade-Fite).

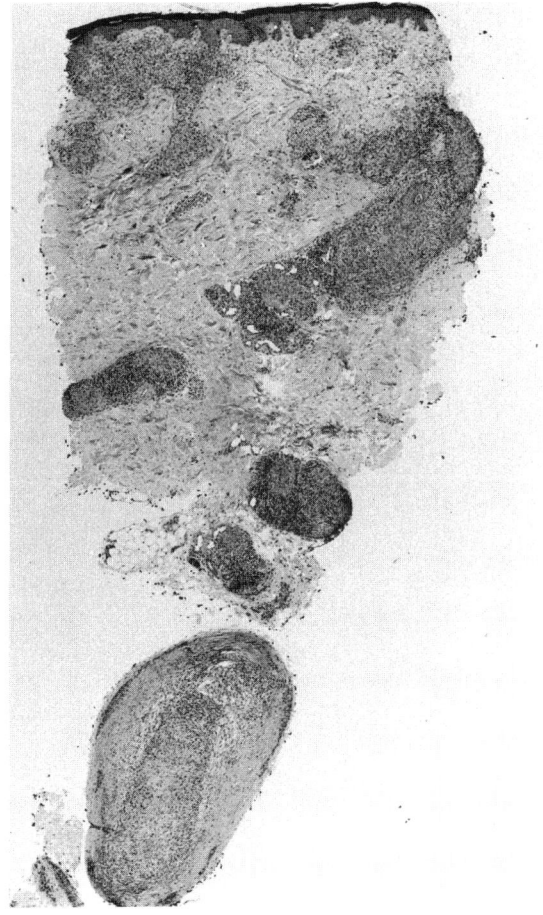

(a)

Figure 13.2   Tuberculoid leprosy. (a) Granulomatous inflammation involving superficial vascular plexus (but not eroding epidermis), and neurovascular bundles throughout the dermis. Not the great expansion of the deep dermal nerve by a granuloma. (b) A deep dermal nerve disrupted by granulomatous infiltrate. The residual Schwann cells and axons are arrowed. (Cont.)

entities to exclude are dermatophytosis, syphilis and drug rashes. If the diagnosis is in doubt, often a superficial cutaneous nerve biopsy will confirm leprosy. Current immunological tests will neither diagnose nor exclude leprosy.

Determined leprosy

If early leprosy does not heal but progresses, two main clinico-pathological patterns emerge: if the patient has cell mediated hypersensitivity

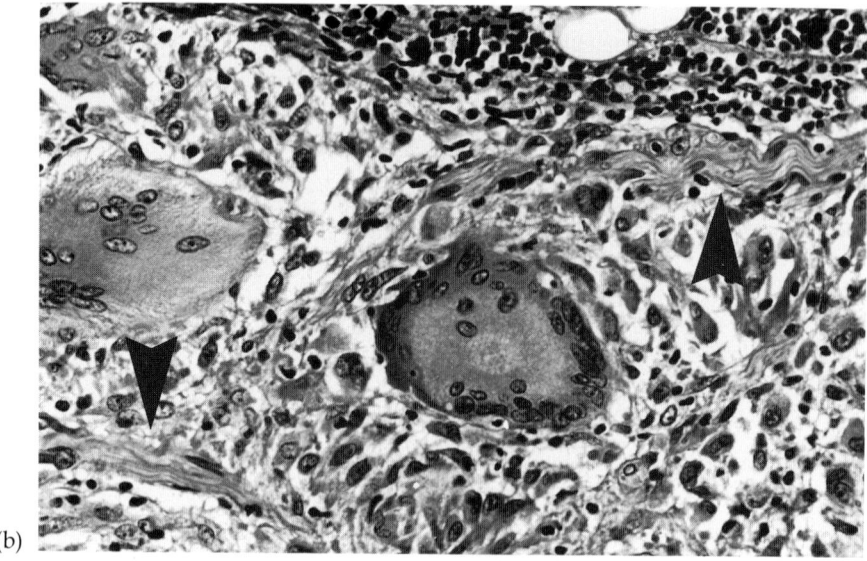

(b)

Figure 13.2 (Cont.)

to *M. leprae* antigens, the lesions are granulomatous and bacilli tend to be scanty; but if there is minimal or no hypersensitivity, epithelioid cell granulomas do not develop and AFB are plentiful within the macrophages, and in Schwann cells of dermal nerves. The first pattern is *tuberculoid* and the second *lepromatous*, but, in reality, these are two poles of a continuous immunopathological spectrum; intermediate positions are described and patients frequently move from one point to another with or without treatment. Outside specialist centres, the precise categorization of leprosy is less important than its basic diagnosis.

(*a*) *Tuberculoid leprosy* This is characterized by epithelioid cell granulomas, with or without Langerhans giant cells, and with variable densities of surrounding lymphocytes. They are seen along neurovascular bundles, in and around sweat glands and erector pili muscle, and around the superficial vascular plexus. This latter inflammation may erode into the epidermis. AFB are absent or scanty; the optimal places to search are within the dermal nerves, the erector pili muscles, and granuloma macrophages. Necrosis is uncommon (Reactions, p. 311).

The differential diagnosis of epithelioid cell granulomas in skin is huge. A crucial aspect for leprosy is, of course, compatibility with the clinical features. Occasionally, AFB will be demonstrated in non-leprosy granulomatous mycobacterioses, but nerves are not specifically involved in them. Whilst many inflammatory conditions produce a mild, lymphocytic infiltrate within the endoneurium of dermal nerves, only in

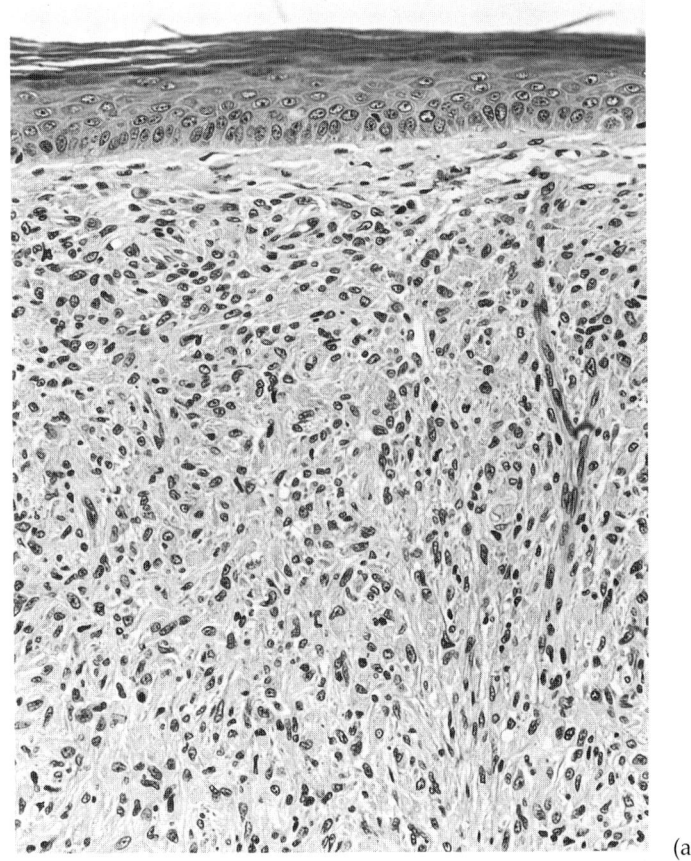

(a)

Figure 13.3   Lepromatous leprosy. (a) Beneath the subepidermal zone, a mass of macrophages, and (b) numerous AFB within the macrophges. (Cont.)

leprosy is granulomatous inflammation to be seen there, with disruption and splaying of the nerve fibres and Schwann cells. Even in the absence of AFB, this feature is diagnostic of tuberculoid leprosy.

(b) *Lepromatous leprosy* is diagnostically straightforward once the possibility is considered, since AFB are plentiful. Macrophages, not organized into granulomas, are located around neurovascular bundles and skin appendages, and this infiltrate progressively expands to fill the dermis. The subepithelial zone is typically clear of inflammation. The macrophages have eosinophilic cytoplasm in the early stages of lepromatous disease, but as mycobacteria accumulate, the cytoplasm becomes more foamy (fatty), and agglomerations of dead and live AFB, staining with haematoxylin, become apparent as globi.

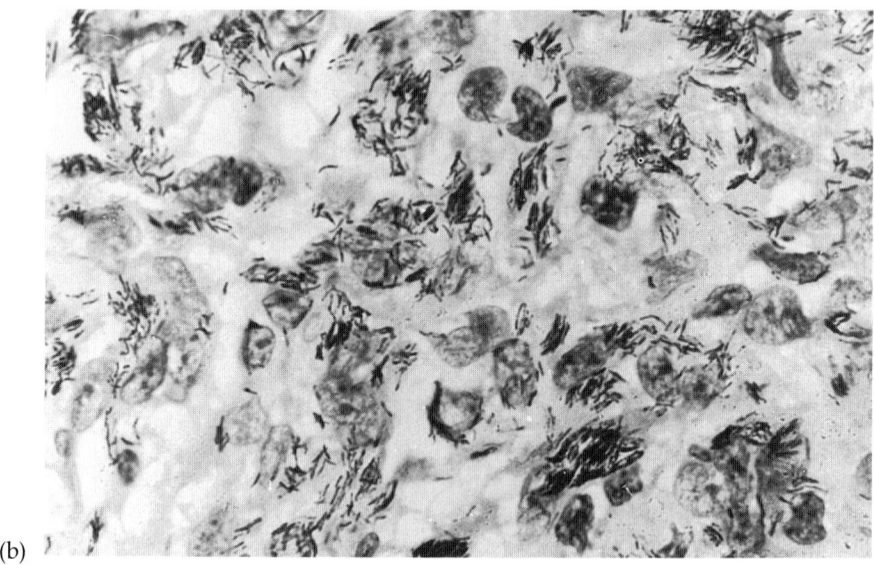

(b)

Figure 13.3   (Cont.)

Plasma cells are usually common in the infiltrate. The density of lymphocytes is variable. In polar lepromatous cases, there are few, but in patients who retain a little hypersensitivity to *M. leprae*, quite large numbers are present amongst the macrophages (known as borderline lepromatous leprosy).

The differential diagnosis of lepromatous leprosy at H and E level is really confined to xanthomas, which do not contain AFB. A histologically similar multibacillary histology is occasionally found in infections with non-leprosy mycobacteria such as *M. avium-intracellulare*; but the AFB will not be seen within nerves and culture will prove a non-leprosy cause. Cases of leprosy that have relapsed may present as exuberant cutaneous nodules with a dermal cellular composition resembling dermatofibroma with a storiform pattern. However, there will be large numbers of AFB; and this hyperactive leproma is known as histoid leprosy. It is important since it signifies possible drug resistance of the infection.

(*c*)   *Borderline leprosy*   The intermediate types of leprosy are termed borderline. Like the polar patterns, they have well-described clinical, histological and immunological (in vitro and skin test) features. Borderline tuberculoid disease is more common than full tuberculoid; it shows smaller Langerhans giant cells and epithelioid cells, and a lesser peri-granuloma cuff of lymphocytes. Mid-borderline leprosy is uncommon since such patients usually become lepromatous without treatment: histologically, it comprises perineurovascular epitheliod cells with a moderate density of AFB (i.e. up to 20 per oil immersion field), poor organization into granulomas, and very scanty lymphocytes.

Leprosy reactions

Reactions in leprosy are acute perturbations in the immune status of the patient, which result in worsening of the lesions. They enlarge, become more erythematous and oedematous, and painful. Two main patterns are recognized:

i.   Reversal (upgrading) reaction. A few borderline tuberculoid patients spontaneously upgrade to full tuberculoid leprosy. About one-third of treated patients from borderline or lepromatous points of the spectrum also demonstrate this reaction. Histologically, the lesions become more tuberculoid (granulomatous) and oedematous. Reversal reactions are the only circumstance where caseous necrosis is seen in leprosy. Usually, it is seen in dermal nerves, which may enlarge to 2 mm or more in diameter; and similar fibrinoid necrosis also occurs within granulomas.

ii. Erythema nodosum leprosum (ENL). This occurs in up to one-half of treated lepromatous patients (and may, occasionally, be a presenting feature of an untreated multibacillary patient). Histologically, it is acute inflammation superimposed on typical lepromatous disease: foamy macrophages with or without globi, polymorphs and oedema are seen. AFB are degenerate, and seen as fragmented and beaded rods. Ulceration and necrotizing vasculitis are features of severe cases. As a practical point, it is worth staining for AFB a dermal infiltrate that manifests foamy macrophages and polymorphs; an undiagnosed leprosy case may be detected.

If multibacillary leprosy is strongly suspected but AFB stains fail to show them, recourse to immunocytochemistry is useful: M. leprae antigens remain for years after the bacteria have disintegrated on treatment, and may be brought out by using a polyclonal antimycobacterial antibody, e.g. to BCG.

13.1.2   Leishmaniasis

Cutaneous leishmaniasis (CL) is a relatively common, imported disease in the UK. It is acquired from the bite of a sandfly found in the

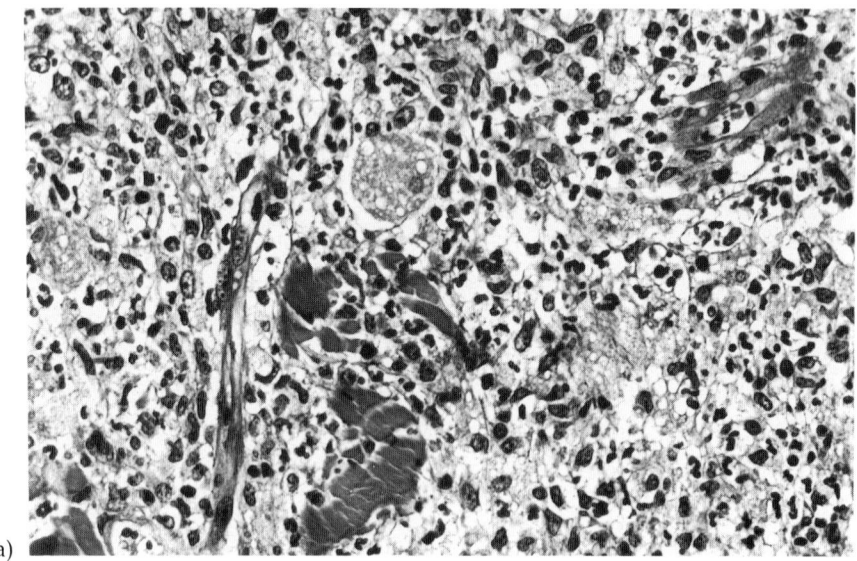

(a)

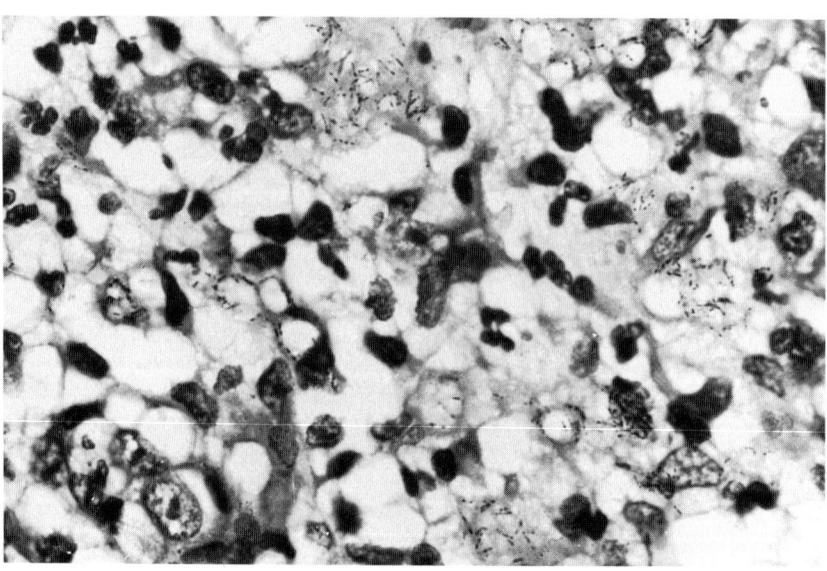

(b)

Figure 13.4 Erythema nodosum leprosum. (a) Foamy macrophages from chronic lepromatous leprosy, with oedema and a diffuse neutrophil polymorph infiltrate. Note the large vacuolated Virchow cell near the centre. (b) Numerous AFB within the macrophages (Wade-Fite).

Mediterranean basin, Middle East, Indian subcontinent, south and central America, and Africa (Ridley and Ridley, 1983).

Infection by many species of the protozoon *Leishmania* result in skin disease; *L. infantum*, which is probably the commonest species identified in the UK, also causes visceral leishmaniasis. In general, most cutaneous cases heal spontaneously, though chemotherapy reduces the time taken and the degree of scarring. Some species spread to mucocutaneous sites after the initial cutaneous lesion, resulting in destructive lesions that may mimic a cancer, e.g. of the nose and nasopharynx.

Under the microscope all *Leishmania* parasites look the same, the species being identified by culture. CL shows a variety of histopathological processes, which may be arranged along an immunological spectrum similar to that of leprosy. Lesions are often multiple. They commence as macrophage accumulations in the dermis containing plentiful intracellular parasites (Leishman-Donovan (LD) bodies). Healing of the lesions occurs by activation of the macrophages and evolution into granulomas, with reduction of the parasite load. Frequently, there is dermal necrosis and ulceration. Plasma cell infiltration is usually dense, and around the foci of macrophage necrosis, epithelioid cell granulomas develop. Dermal fibrosis is prominent. The parasite density drops, and the lesion heals as a non-specific chronic inflammation with scarring.

In practice, CL is usually biopsied in the chronic phase when the aetiology of an ulcerated lesion is unknown. LD bodies are often scanty by then; the sites to search are in the macrophage rim around an ulcer crater, and in granulomas deeper in the dermis. To detect LD bodies, H and E stain is quite adequate: the parasites are 2–4 microns in diameter, with a round haematoxyphilic nucleus, colourless cytoplasm and a rod-shaped haematoxyphilic kinetoplast, though this latter body is often difficult to identify in sections. Immunocytochemistry is not useful in bringing out very small numbers of LD bodies.

In the absence of LD bodies, the histology of CL is similar to that of syphilis, tuberculosis, leprosy, sarcoidosis and silicosis. Confirmation of the diagnosis may come from smears and cultures of a lesion (both of which are more sensitive in detecting parasites than histology) and delayed hypersensitivity skin tests. Obviously, a clinical history of appropriate travel is required.

With the increased numbers of HIV-infected patients with depression of cell-mediated immunity, unusual cases of CL are appearing. Predictably, they tend to be more parasite-laden and less granulomatous than lesions in normal people. Often they may be clinically silent. In a biopsy taken for other reasons, e.g. to diagnose Kaposi's sarcoma,

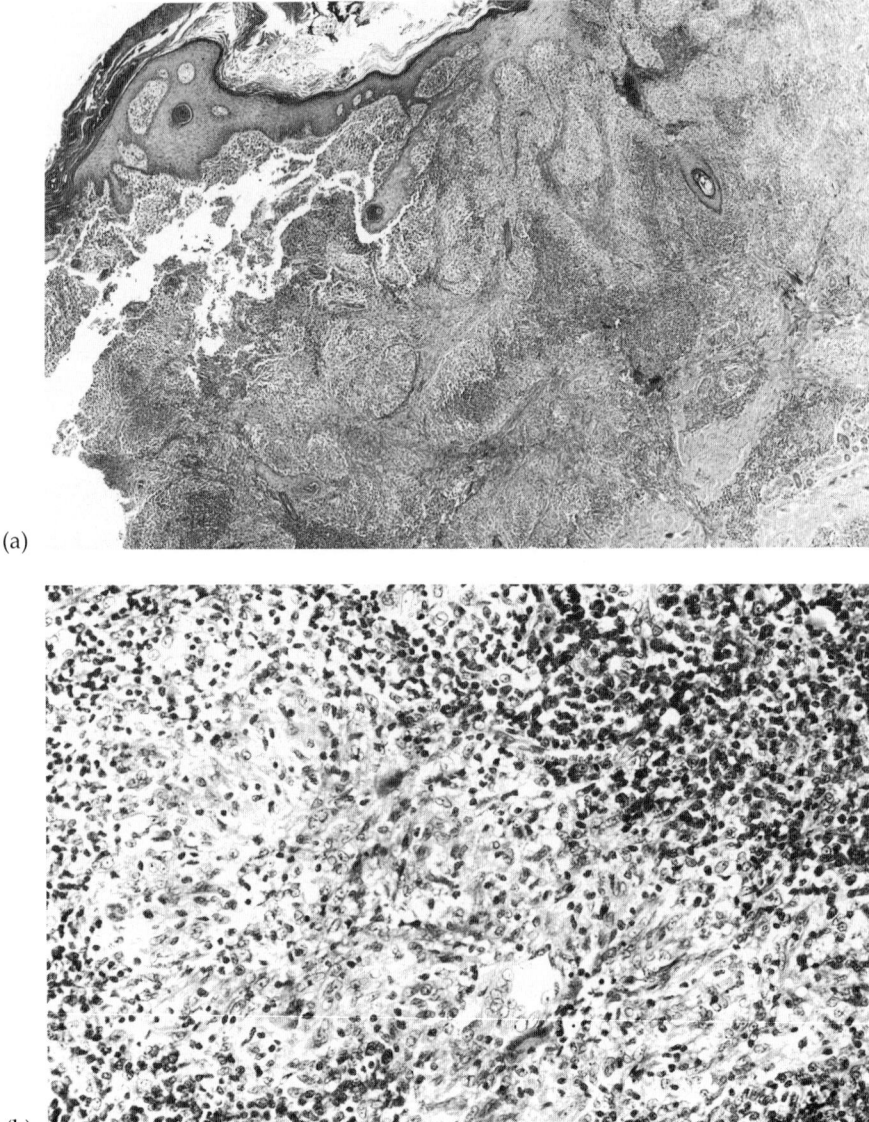

(a)

(b)

Figure 13.5 Cutaneous leishmaniasis. (a) Pandermal granulomas, pseudo-epitheliomatous hyperplasia and ulceration, and (b) typical granuloma with a giant cell and peripheral plasma cells. If no parasites are identified, this appearance is indistinguishable from tuberculosis. (c) Numerous Leishman-Donovan bodies, with colourless cytoplasm, and an eccentric nucleus. Many display the rod-shaped kinetoplast. (Cont.)

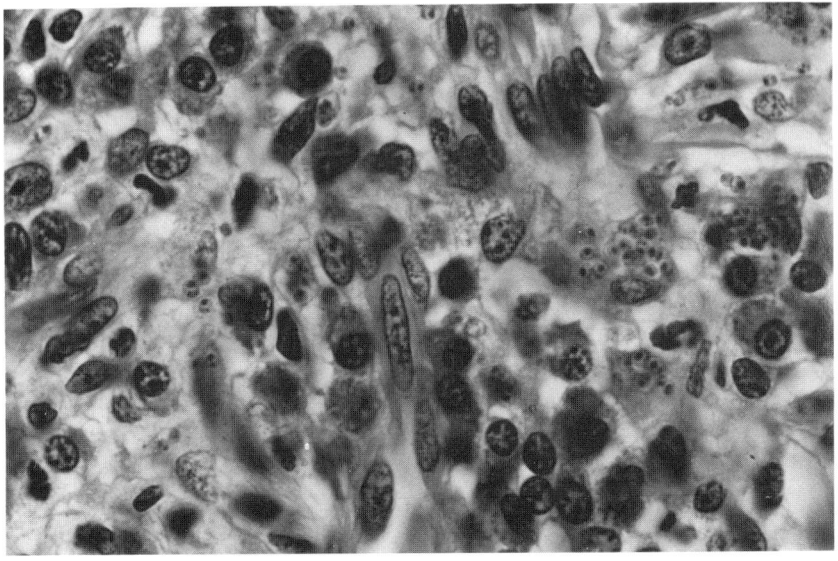

(c)

Figure 13.5   (Cont.)

histology shows a diffuse infiltrate of macrophages containing LD bodies in the dermis.

13.1.3   *Tuberculosis*

Primary cutaneous tuberculosis is relatively rare, but granulomatous lesions are relatively common. They are characterized by granulomas with central caseation and a peripheral rim of lymphocytes, which may lie in the dermis, or may involve the hair follicles. Acid-fast baccili may not be found, so it is always worth culturing part of the fresh biopsy for *M. tuberculosis* and also under appropriate conditions for detection of atypical mycobacteria. If fresh tissue is not available from the initial biopsy and one suspects the diagnosis, then a further biopsy should be taken and submitted for culture (Hruza *et al.*, 1989).

In patients with tuberculosis, the skin biopsy will probably be from skin which has become involved by the underlying inflammation in a lymph node. This may eventually produce a discharging sinus – so-called scrofula.

Atypical mycobacteria get into the skin through minor injuries or abrasions in people who put themselves at risk by undertaking activities such as keeping tropical fish (the fish tank granuloma).

13.1.4   Syphilis

The most likely way for syphilis to present as a biopsy is as an undiagnosed primary chancre or, occasionally, as a lesion of secondary disease. Plasma cells in the dermis are usually held to be indicative of the diagnosis; indeed, they are certainly unusual in the majority of dermal infiltrates. Monoclonal antibodies to spirochaetes are now available and provide an excellent way of identifying the large number of organisms which may be present amongst the plasma cells. In secondary syphylis it is common to find small perivascular naked granulomas, together with plasma cells and overlying epidermal hyperplasia.

13.1.5   Fungal granulomas

In any undiagnosed granulomatous reaction in the dermis or subcutis, it is mandatory to perform a stain for fungi; the authors use Grocott's silver stain, whilst others prefer a PAS stain. Fungi can sometimes be seen on the H and E or AOG stained sections as well.

13.1.6   Fish tank granuloma

Tropical fish can become infected with *Mycobacterium marinum*, which causes a chronic infection that can take up to a year to kill the fish. During that time, organisms will be present not only in the fish but in the water, the sand and on the walls of the tank in which they are kept. Aquarists are at risk of becoming infected if they have open cuts or grazes on their hands or arms when maintaining the inside of the tank. The lesions take the form of necrotizing epithelioid granulomas, which may be solitary at the site of primary infection, or multiple with sporotrichoid spread along lymphatics in the arm.

It may be possible to see acid-fast bacilli in biopsy, but more often than not they will be difficult if not impossible to find. Samples of skin must be cultured at 30°C to confirm the diagnosis (Gray *et al.*, 1990).

13.1.7   Cutaneous toxoplasmosis

Toxoplasmosis, caused by infection with the protozoan *Toxoplasma gondii*, is a familiar cause of painful cervical lymphadenopathy. Occasionally, the skin can become involved. Biopsy of developed papulonodular lesions may show changes similar to those found in lymph nodes. There is a background of lymphoid hyperplasia, within which small epithelioid cell granulomas will be present. The diagnosis can be confirmed by by serological studies (Binazzi, 1986a, b).

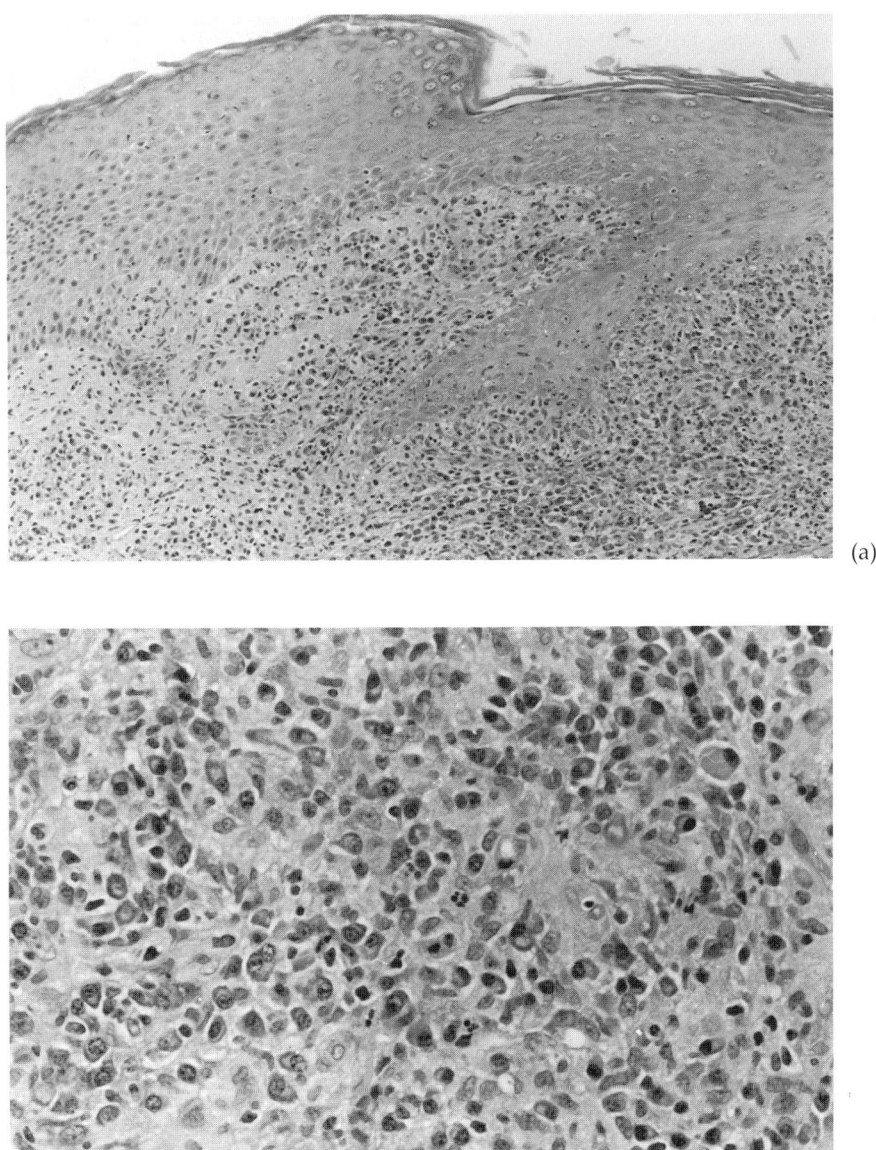
(a)

(b)

Figure 13.6 Syphilitic chancre containing many plasma cells (a and b). This lesion contained vast numbers of spirochetes.

13.2 Non-infective granulomas

13.2.1 Sarcoidosis

The diagnosis of sarcoidosis depends on the clinical and radiologic features, as well as the demonstration in a skin biopsy of the smaller lesions seen in erythrodermic sarcoidosis of multiple, small, discrete, non-caseating granulomas in the dermis, without a prominent rim of lymphocytes. Larger lesions may show the changes of erythema nodosum, and papular lesions may show granulomas throughout the dermis and extend into subcutaneous fat.

A Kveim test may be performed to confirm the diagnosis and these biopsies must, of course, be sectioned at multiple levels before concluding that no granulomas can be found.

The amount of histopathological support needed varies inversely with the confidence with which the pattern of clinical features is recognized. It is essential to exclude other recognized causes of granulomatous disease. A chest X-ray is the easiest way of confirming the diagnosis, although as many as 15% of patients will have a normal film (Jordan et al., 1988).

13.2.2 Crohn's disease

The granulomatous inflammation of Crohn's disease may extend beyond the bowel and manifest as cutaneous lesions: either in the dermis or subcutis. The lesions may show marked necrobiotic changes at the centre of the granulomas (Billings et al., 1986; Sutphen et al., 1984). In addition, purely neutrophilic lesions of Sweet's syndrome may also occur (Kemmett et al., 1988).

13.2.3 Erythema nodosum

Athough considered here, this condition is predominantly a septal panniculitis and represents an inflammatory reaction pattern that is the result of many different causes. It is illustrated in Figures 16.3 to 16.5. It is essential to have a deep biopsy as the changes in the dermis may be relatively mild and non-specific. It has a different pathogenetic mechanism from erythema multiforme (Soderstrom and Krull, 1978).

13.2.4 Granuloma annulare

Granuloma annulare is well named. In a typical biopsy there will be an annular palisade of macrophages, often not very numerous, around a focus of altered collagen which will be weakly haematoxophilic. This

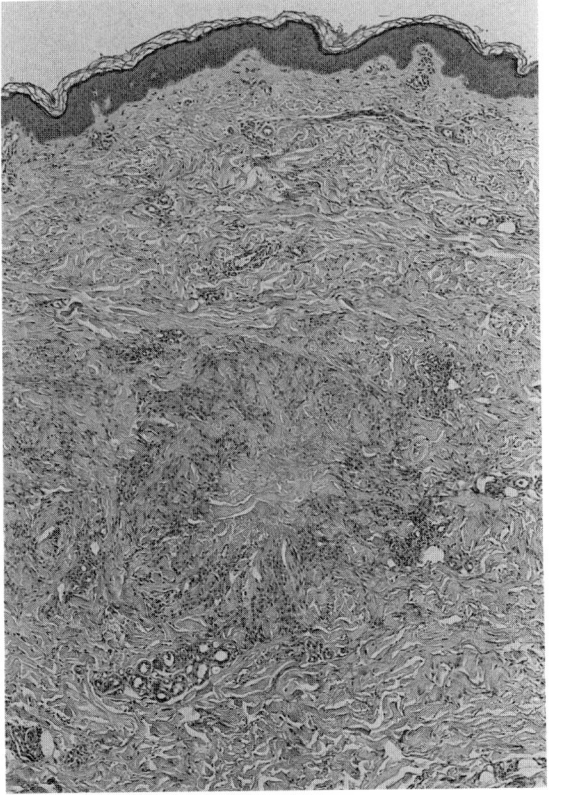

(a)

Figure 13.7   Granuloma annulare (a and b). A small dermal palisaded granuloma with necrobiotic change in the dermis at the centre of the granuloma. (Cont.)

change has sometimes been called collagen necrosis but, of course, collagen cannot undergo necrosis because it is extracellular. Often, biopsies will not be deep enough to include the whole granuloma, or the epithelioid cells may be sparse, making the diagnosis a little more tricky. In case of difficulty, a deeper level or AOG stain will usually assist.

The condition is benign and usually limited to the distal extremities, although generalized, perforating and subcutaneous variants have been described. The pathogenesis remains uncertain, but possibly represents a delayed type hypersensitivity reaction or a response to vascular injury (Muhlbauer, 1980; Dahl *et al.*, 1977). Giant cells may contain phagocytosed elastic material, suggesting that degenerating elastic may promote the granulomatous reaction (Friedman-Birnbaum *et al.*, 1989).

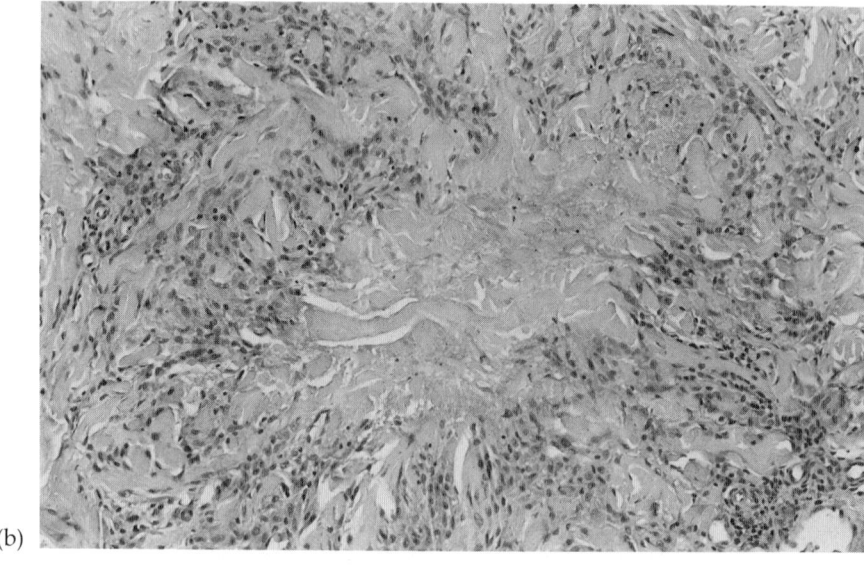

(b)

Figure 13.7   (Cont.)

A related form of dermal granuloma with phagocytosis of elastic fibres has been reported in a 13-year-old girl who had annular erythematous lesions, with central atrophic areas, on the trunk and limbs. These lesions regressed after intradermal injection of corticosteroids (Boneschi et al., 1988).

The subcutaneous lesions of granuloma annulare can occur in otherwise healthy young people, who do not subsequently develop arthritis (Rubin and Lynch, 1966), but the lesions may be confused with the palisading subcutaneous granulomas associated with rheumatoid arthritis. The necrobiotic collagen at the centre of the granulomas is more likely to stain positively for acid mucin with an Alcian blue stain, and to be more palely eosinophilic than in a rheumatoid nodule. On the other hand, rheumatoid lesions are more likely to contain giant cells, show significant stromal fibrosis and stain more strongly and homogeneously with eosin and negatively with Alcian blue (Patterson, 1988).

13.2.5   Necrobiosis lipoidica

There is some doubt about whether granuloma annulare and necrobiosis lipoidica represent truly distinct entities, or merely ends of a spectrum. The latter is probably the truth. The usual description of a lesion is of a large, deep dermal palisaded granuloma, in contrast to the usual description of granuloma annulare as smaller, more superficial and sometimes multiple granulomas.

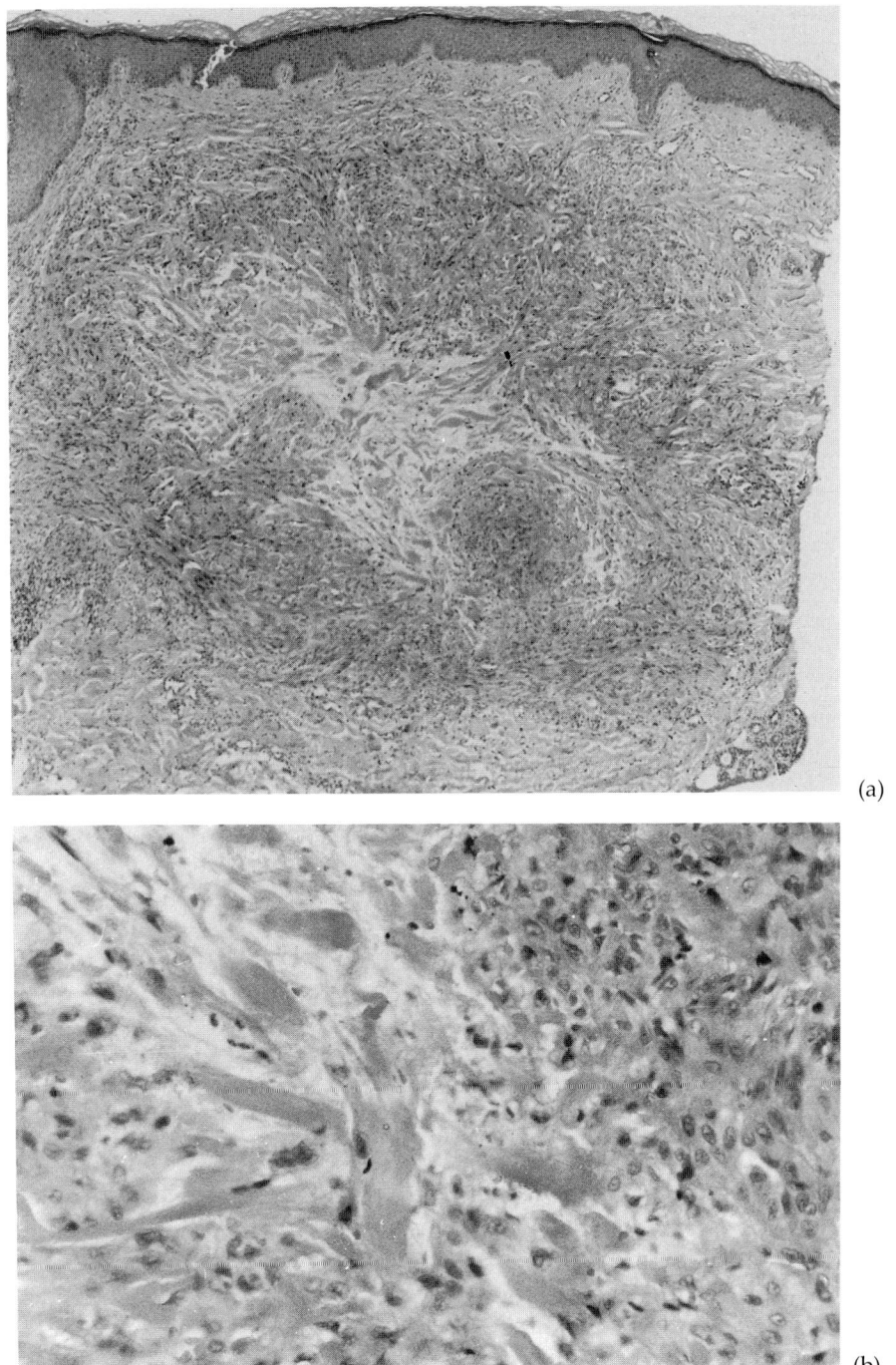

(a)

(b)

Figure 13.8 Granuloma annulare. (a) A large lesion, showing (b) necrobiotic change of collagen in the granuloma.

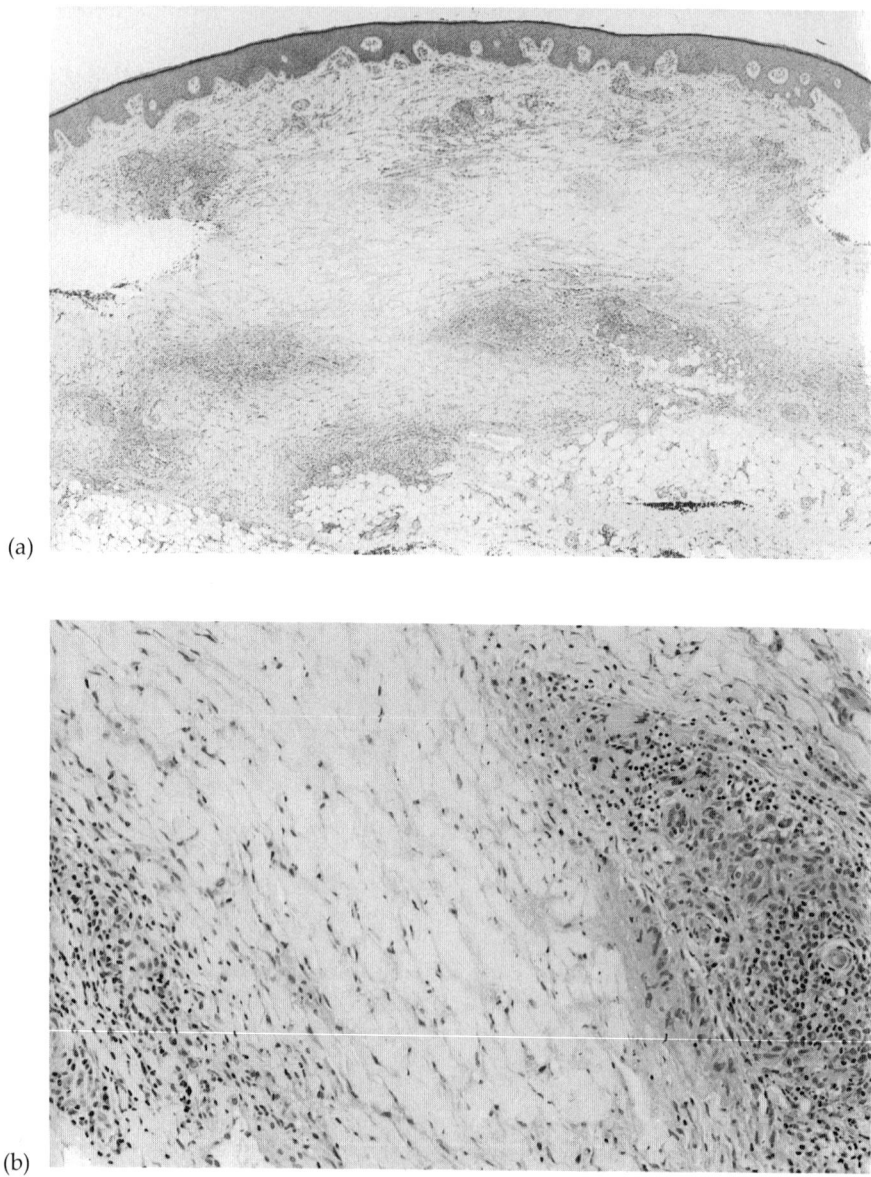

(a)

(b)

Figure 13.9 Necrobiosis lipoidica (a and b). A large, extensive granuloma with extension through the full thickness of the dermis.

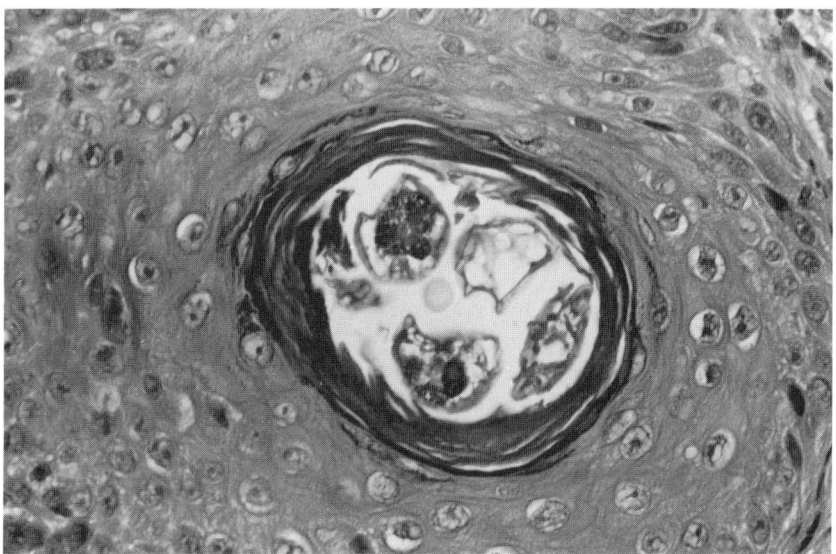

Figure 13.10   Demodex within a hair follicle.

13.2.6   Foreign body granuloma

All sorts of foreign bodies can find their way into the dermis, but amongst the commonest are pieces of suture material, bits of biting insects, splinters of all kinds and keratin from ruptured epidermal cysts. The diagnosis is usually fairly obvious, but it is worth remembering to polarize the section to look for refractile material, which may be present in significant amounts but may be inapparent on the H and E stained section.

13.2.7   Acne agminata

This condition is characterized by multiple small papules, sometimes with purulent, necrotic centres, on the face and sometimes involving the eyelids. The dermis contains well-formed discreet granulomas, with the larger ones showing central caseation. Many of them will be related to pilosebaceous follicles. Some follicles may be seen to be disintegrating. Further investigations to find foreign material, bacteria or fungi will be uniformly negative. Sometimes *Demodex folliculorum* will be found in the follicles, but it seems unlikely that they are the cause of this process (Ecker and Winkelmann, 1979).

   The granulomas may heal within 1 to 2 years, with secondary scarring. The condition is associated with acne rosacea, which about half of

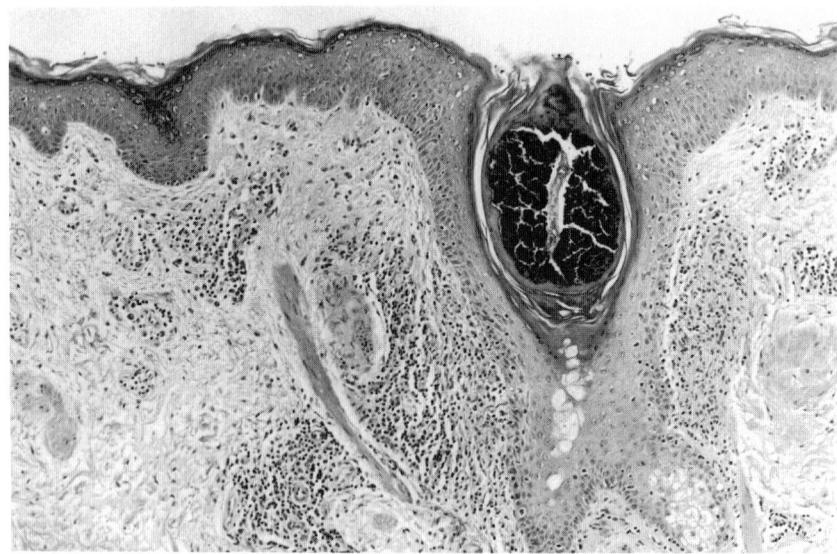

Figure 13.11   Acne agminata. Demodex in a dilated follicle, with a granuloma in the adjacent dermis.

the cases go on to develop (Scott and Calnan, 1967; Mullanex and Kierland, 1970).

13.2.8   Acne rosacea

Rosacea is a relatively common but ill-defined and poorly studied disease, which represents a progression from acne agminata and is usually thought of as a granulomatous process, with granulomas associated with Demodex-bearing hair follicles. This may not be exactly the case. Biopsies usually show elastosis and varying degrees of vasodilatation and lympho-histiocytic infiltration. Sometimes there may be neutrophils around skin appendages, tuberculoid granulomas unrelated to appendages or, rarely, tuberculoid granulomas surrounding follicle-related necrosis.

It has been postulated that *D. folliculorum* is involved in the pathogenesis of rosacea, notably in its granulomatous form, when the acarid may be seen at the centre of the granuloma, but it is also possible that the granulomas result from the destruction and resorption of hair follicles secondary to the dermal inflammation, with the mite being digested more slowly than follicular epithelium (Ramelet and Perroulaz, 1988).

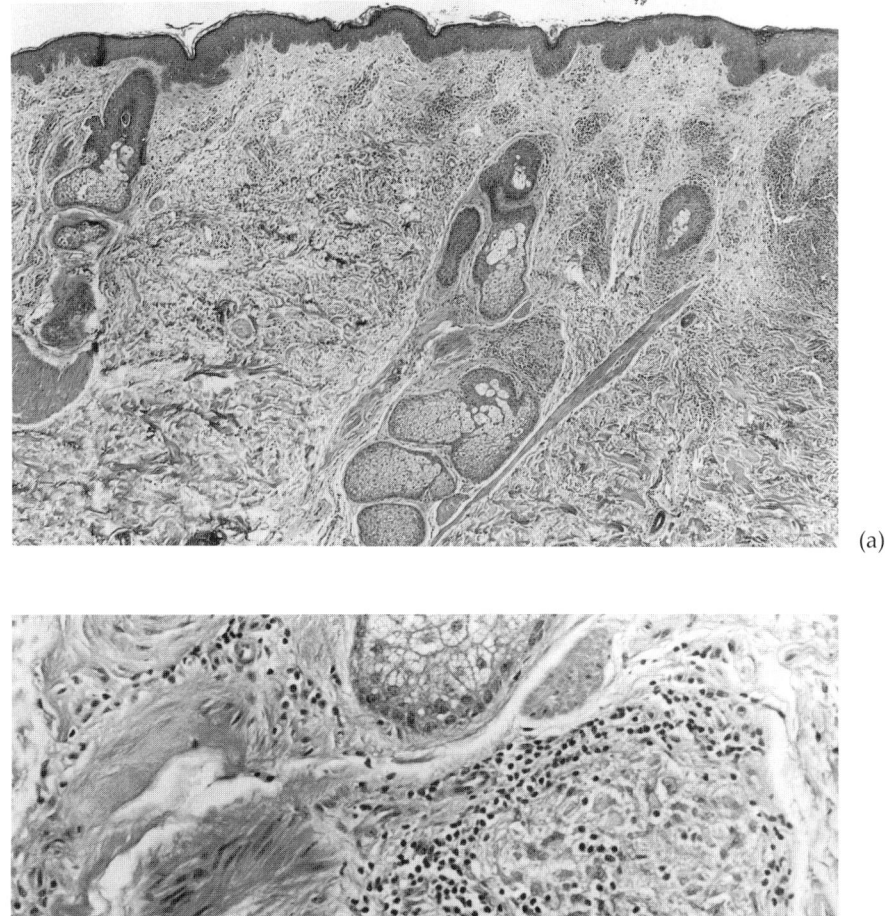

Figure 13.12 (a) Acne agminata showing (b) perifollicular granuloma.

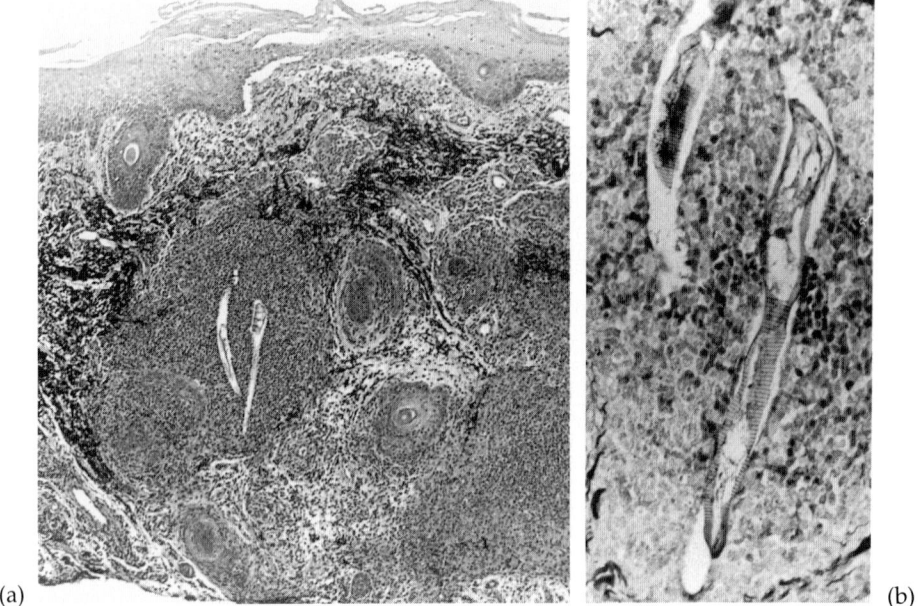

(a)   (b)

Figure 13.13   (a) Extensive granulomatous dermatitis with Demodex at the centre of one lymphoid nodule. (b) The Demodex have a characteristic muscle-like striation.

13.2.9   *Actinic granuloma*

In chronicly sun-damaged skin, a granulomatous reaction to weakly antigenic determinants on altered elastic fibres can occur (McGrae, 1986). This may take the form of epithelioid granulomas in the papillary dermis. A lympho-histiocytic infiltrate around dermal venules is also usually present, in which mast cells may be numerous. It is possible that mediators released by the mast cells lead to the breakdown of collagen and elastic fibres and contribute to the development of the lesions (Lavker and Kligman, 1988).

The description 'chronic heliodermatitis' has been proposed for this condition, which probably represents the underlying lesion of 'redneck': the chronic change seen in the skin of whites subject to chronic sun exposure.

References

Alterman, K., Remmele, W. and Smith, M. (1988) Karl Touton and his "xanthelasmic giant cell". A selective review of multinucleated giant cells. *Am. J. Dermatopathol.*, **10**, 257–69.
Billings, J. K., Ellis, C. N. and Milgraum, S. S. (1986) Cutaneous granuloma

formations in Crohn's disease. *JAMA*, **255**, 2661.

Binazzi, M. (1986a) Profile of cutaneous Toxoplasmosis. *Int. J. Dermatol.*, **25**, 357–63.

Binazzi, M. (1986b) Historical aspects of cutaneous Toxoplasmosis. *Int. J. Dermatol.*, **25**, 401–4.

Boneschi, V., Brambilla, L., Fossati, S., Parini, F. and Alessi, E. (1988) Annular elastolytic giant cell granuloma. *Am. J. Dermatopathol.*, **10**, 224–8.

Dahl, M. V., Ullman, S. and Goltz, R. W. (1977) Vasculitis in granuloma annulare. *Arch. Dermatol.*, **113**, 463–7.

Ecker, R. I. and Winkelmann, R. K. (1979) Demodex granuloma. *Arch. Dermatol.*, **115**, 343–4.

Friedman-Birnbaum, R., Weltfriend, S., Kerner, H. and Lichtig, C. (1989) Elastic tissue changes in generalized granuloma annulare. *Am. J. Dermatopathol.* **11**, 429–33.

Gray, S. F., Smith, R. S., Reynolds, N. J. and Williams, E. W. (1990) Fish tank granuloma. *Br. Med. J.*, **300**, 1069–70.

Hruza, G. J., Posnick, R. B. and Weltman, R. E. (1989) Disseminated lupus vulgaris presenting as granulomatous folliculitis. *Int. J. Dermatol.*, **28**, 388–92.

Jordan, D. R., Anderson, R. L., Nerad, J. A. and Scrafford, D. B. (1988) The diagnosis of sarcoidosis. *Can. J. Ophthalmol.*, **23**, 203–7.

Kemmett, D., Gawkrodger, D. J., Wilson, G. and Hunter, J. A. A. (1988) Sweet's syndrome in Crohn's disease. *Br. Med. J.*, **297**, 1513–14.

Lavker, R. M. and Kligman, A. M. (1988) Chronic heliodermatitis: a morphologic evaluation of chronic actinic dermal damage with emphasis on the role of mast cells. *J. Invest. Dermatol.*, **90**, 325–30.

Lucas, S. and Ridley, D. S. (1989) The uses of histopathology in leprosy diagnosis and research (editorial). *Lepr. Rev.*, **60**, 257–62.

McGrae, J. D. Jr (1986) Actinic granuloma. A clinical, histopathologic, and immunocytochemical study. *Arch. Dermatol.*, **122**, 43–7.

Muhlbauer, J. E. (1980) Granuloma annulare. *J. Am. Acad. Dermatol.*, **3**, 217–30.

Mullanex, M. G. and Kierland, R. R. (1970) Granulomatous rosacea. *Arch. Dermatol.*, **101**, 206–11.

Patterson, J. W. (1988) Rheumatoid nodule and subcutaneous granuloma annulare. A comparative histologic study. *J. Am. Acad. Dermatol.*, **10**, 1–8.

Ramelet, A. A. and Perroulaz, G. (1988) [Rosacea: histopathologic study of 75 cases]. *Ann. Dermatol. Venereol.*, **115**, 801–6.

Ridley, D. S. (1974) Histological classification and the immunological spectrum of leprosy. *Bull. WHO*, **51**, 451–65.

Ridley, D. S. and Ridley, M. W. (1983) The evolution of the lesion in cutaneous leishmaniasis. *J. Pathol.*, **141**, 83–96.

Ridley, D. S. (1985) *Skin Biopsy in Leprosy*, 2nd edn, Documenta Giegy, Basel.

Rubin, M. and Lynch, F. W. (1966) Subcutaneous granuloma annulare. Arch. Dermatol., **98**, 416–20.

Scott, K. W. and Calnan, C. D. (1967) Acne agminata. Trans. St John's Hosp. Dermatol. Soc., **53**, 60–9.

Sutphen, J. L., Cooper, P. H., Mackel, S. E. and Nelson, D. L. (1984) Metastatic cutaneous Crohn's disease. *Gastroenterology*, **86**, 941–4.

Soderstrom, R. M. and Krull, E. A. (1978) Erythema nodosum: a review. *Cutis*, **21**, 806–10.

14 The skin and AIDS

The last decade has been overshadowed by the arrival of the acquired immunodeficiency syndrome (AIDS). At the time of writing, this remains an unremittingly fatal disease. Kaposi's sarcoma is well recognized as a cutaneous complication of the disease, but there is an important and continuing role for skin biopsy in AIDS. Many causes can be found for the lumps and bumps which may arise: they are not all due to Kaposi's sarcoma and many are amenable to treatment (Cockerell and Friedman-Kien, 1989; Cockerell, 1989). All is not always what it seems, e.g. although molluscum contagiosum is relatively common in AIDS cutaneous cryptococcosis can simulate it (Rico and Penneys, 1985). As ever, close liaison between laboratory and clinic is essential. Improvements are increasingly being made in the symptomatic management of the various infections which occur, with consequent improvement in quality, if not in quantity, of life.

A previous generation of doctors were told that to know medicine they should know syphilis in all of its manifestations. A similar case could be made today for AIDS. Every post seem to bring some new development of understanding or some previously unrecognized complication. A survey from Lusaka, Zambia, showed that 98.3% of individuals with AIDS and 53.6% of those with AIDS-related complex had one or more skin lesions. These included Kaposi's sarcoma, necrotic herpes zoster, seborrhoeic dermatitis and pruritic maculopapular rashes. Infections included candidiasis, severe genital herpes, extensive molluscum contagiosum, and tinea corporis. Drug reactions were also common, including the Stevens-Johnson syndrome following therapy with streptomycin, thiacetazone, and rifampicin for pulmonary tuberculosis (Hira et al., 1988). Even in apparently normal skin the tubuloreticular inclusions associated with human immunodeficiency virus (HIV) infection can be found in endothelial cells (Pedersen et al., 1989).

It also seems possible that there may also be an increase in melanomas. Cases of eruptive dysplastic naevi have certainly been identified (Duvic et al., 1989).

14.1   Kaposi's sarcoma

The curious appearance of disseminated Kaposi's sarcoma in young homosexual men was one of the earliest intimations of the arrival of AIDS (Gottlieb and Ackerman, 1982). The lesions which are seen in various contexts, such as idiopathic cases in Europe, in Africa and those seen in persons with AIDS are morphologically identical (Templeton, 1981; Leu and Odermatt, 1985). The biopsy appearances depend upon the stage of development of the lesion, which progress from the early patch stage through to a fully developed nodular tumour. The earliest lesions may show quite subtle changes but, irrespective of size, all contain a combination of vascular proliferation, stromal cell proliferation, stromal haemorrhage and haemosiderin deposition (Francis et al., 1986).

The macroscopic appearance of the unfixed biopsy is quite characteristic: the lesion can be seen as a red-pink, circumscribed flush, different to the dark red of a haemangioma or the brown-black of a naevus or melanoma. The vascular proliferation takes two forms which can be summarized as dermal dissection and perivascular proliferation.

Around what are probably pre-existing vascular bundles, thin-walled ectatic vessels predominate. These are often very closely applied to each other without much in the way of intervening stroma: the so-called 'back-to-back' appearance. The reticular dermis, on the other hand, shows a varying degree of dissection of collagen bundles by spindle cells, which form small vascular spaces whose presence is often only given away by the red cells within them. This feature corresponds to the flushed macroscopic appearance of the tumours. As the tumour invades the dermis, pre-existing collagen is broken down and new collagen is laid down by the advancing tumour (Becker et al., 1987).

Some of the blood becomes extravasated and broken down, with the resulting development of haemosiderin granules. This alone is a worrying finding in a skin biopsy, as even in purpura haemosiderin it is not a common feature. Acroangiodermatitis is usually related to venous insufficiency of the lower limbs, but may mimic some of the features of Kaposi's sarcoma, both clinically and pathologically (Strutton and Weedon, 1987).

The second component of the lesions is the variable number of stromal spindle cells. The number of spindle cells is related to the size of the lesion: there are few in a patch, whilst they constitute a large part of a nodule. Irrespective of the size of the tumour, a small number of mitoses are likely to be found.

Immunohistochemical studies have been used to try and resolve the argument about whether the vascular proliferation is of blood vessel or lymphatic origin, using comparative staining with antibodies to markers

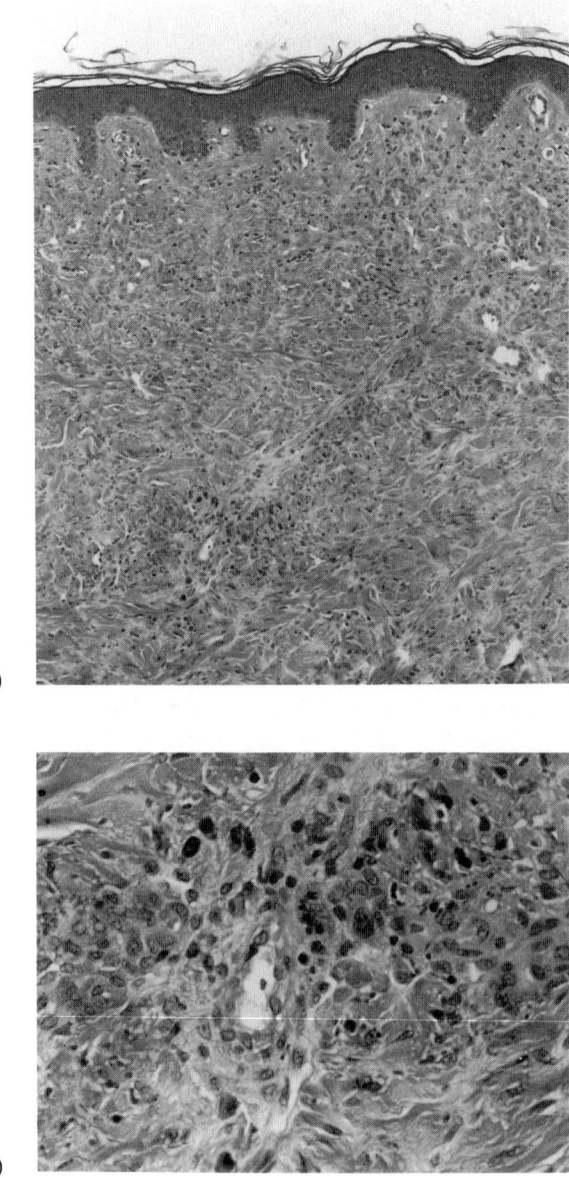

(a)

(b)

Figure 14.1 Kaposi's sarcoma (a and b). An early lesion with sparse cellularity.

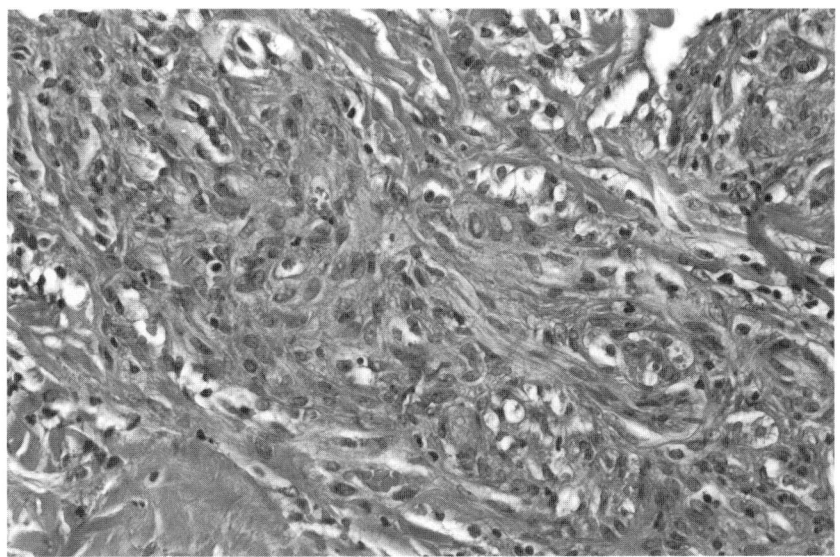

Figure 14.2 Kaposi's sarcoma. Spindle cell proliferation in the dermis.

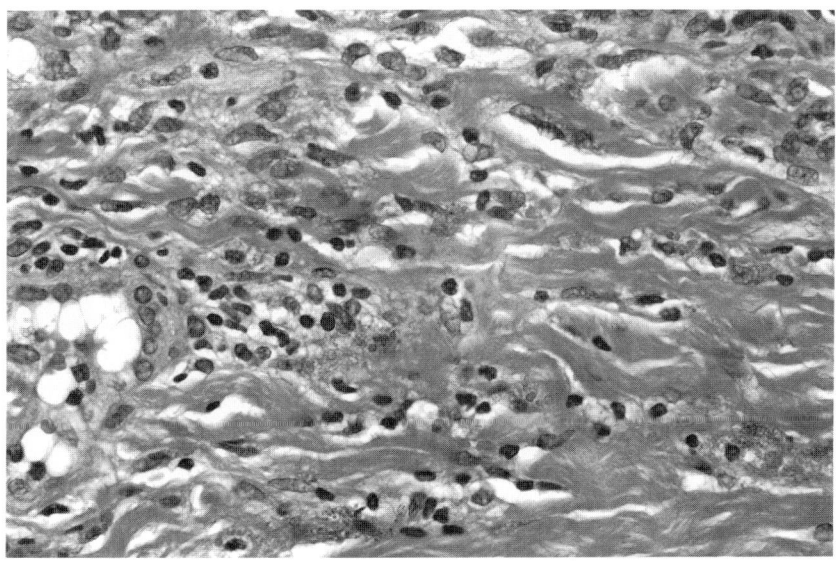

Figure 14.3 Kaposi's sarcoma. Dissection of dermal collagen bundles with occasional granules of haemosiderin present.

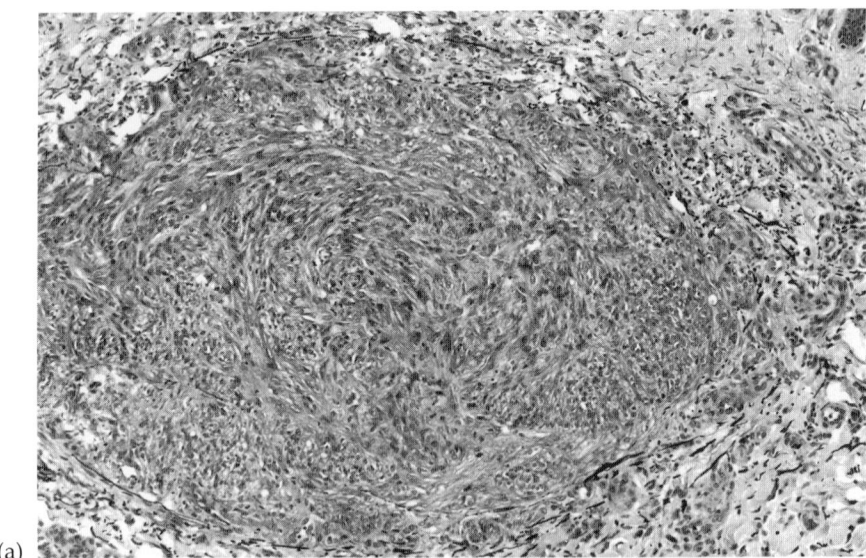

(a)

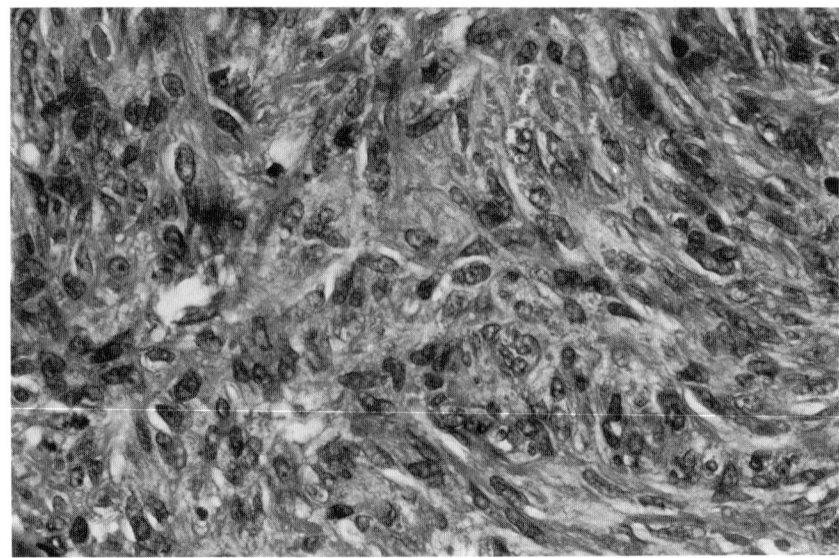

(b)

Figure 14.4 Kaposi's sarcoma (a and b). Nodular lesion with tumerous proliferation of spindle cells.

such as factor VIII-related antigen and *Ulex europeus* (Ordonez and Batsakis, 1984). These studies have failed to resolve the question, although other monoclonal antibody studies point towards an origin from vascular endothelium (Scully *et al.*, 1988). The spindle cells show factor XIIIa immunoreactivity: a marker of dermal dendrocytes, which are a component of the reticulo-endothelial system (Nickloff and Griffiths, 1989). Vimentin can be used as a non-specific mesenchymal marker of all of the cells in the lesions.

This puzzling condition has undergone a considerable reappraisal in recent years, because of its association with AIDS. It is found in up to 50% of AIDS patients, either before or after death, but whilst it is well recognized in homosexuals with HIV infection, it is rarely seen in haemophiliacs who have gained their infection by transfusion. In homosexuals, the development of the lesions of Kaposi's sarcoma usually presages the further deterioration of the patient, with death often no more than 6 months away.

The relationship with HIV infections remains unclear. At the time of writing, no HIV genes or gene products have been found in Kaposi lesions. On the other hand, the incorporation of one of the nine known HIV genes into the genome of mice resulted in the development of Kaposi-like lesions in some of the male animals (Vogel *et al.*, 1988). Similar lesions have also been induced in nude mice after long-term culture of tumour cells: in this system, the tumours appear to be caused by growth-stimulating factors (Salahuddin *et al.*, 1988). The Tat protein of HIV-1 is a candidate for this role, and does appear to stimulate growth in cells derived from lesions of Kaposi's sarcoma (Ensoli *et al.*, 1990).

The epidemiological evidence is very strongly in favour of a sexually transmitted infection. In the USA, Kaposi's sarcoma is 20000 times commoner in persons with AIDS than in the general population. Furthermore, amongst those with AIDS it has been suggested that it is commoner in those who acquired the infection sexually, although this may be a statistical artefact and the prevalence may be the same in both sexually and transfusion acquired disease (Couturier *et al.*, 1990). There remains the possibility of an unidentified infectious agent as the cause (Beral *et al.*, 1990). This may be a retrovirus. Avian haemangiomatosis is a similar condition from a histological point of view, and has been shown to be due to a retrovirus of the avian leukosis group (Dictor and Jarplid, 1988).

14.2 Bacillary angiomatosis

More recently, there have been reports of a further complication of HIV infection, known variously as bacillary angiomatosis, epithelioid angiomatosis and bacillary ailuronosis (Cockerell *et al.*, 1987; Knobler *et al.*, 1988; Axiotis *et al.*, 1989; LeBoit *et al.*, 1989; Walford *et al.*, 1990). The lesions resemble Kaposi's sarcoma or pyogenic granulomas clinically, and contain lobular vascular proliferations with prominent epithelioid endothelial cells, surrounded by an infiltrate which includes neutrophils and is characterized by large macrophages, which contain aggregates of Gram-negative bacteria (Figure 14.5). Organisms are also present in amorphous amphophilic interstitial clusters. Ultrastructural studies show that they have a tuft of flagellae at one pole (Cockerell, 1990).They stain with the Warthin-Starry stain, and it had, therefore, been suggested that they were similar, if not identical, to the organisms of cat scratch disease (LeBoit *et al.*, 1988; Cockerell and Friedman-Klein, 1988). More recently, however, it has been suggested that this condition is none other than Carrion's disease. The clinical and histological features of Bartonellosis seem very similar, and the infection may well have been imported from South to North America (Goldman, 1989; Berger *et al.*, 1989; Arias-Stella *et al.*, 1986).

Cases have been diagnosed both clinically and pathologically as Kaposi's, but accurate diagnosis is important because this condition responds to treatment with erythromycin, with resolution of the lesions and associated systemic symptoms (Koehler *et al.*, 1988).

14.3   Acute virus exanthema

Acute HIV infection may be associated with a roseola-like rash, of sudden onset and lasting 1 to 2 weeks. The rash is macular and occurs on the upper trunk, neck and face (Lindskov *et al.*, 1986; Ludlam *et al.*, 1985; Cooper *et al.*, 1985; Wanzin *et al.*, 1985). Biopsies show little epidermal change and slight lymphocytic and histiocytic infiltration around upper dermal vessels (Balslev *et al.*, 1990). Tubulo-reticular structures have been identified in venular endothelial cells within the lesions (Berk *et al.*, 1988).

14.4   Seborrhoeic-like dermatitis

As many as 46% of HIV-positive patients develop a skin rash with clinical features similar to seborrhoeic dermatitis (Eisenstat and Wormser, 1984; Soeprono *et al.*, 1986; Berger *et al.*, 1988). The biopsy appearances consist of a complex of a superficial perivascular infiltrate of lymphocytes, plasma cells and neutrophils, which may show leukocytoclasis. The overlying epidermis shows spotty keratinocyte necrosis and exocytosis, as a result of lymphocytes moving into the epidermis and obliterating the dermoepidermal junction. Hyperkeratosis is seen in

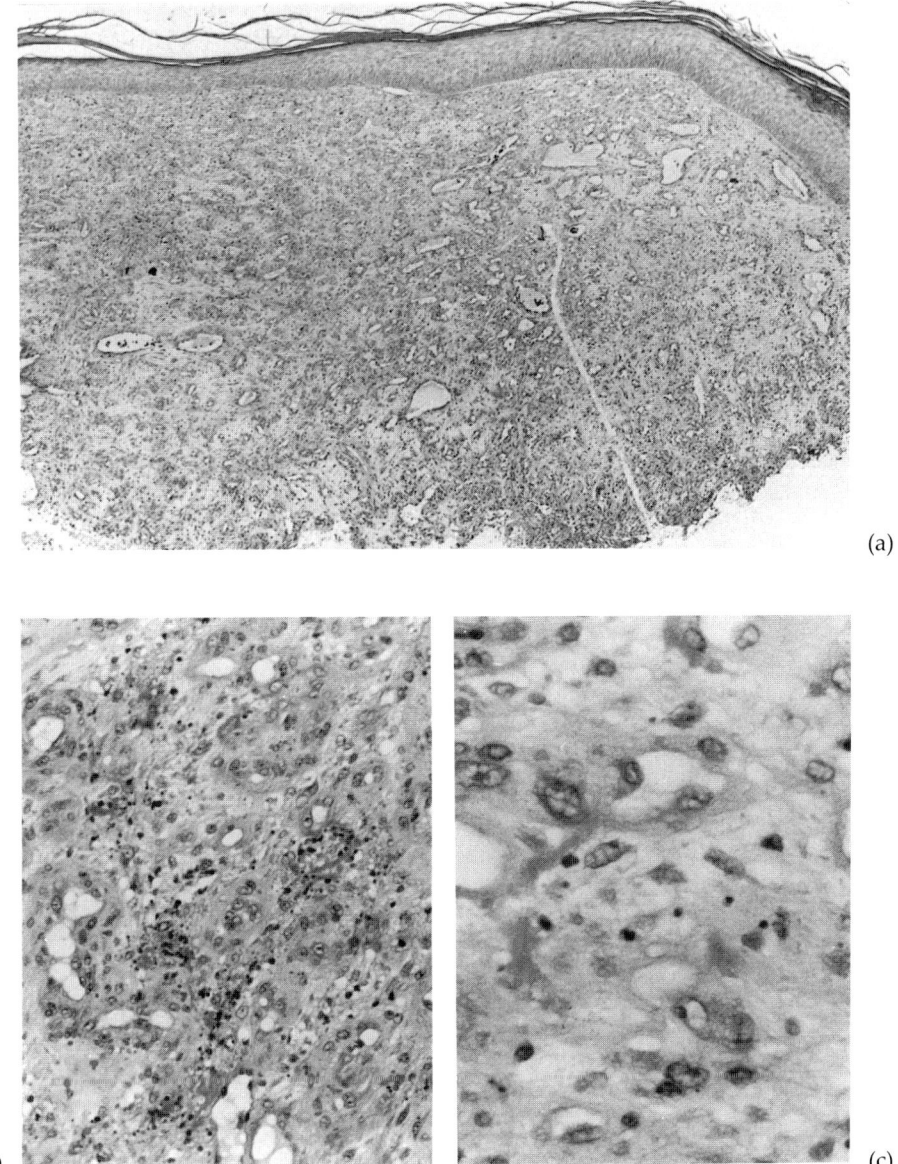

Figure 14.5 Bacillary angiomatosis. (a) Dermal vascular proliferation, (b) multiple interstitial nuclear fragments, and (c) smudged stromal aggregates of organisms. (Courtesy of Dr T. Krausz)

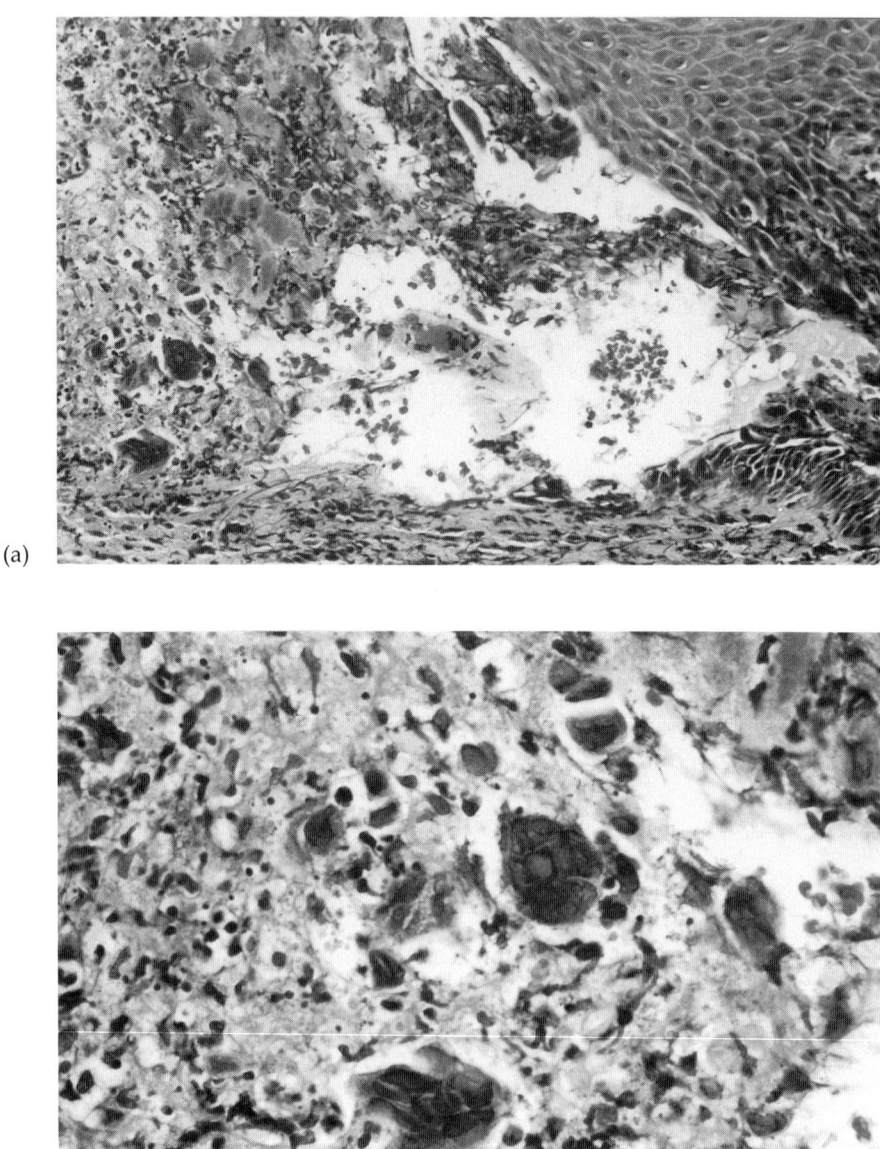

(a)

(b)

Figure 14.6 (a) Herpetic ulcer with necrotic base, and (b) multinucleated cells with nuclear inclusions within the reaction at the base of the ulcer.

long-standing lesions. The presence of this rash appears to correspond to a low helper T-cell count (Sindrup *et al.*, 1988).

14.5   Other infections

The number of infections that have been described as complications of AIDS is ever increasing (Figure 14.6). The disease renders the patient liable to any number of infections, many of which can present in the skin, including *Pneumocystis carinii*, *Cryptococcus*, *Histoplasma* and cytomegalovirus. Cytomegalovirus (CMV) is a rare complication in contrast to the relatively high level of ocular and visceral disease reported, but has been described in ulcers, especially those in the ano-genital region (Kwan and Kaufman, 1986), and in keratotic lesions (Bournerias *et al.*, 1989).

Biopsies from these patients must always be examined with the possibility of multiple infections in mind and appropriate special stains done to exclude or confirm them. The presence of macrophages or neutrophils in the skin, in the absence of demonstrable organisms, should still raise the possibility of infection (Cockerell, 1989). Furthermore, one cannot rest after finding one kind of organism; for instance, CMV may co-exist with herpes simplex virus (Lee and Peel, 1989), fungi with atypical mycobacteria (Kwan and Kaufman, 1986) and spirochetal organisms can be found in the same lesion with *Cryptococcus neoformans* and other fungi (Pierard *et al.*, 1990).

References

Arias-Stella, J., Lieberman, P. H., Erlandson, R. A. and Arias-Stella, J. Jr (1986) Histology, immunohistochemistry, and ultrastructure of the verruga in Carrion's disease. *Am. J. Surg. Pathol.*, **10**, 595–610.

Axiotis, C. A., Schwartz, R., Jennings, T. A. and Glaser, N. (1989) AIDS-related angiomatosis. *Am. J. Dermatopathol.*, **11**, 177–81.

Balslev, E., Thomsen, H. K. and Weismann, K. (1990) Histopathology of acute human immunodeficiency virus exanthema. *J. Clin. Pathol.*, **43**, 201–2.

Becker, J., Schuppan, D. and Reichart, P. (1987) The extracellular matrix in oral Kaposi sarcoma (AIDS): the immunohistochemical distribution of collagens type IV, V, VI, of procollagens type I and III, of laminin and of undulin. *Virchows Arch. A.*, **412**, 161–8.

Beral, V., Peterman, T. A., Berkelman, R. L. and Jaffe, H. W. (1990) Kaposi's sarcoma among persons with AIDS: a sexually transmitted infection? *Lancet*, **335**, 123–8.

Berger, R. S., Stoner, M. F., Hobbs, E. R., Hayes, T. J. and Boswell, R. N. (1988) Cutaneous manifestations of early human immunodeficiency virus exposure. *J. Am. Acad. Dermatol.*, **19**, 298–303.

Berger, T. G., Tappero, J. W., Kaymen, A. and LeBoit, P. E. (1989) Bacillary (epithelioid) angiomatosis and concurrent Kaposi's sarcoma in acquired immunodeficiency syndrome. *Arch. Dermatol.*, **125**, 1543–7.

Berk, M. A., Medenica, M. and Laumann, A. (1986) Tubuloreticular structures in a papular eruption associated with human immunodeficiency virus disease. *J. Am. Acad. Dermatol.*, **18**, 452–6.

Bournerias, I., Boisnic, S., Patey, O., Deny, P., Gharakhanian, S., Duflo, B. and Gentilini, M. (1989) Unusual cutaneous cytomegalovirus involvement in patients with acquired immunodeficiency syndrome. *Arch. Dermatol.*, **125**, 1243–6.

Cockerell, C. J., Whitlow, M. A., Webster, G. F. and Friedman-Kien, A. E. (1987) Epithelioid angiomatosis: a distinct vascular disorder in patients with the acquired immunodeficiency syndrome or AIDS-related complex. *Lancet*, **ii**, 654–6.

Cockerell, C. J. and Friedman-Klein, A. E. (1988) Epithelioid angiomatosis and cat scratch disease bacillus. *Lancet*, **i**, 1334–5.

Cockerell, C. J. and Friedman-Kien, A. E. (1989) Skin manifestations of HIV infection. *Primary Care*, **16**, 621–44.

Cockerell, C. J. (1989) The dermatopathologist and human immunodeficiency virus infection. *Arch. Dermatol.*, **125**, 1565–7.

Cockerell, C. J. (1990) Bacillary epithelioid angiomatosis. *Sixth Zagazig International Conference of Dermatology and Venereology*, Cairo, Egypt.

Cooper, D. A., Gold, J., MacLean, P., Donovan, B., Finlayson, R., Barnes, T. G., Michelmore, H. M., Brooke, P. and Penny, R. (1985) Acute AIDS retrovirus infection. Definition of a clinical illness associated with seroconversion. *Lancet*, **i**, 537–40.

Couturier, E., Ancelle-Park, R. A., De Vincenzi, I., Downs, A. M. and Brunet, J. B. (1990) Kaposi sarcoma as a sexually transmitted disease. *Lancet*, **335**, 1105.

Dictor, M. and Jarplid, B. (1990) The cause of Kaposi's sarcoma: an avian retroviral analogue. *J. Am. Acad. Dermatol.*, **18**, 398–402.

Duvic, M., Lowe, L., Rapini, R. P., Rodriguez, S. and Levy, M. L. (1989) Eruptive dysplastic nevi associated with human immunodeficiency virus infection. *Arch. Dermatol.*, **125**, 397–401.

Ensoli, B., Barillari, G., Salahuddin, S. Z., Gallo, R. C. and Wong-Staal, F. (1990) Tat protein of HIV-1 stimulates growth of cells derived from Kapsi's sarcoma lesions of AIDS patients. *Nature*, **345**, 84–6.

Eisenstat, B. A. and Wormser, G. P. (1984) Seborrheic dermatitis and butterfly rash in AIDS. *N. Engl. J. Med.*, **311**, 189.

Francis, N. D., Parkin, J. M., Weber, J. and Boylston, A. W. (1986) Kaposi's sarcoma in aquired immunodeficiency syndrome. *J. Clin. Pathol.*, **36**, 469–74.

Goldman, L. (1989) Bartonellosis and Kaposi sarcoma of AIDS [letter]. *Lancet*, **i**, 852.

Gottlieb, G. J. and Ackerman, A. B. (1982) Kaposi's sarcoma: an extensively disseminated form in young homosexual men. *Hum. Pathol.*, **13**, 882–92.

Hira, S. K., Wadhawan, D., Kamanga, J., Kavindele, D., Macuacua, R., Patil, P. S., Ansary, M. A., Macher, A. M. and Perine, P. L. (1988) Cutaneous manifestations of human immunodeficiency virus in Lusaka, Zambia. *J. Am. Acad. Dermatol.*, **19**, 451–7.

Knobler, E. H., Silvers, D. N., Fine, K. C., Lefkowitch, J. H. and Grossman, M. E. (1988) Unique vascular skin lesions associated with human immunodeficiency virus. *JAMA*, **260**, 524–7.

Koehler, J. E., LeBoit, P. E., Egbert, B. M. and Berger, T. G. (1988) Cutaneous vascular lesions and disseminated cat-scratch disease in patients with the acquired immunodeficiency syndrome (AIDS) and AIDS-related complex. *Ann. Intern. Med.*, **109**, 449–55.

Kwan, T. and Kaufman, H. (1986) Acid-fast bacilli with cytomegalovirus and herpes virus inclusions in the skin of an AIDS patient. *Am. J. Clin. Pathol.*, **85**, 236–8.

LeBoit, P. E., Berger, T. G., Egbert, B. M., Benedict, Yen, T. S., Stoler, M. H., Bonfiglio, T. A., Strauchen, J. A., English, C. K. and Wear, D. J. (1988) Epithelioid haemangioma-like vascular proliferation in AIDS: manifestation of cat scratch disease bacillus infection? *Lancet*, **i**, 960–3.

LeBoit, P. E., Berger, T. G., Egbert, B. M., Beckstead, J. H., Benedict Yen, T. S. and Stoler, M. H. (1989) Bacillary angiomatosis. The histopathology and differential diagnosis of a pseudoneoplastic infection in patients with human immunodeficiency virus disease. *Am. J. Surg. Pathol.*, **13**, 909–20.

Lee, J. Y.-Y. and Peel, R. (1989) Concurrent cytomegalovirus and *Herpes simplex* virus infections in skin biopsy specimens from two AIDS patients with fatal CMV infection. *Am. J. Dermatopathol.*, **11**, 136–43.

Leu, H. J. and Odermatt, B. (1985) Multicentric angiosarcoma (Kaposi's sarcoma). Light and electron microscopic and immunohistochemical findings of idiopathic cases in Europe and Africa and of cases associated with AIDS. *Virchows Arch. A.*, **408**, 29–41.

Lindskov, R., Orskov Lindhardt, B., Weismann, K., Ulrich, K. and Wanzin, G. L. (1986) Acute HTLV III infection with roseola-like rash. *Lancet*, **i**, 447.

Ludlam, C. A., Tucker, J., Steel, C. M., Tedder, R. S., Cheingsong-Popov, R., Weiss, R. A., McClelland, D. B. L., Philip, I. and Prescott, R. J. (1985) Human T-lymphotrophic virus type III (HTLV III) infection in seronegative haemophiliacs after transfusion of factor VIII. *Lancet*, **ii**, 233–6.

Nickoloff, B. J. and Griffiths, C. E. M. (1989) The spindle-shaped cells in cutaneous Kaposi's sarcoma. *Am. J. Pathol.*, **135**, 793–800.

Ordonez, N. G. and Batsakis, J. G. (1984) Comparison of *Ulex europaeus I* lectin and factor VIII-related antigen in vascular lesions. *Arch. Pathol. Lab. Med.*, **108**, 129–32.

Pedersen, C., Horn, T., Junge, J., Haahr, S. and Nielsen, J. O. (1989) Tubuloreticular inclusions in skin biopsies from patients with HIV infection. *APMIS*, **97**, 249–52.

Pierard, G. E., Pierard-Franchimont, C., Estrada, J. A., Rurangirwa, A. and Dosal, F. L. (1989) Cutaneous mixed infections in AIDS. *Am. J. Dermatopathol.*, **12**, 63–6.

Rico, N. J. and Penneys, N. S. (1985) Cutaneous cryptococcosis resembling molluscum contagiosum in a patient with AIDS. *Arch. Dermatol.*, **121**, 901–2.

Salahuddin, S. Z., Nakamura, S., Biberfeld, P., Kaplan, M. H., Markham, P. D., Larsson, L. and Gallo, R. C. (1988) Angiogenic properties of Kaposi's sarcoma-derived cells after long-term culture in vitro. *Science*, **242**, 430–3.

Scully, P. A., Steinman, H. K., Kennedy, C., Trueblood, K., Frisman, D. M. and Voland, J. R. (1988) AIDS-related Kaposi's sarcoma displays differential expression of endothelial surface antigens. *Am. J. Pathol.*, **130**, 244–51.

Sindrup, J. H., Weismann, K., Sand Petersen, C., Rindum, J., Pedersen, C., Mathiesen, L., Worm, A. M., Kroon, S., Sondergaard, J. and Lange Wantzin, G. (1988) Skin and oral mucosal changes in patients infected with human immunodeficiency virus. *Acta. Derm. Venereol. (Stockh.)*, **68**, 440–3.

Soeprono, F. F., Schinella, R. A., Cockerell, C. J. and Comite, S. L. (1986)

Seborrheic-like dermatitis of acquired immunodeficiency syndrome. *J. Am. Acad. Dermatol.*, **14**, 242–8.

Strutton, G. and Weedon, D. (1987) Acro-angiodermatitis. A simulant of Kaposi's sarcoma. *Am. J. Dermatopathol.*, **9**, 85–9.

Templeton, A. C. (1981) Kaposi's sarcoma. *Pathol. Annu.*, **17**, 315–36.

Vogel, J., Hinrichs, S. H., Reynolds, R. K., Luciw, P. A. and Jay, G. (1988) The HIV *tat* gene induces dermal lesions resembling Kaposi's sarcoma in transgenic mice. *Nature*, **335**, 606–11.

Walford, N., Van der Wouw, P. A., Das, P. K., Ten Velden, J. J. and Hulsebosch, H. J. (1990) Epithelioid angiomatosis in the acquired immunodeficiency syndrome: morphology and differential diagnosis. *Histopathology*, **16**, 83–8.

Wanzin, G. L., Orskov Linhardt, B., Weismann, K. and Ulrich, K. (1985) Acute HTLV III infection associated with exanthema, diagnosed by seroconversion. *Br. J. Dermatol.*, **115**, 601–6.

15 Vasculitis

Cutaneous vasculitis is yet another area where imprecise terminology and a proliferation of eponyms has tended to confuse the innocent (Fauci, 1979; Ryan, 1985; Ryan and Burge, 1985). It is perhaps best to start at the end rather than the beginning. The biopsy is on the microscope stage has been performed to establish the nature and likely extent of disease, and to give a guide to appropriate further investigations and treatment. In many ways, the precise diagnosis is a nicety.

Vasculitis is the process of inflammation of blood-vessel walls. It is not an appropriate term to describe simple outpourings of lymphocytes into the tissues surrounding the vessels. Vasculitis is due to a variable combination of cellular and humoral factors, associated in a varying degree of severity and extent of the lesions.

The minimum definition of vasculitis is something of a problem. In the past, there has been a tendency to call any process with prominent perivascular lymphocytic infiltration 'vasculitis'. However, to make the diagnosis there must be evidence of inflammation, and probably also tissue damage, actually involving the vessel walls. This is best characterized by definite fibrinoid change, which is almost always accompanied by some degree of leukocytoclasis in the surrounding dermis.

When looking at the biopsy, the features to look for are vessel wall inflammation, red cell extravasation, the depth of the infiltrate in the dermis, the presence or absence of leukocytoclasis, fibrinoid necrosis, epidermal necrosis and fibrin thrombi.

What the dermatologist wants to know is, first, whether the disease is trivial or severe in degree and, second, whether it is a localized disease or is more likely to be a manifestation of a multi-system or systemic process. If the first priority is given to answering these questions, then the difficulties associated with trying to fit the biopsy into one of the compartments of the available classifications start to melt away.

15.1 Leucocytoclastic vasculitis

The activation of complement and consequent cell lysis lead to the development of a characteristic appearance of leukocytoclasis, with fragments of haematoxophilic nuclear material scattered around the vessels and between the remaining inflammatory cells. The process must be stimulated by some form of antigen. In the majority of cases this is not identified. In some cases retinoids, have been shown to play a causative role (Dwyer *et al.*, 1989).

The vasculitis itself is manifested by swelling of endothelial cells, variable degrees of fibrin deposition and sometimes actual necrosis of the vessel walls, probably associated with a variable degree of extra-vasation of erythrocytes into the surrounding dermis. Neutrophil poly-morphs predominate in the dermal infiltrate around the inflamed vessels. This sort of reaction usually takes place in the papillary der-mis, only occasionaly extending down into the reticular dermis. In more severe cases, fibrin thrombi may be present in vessels. The process may even extend to cause necrosis of the overlying epidermis. The severity of the changes in the biopsy are a good predictor of the severity of the clinical disease, but do not correlate with the presence or absence of systemic vasculitis (Hodge *et al.*, 1987). Lesser degrees of change overlap with the changes seen in severe urticaria (Peters and Winklemann, 1972; Jones, *et al.*, 1983; Winklemann, 1988).

Many cases of leukocytoclastic vasculitis have perivascular deposits of IgA as a manifestation of Henoch-Schonlein purpura. Occasionally, granulomas may also be present, perhaps representing a link to the more overt stage of palisading granuloma formation seen in rheumatoid disease (Smith *et al.*, 1989).

15.2 Necrotizing vasculitis

Necrotizing vasculitis more often than not presages some form or other of severe underlying systemic disease. Both Wegener's granulomatosis and the Churg-Strauss syndrome can present in this way in the skin, as can the condition formerly called lymphomatoid granulomatosis, but which is now recognized to be a T-cell lymphoma. Other associations include necrotizing vasculitis of small- and medium-sized dermal ves-sels with enteropathy associated T-cell lymphoma (Alegre *et al.*, 1988). A non-causal association has been reported with severe atherosclerosis, where each disease exacerbated the other (Alegre *et al.*, 1988).

15.3 Wegener's granulomatosis

The condition which we know as Wegener's granulomatosis was first described in 1931 by Klinger and takes the form of a triad of (1)

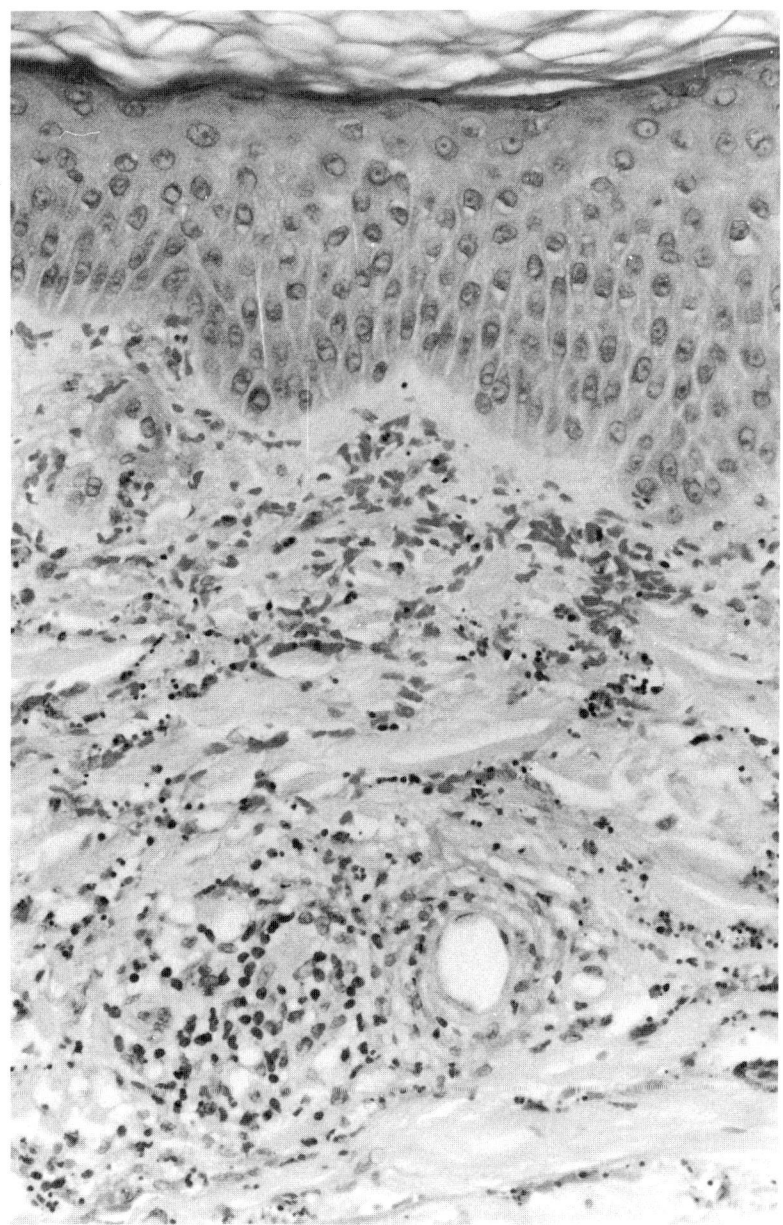

Figure 15.1 Leukocytoclastic vasculitis. The dermis contains many leukocytoclastic nuclear fragments and also shows haemorrhage.

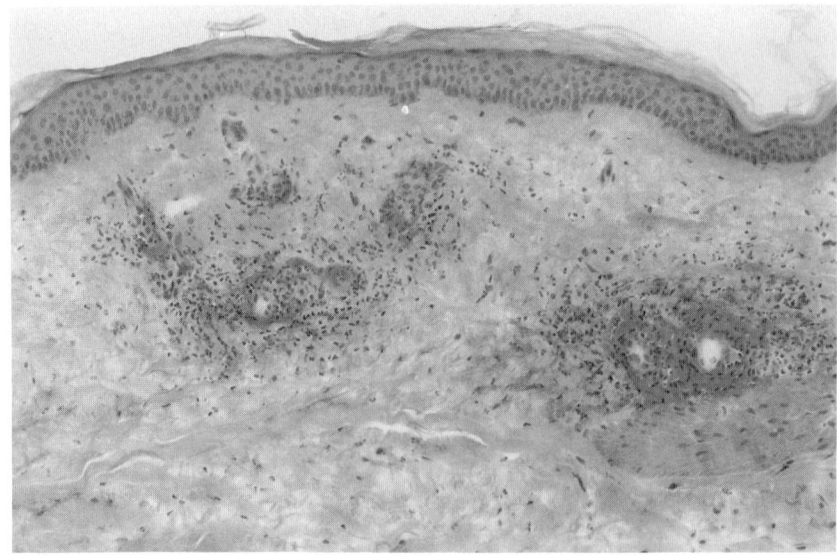

(a)

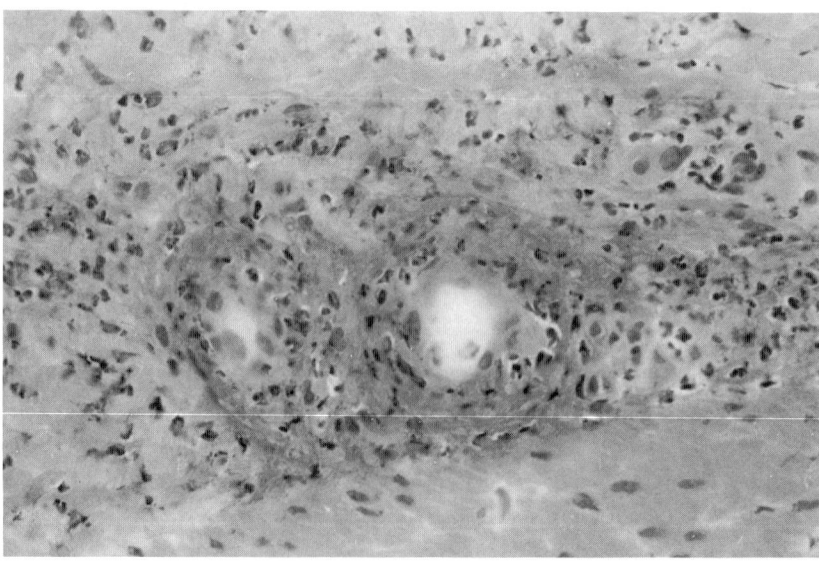

(b)

Figure 15.2 Henoch-Schonlein purpura (a and b). An example of an acute leukocytoclastic vasculitis, also showing eosinophilic fibrinoid change in these frozen sections.

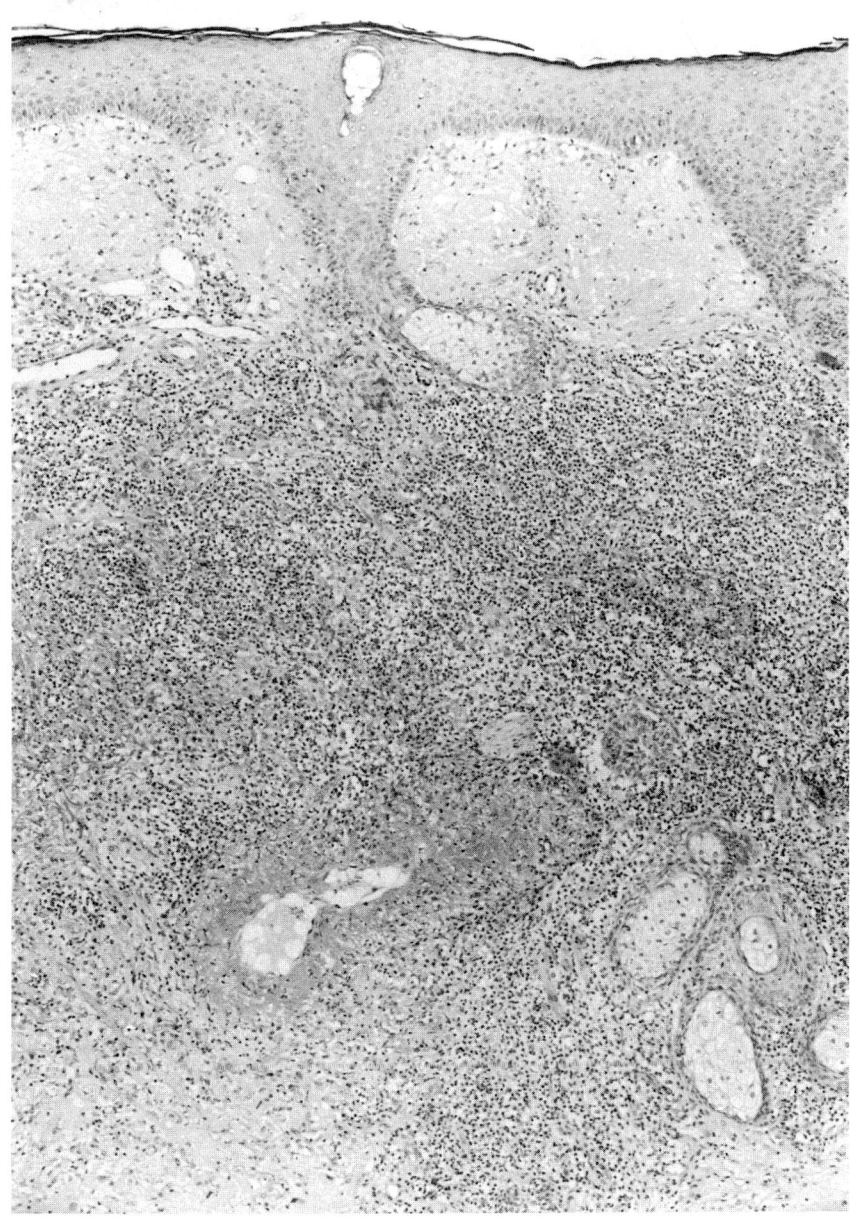

Figure 15.3 Necrotizing vasculitis. The dermis is filled with an infiltrate, with a necrotic dermal artery at its centre.

necrotizing granulomatous lesions in the upper and lower respiratory tract, (2) a generalized focal necrotizing vasculitis, and (3) a focal necrotizing or granulomatous glomerulonephritis (Klinger, 1931; Wegener, 1936; Godman and Churg, 1954; Norris *et al.*, 1988). Only one or two parts of the triad may be present if the patient presents during the early phase of the disease (Cassan *et al.*, 1970). Skin lesions are reasonably common (Reed et al., 1963; Hansen *et al.*, 1985), but diagnosis may be difficult because of tissue destruction and the possible problems of differentiating it from 'lymphomatoid granulomotosis' (Liebow *et al.*, 1972).

The commonest skin lesion is a necrotizing vasculitis presenting clinically with purpuric and haemorrhagic lesions. Medium-sized dermal vessels show fibrinoid material in a cuff around their walls and sometimes also in the lumen. The vessel walls are infiltrated with neutrophil polymorphs, with associated leukocytoclasis. Associated with this necrobiosis and fibrinoid change is extravasation of red cells: the whole complex having the appearance of a kind of infarct.

In less severely affected areas, endothelial cell swelling and angioectasia may be seen. The process may extend from the dermis to the subcutis. In severe lesions, the epidermis will become involved by the underlying dermal infarction, resulting in vesicle formation or actual ulceration.

In other patients, palisading granulomas or granulomatous vasculitis may be seen and which make interpretation more difficult. Coexisting lymphomatoid granulomatosis and Wegener's granulomatosis has also been described, although if a similar case were to be published today, no doubt ways would be found of deciding which of the two conditions was actually the true diagnosis (Hu *et al.*, 1977).

In short, classic Wegener's granulomatosis involves both the upper and lower respiratory systems and the kidneys, with renal involvement as a major cause of morbidity and mortality. It is mainly a necrotizing granulomatous reaction with neutrophil polymorphs predominating in the infiltrate, together with plasma cells and macrophages, compared with the eosinophilic granulomas of Churg-Strauss syndrome and the atypical lymphocytic reaction of lymphomatoid granulomatosis (Yevich, 1988).

15.4 Churg-Strauss syndrome

This syndrome was originally described as 'allergic granulomatosis': a systemic clinical and pathological syndrome with frequent skin involvement (Strauss *et al.*, 1951). It is commonly associated with maturity onset asthma, which may precede the skin lesions, perhaps by years.

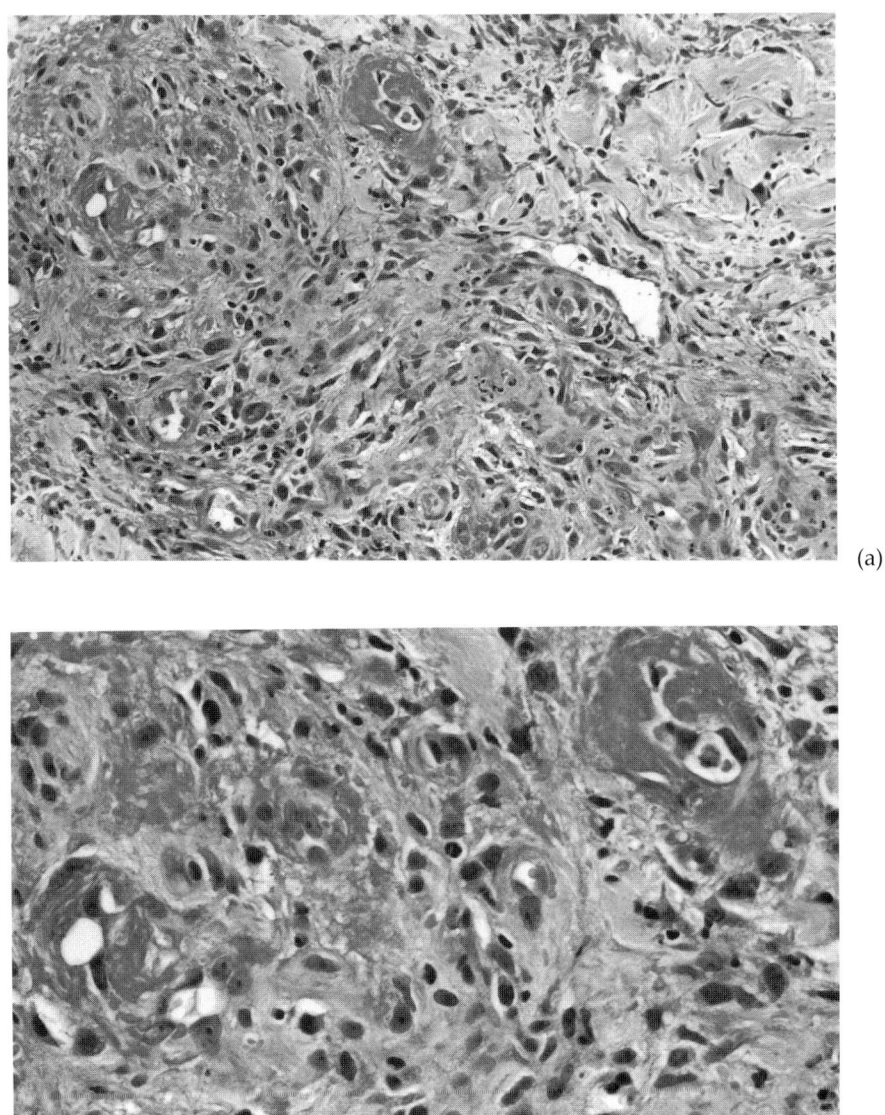

(a)

(b)

Figure 15.4 Diabetic dermopathy (a and b). Fibrinoid change in vessel walls in the dermis of a diabetic with necrotizing skin lesions.

The biopsy shows a leukocytoclastic vasculitis, with many eosinophils present in the infiltrate, which is the main differential point in distinguishing it from Wegener's granuloma and lymphomatoid granulomatosis.

15.5   Lymphomatoid granulomatosis

This is a multisystem disorder involving skin, lungs and central nervous system (Liebow *et al.*, 1972). Although still sometimes considered to be a form of reactive vasculitis, it has been shown repeatedly to be a form of malignant peripheral T-cell lymphoma, and should be treated as such, and is therefore described in Chapter 11 (Troussard *et al.*, 1990; Isaacson,1990).

15.6   Pyoderma gangrenosum

Pyoderma gangrenosum is a potentially destructive disorder which is easier to treat early rather than late, usually with high-dose corticosteroids, but must be given with care as there is a danger of death from the complications of steroid therapy (Holt *et al.*, 1980). The lesions occur both in the legs, where they may be associated with trauma, and in the head and neck where they probably will not be (Snyder, 1986).

They start as tender pustules, papules, nodules, vesicles or bullae and extend laterally, with central necrosis to produce ulcers with raised, purple borders, irregular margins and purulent bases. They may evolve quickly, over just a few hours, or more slowly (Holt *et al.* 1980).

Pyoderma gangrenosum has been associated with several systemic diseases including ulcerative colitis, Crohn's disease, rheumatoid arthritis, polyarthritis, monoclonal gammopathy and myeloproliferative diseases (Perry and Winklemann, 1972; Hickman and Lazarus, 1980). The systemic disease usually comes first, and can be present for between 1 and 25 years before the development of pyoderma gangrenosum (Holt *et al.*, 1980), and, indeed, an underlying systemic disease may not be found in up to 50% of cases (Hickman and Lazarus, 1980).

In younger lesions, there may be a predominantly neutrophil polymorph infiltrate in the papillary dermis, extending into the reticular dermis. Endothelial cells may be swollen and fibrinoid necrosis and leukocytoclasis may be seen in and around vessels, but this is not an angiocentric process. Although immune complexes, have been reported around vessels at the periphery of lesions (Powell *et al.*, 1983), other studies have failed to find complexes and so their presence or absence has no apparent part to play in the differential diagnosis (Snyder, 1986). Immune complexes found at the periphery correspond to the

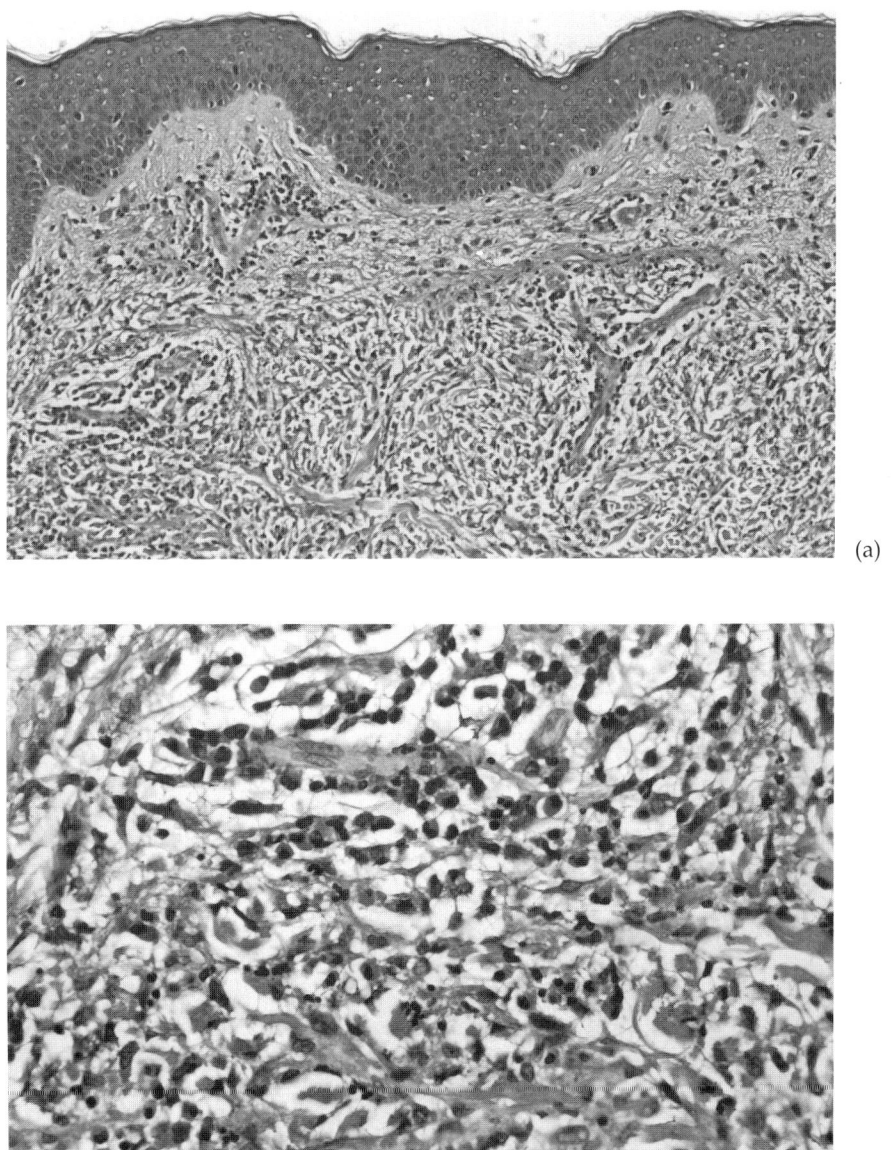

Figure 15.5 Churg-Strauss syndrome (a and b). The dermal infiltrate contains large numbers of eosinophils.

zone of active damage. Loss of complexes at the centre may be due to destruction of immune complexes during the inflammatory process (Powell *et al.*, 1985).

The diagnosis is mainly a clinical one. The biopsy is useful in excluding other possible diagnoses, such as necrotizing vasculitis, or mycobacterial or fungal infection. Biopsies from the edge of an established ulcerated lesion will show epidermal hyperplasia and non-specific chronic dermal lymphohistiocytic infiltration, usually without evidence of vascular damage.

Like pyoderma gangrenosum, Sweet's syndrome is also associated with leukaemia, with granulocytic leukaemia being commoner than lymphocytic or monocytic leukaemia, where the association is usually with a poor prognosis. There appears to be a wide spectrum of acute neutrophilic dermatoses, with typical Sweet's syndrome at one end and pyoderma gangrenosum at the other. In the middle there is an overlap of blistering and ulcerative skin lesions which are difficult to classify into one or the other spectrum ends (Dereure *et al.*, 1988).

It can often be difficult to differentiate the necrosis and inflammation of the pyoderma from a possible malignant infiltrate. A good biopsy is essential to have a chance of being able to say whether the lesion is directly infiltrated by tumour, or is merely an associated manifestation of disease. In the case of lymphoma, the tumour may be identifiable around the margins of the main lesion (Vose *et al.*, 1988).

15.7   Granuloma faciale

This condition presents as patches or nodules on the face and ears. The process is not strictly speaking granulomatous, but takes the form of a leukocytoclastic infiltrate around superficial and deep dermal vessels, and with an essentiallly normal epidermis above an uninvolved Grenz zone in the papillary dermis. The infiltrate contains eosinophils and neutrophils in the early lesion. Fibrinoid change may be present around dermal vessels. As the lesions heal, the infiltrate first of all changes to a predominantly lymphocytic one. This is eventually replaced by a fibrous scar, with variable numbers of lymphocytes, macrophages and plasma cells, together with haemosiderin (Frost and Heenan, 1984).

15.8   Cryoglobulinaemia

The hyperviscosity syndromes associated with paraproteinaemia and, in particular, with cryoglobulinaemia can be associated with cutaneous lesions. The manifestations can be variable and include urticaria and angio-oedematous lesions, as well as erythema elevatum diutinum,

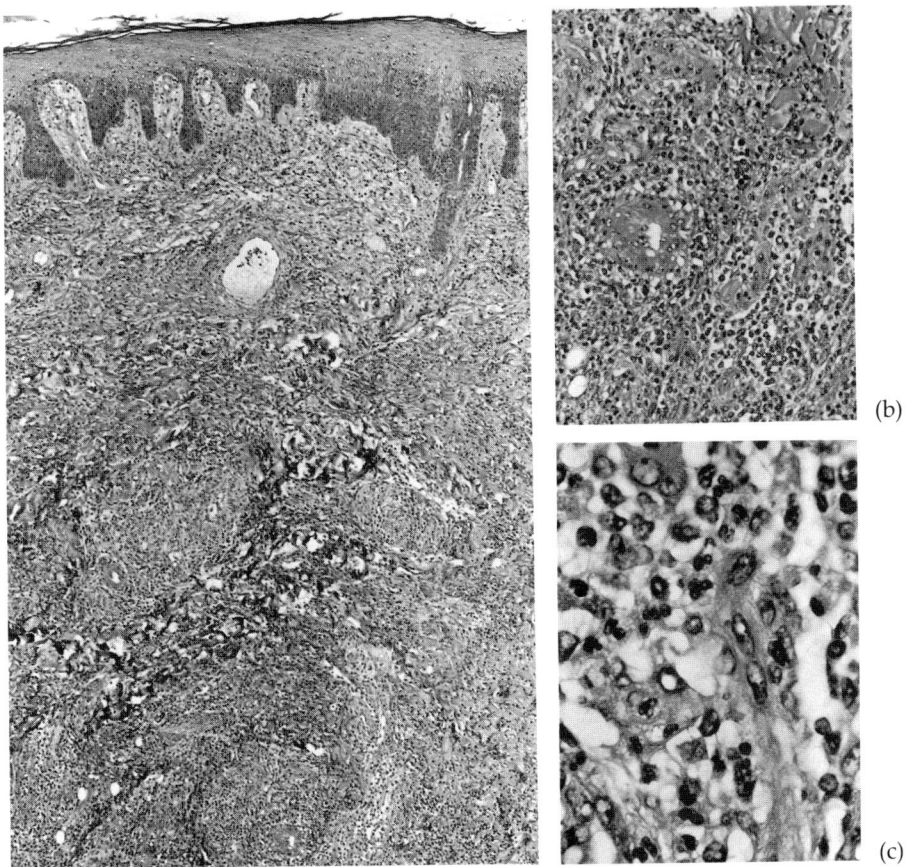

Figure 15.6 Granuloma faciale. (a) The dermis is filled with a dense infiltrate which does not invade the epidermis, (b) dermal vessels are dilated, and (c) the infiltrate includes many neutrophils. (Courtesy of Dr A. Macdonald)

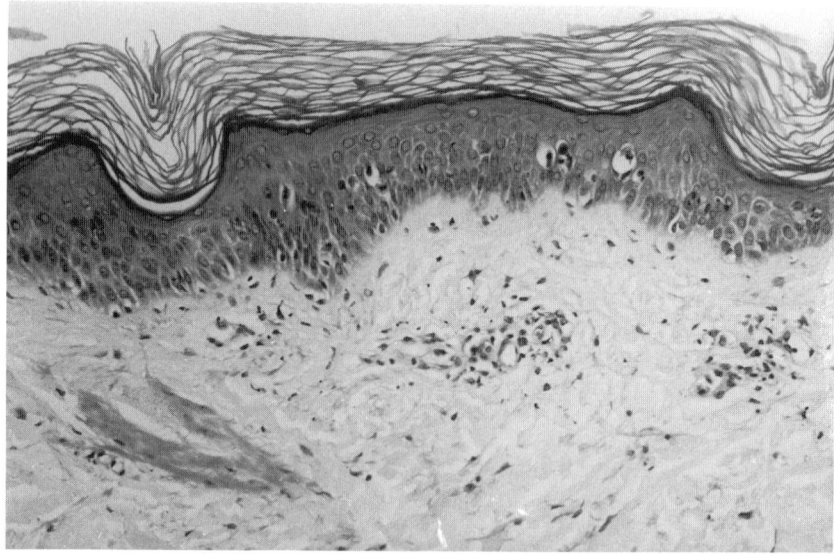

Figure 15.7 Pigmented purpuric eruption. A sparse, superficial perivascular infiltrate with associated haemosiderin deposition and, in the acute lesion, extravasated erythrocytes.

with associated leukocytoclasis around dermal vessels and with IgA deposition (Jones, 1980).

15.9 Pigmented purpuric eruptions

There is a small spectrum of conditions which differ in their clinical appearance and in their eponyms, but which usually affect the legs and are characterized by an irritating purpuric or pigmented rash. The biopsy, however, shows a constant pattern of a thin but intact epidermis, and diffuse extravasation of erythrocytes in the papillary dermis, with associated haemosiderin deposition. There is usually only a sparse, lymphocytic infiltrate around dermal vessels. Neutrophils and macrophages may also be present in the infiltrate (Gougerot and Blum, 1925; Fishman, 1982; Solomon, 1985).

15.10 Erythema elevatum diutinum

This condition is a form of chronic leukocytoclastic vasculitis which may be exacerbated by cold. IgA paraproteins have been reported (Katz *et al.*, 1977). It is characterized clinically by plaques and nodules, often symmetrical, which are often found over the interphalangeal joints of the hands and on the backs of the hands, elbows and knees. The infiltrate usually contains lymphocytes, eosinophils and macrophages, as well as the predominant neutrophil polymorphs.

15.11 Behçet's disease

Behçet's disease is a form of vasculitis with mucocutaneous involvement including recurrent aphthous ulcers of the mouth and genitalia, cutaneous folliculitis and nodular lesions on the limbs (Touraine, 1988). The mucocutaneous involvement and presence of vasculitis can be used to differentiate Behçet's disease from Sweet's syndrome, which otherwise has clinical similarities (Cho et al., 1989). The problems of defining the disease have been eased by a new set of diagnostic criteria, which require oral ulceration plus two other manifestations from the list of genital ulceration, eye lesions, skin lesions or a positive pathergy test (International Study Group for Behçet's Disease, 1990).

The cause remains uncertain. There is evidence of a genetic predisposition. Human lymphocyte antigens HLA-Bw51, HLA-B27, and HLA-B12 have each been associated with various manifestations of the disease. Viral infection may also be important, with suggestions that herpes simplex may be involved (Arbesfeld and Kurban, 1988; Editorial, 1989).

References

Alegre, V. A. and Winkelmann, R. K. (1988) Necrotizing vasculitis and atherosclerosis. Br. J. Dermatol., 119, 381–4.

Alegre, V. A., Winkelmann, R. K., Diez-Martin, J. L. and Banks, P. M. (1988) Adult celiac disease, small and medium vessel cutaneous necrotizing vasculitis, and T cell lymphoma. J. Am. Acad. Dermatol., 19, 973–8.

Arbesfeld, S. J. and Kurban, A. K. (1988) Bahçet's disease. New perspectives on an enigmatic syndrome. J. Am. Acad. Dermatol., 19, 767–79.

Cassan, S. M., Coles, D. T. and Harrison, E. G. Jr (1970) The concept of limited forms of Wegener's granulomatosis. Am. J. Med., 49, 366–79.

Cho, K. H., Shin, K. S., Sohn, S. J., Choi, S. J. and Lee, Y. S. (1989) Bahçet's disease with Sweet's syndrome-like presentation – a report of six cases. Clin. Exp. Dermatol., 14, 20–4.

Dereure, O., Guillot, B., Bareon, G., Zabarino, P. and Guilhou, J. J. (1988) [Acute febrile neutrophilic dermatosis and malignant hematologic diseases: report of a new bullous case and review of the literature]. Ann. Dermatol. Venereol., 115, 689–701.

Dwyer, J. M., Kenicer, K., Thompson, B. T., Chen, D., LaBraico, J., Schiefferdecker, R. and Winkelmann, R K (1989) Vasculitis and retinoids. Lancet, ii, 494–6.

Editorial. (1989) Bahçet's disease, Lancet, i, 761–2.

Fauci, A. S. (1979) Vasculitis: new insights amid old enigmas. Am. J. Med., 67, 916–18.

Frost, F. A. and Heenan, P. J. (1984) Facial granuloma. *Aust. J. Dermatol.*, **25**, 121–4.

Fishman, H. C. (1982) Pigmented purpuric lichenoid dermatitis of Gougerot-Blum. *Cutis*, **29**, 260–4.

Godman, G. C. and Churg, J. (1954) Wegener's granulomatosis: pathology and review of the literature. *Arch. Pathol.*, **58**, 533–53.

Gougerot, H. and Blum, P. (1925) Purpura angiosclereux prurigineux avec elements lichenoides. *Bull. Soc. Fr. Dermat. Syph.*, **32**, 161–3.

Hansen, L. S., Silverman, S., Pons, V. G., Hales, M., Greenspan, J. S., Sagebiel, R. W. and Tuffanelli, D. C. (1985) Limited Wegener's granulomatosis. Report of a case with oral, renal, and skin involvement. *Oral. Surg. Oral. Med. Oral. Pathol.*, **60**, 524–31.

Hickman, J. G. and Lazarus, G. S. (1980) Pyoderma gangrenosum: a reappraisal of associated systemic diseases. *Br. J. Dermatol.*, **102**, 235–7.

Hodge, S. J., Callen, J. P. and Ekenstam, E. (1987) Cutaneous leukocytoclastic vasculitis: correlation of histopathological changes with clinical severity and course. *J. Cut. Pathol.*, **14**, 279–84.

Holt, P. J. A., Davies, M. G., Saunders, K. L. and Nuki, G. (1980) Pyoderma gangrenosum: Clinical and laboratory findings in 15 patients with special reference to polyarthritis. *Medicine*, **59**, 114–33.

Hu, C.-H., O'Loughlin, S. and Winkelmann, R. K. (1977) Cutaneous manifestations of Wegener's granulomatosis. *Arch. Dermatol.*, **113**, 175–82.

International Study Group for Bahçet's Disease (1990) Criteria for diagnosis of Bahçet's disease. *Lancet*, **335**, 1078–80.

Isaacson, P. G. (1990) Lymphomatoid granulomatosis. *Br. Med. J.*, **300**, 612.

Jones, R. R. (1980) The cutaneous manifestations of paraproteinaemia. I. *Br. J. Dermatol.*, **103**, 335–45.

Jones, R. R., Bhogal, B., Dash, A. and Schifterli, J. (1983) Urticaria vasculitis: a continuum of histological and immunopathological changes. *Br. J. Dermatol.*, **108**, 695–703.

Katz, S. I., Gallin, J. I., Hertz, K. C., Fauci, A. S. and Lawley, T. J. (1977) Erythema elevatum diutinum: skin and systemic manifestations, immunological studies and successful treatment with dapsone. *Medicine (Baltimore)*, **56**, 443–55.

Klinger, H. (1931) Grenzformen der Periarteriitis nodosa. *Frankfurt Z. Pathol.*, **42**, 455–80.

Liebow, A. A., Carrington, C. R. B. and Friedman, P. J. (1972) Lymphomatoid granulomatosis. *Hum. Pathol.*, **3**, 457–8.

Norris, M. J., Tomecki, K. J., Bergfeld, W. F. and Wilke, W. S. (1988) Cutaneous Wegener's granulomatosis. Report of a case and review of the literature. *Cleve. Clin. J. Med.*, **55**, 181–4.

Perry, H. O. and Winklemann, R. K. (1972) Bullous pyoderma gangrenosum and leukaemia. *Arch. Dermatol.*, **106**, 901–5.

Peters, M. S. and Winklemann, R. K. (1985) Neutrophilic urticaria. *Br. J. Dermatol.*, **113**, 25–30.

Powell, F. C., Schroeder, A. L., Perry, H. O. and Su, W. P. D. (1983) Direct immunofluorescence in pyoderma gangrenosum. *Br. J. Dermatol.*, **108**, 287–93.

Powell, F. C., Schroeder, A. L. and Su, W. P. D. (1985) Pyoderma gangrenosum: a review of 86 patients. *Q. J. Med.*, **55**, 173–86.

Reed, B. W., Jensen, A. K. and Konwaler, B. E. (1963) The cutaneous manifestations of Wegener's granulomatosis. *Acta. Derm. Venereol. (Stockh.)*, **43**, 250–64.

Ryan, T. J. (1985) Cutaneous vasculitis. *J. Cut. Pathol.*, **12**, 381–7.

Ryan, T. J. and Burge, S. M. (1985) Cutaneous vasculitis. In *Dermatopathology, Current Topics in Pathology 74* (ed. C. L. Berry), Springer-Verlag, Berlin, Heidelberg, pp. 58–102.

Smith, M. L., Jorizzo, J. L., Semble, E., Arrington, J. H. and White, W. L. (1989) Rheumatoid papules: lesions showing features of vasculitis and palisading granuloma. *J. Am. Acad. Dermatol.*, **20**, 348–52.

Solomon, A. R. Jr (1985) The histologic spectrum of the reactive inflammatory vascular dermatoses. *Dermatol. Clin.*, **3**, 171–83.

Snyder, R. A. (1986) Pyoderma gangrenosum involving the head and neck. *Arch. Dermatol.*, **122**, 295–302.

Strauss, L., Churg, J. and Zak, F. G. (1951) Cutaneous lesions of allergic granulomatosis: a histopathologic study. *J. Invest. Dermatol.*, **17**, 349–59.

Touraine, R. (1988) [Mucocutaneous involvement in Bahçet's disease]. *J. Mal. Vasc.*, **13**, 220–1.

Troussard, X., Galateau, F., Gaulard, P. Reman, O., Henni, T., Le Couedic, J.-P. and Leporpier, M. (1990) Lymphomatoid granulomatosis in a patient with acute myeloblastic leukemia in remission. *Cancer*, **65**, 107–11.

Vose, J. M., Armitage, J. O., Duggan, M. and Braddock, S. W. (1988) Pyoderma gangrenosum or cutaneous lymphoma: a difficult clinical diagnosis. *Cutis*, **42**, 335–7.

Wegener, F. (1936) Uber generalisierte, septische Gefasser-Krankungen. *Vehr. Dtsch. Ges. Pathol.*, **29**, 202–8.

Winkelmann, R. K. and Reizner, G. T. (1988) Diffuse dermal neutrophilia in urticaria. *Hum. Pathol.*, **19**, 389–93.

Yevich, I. Necrotizing vasculitis with granulomatosis. *Int. J. Dermatol.*, **27**, 540–6.

16 Panniculitis

The subcutaneous fat, or panniculus adiposus, is an orphan organ, although in the more obese person it can stake a claim to be the largest organ in the body. It is too deep to be really dermatological, and not quite fitting into the domains of rheumatology or general medicine. Soft-tissue pathology specialists have described its tumours and they will not be considered here. Its inflammatory conditions are of two main types. The first group are localized and relatively benign, whilst the second group are cutaneous manifestations of systemic diseases, which may often be quite severe.

The task of the pathologist is to try and decide which of these major categories the biopsy belongs to, and then to try and be more specific in differential diagnosis. This is, of course, not always easy and depends to a large extent upon the degree to which the patient has been examined and investigated before biopsy, and how many of the results of those investigations have been made known to you.

16.1 Approach to diagnosis

There are five items of anatomy which must be taken into account when analysing the biopsy. First, the arteries, which vary in size from 500 to 20 microns and have muscular walls with internal and external elastic laminae, visible especially on AOG stained sections. They run in the fibrous septae between the lobules of adipocytes.

Second, veins are also present in the septae, but tend to be slightly larger than the nearest artery, to have less muscle in their media, to lack an internal elastic lamina, and to be more oval than round in profile.

Third, the fibrous septae themselves, which are thin in the normal state, but may become expanded by differing proportions of oedema, cellular infiltration and fibrosis, in inflammatory conditions.

The fourth component is the adipocytes, which are arranged in

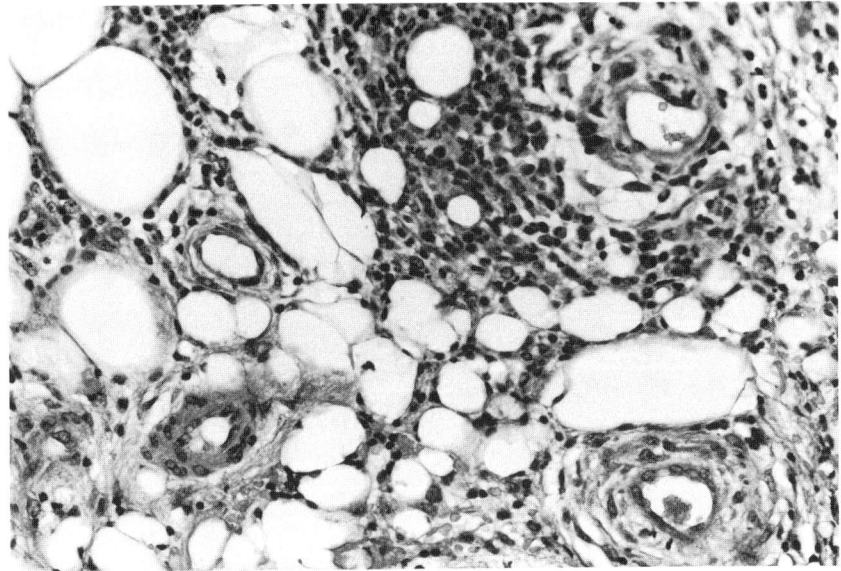

Figure 16.1   Septal panniculitis without vasculitis. The infiltrate includes lymphoctes, neutrophils and macrophages. Vessel walls are not damaged.

lobules, surrounded by fibrous septae and with arterioles and venules extending into each lobule.

Finally, one must not forget the deep fascia. An inflammatory process may involve the fascia as well as the fat, and so fasciitis will be considered together with panniculitis.

In the biopsy diagnosis of panniculitis it is vital to have a deep enough biopsy. In many cases, the lesion will not extend into the overlying dermis, so unless the biopsy is deep it will not be diagnostic. It may be necessary for the dermatologist to refer the patient to a surgeon for biopsy so that an adequate specimen can be obtained, probably taken under general anaesthetic.

In analysing the biopsy, it is then essential to decide to what extent each of the components is involved, and what special features of inflammation are present in the lesion. Thus panniculitis may be predominantly septal or predominantly lobular and may, or may not, be associated with vasculitis. The vasculitis may involve either the arteries or the veins, and may predominantly involve either the small or the larger vessels.

The infiltrate varies in character from one condition to another. For instance, it may consist mainly of neutrophils, or of other lymphoid cells, may include eosinophils, may feature leukocytoclasis, or necrosis

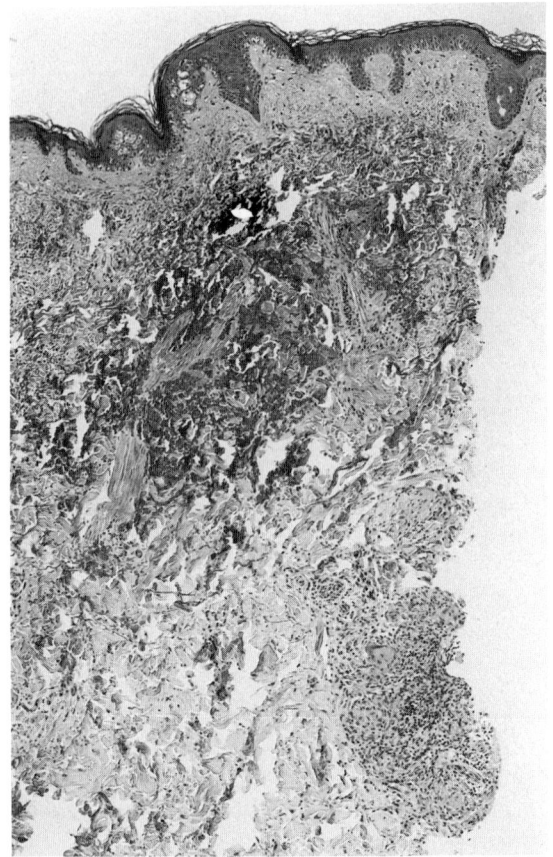

Figure 16.2   Biopsy showing granulomatous panniculitis, with giant cell formation: the biopsy only extends to the base of the dermis, making assessment of the subcutis impossible.

and may include granulomas. By considering what the characteristics of a particular lesion are, one can start to make a sensible statement about the likely diagnosis and the likelihood of the process being a manifestation of a localized or a systemic disease.

16.2   Erythema nodosum

These lesions occur typically as painful nodules on the shins of young women. They do not usually ulcerate, and heal without forming a scar. In some cases, they may be associated with infection, for instance with beta-haemolytic streptococci, with deep fungal infections, or Lyme

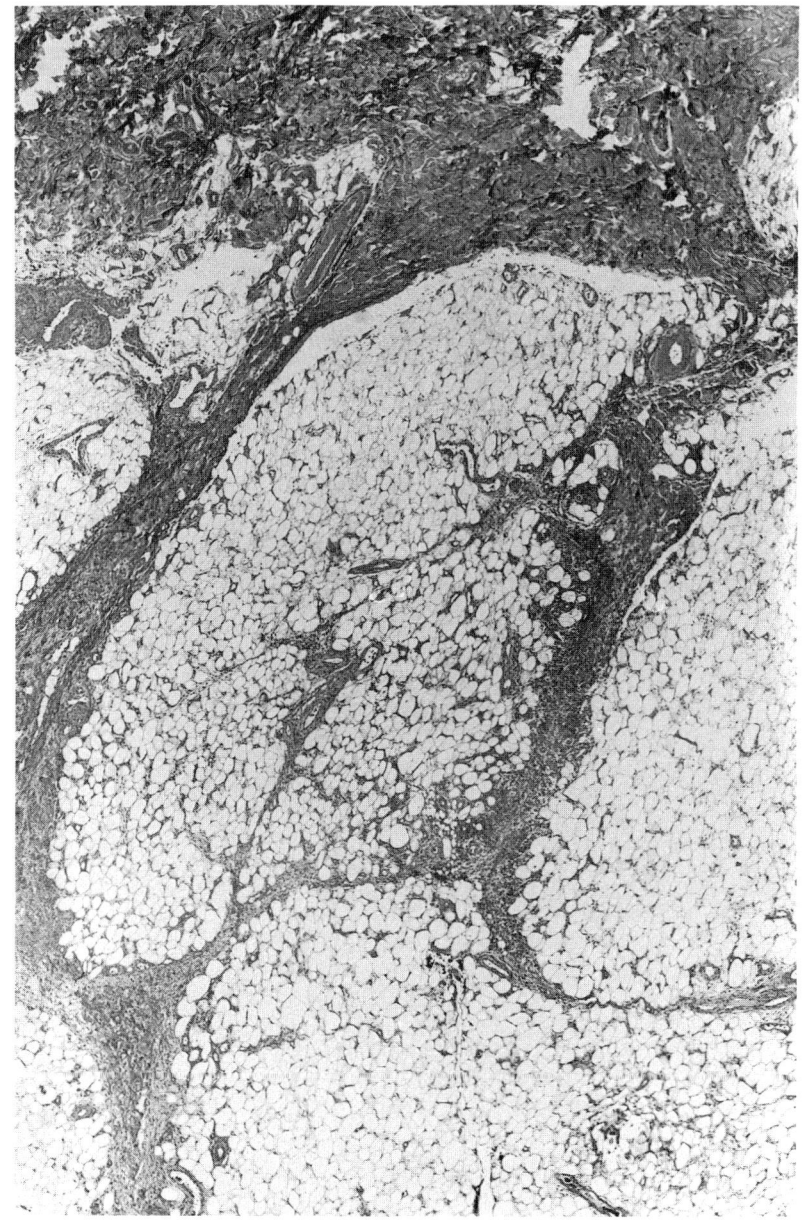

Figure 16.3 Erythema nodosum. Lymphohistiocytic infiltration of the reticular dermis extending to form a septal panniculitis with focal extension into lobules of fat.

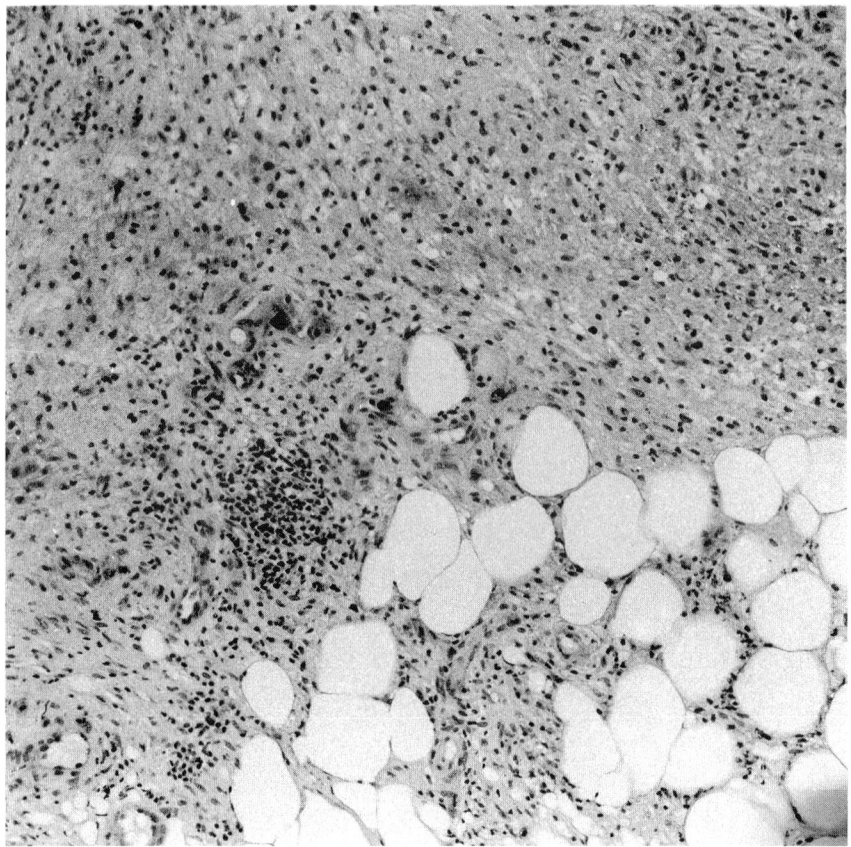

Figure 16.4   Junction of septum and lobule. The infiltrate contains lymphocytes, macrophages and occasional multinucleate cells. Few adipocytes are lost.

disease (Kramer *et al.*, 1986). Other associations include sarcoidosis and some drug reactions.

In the early stages, the infiltrate consists of neutrophils and eosinophils around septal vessels, but in time the process expands the septae and extends into the fat with the subsequent development of granulomas and a variable degree of fat necrosis, but with little loss of adipocytes.

Whilst the lesions are idiopathic in most cases, it is always worth examining multiple levels and sections stained for bacteria and fungi, to try and identify an underlying cause.

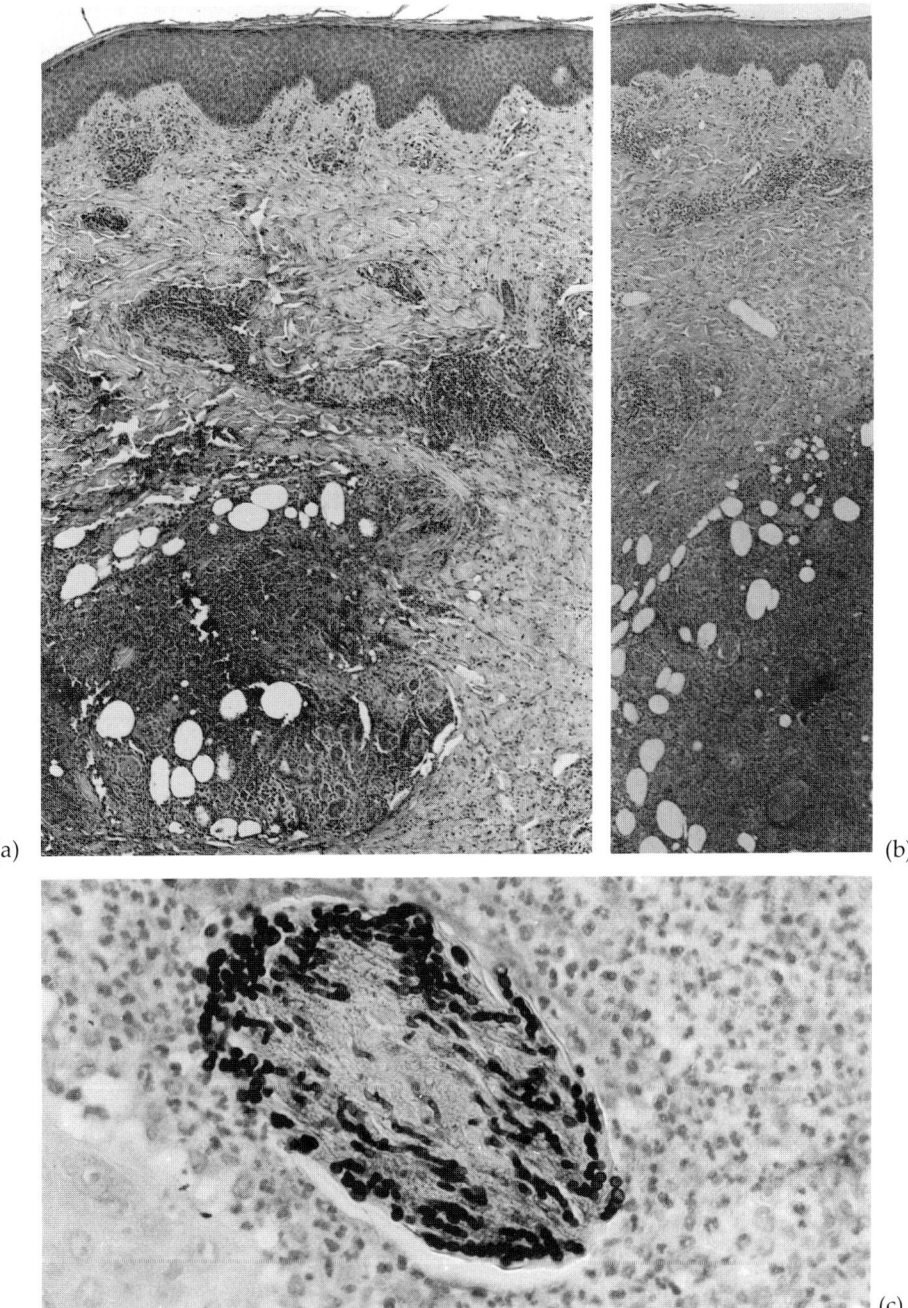

Figure 16.5 Nodular panniculitis. (a) The fat in a lobule is largely obliterated by an infiltrate which includes many neutrophils. (b) Deeper levels on the same block revealed a circumscribed abnormality, and (c) Grocott's methanamine silver stain confirms the diagnosis of deep fungal infection.

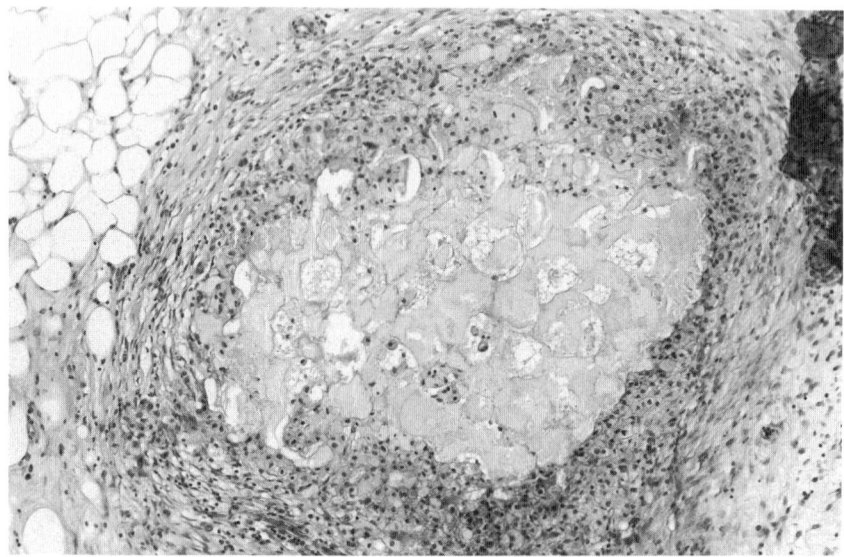

Figure 16.6 Pancreatic fat necrosis showing a central zone of enzymic necrosis with a surrounding reactive infiltrate.

16.3 Pancreatic fat necrosis

In both inflammatory and neoplastic pancreatic disease, serum lipase levels may be elevated. This may lead to the development of localized foci of subcutaneous nodular fat necrosis, usually in the legs, which is clinically indistinguishable from erythema nodosum. The lesions may break down and ulcerate producing a discharge of oily material.

The lesions show central zones of enzymic necrosis, with adipocytes showing typical changes of necrosis, including loss of nuclei, pale-staining cytoplasm, basophilia and calcification. Around the necrosis there is an inflammatory cell reaction containing varying proportions of neutrophils, lymphocytes, macrophages, giant cells, plasma cells and extravasated red cells, depending upon the age and extent of the necrosis (Schumacher *et al.*, 1989).

16.4 Lupus panniculitis

Some cases of systemic and, to a lesser extent, discoid lupus erythematosus are associated with lesions which occur mainly on the face, upper arms and buttocks. They present as indurated plaques or nodules which heal to leave depressed scars. The disease tends to run a chronic course.

The overlying epidermis and papillary dermis may, or may not,

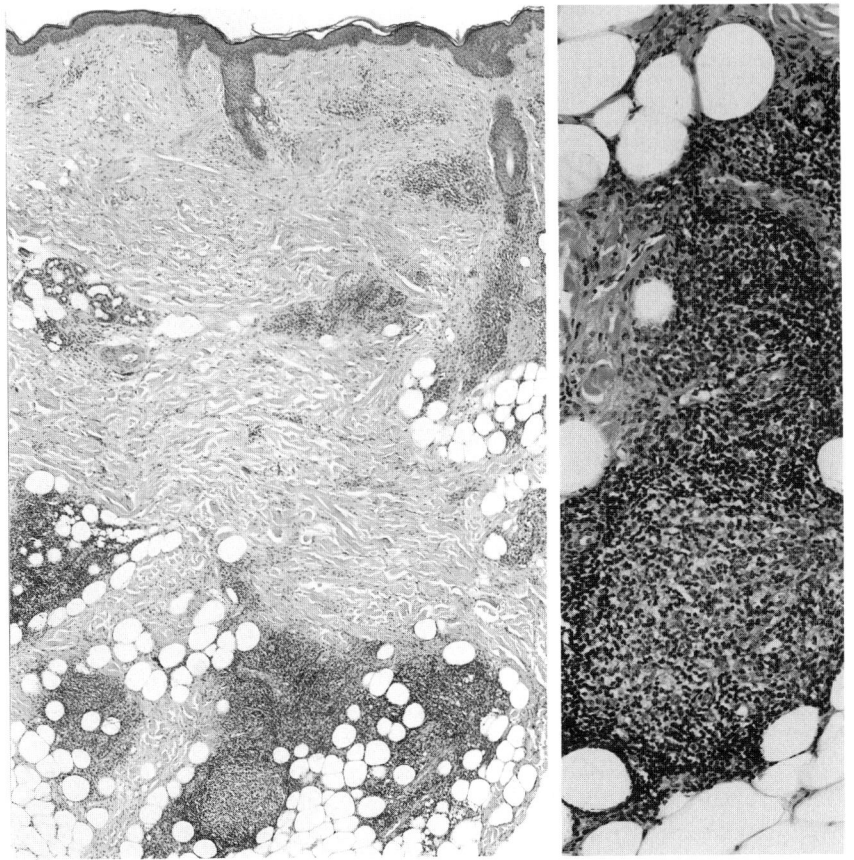

(a)   (b)

Figure 16.7   Lupus panniculitis (a and b). A lobular panniculitis with germinal centre formation.

show changes of lupus erythematosus. The early lesions show perivascular lymphocytic infiltration in the lower dermis and fat. Established lesions show hyaline fat necrosis within lobules, together with a lymphocytic and fibrosing reaction associated with inflamed blood vessels and, possibly, with the formation of lymphoid follicles with germinal centres. Granular deposits of IgG and C3 may be present in the epidermal basement membrane zone, which will, of course, help in supporting the diagnosis (Peters and Su, 1989).

16.5   Eosinophilic panniculitis

A variety of factors including insect bites, drug injections, lymphoma and autoimmune diseases, and chronic parotitis have been associated with a localized lobular panniculitis in which eosinophils predominate (Glass *et al.*, 1989). The clinical picture is similar to erythema nodosum, with lesions presenting on arms or legs. In most cases, it is self-limiting, but may respond to steroids if it persists (Winklemann and Frigas, 1986).

16.6   Cytophagic histiocytic panniculitis

Cytophagic histiocytic panniculitis is a form of regional histiocytosis, which involves the subcutaneous tissue predominantly, to produce a chronic lobular panniculitis. It is midway in the spectrum of the cytophagic histiocytoses, which range from totally benign conditions to outright malignant ones. Histologically, the infiltrate in the lobular panniculitis includes large, so-called 'beanbag' histiocytes (Peters and Winklemann, 1985).

As well as making the diagnosis, the problem is to predict the likely prognosis. Benign-looking macrophages which phagocytose erythrocytes, nuclear debris, and platelets are the most typical feature of the disease. The phagocytosis tends to be massive in the subcutaneous tissue. The course is chronic in the benign form. Potentially malignant cases show visceral involvement and multisystem symptoms including fever, hepatosplenomegaly, serosal effusions, ecchymoses, peripheral lymphadenopathy, and mucosal ulcers, together with multiple features of biochemical and haematological dysfunction, including anaemia, leukopaenia, elevated liver enzyme levels, and coagulopathy in most and hypocalcaemia in many cases (White and Winklemann, 1989). Furthermore, non-histiocytic malignancy has been reported in a chronic case (Peters and Winklemann, 1985).

16.7   Panniculitis artefacta

There remain a small number of cases in which panniculitis is induced by self-injection of drugs or other foreign material. The material, if not immediately apparent on H and E staining, may well be visible in polarized light. In unresolved cases, it is always worth using polarizing filters to examine all the extra sections that have been cut in the search for the cause of the panniculitis (Forstrom and Winklemann, 1974).

16.8   Eosinophilic fasciitis

Fascial inflammation is seen in a number of related conditions, including eosinophilic fasciitis, scleroderma, polymyositis, dermatomyositis, systemic lupus erythematosus and mixed connective tissue disease.

Eosinophilic fasciitis is closely related to the syndromes of localized scleroderma, morphoea profunda and pansclerotic morphoea. It is a rare disease, characterized clinically by pain, swelling and tenderness over the extremities, followed by induration of the skin.

A deep skin biopsy will show relatively little change in the epidermis and dermis. The changes are found in the subcutaneous fat and deep fascia, and depend upon the stage of the disease at the time of biopsy. In the earlier stages, inflammatory cell infiltration and oedema predominate, the infiltrate consisting of lymphocytes, eosinophils and plasma cells, whilst later on fibrosis becomes the main feature. These changes are essentially similar to those seen in scleroderma: the only difference is the level at which they occur.

As well as eosinophilia and fibrosis, the two conditions also have in common hypergammaglobulinaemia, positive anti-nuclear antibodies and rheumatoid factor, and an association with anaemia and other haematological disorders. Unlike scleroderma or systemic sclerosis, eosinophilic fasciitis is not usually associated with significant visceral disease or with Raynaud's phenomenon (Barnes *et al.*, 1979; Amdur and Levin, 1989; Doyle and Ginsburg, 1989).

16.9 Necrotizing fasciitis

Necrotizing fasciitis is an acute, severe, potentially life-threatening condition that is usually associated with streptococcal infection. It may follow some minor surgery or minor penetrating injury, although in many cases no cause can be demonstrated. Surgical debridement and skin grafting is usually needed to control the rapid spread of the necrotizing process in the fascia. Biopsies show an acute necrotizing process without granulomas. It may be possible to identify Streptococci with a Gram stain (Tharakaram and Keczkes, 1988).

References

Amdur, H. S. and Levin, R. F. (1989) Eosinophilic fasciitis during pregnancy. *Obstet. Gynecol.*, **73**, 843–7.

Barnes, L., Rodnan, G. P., Medsger, T. A. and Short, D. (1979) Eosinophilic fasciitis. A pathologic study of twenty cases. *Am. J. Pathol.*, **96**, 493–518.

Doyle, J. A. and Ginsburg, W. W. (1989) Eosinophilic fasciitis. *Med. Clin. North Am.*, **73**, 1157–66.

Forstrom, L. and Winklemann, R. K. (1974) Factitial panniculitis. *Arch. Dermatol.*, **110**, 747–50.

Glass, L. A., Zaghoul, A. B. and Solomon, A. R. (1989) Eosinophilic panniculitis associated with chronic recurrent parotitis. *Am. J. Dermatopathol.*, **11**, 555–9.

Kramer, N., Rickert, R. R., Brodkin, R. H. and Rosenstein, E. D. (1986) Septal panniculitis as a manifestation of Lyme disease. *Am. J. Med.*, **81**, 149–52.

Peters, M. S. and Winklemann, R. K. (1985) Cytophagic panniculitis and B cell lymphoma. *J. Am. Acad. Dermatol.*, **13**, 882–5.

Peters, M. S. and Su, W. P. (1989) Lupus erythematosus panniculitis. *Med. Clin. North Am.*, **73**, 1113–26.

Schumacher, B., Lubke, H. J., Hagen-Aukamp, C., Jungblut, R. M. and Hengels, K. J. (1989) [Necrotizing panniculitis in pancreatitis]. *Z. Gastroenterol.*, **27**, 6–9.

Tharakaram, S. and Keczkes, K. (1988) Necrotizing fasciitis. A report of five patients. *Int. J. Dermatol.*, **27**, 585–8.

White, J. W. Jr and Winkelmann, R. K. (1989) Cytophagic histiocytic panniculitis is not always fatal. *J. Cutan. Pathol.*, **16**, 137–44.

Winklemann, R. K. and Frigas, E. (1986) Eosinophilic panniculitis: a clinicopathologic study. *J. Cutan. Pathol.*, **13**, 1–12.

17 Dermal stromal diseases

A group of dermal stromal abnormalities are considered in this chapter which do not fall easily into the categories of inflammatory and neo-plastic conditions dealt with in earlier chapters. As ever, good clinico-pathological liason is essential to sort out these biopsies: only minimal changes may be present and may be dismissed entirely unless the possible diagnosis is thought of, and special stains done as appropriate. Even then, the changes present in the biopsy may be short of those needed for a confident histopathological diagnosis.

17.1 Morphoea and scleroderma

Scleroderma exist in two main clinical forms: systemic and localized. The biopsy appearances are essentially similar. The early lesions may have an inflammatory component, which diminishes with time. The dermis becomes progressively thickened, with extension of the fibrosing process to involve the septae of the subcutaneous fat. It has been suggested that spirochetal infection, possibly by the Lyme disease organism *Borrelia burgdorferi*, may be important in the development of these lesions (Ross *et al.*, 1990).

In the fully developed sclerosed lesion there may be no residual inflammatory component. The dermal collagen bundles will be thicker and more eosinophilic than normal. Elastic fibres may show thickening, clumping and fragmentation, but the overall dermal content of elastic fibres is not altered (Rustin *et al.*, 1989). Sweat glands will look compressed and atrophic. Occasionally, haemorrhagic bullous lesions may develop (Tosti *et al.*, 1989).

17.2 Lichen sclerosus

Lichen sclerosus mainly affects the genitalia. When it involves the glans penis, it is still usually called balanitis xerotica obliterans. The

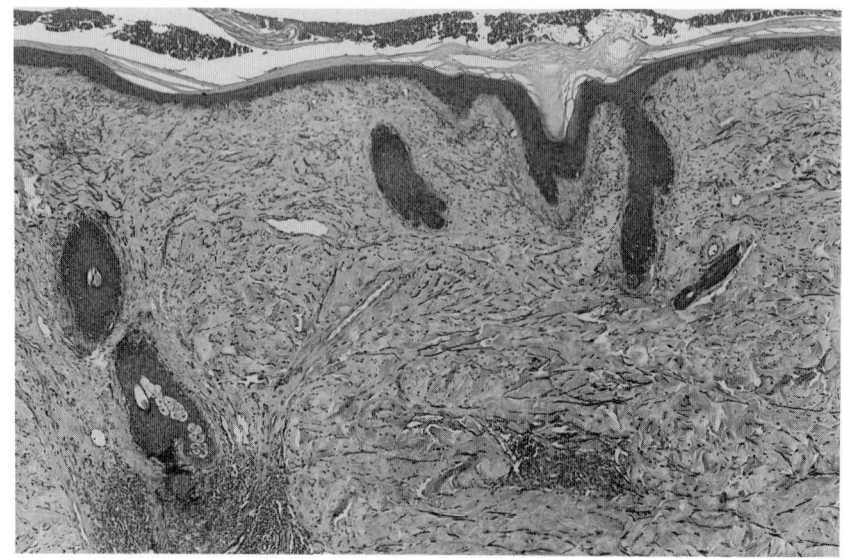

(a)

(b)

Figure 17.1 Morphoea (a and b). Dermal collagen fibres are thickened, with retention of elastic fibres. Lymphocytic infiltration is present around deeper dermal vessels.

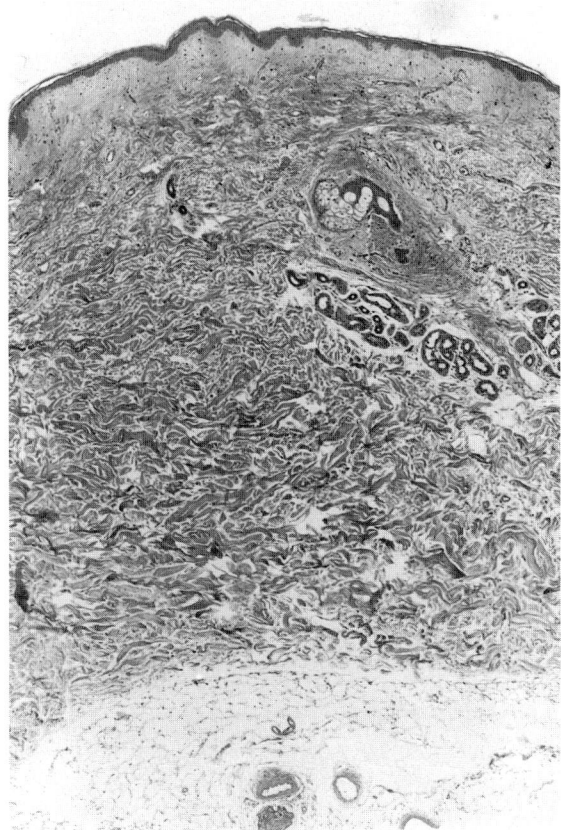

Figure 17.2   Scleroderma. The dermis is increased in thickness, with sweat gland atrophy, but without any lymphocytic infiltration.

biopsy appearances vary depending on the age of the lesion. The epidermis is hyperkeratotic, with associated follicular plugging and with atrophy of the prickle cell layer. The papillary dermis shows oedema and hyalinization of the collagen. Beneath this there is a zone of lymphocytic infiltration. With increasing age, the zone of hyalinization increases and the inflammatory infiltrate migrates downwards and, at the same time, diminishes in intensity.

Similar lesions can occur at non-genital sites, where the differential diagnosis is from morphoea or localized scleroderma. An AOG stained section can help in differential diagnosis, as elastic fibres are retained in scleroderma and lost in lichen sclerosus (Rahbari, 1989).

Recent evidence suggests that infection with the spirochete of Lyme

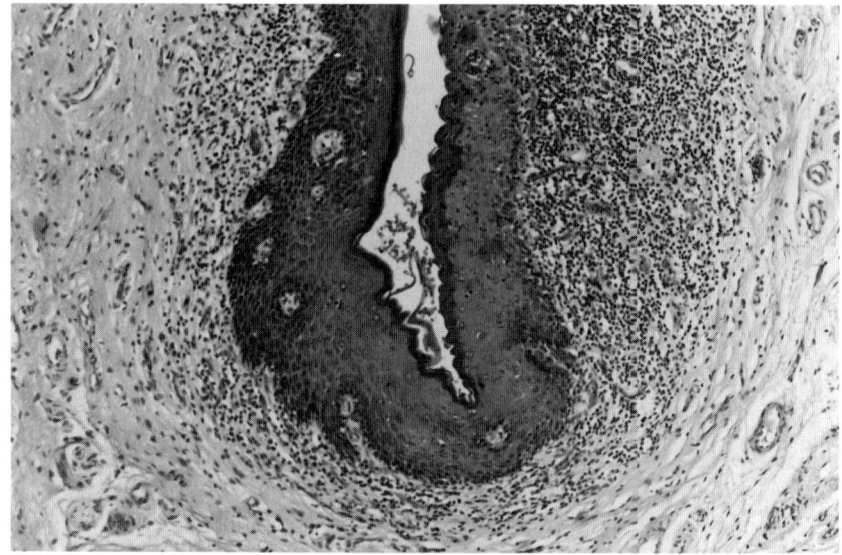

Figure 17.3   Balanitis xerotica obliterans of prepuce, showing hyperkeratosis and lyphocytic infiltration but without dermal hyalinization.

disease may play a role in the aetiology of both conditions, but especially of lichen sclerosus (Aberer and Stanek, 1987; Aberer and Aberer, 1988; Duray, 1989). This is an interesting proposition, as other lines of investigation, including the search for an autoimmune basis, have drawn a blank (Meyrick Thomas *et al.*, 1988).

17.3 Mucinoses

There is a group of rare conditions in which the biopsy may show an increase of connective tissue mucin (Truhan and Roenigk, 1986). This acid mucin can be stained with Alcian blue at pH 2.5, but will not be seen with staining after hyaluronidase incubation or at the lower pH of 0.5 (Johnson and Helwig, 1966). Giemsa staining may also stain the mucin (Steigleder and Kuchmeister, 1985).

The mucin may be present either focally or diffusely between collagen bundles in the dermis. The amount of mucin present varies and may be quite small. It can be reliably found in pretibial myxoedema, which is usually a complication of thyrotoxicosis. Indeed, massive accumulation of mucin in this condition causes the indurated nodules and plaques on the shins, which characterize the condition (Truhan, 1985). Generalized myxoedema, due to hypothyroidism, shows more subtle changes, with either no detectable mucin or small amounts around hair follicles and blood vessels.

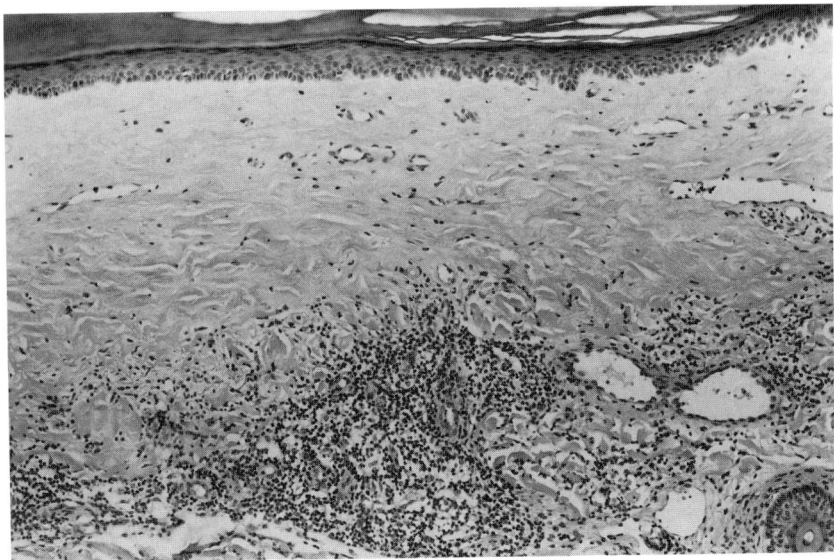

Figure 17.4 Lichen sclerosus. Developed lesion with dermal hyalinization and deep dermal lymphocytic infiltration.

The idiopathic mucinoses may have papular lesions (lichen myxoedematosus and scleromyxoedema), with focal collections of mucin in the papillary dermis, or form macules (reticular erythematous mucinosis), with the mucin around hair follicles and blood vessels. Scleromyxoedema is usually, although not exclusively, associated with a paraprotein (Pravata *et al.*, 1989), and with autoimmune diseases, especially lupus erythematosus (Rongioletti and Rebora, 1986; Bourgeois *et al.*, 1987). The mucin is probably produced as a result of immunological stimulation of dermal fibroblasts (Igarashi *et al.*, 1985). Conversely, it has been suggested that the clinical appearance of rheumatoid disease can be mimicked by scleromyoedema with systemic involvement (Fudman *et al.*, 1986).

Larger collections of mucin, described as focal mucinosis by Johnson and Helwig (1966) are almost certainly the same condition as that described as superficial angiomyxoma by Allen *et al.* (1988).

17.4 Reactive perforating collagenosis

There are a number of related conditions presenting clinically with hyperkeratotic papules, and which have in common the appearance of collagen bundles which appear to perforate from the dermis through the epidermis, usually in the base of a crater. The collagen will usually stain strongly with elastic stains such as orcein. Sometimes, the condi-

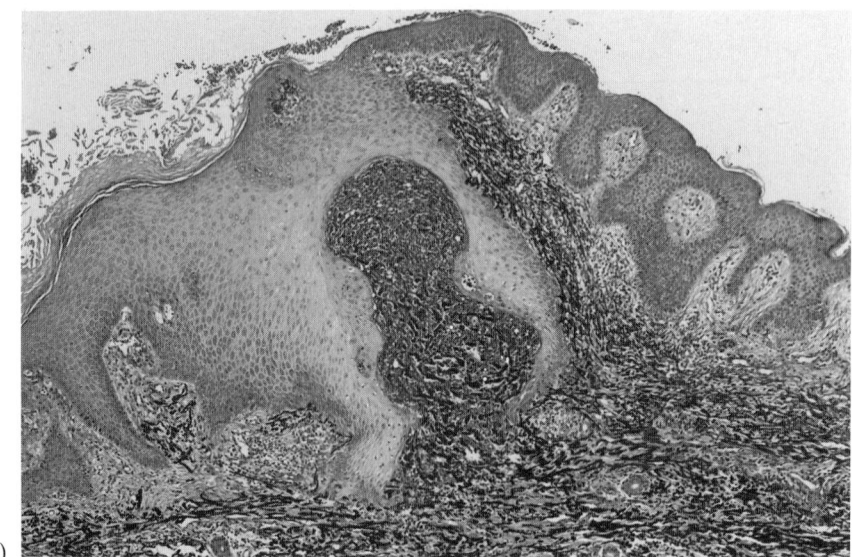

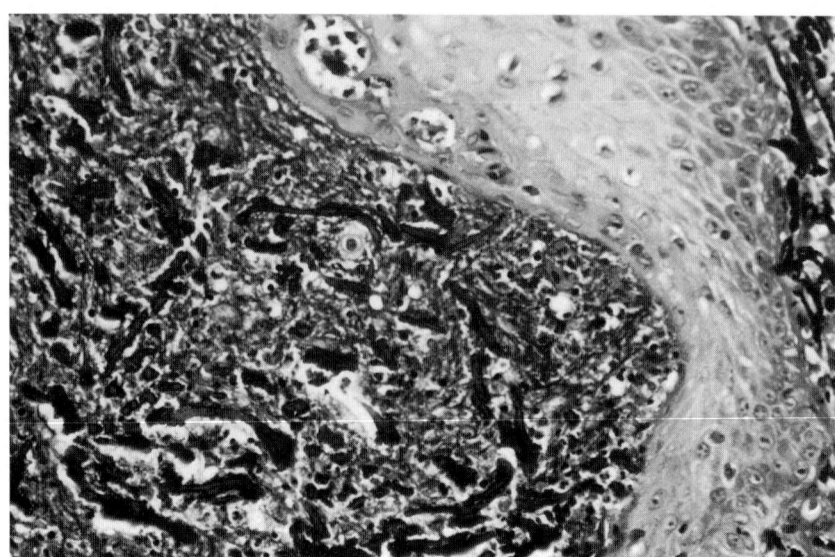

Figure 17.5 Reactive perforating collagenosis. (a) A dense column of elastotic material is being extruded through the epidermis (AOG), and (b) high-power view of elastotic material (AOG).

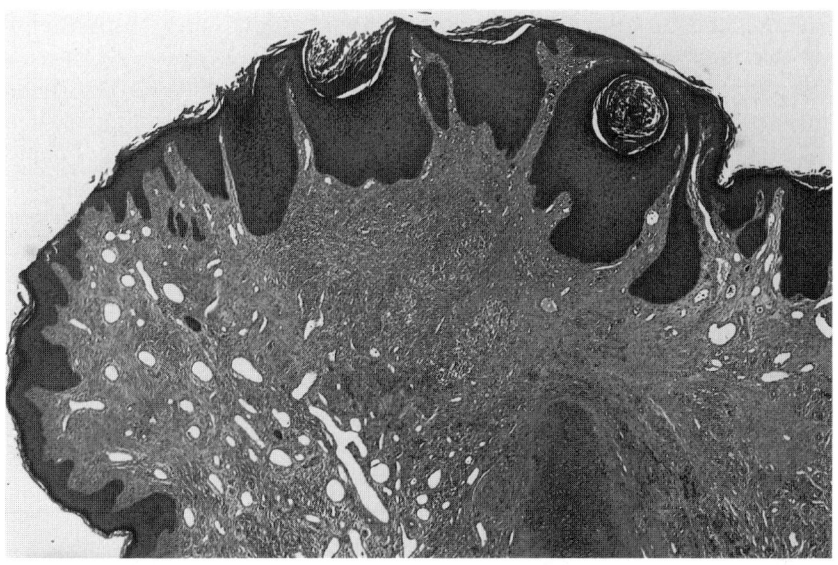

(a)

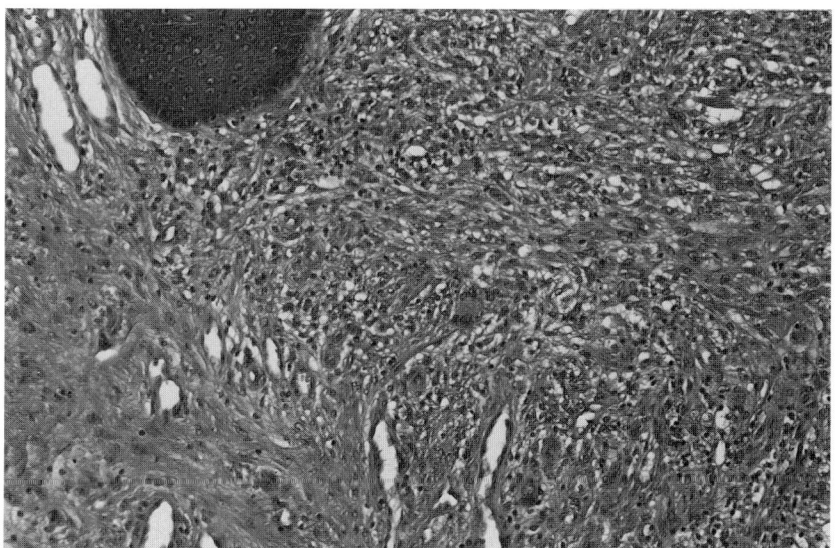

(b)

Figure 17.6 Chondrodermatitis nodularis. (a) The lesion shows epidermal acanthosis, dermal granulation tissue and basophilic change in cartilage, and (b) a closer view of the centre of the lesion.

tion will be of hereditary type, appear in infancy and subsequently resolve spontaneously (Mehregan *et al.*, 1967). The cause is uncertain but may be a consequence of intense scratching, such as the severe pruritis associated with Hodgkin's disease (Pedragosa *et al.*, 1987), or be associated with renal disease (Schamroth *et al.*, 1986), or diabetes mellitus (Poliak *et al.*, 1982).

This appearance has been described variously as reactive perforating collagenosis, elastosis perforans serpiginosa, perforating folliculitis, or Kyrle's disease.It has been suggested that these related conditions could be grouped together under the title of 'acquired perforating dermatosis' (Tappeiner *et al.*, 1969) Different papules from the same patient may show different appearances, so it is difficult to subdivide the possible diagnosis accurately based on random sampling of only a few lesions (Rapini *et al.*, 1989).

17.5   Chondrodermatitis nodularis

Small, firm, painful nodules on the ears of old men are the typical background to these biopsies. The cause is uncertain. Speculation about ischaemia and hard pillows has been largely inconclusive. The biopsy appearances are characteristic; difficulties arise when the biopsy does not extend down to cartilage.

The lesion has three components, forming a circumscribed nodule. The epidermis shows localized acanthosis and hyperkeratosis, sometimes with central ulceration. The underlying dermis contains a reactive proliferation of capillaries, with small numbers of associated lymphoid cells, amounting to a focus of granulation tissue. Both of these features can be found in a typical biopsy. In larger specimens, part of the cartilage will be included and will usually show a characteristic basophilic degenerative change. The absence of cartilage in the biopsy sometimes leads to confusion, but the overlying complex of dermal and epidermal hyperplasia usually suffice for diagnosis.

References

Aberer, E. and Stanek, G. (1987) Histological evidence for spirochetal origin of morphoea and lichen sclerosus et atrophicus. *Am. J. Dermatopathol.*, **9**, 374–9.

Aberer, E. and Aberer, W. (1988) [The spectrum of Lyme borreliosis from the dermatologic viewpoint]. *Derm. Beruf. Umwelt.*, **36**, 39–44.

Allen, P. W., Dymock, R. B. and MacCormac, L. B. (1988) Superficial angiomyxomas with and without epithelial component. *Am. J. Surg. Pathol.*, **12**, 519–30.

Bourgeois, P., Bard, H., Bourgeois-Droin, C. and Kahn, M. F. (1987) Papular mucinosis. Associated dermatologic and dysimmune aspects. *Rev. Rhum. Mal. Osteoartic.*, **54**, 109–12.

Duray, P. H. (1989) Clinical pathological correlations of Lyme disease. *Rev. Infect. Dis.*, **11** (suppl. 6P), S1487–93.

Fudman, E. J., Golbus, J. and Ike, R. W. (1986) Scleromyxedema with systemic involvement mimics rheumatic diseases. *Arthritis Rheum.*, **29**, 913–17.

Igarashi, M., Aizawa, H., Tokudome, Y. and Tagami, H. (1985) Dermatomyositis with prominent mucinous skin change. Histochemical and biochemical aspects of glycosaminoglycans. *Dermatologica*, **170**, 6–11.

Johnson, W. C. and Helwig, E. B. (1966) Cutaneous focal mucinosis. *Arch. Dermatol.*, **93**, 13–20.

Mehregan, A. H., Schwartz, O. D. and Livingood, C. S. (1967) Reactive perforating collagenosis. *Arch. Dermatol.*, **96**, 277–82.

Meyrick Thomas, R. H., Ridley, C. M., McGibbon, D. H. and Black, M. M. (1988) Lichen sclerosus et atrophicus and autoimmunity – a study of 350 women. *Br. J. Dermatol.*, **118**, 41–6.

Pedragosa, R., Knobel, H. J., Huguet, P., Oristrell, J., Valdes, M. and Bosch, J. A. (1985) Reactive perforating collagenosis in Hodgkin's disease. *Am. J. Dermatopathol.*, **9**, 41–4.

Poliak, S. C., Lebwohl, M. G., Parris, A. and Ptioleau, P. G. (1982) Reactive perforating collagenosis associated with diabetes mellitus. *New Engl. J. Med.*, **306**, 81–4.

Pravata, G., Noto, G. and Arico, M. (1989) Scleromyedema without paraproteinemia. *G. Ital. Dermatol. Venereol.*, **124**, 85–8.

Rahbari, H. (1989) Histochemical differentiation of localized morphoea-scleroderma and lichen sclerosus et atrophicus. *J. Cutan. Pathol.*, **16**, 342–7.

Rapini, R. P., Herbert, A. A. and Drucker, C. R. (1989) Acquired perforating dermatosis. Evidence for combined transepidermal elimination of both collagen and elastic fibers. *Arch. Dermatol.*, **125**, 1074–8.

Rongioletti, F. and Rebora, A. (1986) Papular and nodular mucinosis associated with systemic lupus erythematosus. *Br. J. Dermatol.*, **115**, 631–6.

Ross, S. A., Sanchez, J. L. and Taboas, J. O. (1990) Spirochetal forms in the dermal lesions of morphoea and lichen sclerosus et atrophicus. *Am. J. Dermatopathol.*, **12**, 357–62.

Rustin, M. H. A., Papadaki, L., Rode, J. and Dowd, P. M. (1989) Elastic fibres in patients with systemic sclerosis. A morphological study. *Virchows Arch. A.*, **416**, 115–20.

Schamroth, J. M., Kellen, P. and Grieve, T. P. (1986) Elastosis perforans serpiginosa in a patient with renal disease. *Arch. Dermatol.*, **122**, 82–4.

Steigleder, G. K. and Kuchmeister, B. (1985) Cutaneous mucinous deposits. *J. Cut. Pathol.*, **12**, 334–7.

Tosti, A., Melino, M. and Bardazzi, F. (1989) Hemorrhagic bullous lesions in morphea. *Cutis*, **44**, 118–19.

Truhan, A. P. (1985) Pretibial myxedema. *Am. Fam. Physician.*, **31**, 135–8.

Truhan, A. P. and Roenigk, H. H. Jr (1986) The cutaneous mucinoses. *J. Am. Acad. Dermatol.*, **14**, 1–18.

Tappeiner, J., Wolff, K. and Schreiner, E. (1969) Morbus Kyrle. *Hautarzt*, **20**, 296–310.

18 Artefact *et al.*

In the preceding description of varying types of inflammatory skin disease, it has been assumed in most cases that the cause is unknown. There remain two areas in which a cause may be more clearly identified. Cutaneous drug reactions are many and varied. Indeed, they really recapitulate the spectrum of inflammatory disease: some examples are given by way of illustration, but it would be an impossible task to list them all here.

Finally, there are those conditions which are inflicted on the skin by the patient, the doctor, or some other third party. These also cover quite a range of possibilities and so illustrative examples are given.

18.1 Drug reactions

The archetypal drug reaction is the fixed type, where the biopsy shows an eosinophilic perivascular infiltrate often of quite mild degree. The underlying mechanism of fixed drug eruptions remains largely unexplained, but may be related to a localized misregulated expression of the intercellular adhesion molecule-1 (ICAM-1) by the keratinocytes in the epidermis of the lesion (Shiohara *et al.*, 1989).

There are now so many drugs on the market that reactions can take many forms (Rehman, 1986). The mechanism will determine the appearance and will either be immune or non-immune in type. Non-immune reactions may be due to overdosage, toxicity or interaction. Immune reactions will vary depending upon whether the process is IgE dependent, immune complex mediated, cytotoxic or cell mediated (Wintroub and Stern, 1985). Furthermore, a particular type of drug, for instance non-steroidal anti-inflammatories, may produce a spectrum of reactions (Stern and Bigby, 1984; O'Brien and Bagby, 1985).

The commoner reactions include urticaria, which is seen with many drugs, including aspirin, penicillin and blood products; morbilliform rashes classically seen 10 days after an injection of ampicillin; photo-

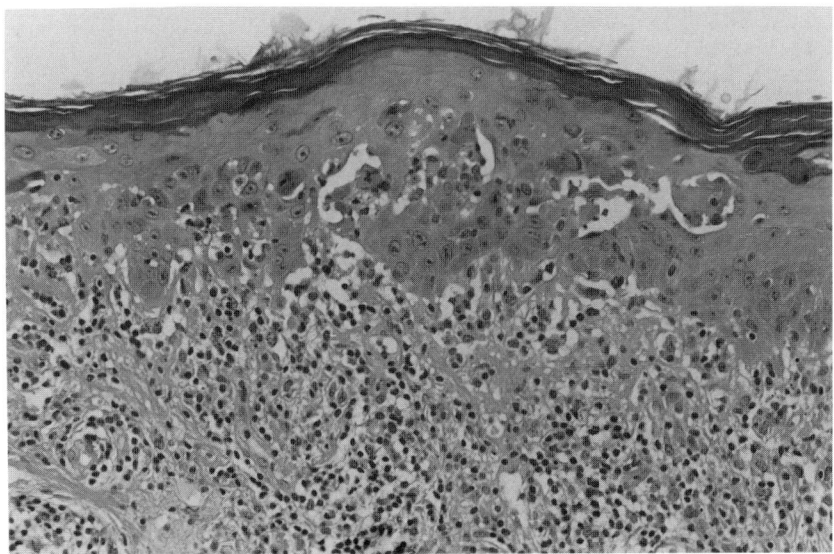

Figure 18.1 Lichenoid drug eruption. A vigorous reaction at the dermal–epidermal interface with many Civatte bodies.

sensitive eruptions caused by non-steroidal, anti-inflammatory drugs, chlorpromazine, tetracycline and thiazides; drug induced photosensitive diseases such as the development of lupus erythematosus after procainamide therapy; and erythema multiforme induced by drugs such as phenylbutazone or diphenylhydantoin (Wintroub and Stern, 1985).

Other examples include aspirin induced erythema nodosum (Abrishami and Thomas, 1977), pseudolymphomas due to mexiletine, thioridazine or D-penicillamine (Kardaun *et al.*, 1988), cutaneous necrosis after coumarin (Grimaudo *et al.*, 1989), and a variety of rashes in the elderly on beta blockers (Clerens, 1981). Existing conditions may be exacerbated when a new treatment is started, for instance, by etretinate in psoriatic patients (David *et al.*, 1986).

These examples must be taken as such. The list is long and ever changing. Some of those listed are now less fashionable, whilst their replacements may produce reactions of their own. At the time of writing a brief epidemic of an acute eosinophilic dermatomyositis-like syndrome related to the consumption of L-tryptophan containing diet aids has just come and gone (Eidson *et al.*, 1990).

In case of doubt, one should consult the librarian or drug information pharmacist for the latest news on the ever expanding range of reported

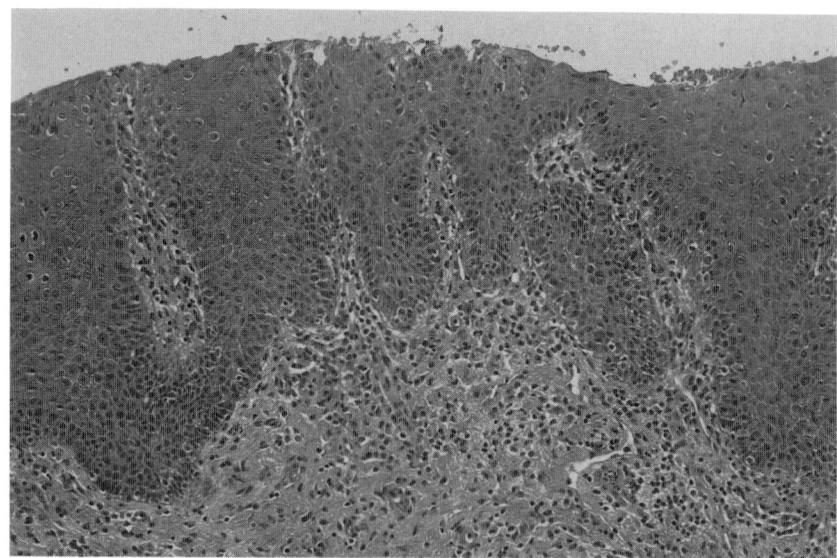

Figure 18.2   A florid nappy rash, with loss of the epidermal surface and reactive dermal infiltrate.

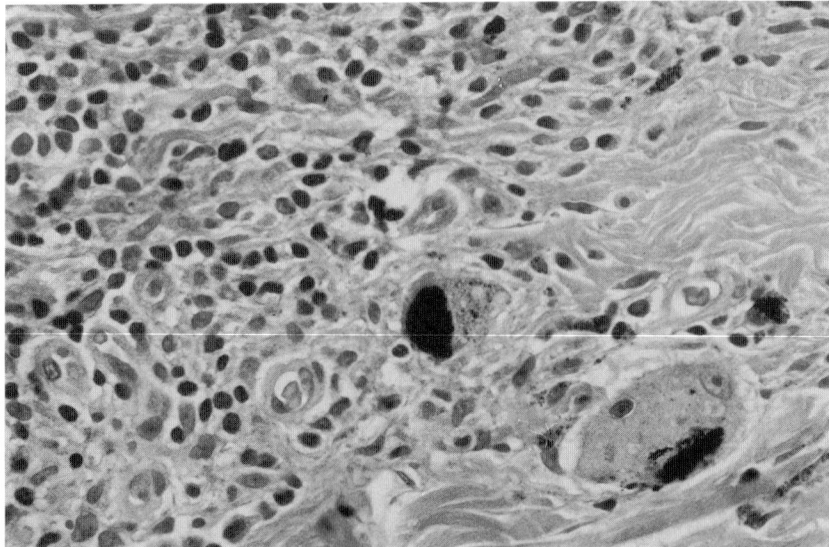

Figure 18.3   Tattoo. Pigment phagocytosed within giant cells must be distinguished from melanin.

drug reactions. In confirmed cases, one should also make sure that the details are reported to the appropriate authority, so that one's findings will be more generally available. This is particularly important for newly introduced agents, where rapid dissemination of news of novel reactions is important.

18.2   Dermatitis artefacta

When all of the process described in the earlier parts of this book have been considered and still no reasonable explanation has been found, then the possibility must be considered that the lesion is self-inflicted.

This conclusion must not be reached easily. One must always be especially careful before saying that the patient is producing the lesion for which medical care is being sought. First, because such a suggestion may hinder the diagnosis of an organic disease and, second, because the treatment of dermatitis artefacta can be so difficult. Dermatitis artefacta is a difficult subject from the clinical point of view, but must always be born in mind when the biopsy does not seem right or does not seem to fit with the other clinical information available.

Artefactual lesions are of two main types. The first is produced by simple physical rubbing or scratching, which produces a reaction characterized by epidermal hyperplasia, possibly with a component of dermal scarring. This is the appearance of lichen simplex. Heavy scratching may lead to excoriation. However, excoriation alone should not be taken as evidence of artefact. So many skin conditions are irritating or painful that changes due to scratching may be found superimposed upon a number of perfectly respectable dermatoses.

The second type is that more usually recognized as dermatitis artefacta, and caused by the application of some form of noxious substance to the skin by the patient. A variety of appearances may be seen, but they are characterized by changes which are often described as being 'outside in'. Often the lesion will have been caused by the use of some form of caustic or thermal injury. The epidermis will be more severely affected than the dermis, with the outer part of the epidermis more markedly affected than the basal layers. Indeed, the dermis will often show little change at all. Whatever dermal change is seen, it will usually be disproportionately mild in comparison to the epidermal changes.

Various foreign bodies may turn up, and in case of doubt it is always worth examining the section under polarized light in order to detect otherwise invisible material.

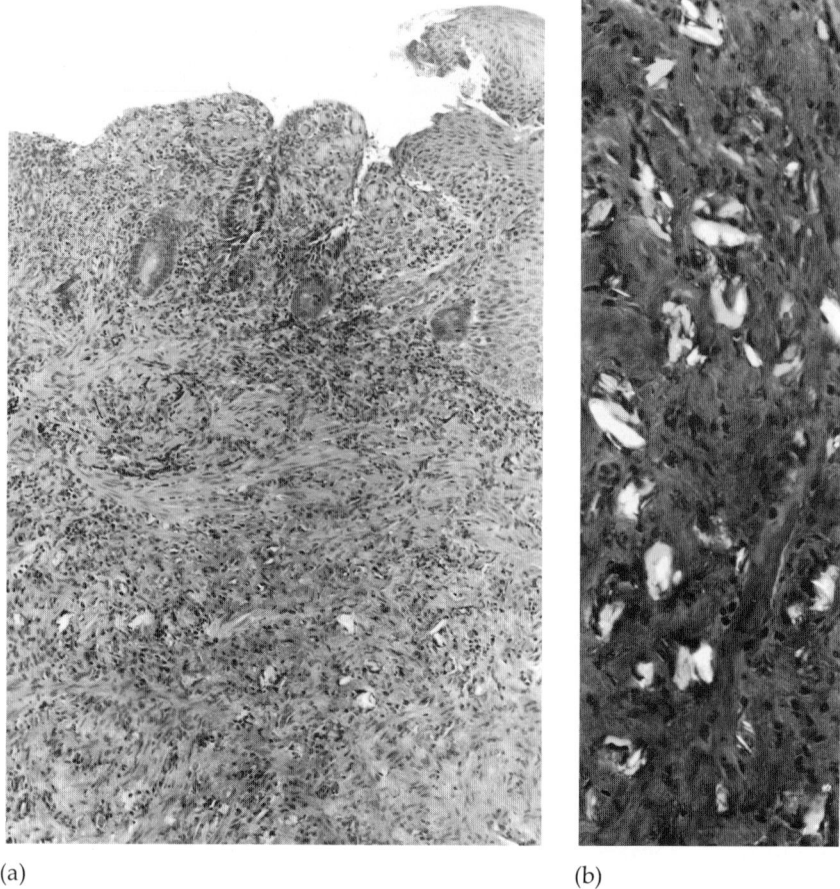

(a)   (b)

Figure 18.4 Umbilical omphalomesenteric duct polyp (a). Polarized light (b) shows large amounts of baby powder within the granulation tissue associated with this ulcerated congenital abnormality.

18.3 Panniculitis artefacta

Most forms of organic panniculitis involve the legs. When unusual sites, such as the breasts or genitalia are involved, or the character of the reaction is unusual, then the possibility of artefact should be considered. The cause is usually some form of injected material, whose presence may be revealed by polarized light. The agent may have been injected legitimately. Some drugs, such as pentazocine, can cause a sclerosing reaction at the injection site. The vehicle used in depot

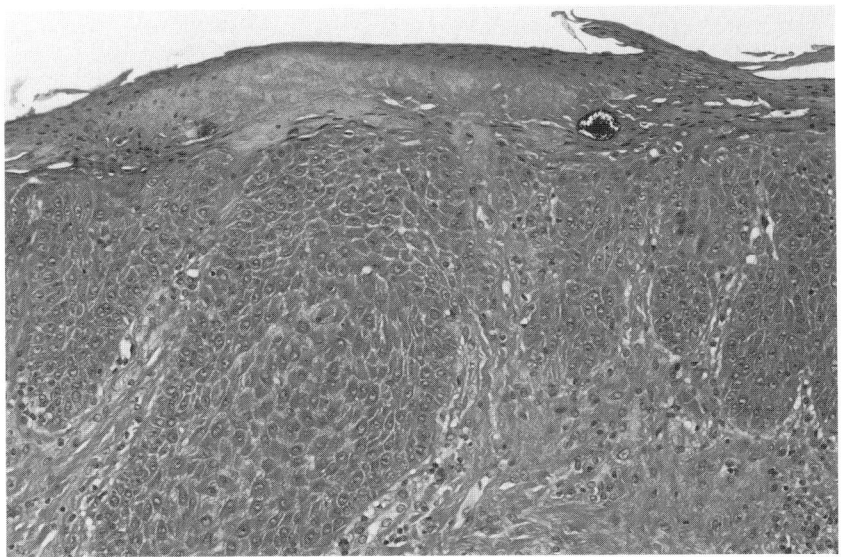

Figure 18.5 Cryotherapy failed to penetrate this viral wart so the remainder was excised. The superficial part shows coagulative necrosis.

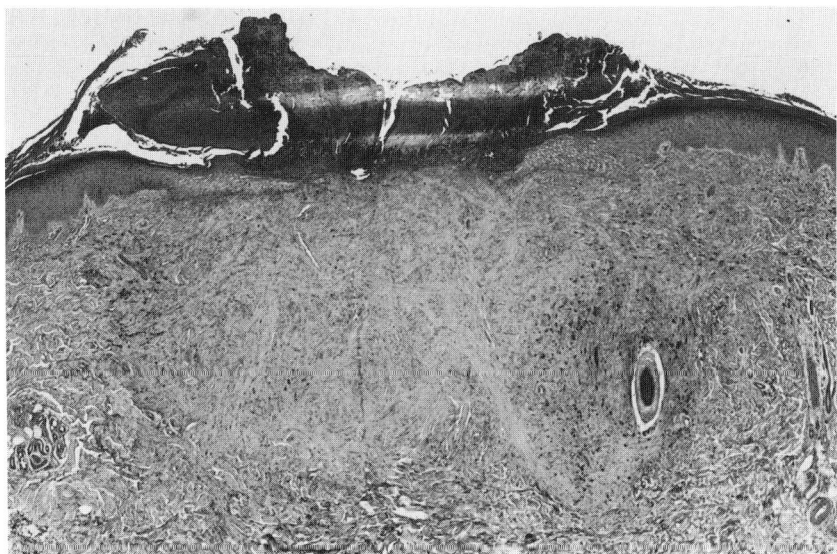

Figure 18.6 Dermatitis artefacta. This excision biopsy of a blue naevus shows superficial excoriation as a result of the patient 'picking' at the lesion.

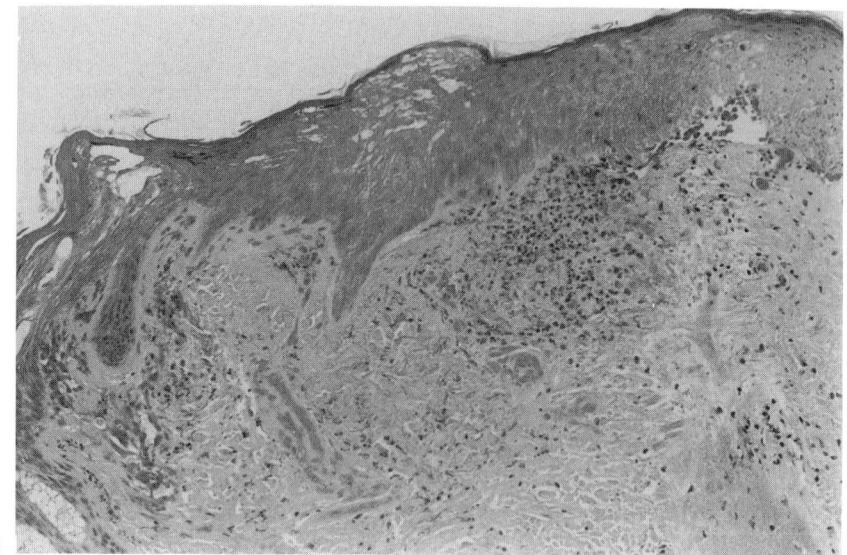

(a)

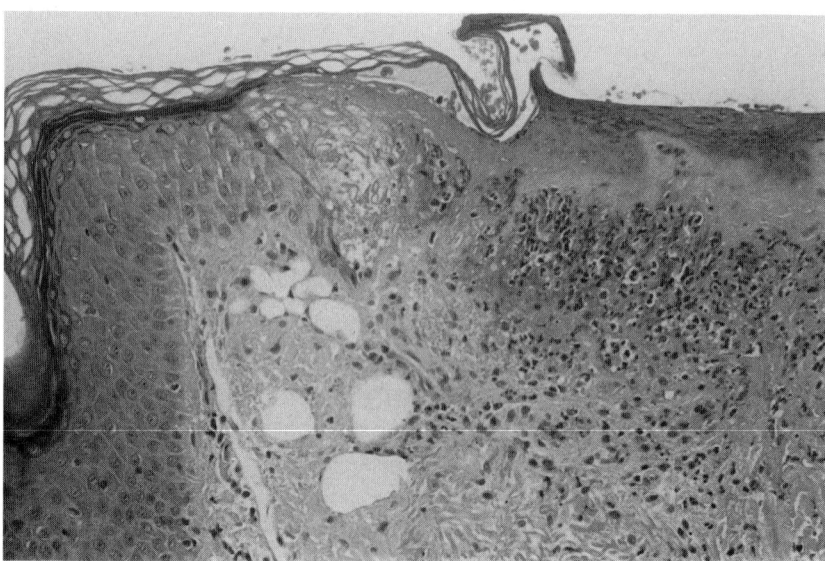

(b)

Figure 18.7   Dermatitis artefacta. Although there is a dermal lymphocytic infiltrate in this biopsy (a), a higher power view (b) shows coagulative necrosis which is maximal on the surface of the epidermis.

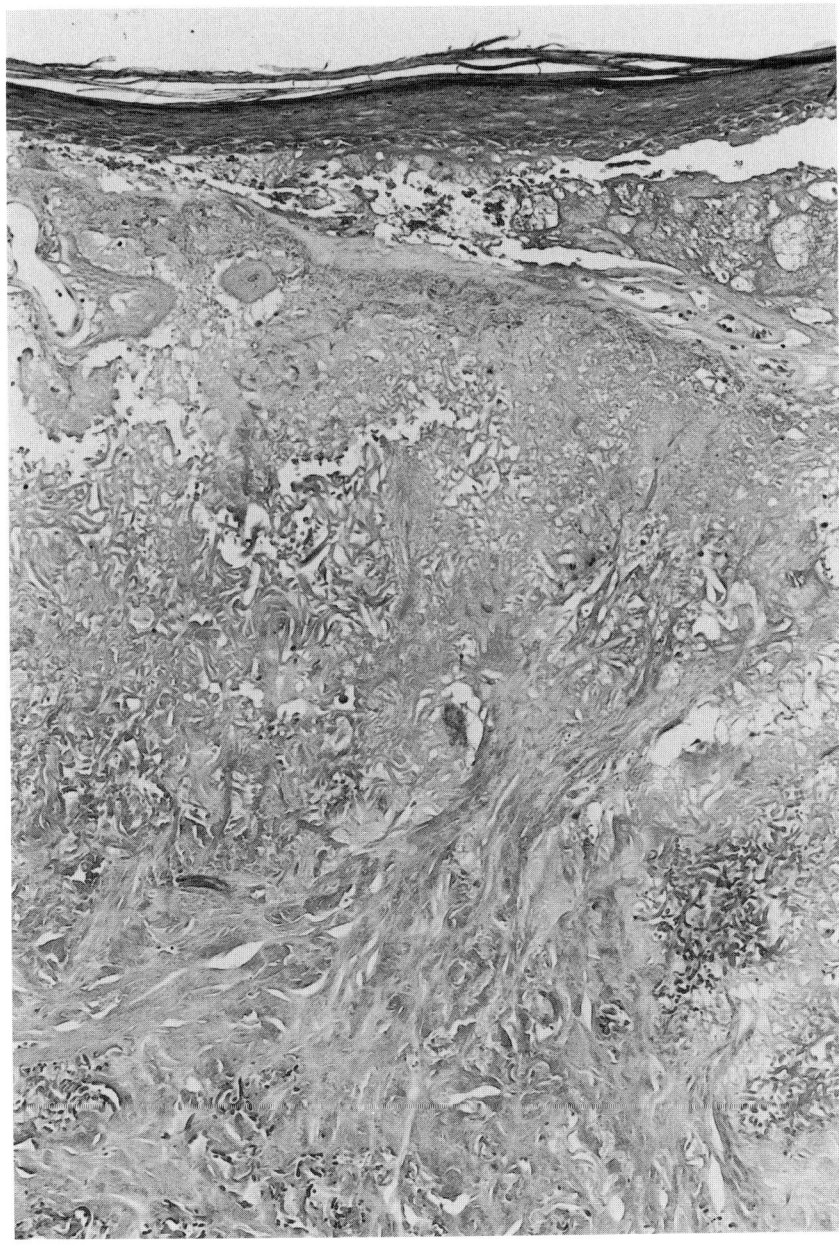

Figure 18.8 Previous radiotherapy. Severe disruption of normal dermal architecture, with stromal changes resembling severe solar elastosis, caused by the long-term effects of radiotherapy.

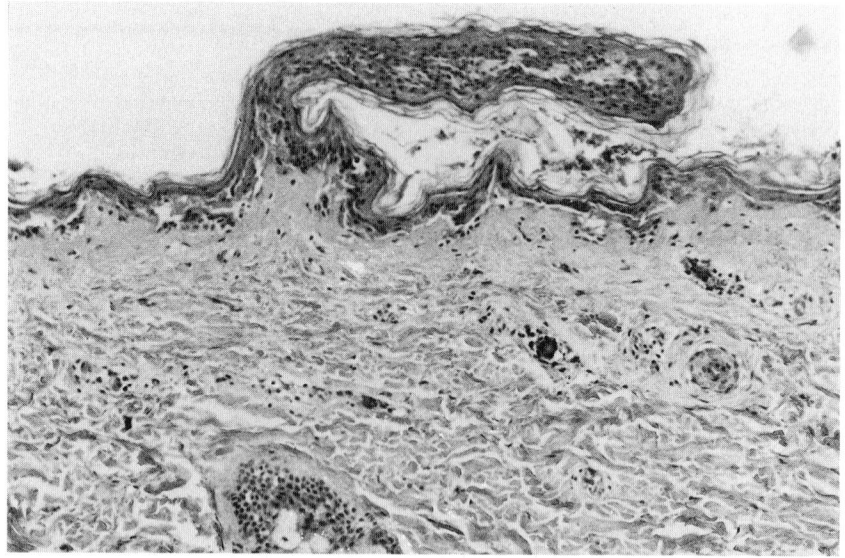

Figure 18.9   Clefting at the base of the epidermis, without cellular reaction in an acute burn.

injections can sometimes turn up as a firm subcutaneous nodule at a later date (Forstrom and Winkelmann, 1974).

18.4   Effects of heat and cold

Coagulative necrosis of the skin may be caused accidentally or therapeutically, the depth of involvement depending on the extent of the insult. The long-term effects of radiotherapy may also present in biopsies, as extensive elastosis, with abnormal collagen and increased fragility.

Finally it is worth reiterating the need for full information to be available – for the clinician to take a full history. We live in changing times, where political fortunes ebb and flow at an ever increasing rate and 'new' lesions may turn up in the clinic, such as the long-term physical effects of torture (Karlsmark *et al.*, 1989), and as travel becomes ever cheaper and easier, holiday-makers returning from exotic vacations on tropical sands may be well and truly jiggered.

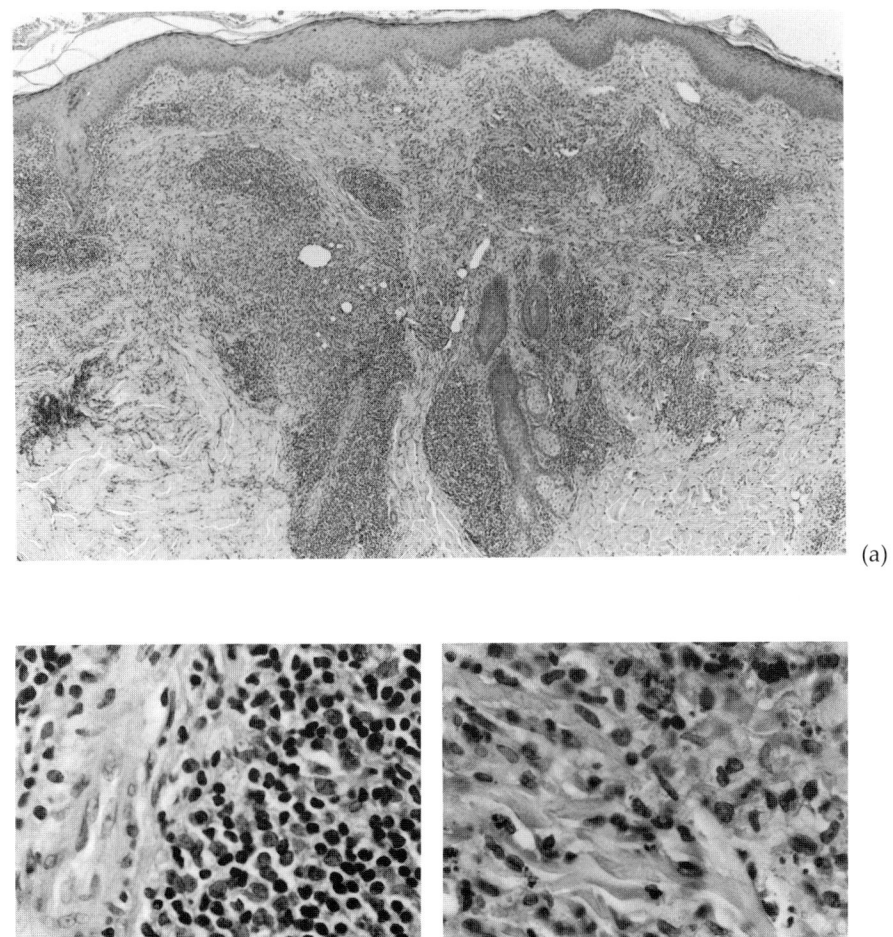

(a)

(b)

(c)

Figure 18.10 Persistent insect bite. (a) An infiltrate tapering towards the base, with (b) peripheral lymphocytic aggregates, and (c) central leukocytoclastic change.

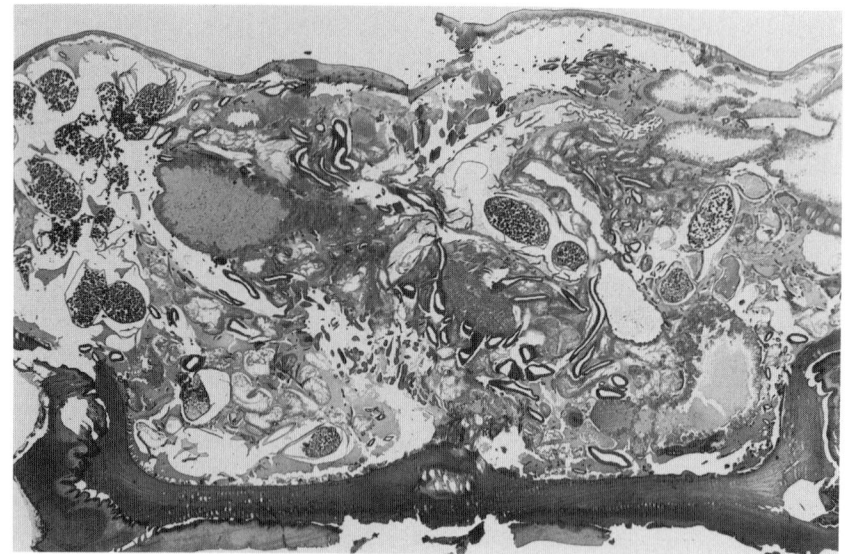

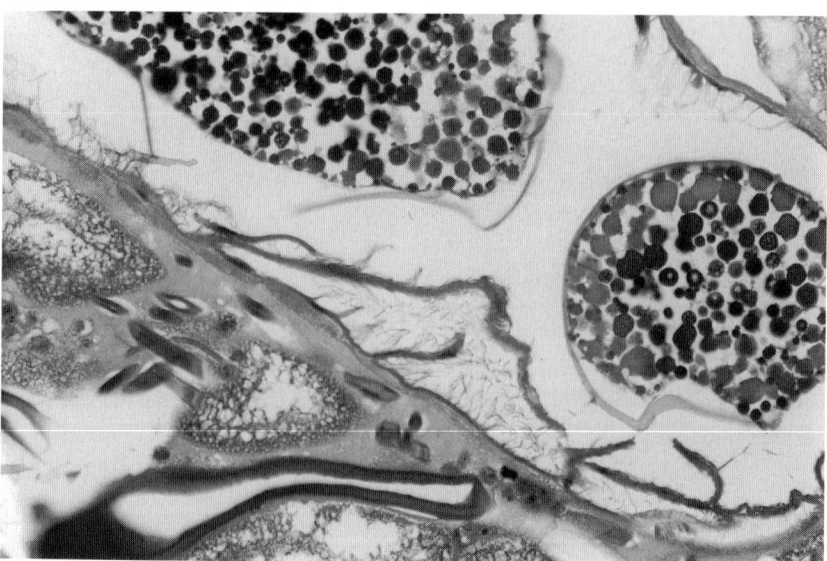

Figure 18.11 A limited local excision of a nodule on the foot, noticed after the patient had been on a beach holiday in East Africa. The biopsy shows (a) a jigger, with (b) the internal structure shown at higher power.

(a)

(b)

References

Abrishami, M. A. and Thomas, J. (1977) Aspirin intolerance: a review. *Ann. Allergy*, **39**, 28–37.

Clerens, A., Guilmot-Bruneau, M. M., Defresne, C. and Bouland, T. (1981) Revue: a propos des beta-bloquants en dermatologie. *Dermatologica*, **163**, 5–11.

David, M., Ginzburg, A., Hodak, E. and Feuerman, E. J. (1986) Palmoplantar eruption associated with etretinate therapy. *Acta. Derm. Venereol. (Stockh.)*, **66**, 87–9.

Eidson, M., Philen, R. M., Sewell, C. M., Voorhees, R. and Kilbourne, E. M. (1990) L-tryptophan and eosinophilia-myalgia syndrome in New Mexico. *Lancet*, **335**, 645–8.

Forstrom, L. and Winkelmann, R. K. (1974) Factitial panniculitis. *Arch. Dermatol.*, **110**, 747–50.

Grimaudo, V., Gueissaz, F., Hauert, J., Sarraj, A., Kruithof, E. K. and Bachmann, F. (1989) Necrosis of skin induced by coumarin in a patient deficient in protein S. *Br. Med. J.*, **298**, 233–4.

Kardaun, S. H., Scheffer, E. and Vermeer, B. J. (1988) Drug-induced pseudolymphomatous skin reactions. *Br. J. Dermatol.*, **118**, 545–52.

Karlsmark, T., Danielsen, J., Thomsen, H. K., Aalund, O., Nielsen, O., Nielsen, K. G., Johnson, E. and Genefke, I. K. (1983) Tracing the use of torture: electrically induced calcification of collagen in pig skin. *Nature*, **301**, 75–8.

Linberg, M. (1986) Dynamic changes in the epidermal OKT6 positive cells at mild irritant reactions in human skin. *Acta. Derm. Venereol. (Stockh.)*, **66**, 117–20.

O'Brien, W. M. and Bagby, G. F. (1985) Rare adverse reactions to nonsteroidal anti-inflammatory drugs. *J. Rheumatol.*, **12**, 13–20.

Rehman, R. S. (1986) Histology of adverse cutaneous drug reactions. *Clin. Dermatol.*, **4**, 23–9.

Shiohara, T., Nickoloff, B. J., Sagawa, Y., Gomi, T. and Nagashima, M. (1989) Fixed drug eruption. Expression of epidermal keratinocyte intercellular adhesion molecule-1 (ICAM-1). *Arch. Dermatol.*, **125**, 1371–6.

Stern, R. S. and Bigby, M. (1984) An expanding profile of cutaneous reactions to nonsteroidal anti-inflammatory reactions. *JAMA*, **252**, 1433–7.

Wintroub, B. G. and Stern, R. (1985) Cutaneous drug reactions: pathogenesis and clinical classification. *J. Am. Acad. Dermatol.*, **13**, 167–79.

Index

Page numbers in *italics* refer to figures and to Colour Plates *(Pl)*, page numbers in **bold** refer to main entries.

Acanthocytes, normal 5
Acantholytic keratosis, transient focal 47
Acanthoma, large cell **40–2**, *41*
Acanthosis 25
Acanthosis nigricans **51**
Accretive growth, in naevus 90
Acid orcein Giemsa stain 5, 26, *29*
Acne agminata **323–4**, *324–6*
Acne rosacea 323, **324**
Acquired immunodeficiency syndrome (AIDS) 328
  acute virus exanthema **334**
  Cryptococcus infection 337
  Cytomegalovirus infection 337
  Herpes infection *336*
  Histoplasma infection 337
  Pneumocystis infection 337
  seborrhoeic-like dermatitis **334–7**
Acrosyryngeal naevus 136
Acrosyryngium *4*
Actinic granuloma **326**
Acute burn *384*
Adenosquamous carcinoma **87**
Adnexal tumours
  as markers of internal malignancy 130
  fifth category 131
  splitting or lumping 130
Alcian blue, stain for mucin 26
Alopecia, transverse sectioning of biopsy **255–8**

Alopecia, scarring **259–60**, *259*
Alopecia areata **258–9**
Amyloidosis, bullous **300**
Anagen, phase of hair follicle growth 8
Anchoring fibrils 5
Angiocentic lymphoma **272–3**, 348
Angioendothelioma, malignant endovascular papillary 195
Angiokeratoma *191*
Angioleiomyoma **203**, *209*
Angiomyxoma, superficial 371
Angiosarcoma **195**
Annual workload, analysis of 2
Apocrine gland tumours **142–4**
  carcinoma **144**
  fibroadenoma **144**
  papillary hidradenoma **144**, *145*
  papillary syringoadenoma **144**
Artefact, dermatitis **379**, *381*, *382*
Artefact, panniculitis **364**
Atrial myxoma, metastatic 188
Audit, feedback on performance 2
Avian haemangiomatosis 333

B-cell lymphoma, cutaneous **277–8**, *278–9*
B-K mole syndrome *105*
Bacillary angiomatosis **333–4**, *335*
Bacillary angiomatosis, Bartonellosis as cause 334

Balanitis xerotica obliterans 370
Baldness, marker of unstoppable
    march of time 255
Bartonellosis 334
Basal cell carcinoma **70–7**
  adenoid *71*
  aggressive growth pattern 75, *74,*
      Pl 13 a and b
  differentiation from
      trichoepithelioma 161
  follow up 76
  form of excision 76
  likelihood of recurrence 76
  metastasis 67, 77
  metatypical *73, Pl 14 a*
  neuroendocrine differentiation in 72
  nodular *69, 75*
  sclerosing growth pattern 75, *74,*
      Pl 13 a and b
  superficial multicentric *68*
Basal cells, normal **4**
Basement membrane, epidermal **4**
Basosquamous carcinoma **85–7,** *86*
Behcet's disease **353**
  clinical overlap with Sweet's
      syndrome 353
  criteria for diagnosis 353
Biopsy
  examining **22–30**
  excisional 17
  fixation 19–20
  incisional 17
  punch 17–18
  reasons for 15–17
  shave 19, *20*
  snip 19
  techniques of 17–20
  trimming of **21**
  types of **15**
Birbeck granules, in Langerhans cells
    7
Blood vessels **6**
Blue naevus **98,** *100*
  cellular **98–102,** *101*
  combined *102–3*
Borst-Jadassohn phenomenon 42
Bowen's disease **34–5,** *35*
Bowenoid papulosis 35, *36*

Breslow tumour thickness, of
    melanoma 111
Bullous amyloidosis **300**
Bullous pemphigoid **291–4,** *288*
Burn, acute *384*

Calcifying epithelioma of Malherbe
    152–5, *156*
Carcino-embryonic antigen (CEA),
    staining in sweat gland tumours
    132–3
Carcinoma, basosquamous **85–7,** *86*
Carcinoma, basal cell, *see* basal cell
    carcinoma
Carcinoma, squamous cells, *see*
    squamous cell carcinoma
Carcinoma, adenosquamous **87**
Carney's complex 130, 185
Catagen, phase of hair follicle growth
    8
CD1 positivity, in Langerhans cells 7
Cellular blue naevus **98–102**
Chondrodermatitis nodularis **374,** *373*
Churg-Strauss syndrome **346–8,** *349*
Cicatricial pemphigoid 291, **294**
Cirsoid aneurysm **188–92,** *194*
Clark's levels of invasion 111
Clark's naevus 108
Clear cell acanthoma, **40,** *39,*
    Pl 4 a and b
Clinical information, necessary for
    pathologist 20
Cold, effects of **384**
Collagen, necrobiotic 320
Collagen, phagocytosis 320
Collagenosis, reactive perforating
    371–4, *372*
Combined naevus *102–3*
Conjunctival naevus 94
Cowden's syndrome 130
Crohn's disease **318**
Cryoglobulinaemia **350–2**
Cryotherapy, effects of *381*
Curettage, 18, *18, 19*
Cutaneous lymphoma
    phenotypic analysis of 266
    monoclonality in 266
Cutaneous T-cell lymphoma **267–72,**

268–72, Pl 22 b, 23 a and b
antigen loss 270, 277
eczema in differential diagnosis 268
multiple biopsies needed for
    diagnosis 268
Pautrier's microabscess in 268
psoriasis in differential diagnosis
    270
stages of 268
transformation to high grade 270
Cysts **165**
    ciliated 171, *170*
    epidermal 165, *168*
    external angular dermoid 171, *169*
    keratin granuloma and rupture 165,
        169
    pilar **149**, *168*
    steatocystoma multiplex *170*
    tricholemmal **149**, *168*
Cytokeratin, staining in sweat gland
    tumours 132–3
Cytology, place in diagnosis 67
Cytomegalovirus infection
    in AIDS 337
    mimicking SLE 238
Cytophagic histiocytic panniculitis **364**

Dabska tumour **195**
Darier's disease **47**, *48*
Deep penetrating naevus **95–6**, *95*
Degos, clear cell acanthoma of **40**, *39*
Demodex folliculorum 323, *323*
Dendrocyte dermal 6
Dermal dendrocyte 6
Dermal duct tumour 132, 133
Dermatitis artefacta **379**
Dermatitis herpetiformis **297–9**, *297–
    8*
Dermatofibroma **176–9**, *177, 178*
Dermatofibrosarcoma protuberans
    180–2, *183*
Dermatologist and pathologist work
    together 1
Dermis **5**
Desmoplastic melanoma **124–5**
Diabetic dermopathy *347*
Digital fibroma **184**
Drug reactions **376–9**, *377*
Dyskeratoma, warty **51**, *49*

Dysplastic naevus **102–8**, *106–9*
Dystrophic epidermolysis bullosa
    296–7

Eccrine gland, normal 8
Eccrine sweat gland tumours **131–42**
    classification 131
    dermal duct tumour 132, 133
    hidradenoma, clear cell *138*
    spiradenoma **136–9**, *140–1*
    hidroacanthoma simplex 132, *133*
    hidroadenoma **139**, *134–5*
    mixed dermal tumour **139–42**, *143*
    poroma 132
    poromatosis 132
    spiradenoma, giant vascular **139**
    syringoacanthoma 136
    syringofibroadenoma 136
    syringoma **136**, *137*
Eczema *23*, **218–21**, *219–21*
Elastic fibres, dermal 5
Elastic fibres, phagocytosis 326
Elastosis *32*
Eosinophilic fasciitis **364–5**
Eosinophilic panniculitis **363–4**
Eosinophils 28
    in bullous skin disease 286
    in dermatitis herpetiformis 297
    in pemphigus 287
Epidermal basement membrane 4
Epidermis **4**
Epidermolysis bullosa, dystrophic
    296–7
Epidermolysis bullosa acquisita
    295–6, *296*
Epithelial membrane antigen (EMA),
    staining in sweat gland tumours
    132–3
Erosive pustular dermatosis of scalp
    260
Erythema annulare centrifugum 247
Erythema chronicum migrans **247**, *250*
Erythema elevatum diutinum **352**
Erythema gyratum repens, as marker
    of internal malignancy 247
Erythema gyratum repens *211*
Erythema multiforme **242**, *243*
Erythema nodosum *318*, **358–60**,
    359–60

Fasciitis, necrotizing, Streptococcal infection in 365
Fasciitis, eosinophilic **364−5**
Fasciitis, necrotizing **365**
Fibroblast 6
Fibroepithelioma of Pinkus *72*
Fibrous histiocytoma, angiomatoid **179**
Fibrous papule of nose **184**, *186*
Fibroxanthoma, atypical **180**, *181*
Fish tank granuloma **316**
Fixation, FMA method 19−20
Flegel's disease **35−7**, *37*
Follicle centre lymphoma
   primary cutaneous 277, *278−9*
   secondary cutaneous involvement **278−80**
Follicular mucinosis **260**
Foreign body granuloma **323**
Fungal infection, superficial *226*
Fungi, special stains for 10

Gardner's syndrome 130, 171
Giant calcifying epithelioma of Malherbe **155**
Giant cells, Langhans 304
Giant cells, Touton 304
Giant cells 304
Glomus tumour **195−7**, *197*
   multiple tumours 197
   myofibroma, related to 197
Glucagonoma, and necrolytic migratory erythema *212*
Gluten sensitive enteropathy 297
Glycogen, PAS stain for 10
Graft versus host disease **254−5**
Granular cell tumour **182**, *184*
Granuloma
   actinic **326**
   annulare, diffentiation from rheumatoid granuloma 320
   annulare **318−20**, *319−21*
   fish tank **316**
   foreign body **323**
   fungal **316**
   types of 304
   faciale **350**, *351*
Granulomatosis
   Lymphomatoid 272−3, **348**

Wegener's **342−6**
Grocott's stain 10
Grover's disease **47**, *45*, *46*
Gyrate erythema **247**

Haemangioendothelioma
   epithelioid **192**
   vegetant intravascular of Masson **188**, *193*
Haemangioma **188**
   cavernous *190*
   verrucous *191−2*
Hailey-Hailey disease **47**
Hair follicle, transverse section *7*
Hair follicle tumours **146−61**
   classification 146
   dilated pore of Winer **148**, *150*
   intrepidermal pilar epithelioma 148
   inverted follicular keratosis **148**, *148, Pl 8 a and b*
   perifollicular fibroma **157**
   pilomatrixoma **152−5**, *156*
   proliferating pilar tumour **149**
   proliferating tricholemmal tumour **149**
   trichoadenoma *153, 154*
   trichoblastic fibroma **155**, *159*
   trichoblastoma **155**
   trichoepithelioma, diagnosis in curetting 161
   trichoepithelioma, giant 161
   trichoepithelioma **157**, *163, Pl 15 a and b*
   trichoepithelioma, differentiation from basal cell carcinoma 161
   trichoepithelioma adenoides sebaceum *158*
   trichofolliculoma **149**
   trichogenic trichoblastoma **155−7**, *160−1*
   tricholemmal carcinoma **151**
   tricholemmoma **149−51**, *151−2*
Hair follicles 8, *9*
Halo naevus **115**, *117, 118*
Heat, effect of **384**
Heliodermatitis, chronic 326
Hemidesmosomes 5
Hen's teeth, rarity of 3
Henoch-Schonlein purpura 342, *344*
Herpes **65**, *65*

Herpes gestationis 294
Herpes simplex 65
Herpes zoster 65
Hidroacanthoma simplex 132, *133*
Hidroadenoma **139**, *134–5*
Histiocyte 6
Histiocytoma, epithelioid **180**
Histiocytoses, non-X 277
Histiocytosis, regressing atypical **276**
Histiocytosis X **277**
History, need for clinical 384
Hodgkin's disease, primary
    cutaneous 276
Hydropic degeneration 25
Hyperkeratosis 24
Hyperkeratosis lenticularis perstans
    35–7, *37*

Immunohistochemical methods **11**
Immunohistochemical staining of
    bullous skin disease 286
Impetigo *254*
Incontinentia pigmenti **254**, *258*
Inflammatory dermatoses, cell types
    in infiltrate 238
Infundibulum, hair follicle 8
Insect bite, persistent *385*
Intraepidermal epithelioma **42**, *42, 43*
Inverted follicular keratosis **148**,
    Pl 8 a and b

Jessner's lymphocytic infiltrate
    239–42, *241*
Jiggered 384, *386*
Juvenile xanthogranuloma **185**

Kaposi's sarcoma **329–33**, *330–2*
Keratin, immunohistochemical
    staining for 11
Keratinocytes, normal 5
Keratoacanthoma **78–83**, *82–5*,
    Pl 10 and 11
Keratosis
    acantholytic 34, *Pl 3 a*
    actinic **33**, *33, Pl 1 a and b*
    Bowenoid *Pl 2 a and b*
    florid 34
    inverted follicular **148**, *Pl 8 a and b*

Kogoj, spongiotic pustule of 223
Kyrle's disease 37

Lamina densa 5
Lamina lucida 5
Langerhans cells,
    immunohistochemical staining
    for 11
Langerhans cells 7
Langhans giant cells 304
Large cell acanthoma **40–2**, *41*
Leiomyoma **203**, *208*
Leiomyosarcoma **205**
Leishman-Donovan bodies 313
Leishmaniasis **311–15**, *314–15*
Lentigo maligna **119**, *120*
Lentigo maligna melanoma 119
Lentigo senilis *119*
Leprosy **304–11**, *306–10*
    borderline **310–11**
    determined **307–8**
    erythema nodosum leprosum 311,
        312
    indeterminate **305–7**, *306*
    lepromatous **309–10**
    reactions **311**
    reversal reaction 311
    tuberculoid **308**, *307*
Leser Trelat, sign of *211*
Leukaemia, cutaneous involvement
    280
Leukocytoclastic vasculitis **342**, *343*
Lichen myxoedematosus 371
Lichen plano-pilaris **232**, *Pl 21 b*
Lichen planus **229–32**, *228–32*,
    Pl 21 a
    Civatte bodies in *230–1*
    pigmentary incontinence in *232*
Lichen sclerosus **367–70**, *370, 371*
    elastic fibres lost 369
Lichen simplex **227**, *227*
Lichenoid drug eruption 229, *230*, 377
Linear IgA disease **295**
Lupus erythematosus 23, **238**, *235–7*
    immunohistochemical staining of
        238, *235–7*
    mimicked by cytomegalovirus
        infection 238

Lupus panniculitis **362–3**
Lyme disease **247–50**, *250*
  cause of lichen sclerosus and
    scleroderma? 369
  erythema nodosum in 248
  granuloma annulare in 248
  Henoch-Schonlein purpura in 248
  morphoea in 249
  papular urticaria in 249
Lymph node metastasis, in blue
    naevus 98
Lymphangioma
  circumscriptum *200*
  circumscriptum superficialis **195**
  solitary circumscribed *199*
Lymphatics **6**
Lymphocytes
  immunohistochemical staining for
    11
  normal 7
Lymphocytoma cutis **242–4**, *244*
Lymphomatoid granulomatosis **348**
  synonym for angiocentric
    lymphoma 348
Lymphomatoid papulosis **273–6**, *274*
  CD30 positive cells in 275
  immunophenotype 275
  types of 273

Macrophages, immunohistochemical
    staining for 11
Malignancy, non-metastatic
    manifestations of 207
Malignant melanoma **108–15**, *109–12,
    114, 116, 118*, Pl 17, *19, 20*
Malpighian layer, normal 5
Mast cells 28
Mastocytoma, cutaneous 257
Mastocytosis **252–3**
Melanoacanthoma **63**
Melanoma, malignant **108–15**,
    109–12, 114, 116, 118, Pl 17, *19,
    20*
  balloon cell **125**
  basement membrane staining
    Pl 17 b
  desmoplastic **124–5**
  excision margins 113–14

HMB-45 immunohistochemical
    staining 113
  horizontal growth phase 112
  increased in AIDS 328
  minimal deviation **121**, 113, *122–3*
  neurotropic **124–5**
  prognostic index 115
  radial growth phase 112
  regression **115**
  S 100 immunohistochemical
    staining of *112*, Pl 17 *a*
  signet-ring cell **125**
  spindle cell **121–4**
  vertical growth phase *111*
Meningioma **198–202**
Meningitis, acute erythema of *251*
Mesenchymal tumours **176**
  dermatofibroma **176–9**, *177, 178*
  dermatofibrosarcoma protuberans
    180–2, *183*
  digital fibroma **184**
  fibrous histiocytoma, angiomatoid
    179
  fibrous papule of nose **184**, *186*
  fibroxanthoma, atypical **180**, *181*
  granular cell tumour **182**, *184*
  histiocytoma, epithelioid **180**
  myxoma **185–8**
  xanthelasma 185, *187*
  xanthogranuloma, juvenile **185**
  xanthoma **185**
Metastasis, cutaneous **205–8**, *210*
Microcystic adnexal carcinoma **144–6**,
    147
Milker's nodule **60**, *59*
Minimal deviation melanoma **121**,
    113, *122–3*
Mixed dermal tumour **139–42**, *143*
Molluscum contagiosum **63**, *64*
Morphoea **367**, *368*
Mucinoses **370**
Mucinosis, focal 371
Munro
  microabscess of 223
  pyknotic neutrophils and 223
Myeloproliferative disease, associated
    with Sweet's disease 252
Myofibroblast **6**

Myofibroma 197
Myxoedema 370
Myxoma **185–8**
  atrial metastatic 188

Naevus **90**
  blue naevus **98**, *100*
  cells, types of 90
  cells, in lymph node 98
  cellular blue **98–102**, *101*
  Clark's 108
  combined true and blue *102–3*
  conjunctival *94*
  deep penetrating **95–6**, *95*
  dysplastic **102–8**, *106–9*
  halo **115**, *117, 118*
  lipomatosus superficialis **205**
  Meischer's *92–3*
  organoid **162**
  pigmented spindle cell **98**, *99–100*,
    Pl 18 a and b
  sebaceous 162
  Spitz **96**, *97*
  true and blue *102–3*
  Unna's *91*
Nappy rash *378*
Necrobiosis lipoidica **320**, *322*
Necrolytic migratory erythema *212*
Necrotizing fasciitis **365**
  Streptococcal infection in 365
Necrotizing vasculitis **342**, *345*
Nerves *9*
Neural tumours **197**
  meningioma **198–202**
  neurilemmoma **198**
  neurofibroma **197–8**, *201, 202*
  neuroma, solitary circumscribed
    204
  neuroma solitary circumscribed **198**
  neurothekeoma, cellular **198**
Neurilemmoma **198**
Neuroendocrine carcinoma **202–3**,
  206
Neurofibroma **197–8**, *201, 202*
Neuroma, solitary circumscribed *204*
Neuroma solitary circumscribed **198**
Neurothekeoma, cellular **198**
Neutrophilic dermatosis, of Sweet
  250–2, *253*

Normal skin **3**
Notalgia paraesthetica *3*

Omphalomesenteric duct polyp *380*
Organoid naevus **162**, *164*

Paget's disease *27, 43, 44*
Pagetoid reticulosis 276–7, *Pl 22 b*
Pancreatic fat necrosis **362**
Panniculitis
  artefacta **364**, **380**
  classification 356
  cytophagic histiocytic **364**
  deep fungal infection *361*
  diagnosis of **356–8**
  enzymatic 362, *362*
  eosinophilic **363–4**
  granulomatous *358*
  lobular *361, 363*
  lupus **362–3**
  septal *357*
Papillary dermis 5
Papilloma, squamous cell **63**
Papular urticaria **252–3**, *255*
Parakeratosis 25
Pemphigoid **291–4**, *288*
  antigen 293
  as non-metastatic manifestation of
    malignancy 293
  gestationis, pathogenesis 295
  gestationis **294–5**
  polymorphic 293
Pemphigus *27, 50*, **287–91**, *289–98*
  benign familial **47**
  drug induced 287
  erythematosus 287
  foliaceus 287, *292*
  immunohistochemical staining 291
  neonatal 287
  vegetans 287
  vulgaris 287
Perifollicular fibroma **157**
Pigmented purpuric eruption **352**, *352*
Pigmented spindle cell naevus **98**,
  99–100, Pl 18 a and b
Pilomatrixoma **152–5**, *156*
Pilosebaceous unit 8
Pityriasis
  lichenoides acuta **244**, *246*

lichenoides chronica **245−7**, *248*
  rubra pilaris **247**
Polarized light
  identification of foreign bodies 26,
    30
  in examination of collagen 26, *30*
Polymorphic light eruption **238−9**,
    240
Polyp, omphalomesenteric duct *380*
Pore of Winer **148**, *150*
Porokeratosis **37−40**
  disseminated superficial actinic **38**,
    38, Pl 3b
  of Mibelli **38−40**
Porphyria cutanea tarda **299**, *299*
Prickle cell layer, normal 5
Proliferating pilar tumour **149**, *148*
Proliferating tricholemmal tumour
    149, *148*
Pseudoepitheliomatous hyperplasia
    81, Pl 9 a and b
Pseudoporphyria **299−300**
Psoriasis *26*, **221−5**, *222−4*, Pl 22 a
Pustular dermatosis
  of scalp, erosive **260**
  subcorneal **260**
Pyoderma gangrenosum **348−50**
  association with Crohn's disease
    348
  association with many systemic
    diseases 348
  association with ulcerative colitis
    348
  overlap with Sweet's syndrome
    252, 350
Pyogenic granuloma **192**, *196*

Quick diagnosis of herpes 65

Radiotherapy, long term effects of *383*
Reactive perforating collagenosis
    371−4, *372*
Red-neck 326
Reporting, strategies for **21−2**
Rete Malpighii, normal 5
Reticular dermis 5
Reticulin stain 6

S100, staining in sweat gland tumours
    132−3

Sarcoidosis **318**
Scabies Pl 24 a and b
Scleroderma **367**, *369*
  elastic fibres retained 369
Scleromyxoedema **371**
Sebaceous tumours **161**
  adenoma 162, *166*
  carcinoma **165**
  epithelioma 162, *167*
  hyperplasia 162, *165*
  naevus 162
  organoid naevus 162, *164*
Seborrhoeic dermatitis **225**
Senile lentigo *119*
Septal panniculitis *357*
Signet-ring cell lymphoma, histiocytic
    276
Skin, largest organ 3
Skin associated lymphoid tissue
    (SALT) **7**
Smooth muscle tumours **203**
  angioleiomyoma **203**, *209*
  leiomyoma **203**, *208*
  leiomyosarcoma **205**
Sneddon-Wilkinson disease 260
Solitary circumscribed neuroma **198**
Special stains **10**
Spindle cell
  melanoma **121−4**
  squamous cell carcinoma **85**
Spinous cell layer, normal 5
Spiradenoma **136−9**, *140−1*
Spitz naevus **96**, *97*
Spongiosis 25
Squamous cell carcinoma **77−8**, *77*,
    79, *80*, Pl 12
  metastasis 67
  spindle cell 85
Squamous cell papilloma **63**
Squirting papilla, in psoriasis 223
St. Elsewheres
  disappointed by reply from 22
  expert at 22
Subcorneal pustular dermatosis 260
Sweat glands **8**, *10*
Sweet's syndrome **250−2**, *253*
  criteria for diagnosis 252
  stages of 252
Synonyms, epidermal 5

Syphilis **316**, *317*
Syringoacanthoma 136
Syringofibroadenoma 136
Syringoma **136**, *137*

T-lymphocytes 7
Tattoo *378*
Telogen, phase of hair follicle growth
    8
Torture, effects of 384
Touton giant cells 304
Toxoplasmosis, cutaneous **316**
Trichoadenoma *153, 154*
Trichoblastic fibroma **155**, *159*
Trichoblastoma **155**
Trichoepithelioma, diagnosis in
    curetting 161
Trichoepithelioma, giant 161
Trichoepithelioma **157**, *163*,
    Pl 15 a and b
Trichoepithelioma adenoides
    sebaceum *158*
Trichofolliculoma **149**
Trichogenic trichoblastoma **155–7**,
    160–1
Tricholemmal cells *7*
Tricholemmoma **149–51**, *151–2*
Trichotillomania **259**
Tuberculosis **315**
Tzanck smear, in rapid diagnosis of
    herpes 65

Urticaria, tantalizingly normal biopsy
    in 16
Urticaria pigmentosum *256*

Vaculitis, clinical types 341
Vascular tumours **188**
    angioendothelioma, malignant
        endovascular papillary 195
    angiokeratoma *191*
    angioleiomyoma **203**, *209*
    angiomyxoma, superficial 371
    angiosarcoma **195**

cirsoid aneurysm **188–92**, *194*
Dabska tumour **195**
glomus tumour **195–7**, *197*
haemangioendothelioma,
    epithelioid **192**
haemangioendothelioma, vegetant
    intravascular of Masson **188**, *193*
haemangioma, cavernous *190*
haemangioma, verrucous *191–2*
haemangioma **188**
lymphangioma, circumscriptum *200*
lymphangioma, circumscriptum
    superficialis **195**
lymphangioma, solitary
    circumscribed *199*
Vasculitis *28*
    definition 341
    histopathological features of 341
    leukocytoclastic **342**, *343*
    necrotizing **342**, *345*
    thorny problem of 234

Warts
    combined 62
    seborrhoeic **60–3**, *61*, *Pl 6 and 7*
    viral **54–8**, *55–7*, *Pl 5 a and b*
    viral in allograft recipients 58, *58*
Warty dyskeratoma **51**, *49*
Wegener's granulomatosis
    dermal infarction 346
    necrotizing vasculitis 346
    palisading granulomas 346
Winer, dilated pore of **148**, *150*
Woringer-Kolopp disease **276–7**

Xanthelasma 185, *187*
Xanthogranuloma, juvenile **185**
Xanthoma **185**

Yuletide, cold injury and 384

Zoonoses 247, 311
Zoster, Herpes 65